The Evidence-Based Foundations of Existential–Humanistic Therapy is a milestone in the annals of psychotherapy research. Not since Carl Rogers and colleagues' landmark studies of client-centered therapy has a treatise more convincingly upheld the centrality of existential–humanistic principles of practice to our profession than this trail-blazing volume. As this book demonstrates, it is high-time that existential–humanistic researchers speak for themselves about the relevance of their purview for a rapidly diversifying psychotherapeutic discipline. Even a cursory perusal of this volume makes clear that existential–humanistic and existential–integrative therapies are at the frontier of psychotherapy effectiveness research as well as the broader cultural shifts out of which this research emerges. Given the upheaval of our times, I predict that existential–humanistic and existential–integrative therapies will soon be at the vanguard of a new emphasis in professional training and practice, and this book will be at its hub.

–KIRK J. SCHNEIDER, PhD, AUTHOR OF *THE PSYCHOLOGY OF EXISTENCE* (WITH ROLLO MAY), *EXISTENTIAL-HUMANISTIC THERAPY* (WITH ORAH KRUG), *EXISTENTIAL-INTEGRATIVE PSYCHOTHERAPY*, AND *LIFE-ENHANCING ANXIETY: KEY TO A SANE WORLD*

This edited volume is the first of its kind; that is, it is the first systematic attempt to demonstrate the evidence-base for existential–humanistic therapy (EHT) based on the model of evidence-based practice in psychology. The editors have accomplished a challenging task of threading the needle between a conception of evidence-based psychotherapy that is too rigid and narrow to accommodate EHT, on the one hand, and demonstrating that EHT is on solid ground in terms of empirical support, on the other. This is a book that will be of great interest to any practitioners of EHT, as it not only provides evidential support for their practice but also highlights basic skills that require ongoing development as well as important multicultural competencies that are increasingly relevant in our multicultural and increasingly global world. The volume will also be essential reading in graduate courses that train students in existential and humanistic approaches to therapy.

–BRENT ROBBINS, PhD, PROFESSOR AND PSYD PROGRAM DIRECTOR, DEPARTMENT OF PSYCHOLOGY, POINT PARK UNIVERSITY, PITTSBURGH, PA, UNITED STATES; PRESIDENT, SOCIETY FOR THEORETICAL AND PHILOSOPHICAL PSYCHOLOGY (AMERICAN PSYCHOLOGICAL ASSOCIATION DIVISION 24); AUTHOR OF *THE MEDICALIZED BODY AND ANESTHETIC CULTURE: THE CADAVER, THE MEMORIAL BODY, AND THE RECOVERY OF LIVED EXPERIENCE*

Wow, this is a fantastic book! It offers a solid case for the fact that existential–humanistic (EH) therapy is a valid, scientific, and empirically valid way of doing therapy. This is something we as EH practitioners have known forever, but it is good to see it in this way to support our claims and to be able to use as a touchpoint for those who fail to understand the power of a relational approach.

This book describes existential–humanistic therapy (EHT) in an encouraging and hopeful tone for psychologists who seek to defend and understand it. The research presented throughout the manuscript is impeccable. The contributing authors collectively provided high-quality research that reflects both seminal studies that have been foundational to the field and studies that reflect the evolving dialogue of these topics in the literature. When such research was not available, the authors transparently identified the gap and, as is indicated in the guidelines for evidence-based practice in psychology, provided the best available research from closely aligned therapies.

Hoffman and Lac are leaders in the renaissance of contemporary existential–humanistic psychotherapy, which honors the virtues of this rich tradition but extends the concepts and practices to a greater diversity of people. This text shines bright in this same light, combining evidence-based and culturally responsive practices with the perennial wisdom shared across various existential–humanistic therapies.

There is an urgent need to establish the evidential foundations for existential–humanistic therapy. Not only does this text take a first, giant step forward in this endeavour, but it lays the necessary foundations for further development of this evidence base. This is an essential text for those interested in existential–humanistic practice and its evolution.

THE EVIDENCE-BASED FOUNDATIONS OF EXISTENTIAL-HUMANISTIC THERAPY

THE EVIDENCE-BASED

FOUNDATIONS OF

EXISTENTIAL-

HUMANISTIC THERAPY

EDITORS

LOUIS HOFFMAN &
VERONICA LAC

 AMERICAN PSYCHOLOGICAL ASSOCIATION

Published by
American Psychological Association
750 First Street, NE
Washington, DC 20002
https://www.apa.org

Order Department
https://www.apa.org/pubs/books
order@apa.org

Typeset in Meridien and Ortodoxa by TIPS Publishing Services, Carrboro, NC

Printer: King Printing Co., Inc., Lowell, MA
Cover Designer: Mark Karis

Library of Congress Cataloging-in-Publication Data

Names: Hoffman, Louis, editor. | Lac, Veronica, editor.
Title: The evidence-based foundations of existential-humanistic therapy / by Louis Hoffman & Veronica Lac.
Description: Washington, DC : American Psychological Association, [2025] | Includes bibliographical references and index.
Identifiers: LCCN 2024045363 (print) | LCCN 2024045364 (ebook) | ISBN 9781433842924 (paperback) | ISBN 9781433842931 (ebook)
Subjects: LCSH: Evidence-based psychotherapy. | Existential psychotherapy. | Humanistic psychotherapy.
Classification: LCC RC455.2.E94 E93 2025 (print) | LCC RC455.2.E94 (ebook) | DDC 616.89--dc23/eng/20250205
LC record available at https://lccn.loc.gov/2024045363
LC ebook record available at https://lccn.loc.gov/2024045364

https://doi.org/10.1037/0000446-000

Printed in the United States of America

10 9 8 7 6 5 4 3 2 1

For Donna Rockwell—always a friend, colleague, and witness to a mindful, compassionate life and "One Love."

For Ilene A. Serlin—a friend, colleague, and ever-present force for humanizing psychology who witnessed that "to move is to live."

We miss you both.

CONTENTS

CONTRIBUTORS

Andrew M. Bland, PhD, Millersville University, Millersville, PA, United States

Arthur C. Bohart, PhD, California State University Dominguez Hills, Dominguez Hills, CA; Santa Clara University, Santa Clara, CA, United States

Chris Bradshaw, PhD, LPC, Fully Human Psychology, Tucson, AZ; Existential–Humanistic Institute, San Francisco, CA, United States

Vanessa Brown, PsyD, Saybrook University, Pasadena, CA, United States

Gayle Byock, MA, MBA, Antioch University Graduate School of Leadership and Change, Yellow Springs, OH, United States

Roxanne Christensen, PsyD, LP, Independent Scholar, Rochester Hills, MI, United States

Trey Cole, PsyD, ABPP, DAAETS, University of Denver, Denver, CO, United States

Rainbow Tin Hung Ho, PhD, University of Hong Kong, Hong Kong, China

Louis Hoffman, PhD, Rocky Mountain Humanistic Counseling and Psychological Association, Colorado Springs, CO, United States

Anne Y. J. Hsu, PhD, Sofia University, Costa Mesa, CA, United States

O'Dell O. Johnson, PhD, Saybrook University, Pasadena, CA; University of Washington Tacoma, Tacoma, WA; University of Arkansas for Medical Sciences, Little Rock, AR, United States

J. Ryan Kennedy, PsyD, LP, CIGT, BC-DMT, CLMA, RSME/T, Center for Professional Development, Noeticus Counseling Center and Training Institute, Denver, CO, United States

Orah T. Krug, PhD, Krug Counseling, Oakland, CA; Existential–Humanistic Institute, San Francisco, CA, United States

Fulya Kurter Musnitsky, MA, Expressive Arts Institute Istanbul, Istanbul, Turkey

Veronica Lac, PhD, The HERD Institute, Orlando, FL, United States

Zenobia Morrill, PhD, William James College, Newton, MA, United States

Marguerite Pintauro, MA, MSW, Saybrook University, Pasadena, CA, United States

Juanita Ratner, PhD, LPC, Private Practice, Westminster, CO, United States

Donna Rockwell, PsyD, (deceased), Saybrook University, Pasadena, CA, United States

Almudena Sánchez-Mazarro, MS, European Institute of Existential–Humanistic Psychotherapy, Madrid, Spain; Existential–Humanistic Institute, San Francisco, CA, United States; Comillas Pontifical University, Madrid, Spain

Shea Scharding, MPA, PhD Student, Saybrook University, Pasadena, CA, United States

Derrick Sebree Jr., PsyD, Michigan School of Psychology, Farmington Hills, MI, United States

Ilene A. Serlin, PhD, BC-DMT, (deceased), Serlin Institute of the Healing Arts, San Francisco, CA; California Institute of the Healing Arts and Sciences, Sacramento, CA, United States

Jerrold Lee Shapiro, PhD, Santa Clara University, Santa Clara, CA, United States

Drake Spaeth, PsyD, Saybrook University, Pasadena, CA, United States

Justin J. Underwood, PsyD, Pepperdine University, Los Angeles, CA, United States

Joseph Alexander Vanderhoff, MA, LPCC, Center for Humanistic and Interpersonal Psychotherapy, Colorado Springs, CO, United States

Brittany Varisco, MA, University of Denver, Denver, CO, United States

Aviva Vincent, PhD, LSW, Cleveland State University, Cleveland, OH, United States

Joel Vos, PhD, MSc, MA, CPsychol, FHEA, Metanoia Institute, London, United Kingdom

ACKNOWLEDGMENTS

We would like to thank APA Books, especially Susan Reynolds, who stayed in regular contact and was always supportive and enthusiastic about the project. We are also indebted to Ed Meidenbauer, who made the initial contact with Louis about writing a book for APA Books. We have great respect and appreciation for the many contributors to this volume and are thankful for their patience as we encountered delays due to workloads and the impact that so many felt from the COVID-19 pandemic.

We want to mention special appreciation for Donna Rockwell, who died on October 7, 2023, in the midst of finishing this book and the chapter she was coauthoring. Donna was an inspiration to many of the contributors to this book and to both of us. Her death was a terrible loss that we are still recovering from. We appreciate too that her coauthors, O'Dell O. Johnson and Shea Scharding, persevered to finish the chapter in the midst of their grief. Many in the humanistic community will continue to miss Donna for many years to come.

We also want to give special appreciation to Ilene A. Serlin, who died on November 26, 2024, during the final stages of production for this book. Ilene impacted many people from around the globe. Her contributions were diverse, including expressive arts therapy, dance and movement therapy, whole person health care, trauma, and feminist psychology, among others. Her loss left us and many others in the existential–humanistic community in shock. We are grateful to her coauthors, Rainbow Tin Hung Ho, Fulya Kurter Musnitsky, and J. Ryan Kennedy, who finished the final edits of the chapter while grieving the loss of their friend and colleague. Ilene will be greatly missed.

Louis would like to thank Michael Moats, who provided encouragement when he reconsidered, multiple times, if he could find the time for this book. Without Michael's encouragement, the book proposal may not have been finished. He would also like to thank Veronica, his coeditor, who is a wonderful scholar and collaborator. The entire board of the Rocky Mountain Humanistic Counseling and Psychological Association has been a constant source of support, encouragement, and inspiration. In particular, Louis wants to acknowledge Nathaniel Granger, Jr., H. Luis Vargas, Shawn Rubin, and Francis J. Kaklauskas, whose friendship and encouragement, including encouragement to say "no" to interesting projects that could have distracted from this one, are always appreciated. His appreciation also goes out to Kirk Schneider and Luisa Xochitl Vallejos, who are regular sources of consultation and encouragement. Lastly, he owes deep gratitude to his family, Heatherlyn, Lakoda, Lukaya, and Lyon, for their support and patience with him taking on yet another large project.

Veronica would like to thank her herd of horses and humans who continue to inspire her to share the work they do. She is particularly grateful to Aviva Vincent who leaned into coauthoring two of the chapters in this volume. Veronica feels that, as always, as educators and practitioners, we are continuously inspired and stretched by our students and colleagues to explore different ways of sharing our knowledge and skills. More importantly, we are often called upon to challenge ourselves, our assumptions, biases, and blind spots. Veronica is forever grateful for Louis's mentorship and support for her leaning into her growing edges.

THE EVIDENCE-BASED
FOUNDATIONS OF
EXISTENTIAL-
HUMANISTIC THERAPY

Introduction: Evidence-Based Psychological Practice in Existential–Humanistic Psychotherapy

Louis Hoffman and Veronica Lac

For many years, we have heard misinformation about existential–humanistic (EH) psychotherapy suggesting that it cannot be practiced consistent with evidence-based practice in psychology (EBPP). In particular, students have informed us that they have been told this by professors, supervisors, practicum sites, and internships. This misinformation has led to restrictions inhibiting students' ability to learn EH psychotherapy in graduate schools, practicums, and internships while also restricting professionals' freedom to practice EH psychotherapy in some settings and creating barriers to seeking reimbursement from insurance companies. These factors have also created unfortunate obstacles to clients seeking this type of psychotherapy. This book sets the record straight and, hopefully, will open doors for students, professionals, and clients.

In his review of *Existential–Integrative Psychotherapy: Guideposts to the Core of Practice* by Kirk J. Schneider (2008), leading outcome researcher Bruce Wampold (2008) wrote

> I have argued that the principles of change in EI [existential–integrative psychotherapy] are as scientific as those of any other psychological treatment (Wampold, 2007); I have no doubt that EI approaches would satisfy any criteria used to label other psychological treatments as scientific. (p. 13)

This is a strong endorsement. This volume compiles the evidence that demonstrates that Wampold was, indeed, correct.

https://doi.org/10.1037/0000446-001
The Evidence-Based Foundations of Existential–Humanistic Therapy, L. Hoffman and V. Lac (Editors)

EH PSYCHOTHERAPY'S PLACE IN PROFESSIONAL PSYCHOLOGY

EH psychotherapy historically has fallen outside of mainstream psychology. Although scholars such as Rollo May and Kirk Schneider have written popular books that have drawn interest beyond humanistic and existential psychology, and in spite of May at one time being one of the most influential U.S. psychologists, EH psychotherapy has long been viewed as an alternative approach falling outside of mainstream psychology. Despite this, its influence has continually been a force. Shahar and Schiller (2016) have even gone as far as saying that EH psychology has taken over the field by stealth, as many of its concepts have been integrated into mainstream approaches. While this may be overly optimistic—especially given that when EH psychotherapy principles are integrated into other approaches, they are frequently simplified and changed—it demonstrates that EH psychology has had a continual impact upon the field in significant and impactful ways.

The growing monoculture in the field of psychology is harmful for the field and the suffering people seeking out mental health treatment (Leichsenring et al., 2016; Levy & Anderson, 2013). Theoretical and clinical diversity is good for the field. Most effective psychotherapists have at least a handful, if not an extensive collection, of stories of clients who previously experienced a different type of therapy with unsatisfactory results. In these cases, after unsuccessful results with other therapists, they found success with a different therapist or modality (see Hoffman, 2024). This does not demonstrate that one modality is superior to the others; it simply demonstrates that a particular modality was the right fit for a particular client. The other extreme of accepting all psychotherapies as valid, bona fide therapies is also dangerous, as evidenced by the death of a child that occurred during rebirthing therapy (Josefson, 2001). Balance is needed.

All psychotherapy modalities need to engage in rigorous reflection, scholarship, and research to continually assess and improve their effectiveness. While EH psychology has consistently engaged in meticulous study and self-examination, it has at times lacked in conducting research on EH psychotherapy. It has been better at utilizing research than conducting original research. We hope this volume will help address this. In the chapters, the contributors reliably engage prior research while also identifying gaps in the current literature. This, we believe, is one of the more important contributions of the current volume: identifying future research needs. We hope this book will inspire professionals engaging in research and students seeking dissertation topics to begin filling the current gaps. This will strengthen the standing of EH therapy beyond its current solid foundation while also identifying areas of growth and change that are needed.

Research should not be the only consideration in identifying appropriate forms of psychotherapy for clients. It is also important to consider client values along with individual and cultural differences. Different approaches to psychotherapy represent different values and desired outcomes. Though some approaches to therapy value rationality and prioritize emotional regulation, others help clients embrace and value their emotions that bring about changes in how emotions are experienced. Some approaches prioritize happiness, whereas others value meaning and view happiness as a byproduct of living a good life. Still more approaches to psychotherapy focus on the individual first, and others prioritize relationships or culture. Of course, these are often differences in degrees rather than absolute distinctions, but they are significant nonetheless.

One of the great errors in the history of psychotherapy is not recognizing the values embedded in different approaches to psychotherapy and imposing them upon clients without consideration for their differences (see Hoffman & Cleare-Hoffman, 2025, Chapter 1). Instead, the appropriateness of fit has been based on outcomes determined by the norms of society and predetermined, acceptable sought outcomes rather than the values of the client. Efficiency, in both time and money, is also prioritized over client preferences and cultural differences. But there are different paths to improved mental health, and what is an ideal approach to mental health may vary between clients. If we are going to truly value diversity in individual and cultural differences, we must move beyond the psychotherapeutic monoculture that is dominating the field and embrace different therapeutic modalities. This also means decolonizing the field through the contributions of practitioners from marginalized spaces. When psychotherapists are able to appreciate the different modalities and embrace a willingness to help clients find the best fit for the client values and preferences, we are better able to serve those seeking mental health services.

EH psychotherapy has a long and vibrant history over the past 60 years. Included in this history is vibrant scholarship and a legacy of providing effective, compassionate psychotherapy services. This volume builds from this history to demonstrate the important place that EH psychotherapy occupies in the contemporary landscape of the mental health professions.

OVERVIEW OF THIS BOOK

The starting point for this book is the 2006 article in the *American Psychologist* by the American Psychological Association Presidential Task Force on Evidence-Based Practice and the three pillars it identified as the foundation of EBPP: (a) the best available research; (b) clinical experience; and (c) client characteristics, culture, and preference. This book was organized in a manner to demonstrate how EH psychotherapy addresses each of these pillars. In Chapter 1, Louis Hoffman begins by providing an overview of EH approaches to EBPP. This includes a history of EBPP and some challenges to specific ways that EBPP has evolved, including privileging certain research methodologies even when they may not be the most appropriate for the research question.

The second pillar of EBPP is clinical experience, which is consistent with psychotherapy competencies. This pillar is addressed separately by Joel Vos in Chapter 2. Vos's chapter discusses existential competencies across the different schools of existential therapy as well as competencies specific to particular schools. In the end, there is more overlap in existential competencies across the schools than differences and, as Vos maintains, there has been a gradual movement toward more convergence among the existential schools. Through addressing the existential competencies across the schools, this chapter provides a foundation for integrating other existential therapies, particularly those with the strongest research support, into EH psychotherapy.

In Chapter 3, Andrew M. Bland reviews the research on EH therapy and related therapies. To date, unfortunately, there has been limited direct research on EH therapy. In part, this is due to EH psychotherapists' resistance to outcome research and randomized clinical trials. However, conducting research also has been challenged by the lack of a structural framework for EH psychotherapy or case formulation. This is being addressed in what is intended as a companion volume to this one: *Case Formulation in Existential–Humanistic Therapy* (Hoffman & Cleare-Hoffman, 2025). In addition to reviewing the research, Bland's chapter helps identify specific needs for future outcome research.

In Part II, Chapters 4–13 review foundations of EH therapy, including presence, empathy, working with emotions, authenticity, self-awareness, facing life directly, working with the here-and-now, meaning, acceptance, genuineness, the real relationship, therapist self-disclosure, and working with the self. These chapters are written by established and emerging leaders in EH psychology, including Orah T. Krug, Arthur C. Bohart, Drake Spaeth, Zenobia Morrill, and others. Each of these chapters consider the other two pillars of EBPP: the best available research and client characteristics, culture, and preference. Therefore, this book provides an in-depth demonstration of how EH psychotherapy can be practiced consistent with the three pillars of EBPP.

The final section, Part III, includes four chapters on integrative strategies, including mindfulness, the creative and expressive arts, experiential techniques, and equine-facilitated psychotherapy. These were selected as examples of approaches that readily fit with EH principles. Each chapter follows the same structure as in Part II with additional considerations about how these approaches may, at times, require some adaptation to be integrated with EH psychotherapy. At the same time, we believe that the contributors to this volume have convincingly demonstrated that EH therapy has a strong research foundation, as supported by the literature.

The chapters were written with an assumption that readers will have at least a foundational knowledge of EH psychotherapy. This will help readers recognize some of the nuances within how EH therapists approach the specific topics covered. With regard to EBPP, there are many variations to how EBPP is understood. Therefore, an overview of the history and current understanding of EBPP is covered in Chapter 1. The book and chapters were not written with any assumptions about the readers' familiarity with EBPP.

CONCLUSION

This book is long overdue. For many years, EH psychotherapists have been bat-
tling to demonstrate effectiveness with no comprehensive resources to support
their arguments. Although the support has long been available, until this current volume, individual researchers and practitioners have had to do the work
themselves of compiling the evidence. *The Evidence-Based Foundations of Existential–Humanistic Therapy* changes that. Practitioners now have the evidence at
hand to demonstrate to the critics and skeptics what we have known for many
years: In terms of EBPP, EH psychotherapy is on solid ground.

REFERENCES

American Psychological Association Presidential Task Force on Evidence-Based Practice.
(2006). Evidence-based practice in psychology. *American Psychologist, 61*(4), 271–285.
https://doi.org/10.1037/0003-066x.61.4.271

Hoffman, L. (2024). The possibilities and slippery slope of evidence-based practice in
psychology: Why humanistic and existential psychologists must engage the conversation. *The Humanistic Psychologist, 52*(3), 318–324. https://doi.org/10.1037/hum0000347

Hoffman, L., & Cleare-Hoffman, H. P. (2025). *Case formulation in existential–humanistic
therapy.* American Psychological Association. https://doi.org/10.1037/0000464-000

Josefson, D. (2001). Rebirthing therapy banned after girl died in 70 minute struggle. *British Medical Journal, 322*(7293), 1014.

Leichsenring, F., Abbass, A., Hilsenroth, M. J., Luyten, P., Munder, T., Rabung, S., & Steinert, C. (2018). "Gold standards," plurality and monocultures: The need for diversity in
psychotherapy. *Frontiers in Psychology, 9,* Article 159. https://doi.org/10.3389/fpsyt.2018.
00159

Levy, K. N., & Anderson, T. (2013). Is clinical psychology doctoral training becoming less
intellectually diverse? And if so, what can be done? *Clinical Psychology: Science and
Practice, 20*(2), 211–220. https://doi.org/10.1111/cpsp.12035

Schneider, K. J. (Ed.). (2008). *Existential-integrative psychotherapy: Guideposts to the core of
practice.* Routledge.

Shahar, G., & Schiller, M. (2016). A conqueror by stealth: Introduction to the special
issue on humanism, existentialism, and psychotherapy integration. *Journal of Psychotherapy Integration, 26*(1), 1–4. http://doi.org/10.1037/int0000024

Wampold, B. E. (2008, February 4). Existential–integrative psychotherapy: Coming of
age [Review of the book *Existential–integrative psychotherapy: Guideposts to the core of
practice,* by K. J. Schneider]. *PsycCritiques 53*(6). https://doi.org/10.1037/a0011070

FOUNDATIONAL RESEARCH AND COMPETENCIES IN EXISTENTIAL–HUMANISTIC PSYCHOTHERAPY

1

Approaching Existential–Humanistic Psychotherapy From an Evidence-Based Perspective

Louis Hoffman

When a new paradigm for evidence-based practice in psychology (EBPP) was first introduced in 2006, many humanistic and existential–humanistic (EH) therapists quickly voiced concern about what this could mean (Hoffman, 2024). For many years prior to the introduction of this new paradigm, the dominant approaches to verifying the effectiveness and appropriateness of treatment modalities were strongly biased to manualized and solution-focused approaches. The quick and premature assumption made by many humanistic and EH therapists was that this was another challenge to depth psychotherapy approaches, including humanistic, existential, psychoanalytic, Jungian, and Gestalt therapies (see Elkins 2009, 2015).

Closer investigation demonstrates that this new paradigm of EBPP does not need to be feared (Hoffman, 2024; Hoffman & Bowers, 2016; Hoffman, Vallejos, et al., 2015). Instead, this paradigm has the potential to be a more flexible and inclusive approach to demonstrating the appropriateness and effectiveness of practice. Furthermore, as will be discussed, it shifts away from a singular focus on the manualized modality to a broader focus on the therapist, basic competencies, and adaptability to particular client needs. This approach allows for a more client-centered strategy with greater flexibility for how the therapy is implemented instead of relying upon strict adherence to a manualized structure that many EH therapists believed objectified and dehumanized clients.

Although this new EBPP paradigm shows promise toward being more flexible and inclusive, a lack of agreement remains pertaining to the definition of what constitutes EBPP. While the seminal article in the *American Psychologist*

https://doi.org/10.1037/0000446-002
The Evidence-Based Foundations of Existential–Humanistic Therapy, L. Hoffman and V. Lac (Editors)

(American Psychological Association [APA] Presidential Task Force on Evidence-Based Practice, 2006) provides a detailed description, soon after its publication, Wampold and colleagues (2007) warned that the understanding of EBPP could change over time. Unfortunately, this warning turned out to be prophetic.

When humanistic and EH therapists first began decrying the new paradigm of EBPP, I advocated that therapists needed to engage the conversation to help assure that a broad, inclusive understanding of EBPP was maintained by the field (Hoffman et al., 2012, 2015; Hoffman, Vallejos et al., 2015). After all, as the old adage goes, whoever defines the terms wins the debate. Unfortunately, the voices narrowing the definition spoke louder and more forcefully in their attempts to define EBPP. Now, EH therapy and other depth psychologies are at a crossroads. Do we try to pressure the field to move on from EBPP to something more inclusive? Or do we return to the understanding from the article in the *American Psychologist* and advocate for a broader and more flexible understanding of EBPP? As is evident with the focus of this book, we are advocating for the latter.

In this chapter, I begin with a brief history of outcome research and paradigms for understanding the effectiveness and appropriateness of therapy. Next, an initial formulation of EBPP followed by an EH-informed understanding of EBPP is discussed. Along with the EH-informed contributions, some multicultural, social justice, and liberatory considerations are addressed. From there, the chapter discusses how to approach EH therapy in a manner consistent with EBPP.

BRIEF HISTORY OF APPROACHES TO VERIFYING THE EFFECTIVENESS OF PSYCHOTHERAPY: FROM ROGERS TO EBPP

The lack of consensus on what constitutes EBPP makes evaluating the effectiveness of psychotherapy a difficult topic. Although any categorization of the approaches to EBPP requires some simplification, it can be maintained that most usages of EBPP fall into two definitions. First, a broad understanding of EBPP can be traced to the 1970s and is inclusive of a multitude of approaches to verifying the effectiveness of psychotherapy, including the different paradigms discussed in this section. Second, a narrow understanding of EBPP is a collection of approaches drawing from the 2006 article "Evidence-Based Practice in Psychology" by the APA Presidential Task Force on Evidence-Based Practice. For this book, we are relying on the second understanding of EBPP. In this section, I identify five waves or paradigms of strategies to evaluate the effectiveness of psychotherapy.

The history of outcome and therapy effectiveness research dates back to at least 1952 when Eysenck challenged the field of psychotherapy regarding the lack of outcome research (Lutz et al., 2021). Since this time, research has generally supported that psychotherapy is effective. Lutz and colleagues note that two traditions emerged in regard to psychotherapy research: outcome research and process research. Outcome research focuses on the impact as well as efficacy and effectiveness of psychotherapy. Process research attempts to identify and research the components of therapy that make it effective. This book is rooted in the latter perspective.

Over time, psychotherapy research became increasingly political. Beginning with the second wave, EBPP has been increasingly influenced by economics, including input and demands from managed care (see Levant, 2004; Tanenbaum, 2006). If one is to understand the current iterations of EBPP and debates about what constitutes it, an understanding of the history and politics is necessary. As argued by Norcross and Wampold (2019a), this has often worked against managed care's own best interests, particularly if it is committed to the best possible client care and long-term outcomes.

The First Wave of Evaluating Psychotherapy Effectiveness

Early attempts to examine the effectiveness of psychotherapy were broad and diverse. They included formalized and informal strategies. However, the most important distinguishing factor from contemporary approaches was the less political nature. The motivation was primarily for understanding, improving, and advancing psychotherapy. Though less political, it was not, however, entirely apolitical. There was some jockeying for evidence to claim superiority to other approaches; however, the motivation to demonstrate effectiveness to third party payors, regulating agencies, and the general public was largely absent.

From its outset, psychoanalysis and psychotherapy sought to understand how psychotherapy works for training purposes and to improve its effectiveness. The writings of Sigmund Freud, Carl Jung, and others are replete with case studies, often informal, that were discussed and interpreted. Many of these continue to be discussed, interpreted, and reinterpreted today. Although these did not follow the more structured contemporary guidelines for case studies, they nonetheless were strategic attempts to analyze what was happening in psychotherapy with a client and why it worked or did not work.

Arguably one of the first individuals to begin utilizing systematic approaches to evaluating psychotherapy was Carl Rogers. Lutz and colleagues (2021) note that Rogers's research beginning in the 1950s marked the beginning of process research. According to Goldfried (2007),

> Rogers' emphasis on psychotherapy research has provided a platform on which current outcome and process investigations have been based. Although the field has clearly become much more specialized over the years, Rogers conducted some of the earliest studies to determine whether or not a therapeutic intervention worked. Moreover, his use of wire recordings—which predated the tape recorder—served as ground-breaking methodology by which the process of therapy could be investigated. (p. 249)

Rogers's strategies were intensive, and they changed the way he understood and practiced psychotherapy. He approached research with openness to learn and improve, not just to prove effectiveness or the superiority of his approach.

Though the introduction of new methods and methodologies[1] of investigation is, without doubt, beneficial to the field, there remains much we can learn from this first wave of evaluating and investigating psychotherapy and its effectiveness. Contemporary approaches are often tainted with political, financial, allegiance, and ego motivations. For Rogers and many other earlier researchers, the motivation was to better understand psychotherapy and improve as a psychotherapist, including advancing one's modality. It could be argued that the changing motivations have harmed the ability to evaluate therapy effectiveness by focusing more on the political and financial motivations. Research on psychotherapy should always first and foremost be in the service of the client, not the researcher or practitioner—or theoretical allegiances. It seems this was much more common in the first wave of outcome research then the later iterations.

Interlude: Setting the Context for a New Paradigm

Although psychotherapists often grumble about the realities of evidence-based practice and similar paradigms for evaluating effectiveness, particularly the implications with third party payors, it is important to understand the context for their emergence and the role therapists played. Several factors are important to consider. First, following legislation establishing Medicaid and Medicare in the United States in the 1960s, health care costs dramatically increased (Yates, 2013). In response, the Health Maintenance Organization Act was passed in 1973 in an attempt to contain rising costs. At the same time, accusations of waste on the part of providers emerged (see Tanenbaum, 2006). Although some of this waste was exaggerated and potentially even fabricated, clearly there was waste occurring, including from therapists and mental health providers. In response, mental health providers began considering ways to demonstrate the effectiveness of psychotherapy.

Demonstrating the effectiveness of psychotherapy alone would not address the issue, including the public's growing distrust of health care providers. It was also necessary to contain some of the other problems contributing to the rising costs, including using questionable procedures and charging exuberant prices for treatment. Therefore, problematic and unethical practices by mental health professionals played a critical role in the emergence of managed care and other factors, leading to the Empirically Validated Treatments (EVTs) and Empirically Supported Treatments (ESTs). Mental health professionals must accept some responsibility for increased scrutiny and regulations of mental health treatment.

The Second Wave: EVTs

The first paradigm that emerged for demonstrating effectiveness of psychotherapy after the Health Maintenance Organization Act, the EVTs paradigm, was

---

[1] *Methods* refers to the approach to collecting data (e.g., self-report measures, interviews, biological data) whereas *methodology* refers to the theoretical framework (e.g., phenomenological, grounded theory, the approach to statistical analysis).

short-lived and arguably indistinct from the third wave. This was largely due to language. The second wave uses the word "validated," which was replaced with "supported" in the third wave. I retain this as a separate wave because language is important and a vital part of the debate. According to the Cambridge Dictionary (n.d.), validate means "to prove something is correct" or "to make something officially acceptable or approved, especially after examining it." Thus, claiming that a therapy approach is validated could be interpreted as claiming it is proven, which contradicts common assumptions about the philosophy of science in psychology.

The model for determining the EVTs was established in the APA Division 12 Task Force on Promotion and Dissemination of Psychological Procedures (1995) article, "Training in and Dissemination of Empirically Validated Psychological Treatments." It did not take long for the critiques to emerge. For example, a year after the 1995 task force article, Garfield (1996), who applauded striving in this direction, argued that "validated" was too strong of a term and, instead, suggested "effective." Furthermore, he argued the field was not ready for the EVTs. For therapies to be validated, they must be manualized, offering little variability. Although there were some manualized therapies at this time, they were few. In the end, the primary factor that brought an end to the EVTs was one word: validated. Despite this, the movement lived on in a new language. As will be seen, the problematic assumptions remained after the word changed.

The Third Wave: ESTs

The shift to the language of ESTs brought little, if any, change to what was trying to be accomplished. Initially, the language of EVTs and ESTs was essentially interchangeable in the literature, even within the same articles, before the shift in preferred language solidified into the ESTs. The ESTs established two lists of therapies: (a) Well-Established Treatments and (b) Probably Efficacious Treatments (Levant, 2004). The initial approach for being established as an EST was through a minimum of two adequately rigorous randomized controlled trials (RCTs), which included comparison to a waitlist group or another therapy modality. Later, the option of 10 rigorous case studies could also be used to meet inclusion after widespread criticism of the ESTs. The ESTs beginning to fall out of favor may have been an influential factor in the concession allowing 10 case studies to qualify modalities. Yet this political move seemed to happen too late, as the next paradigm was beginning to emerge.

The momentum around the ESTs allowed for it to move in dangerous directions, including the possibility of sanctions against therapists that used therapy treatments that were not included in the list of ESTs. Furthermore, the ESTs began changing how psychotherapy was practiced, moving toward what Elkins (2009) called "short-term linear treatments" (p. 21). Treatments had to be manualized and carefully followed, especially in clinical trials, even if this did not translate to as rigid of adherence to the manuals in actual practice outside of the trials. Clinical judgment was discouraged and even viewed as dangerous (Levant, 2004).

The rigidity of how approaches needed to be manualized to minimize thera-pist variability favored certain approaches, such as cognitive behavior therapy, that could be readily structured to fit into a manual. Thus, many practitioners from other approaches, such as psychoanalytic, Jungian, humanistic, and exis-tential therapy, were highly concerned about the growing influence of the ESTs. This led to the development of alternatives, which would form the next wave.

Fourth Wave: Alternatives to the ESTs

The fourth wave emerged while the ESTs remained the zeitgeist in the field of psychology. These alternatives never overtook the ESTs in influence before the emergence of the fifth wave, though they likely played an important role in paving the way for the fifth wave. Though there were several alternatives or challenges to the ESTs that emerged, the most influential one was the Empiri-cally Supported Relationships.

In 1999, Norcross (2001) established the APA Division 29 Task Force on Empirically Supported Therapy Relationships. Drawing on the criticisms and limitations of the ESTs, this task force sought to establish relational qualities that have sufficient empirical support. The results were presented in a 2001 special issue of *Psychotherapy*. Similar to the Division 12 (Society of Clinical Psychology) task force, the Division 29 (Society for the Advancement of Psychotherapy) task force categorized aspects of the relationship into three groups: (a) "demonstra-bly effective," (b) "promising or probably effective," and (c) "insufficient research to judge" (p. 349).

The initial results yielded four demonstrably effective elements of the ther-apy relationship (therapeutic alliance, cohesion in group therapy, empathy, and goal consensus and collaboration) and seven promising and probably effective elements (positive regard, congruence/genuineness, feedback, repair of alli-ance ruptures, self-disclosure, management of countertransference, and qual-ity of relational interpretations; Ackerman et al., 2001). Shortly after the special edition of *Psychotherapy*, Norcross (2002) edited the book *Psychotherapy Relation-ships That Work: Therapist Contributions and Responsiveness to Patients*. A second edition was published in 2011 with a noticeable change in the subtitle to *Evidence-Based Responsiveness* (Norcross, 2011). A newer update, published in 2019, expanded to a two-volume set (Norcross & Lambert, 2019; Norcross & Wampold, 2019b). The first volume focused on the component of effective therapy relationships, whereas the second volume focuses on therapist respon-siveness or adaptability. Though the list of factors in volume one is largely con-sistent with original factors identified in 2001 with updated research reviews, additional factors included real relationships (Gelso et al., 2019), emotional expression (Peluso & Freund, 2019), cultivating positive outcome expectations (Constantino, Vîslǎ, et al., 2019), and promoting treatment credibility (Con-stantino, Coyne, et al., 2019).

These factors are often considered part of the *common factors of psychotherapy*, which refers to aspects of psychotherapy that account for substantive portions of psychotherapy change across modalities (Carter, 2006; Norcross & Wampold, 2019a). In particular, these are the relational components of the common factors that, outside of client factors, have been found to account for the greatest amount of psychotherapy change (Wampold & Imel, 2015). It is important to note, too, that there is a great similarity between the relational common factors and what humanistic and existential therapies have long advocated are the primary change factors. However, as Elkins (2009) warns, it is important that this is not taken to indicate that humanistic and existential approaches have been right all along. There remain some differences, including in how some of these factors are applied. Yet the relational common factors do provide strong support for the effectiveness of humanistic therapies, including EH therapy. Therefore, the chapters in Norcross and Lambert (2019) influenced how Part II of this book was developed.

A second alternative focused on identifying principles of change (Beutler & Johannsen, 2006). A joint task force of APA Division 12 (the Society for Clinical Psychology) and the North American Society for Psychotherapy Research advocated for this approach. This approach identified specific components of change without consideration of the therapeutic models they emerged from. The emphasis here was to move away from the treatment models to a more general or universal model of change. Ultimately, this model has been influential, but not to the degree of Evidence-Based Relationships.

Although also not as influential as the Empirically Supported Relationships (later called Evidence-Based Relationships), humanistic psychology had a response of its own. Spearheaded by Arthur C. Bohart and Maureen O'Hara and supported by APA Division 32 (now the Society for Humanistic Psychology), this article developed specific provisions for practicing humanistic psychotherapy (APA Division 32 Task Force for the Development of Guidelines for the Provision of Humanistic Psychosocial Services, 1997). These guidelines were developed primarily in response to the attempts to establish EVTs and treatment guidelines. These guidelines begin with a critique of the EVTs and treatment guidelines before providing a rationale and guidelines for humanistic psychosocial services, including psychotherapy. These were later updated in 2004 (APA Division 32 Task Force for the Development of Practice Recommendations for the Provision of Humanistic Psychosocial Services, 2004).

Although it is difficult to assess how influential the humanistic practice recommendations were in dismantling the ESTs, it is likely that they played at least a modest role through alerting humanistic psychologists to the risks and dangers of the ESTs and energizing their critiques. Even if the impact on dismantling the ESTs was limited, the document remains a valuable guide for humanistic psychologists for training and practice.

The Fifth Wave: EBPP

Although the language of EBPP had been around for many years prior to the seminal article by the APA Presidential Task Force on Evidence-Based Practice in 2006, it was 2006 when a new paradigm of EBPP emerged, replacing the previous paradigms as the new zeitgeist. With this, the ESTs movement faded from influence. The growing criticism of the ESTs, particularly around their rigidity, ultimately contributed to their demise. Though the 2006 task force article established a new paradigm, it did not curtail years of continued debate about what constitutes EBPP.

THE PILLARS OF EBPP: AN EH INTERPRETATION

The 2006 article by the APA Presidential Task Force on Evidence-Based Practice published in the *American Psychologist* clarified the foundations of EBPP. Shortly after its publication, Wampold et al. (2007) warned that the flexibility and inclusivity of EBPP could regress to a more rigid approach similar to the ESTs. Unfortunately, this has occurred to a significant degree.

The article by the APA Presidential Task Force on Evidence-Based Practice (2006) included three pillars of EBPP: (a) best available research evidence; (b) clinical experience; and (c) client characteristics, culture, and preferences. Whereas the ESTs approach focused on the treatment modality and evaluating it, EBPP goes beyond merely evaluating the treatment modality to also include foundational clinical competencies and adjustments based upon the particular client, their social positions, their values, and their preferences. Given this approach, the idea that any therapy modality is an evidence-based practice does not fit with the structure established by the task force.

EBPP is best understood as rooted in the therapist and therapy relationship more than the therapy modality (see Norcross & Lambert, 2006; Wampold, 2006). In this consideration, it could be maintained that EBPP is "a competent therapist using a bona fide therapy vetted in the peer-reviewed literature and through practice-based evidence drawing from the best available research while adjusting for individual and cultural differences and preferences with appropriate cultural humility" (Hoffman, 2024, p. 319). Implicit in this definition is that the therapist is adequately responsive and flexible to the client, their preferences, and their needs. This succinct definition more closely aligns with the APA Presidential Task Force on Evidence-Based Practice's (2006) guidelines than viewing particular modalities as being an evidence-based practice. Instead of saying that an approach is an evidence-based practice, it is more accurate to say that a particular therapist is practicing consistent with the standards of EBPP. As demonstrated in this edited volume, when using this more inclusive understanding of evidence-based practice, EH therapists are on solid ground (Cleare-Hoffman et al., 2013; Hoffman & Bowers, 2016; Hoffman et al., 2012, 2013, 2015).

The later sections of this chapter provide an overview of the three pillars of EBPP, including an EH interpretation and adaptation of each pillar. On the second pillar, we add "competencies" to the section heading for clarification. What was described as "clinical experience" in the article by the APA Presidential Task

Force of Evidence-Based Practice (2006) fits closely with core clinical competencies, as defined by National Counseling of Schools and Programs of Professional Psychology (n.d.). After providing an overview of the three pillars, I consider an EH approach to implementing these pillars to demonstrate the evidence-based foundations of EH therapy.

Best Available Research Evidence

Many earlier approaches to evaluating psychotherapy focus on efficacy, not effectiveness—a distinction often not considered in psychotherapy research. Efficacy evaluates the performance in ideal or laboratory settings, whereas effectiveness refers to the performance in normal or real-world contexts (Singal et al., 2014; van der Lem et al., 2012). Efficacy does not always translate to effectiveness. What was considered appropriate research in the past was narrowly defined in a manner that rendered most psychotherapy clients ineligible (Peterson, 2006; Tanenbaum, 2006), limiting the relevance. The manualized approaches were often rigidly followed in clinical trials, which is frequently not the case in actual practice. This further limited the research's relevance to psychotherapy as typically practiced. Furthermore, these strategies focused on research to the exclusion of other considerations, such as therapist competencies, the common factors, individual and cultural differences, and client preferences. The shift to EBPP not only broadened considerations beyond research, but it also developed a more inclusive understanding of relevant research that can be more applicable to real-world clients.

The article by the APA Presidential Task Force on Evidence-Based Practice (2006) notes, "Best research evidence refers to scientific results related to intervention strategies, assessment, clinical problems, and patient populations in laboratory and field settings as well as to clinically relevant results of basic research in psychology and related fields" (p. 274). Furthermore, it suggests that diverse research methods and methodologies are appropriate. In the list of research approaches, which is not intended to be exhaustive, it lists clinical observation, qualitative research, systemic case studies, single-case experimental designs, public health and ethnographic research, process-outcome studies, RCTs, and meta-analysis. Although, unfortunately, there remains some hierarchy in the value given to these research approaches, there also is increased flexibility. Most importantly, though, it does not necessitate the use of certain methods or methodologies.

From an EH perspective, the flexibility is a significant improvement, whereas the hierarchy retains problematic assumptions. There are at least four significant problems with retaining the hierarchy. First, it suggests that method and methodology are more important than the research question in determining the type of research designed or utilized. Second, it does not take into consideration which method and methodology are most appropriate for the particular type of psychotherapy (see Tanenbaum, 2006). Third, though there is little debate that RCTs and meta-analyses (the two most privileged approaches) can produce useful research, there are a significant number of limitations as well (Lutz et al., 2021; Tanenbaum, 2006). For example, the way therapies must be applied to meet the standards for RCTs typically do not reflect either the clients or the applications in the real world (i.e., efficacy versus effectiveness).[2] Last, Yakushko and colleagues (2016) discuss the problematic cultural implications of overreliance upon Western scientific paradigms, including the potential for *epistemological violence*. Western scientific models focus on individual health over collective or community health, self-actualization over coactualization, and Western views of psychological health to the exclusion of culture-specific understandings of mental health.

Fortunately, only a minor modification is needed for the APA Presidential Task Force on Evidence-Based Practice model to be adapted to better fit with EH therapy and more culturally sensitive approaches: remove the hierarchy. This is not suggesting that all research and forms of evidence are equal; rather, it challenges the notion that a particular hierarchy should be set based solely on Western appraisals of what method or methodology is viewed as superior. Different methods and methodologies are better for different research questions.

Clinical Experience and Competencies

The footnote to the first sentence in the Clinical Experience section of the APA Presidential Task Force on Evidence-Based Practice (2006) article states, "Clinical experience refers to competence attained by psychologists through education, training, and experience that results in effective practice" (p. 275). The focus here is that of a generalist—it is concerned with what the foundational competencies are that are important for all psychologists to develop. The list of competencies developed in the article include

> (a) assessment, diagnostic judgment, systematic case formulation, and treatment planning; (b) clinical decision making, treatment implementation, and monitoring of patient progress; (c) interpersonal expertise; (d) continual self-reflection and acquisition of skills; (e) appropriate evaluation and use of research evidence in both basic and applied psychological science; (f) understanding the influence of individual and cultural differences on treatment; (g) seeking available resources (e.g., consultation, adjunctive or alternative services) as needed; and (h) having a cogent rationale for clinical strategies. (p. 275)

All of these are consistent, or potentially consistent, with an EH approach. A few of these may raise concerns with some EH practitioners, particularly assessment, diagnostic judgment, systematic case formulation, and treatment planning. I will briefly consider each of these.

---

[2]There are many thorough critiques of RCTs and the ESTs. For readers who are interested, I recommend Elkins (2009, 2015), E. S. Freire (2006), Lambert and Archer (2006), Smith (2009), Tanenbaum (2006), the American Psychological Association Division 32 Task Force for the Development of Practice Recommendations for the Provision of Humanistic Psychosocial Services (2004), and Wampold and Imel (2015).

EH therapists tend to be less focused on assessment, particularly as assessment is often embedded in a hierarchical approach in which the therapist is viewed as the expert and the client as the subject. However, Constance Fischer pioneered a collaborative or therapeutic approach to assessment that seeks to address these concerns (see Finn et al., 2012; Fischer, 1984; Pade & Holman, 2026). Therefore, EH assessment competencies emphasize a collaborative approach used with the client.

In a study by Hoffman and Cleare-Hoffman (2017a), 62.5% of EH therapists surveyed preferred not to diagnose but would if it was in the best interest of clients. Just over 6% of the therapists said they would never diagnose. Thus, it is understandable that humanistic psychologists have led the way to developing alternatives to diagnosis (Kamens et al., 2019; Pavlo, 2026). From an EH perspective, it is critical to recognize the limitations of diagnosis, how it is often misused, and how it can be harmful to the client. Still, even if preferring not to give a *Diagnostic and Statistical Manual of Mental Disorders* (5th ed; *DSM-5*; American Psychiatric Association, 2013) or *International Statistical Classification of Diseases and Related Health Problems* (11th ed.; *ICD-11*; World Health Organization, 2019) diagnosis, it is important for psychologists to know diagnosis and know it well. Additionally, it is important to recognize that this competency does not necessitate routinely giving a diagnosis or using the *DSM-5* or *ICD-11*. A nondiagnostic approach could include using the diagnostic alternatives that are being developed.

EH therapists have traditionally avoided and critiqued case formulation and treatment planning. There are several reasons for this, including that they, again, often require a hierarchical approach. EH therapy tends to use a phenomenological approach that focuses on understanding the client apart from theory. There is concern that the use of theory in case formulation will distort the client's experience. Similarly, there is the consideration that treatment planning imposes a therapeutic direction on the client. However, Hoffman and Cleare-Hoffman have been developing an approach to case formulation and treatment planning that seeks to avoid these problems (Cleare-Hoffman & Hoffman, 2017; Hoffman & Cleare-Hoffman, 2017a, 2017b, 2025).

Although clinical experience and competencies may require minor modifications within different theoretical approaches, these are general competencies and not antagonistic to any theoretical orientation, including EH therapy. Furthermore, many of these fit well with the common factors of psychotherapy (see Elkins, 2009, 2015; Wampold & Imel, 2015), which EH therapists often have argued fit well with EH therapy.

Client Characteristics, Culture, and Preferences

The article by the APA Presidential Task Force on Evidence-Based Practice (2006) suggests that the third leg of EBPP was developed in part due to concerns and limitations with the first two legs. However, adaptations for individual and cultural differences and preferences ought to be a primary concern for all psychotherapies. EH therapy has long championed the importance of adaptation for individual differences. However, EH therapy has historically struggled with cultural adaptations, including sometimes suggesting a universality to its approaches. Previously, I noted that although humanistic therapies, including EH therapy, were among the first espousing a valuing of multiculturalism, they have struggled and, until recently, failed in actualizing this value (Hoffman, 2016).

EH therapists have begun deeply embracing multicultural, social justice, and liberatory approaches to psychotherapy in ways that are transforming EH therapy. This is evidenced in a growing number of publications on this topic (see Alexander et al., 2026; Beauregard, 2022; Berry Newton & Jackson, 2026; Chávez et al., 2016; Chigangaidze et al., 2022; Gupta, 2022; Hoffman, 2016, 2019; Hoffman, Cleare-Hoffman, & Jackson, 2014; Hoffman, Cleare-Hoffman, et al., 2019; Lemberger & Hutchison, 2014; Levitt & Whelton, 2023; Lorenz & James, 2026; Perrin, 2013; Vallejos & Johnson, 2019; White & Palacios, 2020). Though this progress is encouraging, it is necessary for it to be an ongoing process rooted in cultural and theoretical humility.

EH also has been advocating for the need for a deeper embracement of what multicultural, social justice, and liberatory frameworks mean. Representation is not sufficient, nor is research on different cultural groups. The field of psychology also needs to consider the implications of multicultural, social justice, and liberatory perspectives for research (James & Lorenz, 2026; Yakushko et al., 2016), epistemology (Hoffman, 2016; James & Lorenz, 2026; Yakushko et al., 2016), and our understanding of the person, including individualist versus collectivist identities (Berry Newton & Jackson, 2026; Ingle, 2021, 2026; Jackson, 2019). This has the potential to be transformative to the entire field of psychology if taken seriously, as it can call into question problematic foundational assumptions that have long shaped the field.

CONFRONTING REGRESSIVE UNDERSTANDINGS OF EBPP

It is no surprise that, as Wampold, Goodheart, and Levant (2007) predicted, the understanding of evidence-based practice has regressed. It is not uncommon to hear in many professional settings, including classrooms, conferences, and conversations with colleagues, that a particular modality, such as cognitive behavior therapy or dialectical behavior therapy, is an evidence-based practice. These can be practiced consistent with evidence-based practice, but they are not, in themselves, evidence based.

Even when the three pillars of EBPP are retained, it is not uncommon for the interpretation of the research to be subtly, or not so subtly, moved in a more conservative direction. For example, in a chapter in the *APA Handbook of Psychotherapy*, Kealy and Ogrodniczuk (2024) state,

> In general, systematic reviews and meta-analyses represent the highest quality of evidence, followed by individual efficacy studies (randomized controlled trials [RCTs]) and effectiveness studies (nonrandomized or cohort designs); case studies and expert consensus are additional, lower options in the hierarchy of evidence when more reliable evidence is unavailable. (p. 153)

Whereas the article by the APA Presidential Task Force on Evidence-Based Practice (2006) did include a hierarchy of research, Kealy and Ogrodniczuk are significantly more forceful in their language regarding this hierarchy without considering the appropriateness of research methods for the particular research question or methodology. They also do not mention what the task force referred to as "clinically relevant results of basic research in psychology" (p. 274), which appears dismissive of the value of other psychological research. Although I appreciate much of Kealy and Ogrodniczuk's perspective, and it retains improvement from the EVTs and ESTs models, the regressive understanding of research is a concern, particularly for models of psychotherapy that do not as easily lend themselves to RCTs.

A great deal is at stake in the fight for a more inclusive understanding of EBPP. Previously, I wrote,

> As we move into a new era of artificial intelligence (AI) with ChatGPT and other new forms of AI, it can be maintained that our humanity is at stake in the fight for a more inclusive and human understanding of EBPP. . . . If we reduce evidence-based practice to being about the modality, techniques, or objective and precise application of these, then we can be assured that a time is coming when AI will replace counselors, psychotherapists, and other mental health professionals. AI is rapidly developing in a manner that allows it to be more flexible in its informed responses to human input. As such, it seems inevitable that in the near future AI will be able to apply psychotherapy with greater technical precision than human psychotherapists. But is this what humanity needs? Maybe technical precision is not as critical to the change process as is the embodied personal and relational qualities of a competent therapist implementing a bona fide therapy with all the human imperfections that are part of the psychotherapy process. (Hoffman, 2024, p. 321–322)

I have been arguing for over a decade now that humanistic and existential therapists should not be afraid of EBPP, but rather that we should be concerned with the narrowing definitions.[3] Furthermore, we should advocate for broader, even broadening, understandings of EBPP. If the evidence does not support what we are doing, we should listen to the evidence and change. However, as we demonstrate in this book, we do not need to be afraid of the evidence. It is strongly and forcefully on our side. Though I am certain that further research into EH therapy and its components will lead to changes and advances in how EH therapy is practiced, especially through further dialogues with indigenous psychologies and research with minoritized clients, I trust that EH is increasingly moving in a direction to work with these adaptations to maintain its general approach while becoming increasingly skilled at adapting when beneficial for the clients being served.

---

[3]As this book was in the final stages of production, an important statement relevant to EBPP was issued by the American Psychological Association Advisory Steering Committee for the development of clinical practice guidelines. This important statement is consistent with and supports many of the critiques and perspectives on EBPP advocated in this chapter and throughout this volume. Although it was published too late to integrate into the content of this chapter, readers are strongly encouraged to read the statement, which is available online (https://www.apa.org/about/offices/directorates/guidelines/evidentiary-basis-statement).

DECOLONIZING AND LIBERATORY APPROACHES TO EBPP

Approaches rooted in scientism[4] claim objectivity while promoting a universalism biased toward the values of the so-called elites, or the most powerful and influential, of the dominant culture. Within psychology, this equates to approaches to psychotherapy that uphold the status quo and norms of the dominant culture. Given the influence of Western thought on psychology, this results in an imposition of the values of European and United States White culture. Any questioning of these values is directly or implicitly pathologized. In other words, psychotherapy can easily become a type of colonization through promoting the values of a minority of people (i.e., White culture) holding the power and influence to determine what is viewed as psychologically healthy and moral. Any approach to therapy, including the EH approach, that considers itself to be universal is at risk of participating in these harms.

In essence, the vast majority of approaches to researching the effectiveness of psychotherapy do so with the implicit, and sometimes explicit, assumption of adjusting to societal norms or the status quo. This includes most approaches to EBPP. From a social justice perspective, this inherently pits social justice against most, if not all, approaches to evaluating therapy effectiveness and EBPP. Adding the third leg of EBPP as adapting to client characteristics, culture, and preferences is not much more than window dressing. Taking individual and cultural factors and preferences into consideration means little if the end goal is still helping all clients become more "normal" (i.e., in line with what the dominant culture has established as normal) and adjusted to the status quo.

Any culturally sensitive approach to EBPP must begin by asking, "Who should be allowed to determine the good life for any individual or group of people?" In essence, the debate for what constitutes EBPP is often a heavily value-laden dispute for the definition of both the good life and upholding the status quo. More concerning, though, is the exclusion of many other voices from this debate. This restriction tramples on the U.S. ideals of self-determinism and freedom. Instead of individuals being allowed to determine how they want to live individually and as part of a cultural group, a particular view of the good life is being imposed on all people regardless of individual and cultural differences.

Arguably, the most prominent values reflected in EBPP are capitalism and economic growth, particularly as understood by a small subset of the population. Tanenbaum (2006) states, "Since the early 1970s, U.S. health policy has been about cost" (p. 241). As a friendly amendment to this statement, I maintain that it is about cost and profit, which are necessarily related.

Most people would agree that efforts to reduce health care costs are necessary; however, disagreement remains about what this means and what is the

---

[4]*Scientism* is an approach to science that believes science is objective, or generally objective, and the only correct way to attain many forms of knowledge, typically denying its limitations and reifying its findings.

most just approach to doing this. The influence of profit, however, is more concerning. Often, it is the providers who are blamed for the exorbitant costs; however, there is significant evidence supporting other factors as the primary reasons for rising costs. As of 2020, over one third of health care costs go to bureaucracy, defined as "insurance company overhead and provider time spent on billing" (Carol, 2020). Additionally, a significant portion of costs goes to health care administrators and insurance providers. Similarly, many large hospital chief executive officers, even at nonprofit hospitals, have salaries of over $1 million (Andrzejewksi, 2019). Another significant contribution to health care costs is the profits of pharmaceutical companies. Erman and Wingrove (2023), for example, report that pharmaceutical companies made billions on selling COVID-19 vaccines and treatments. Similarly, drug prices are increasing at record rates (Beasley, 2022; Hopkins, 2023). The price increases are greater than inflation (Shalal, 2023) at a time when these companies are recording record profits. The result is that most families in the United States pay $20,000 or more per year toward health care (Andrzejewksi, 2019).

Tanenbaum (2006) also points to more direct ways that financial implications affect psychotherapy research. For example, researchers often are influenced by funding sources, which frequently are invested in outcomes. For researchers seeking tenure, job security, or advancement, there is an incentive to find results that will lead to future funding and publications. Similarly, Robert Whitaker (2011) shows the rather pervasive influence of large pharmaceutical companies through their funding and marketing. As Vos (2020) illustrates, the economic values promoted by capitalism have broad implications for mental health.

These economic trends, then, have a profound influence on psychological research. It is more cost effective in the short term to utilize narrowly defined outcomes. Therefore, these models are vigorously pursued. Yet it could be argued that what may save money in the short term is likely to be more expensive in the long term. For example, Whitaker (2011) provides evidence suggesting that reliance upon psychotropic medications as the first line of treatment for mild and moderate symptomology often brings about improvement in the short term whereas, in the long term, results in increased chronicity and severity. Lambert and Archer (2006) similarly note that despite studies showing that psychotherapy is generally as effective as medication for many disorders (regardless of treatment modality), medication remains the first line of treatment. Though medication may be more cost effective in the short run, psychotherapy is significantly less expensive than being on medication for the rest of one's life. Again, values or positions that benefit the few (i.e., pharmaceutical companies) are prioritized over the benefits of the many.

Mental health issues also have a significant impact upon physical health, including cardiovascular health (Henein et al, 2022), immune system functioning (Anisman et al., 2018), and cancer risk (Mohan et al., 2023), among others. Minoritized clients are often disproportionally impacted by stress, which is exacerbated by health care disparities including difficulty finding access to practitioners with appropriate cultural competencies and humility (Rose, 2021). Furthermore, many minoritized individuals struggle with trusting the health care system due to a history of mistreatment (Washington, 2008) and negative experiences with health care providers. Investment in addressing social, systemic, and psychological factors contributing to individual health care costs is not easy nor is it something that can be quickly accomplished; however, in the long run, it is likely to be more economically beneficial while also being more compassionate and humane.

Like most therapists, I have had many clients who have come to me for therapy after failed attempts at therapy with other providers. In my case, most of these clients previously were seen by therapists using cognitive behavioral therapy, dialectical behavior therapy, eye movement desensitization and reprocessing (EMDR), and other short-term therapies. These clients often dropped out of the previous therapy and sought out something different. I do not believe that my success with these clients is necessarily due to me being a better therapist than their previous therapists or that the EH approach I use is a superior modality. Rather, the therapy I offered was effective because it was the right fit for these clients.

The mental health field needs to focus on helping clients find the right fit for them, not imposing one upon them. This is a liberatory approach that values the individual and cultural differences in clients and the diverse approaches to psychotherapy. The pursuit of which therapy modality is best has been, from the outset, the wrong question. We can better meet the unique needs of diverse clients through having varied therapeutic modalities, adjusting the length of treatment to the long-term needs of the client, respecting our differences, helping clients find the right fit for them, and working to improve each modality through vigorous research. Most likely, too, this will be more financially efficient in the long term. I am thankful that, when a client is not the right fit for EH therapy, I can refer them to a cognitive behavioral, EMDR, or psychoanalytic therapist. At times, too, a client may benefit from different therapy modalities at different points of their journey. The debate about which approach to therapy is superior is more about ego, short-term economics, and believing in the superiority of certain value systems than it is about serving our clients.

Clients, however, often do not know that they have options, and frequently they do not know what they want from psychotherapy. Popular culture has shaped how most people understand therapy, including what they should expect or want to get from attending therapy. Typically, clients enter therapy to decrease their emotional suffering and increase pleasure or to cure a mental illness. Although there is nothing wrong with seeking these outcomes, there remains great ambiguity in what these goals mean and how to pursue them. Furthermore, they may not be the preferred outcomes for all clients.

For educator and philosopher Paulo Freire (1968/2018), any liberatory movement must dialogue with the people who are being liberated without imposing a worldview or set of values upon them. Although Freire was applying this principle in a very different context, it is relevant to psychotherapy. Freire sees an essential part of colonization as the imposition of a worldview upon the colonized. Mainstream approaches to psychology tend to value rationalism, individualism, objectivity, improved functionality, and a decrease in symptoms of what is deemed mental illness. Furthermore, mental illness or psychological problems are conceived as meeting a certain number of criteria of a psychological diagnosis regardless of the etiology that has brought about these symptoms. This makes it easier to give a diagnosis but more difficult to adequately understand the problem in context. These values, then, are imposed directly and implicitly upon clients. If they resist this worldview, they are further pathologized by the therapist, often called a "resistant client" or difficult client" when, in fact, it may be that they are taking a healthy stand against having someone else's values imposed upon them.

Drawing from Paulo Freire, I maintain that an essential competency of EBPP should be developing a skillset that helps clients explore and clarify what they see as the good life and the goals they want to pursue in therapy. This should take into consideration cultural values as well as personal values. Critical to this competency, therapists must learn to minimize imposing a value set upon clients, even if it is derived from research.[5] At times, this may entail helping clients recognize the influence of the social context, including recognizing where their values may not fit with the values of the dominant culture in which they live. This, again, is a liberatory framework. It fits with Rollo May's (1981) assertion that "the purpose of psychotherapy is to set people free" (p. 19). Unfortunately, psychology too often, as Paulo Freire (1968/2018) states, "confuse[s] freedom with the maintenance of the status quo" (p. 36).

Consistent with this framework, Viktor Frankl (1946/1984) maintains that happiness is best achieved through a life well-lived. In this conception, which fits with EH approaches, happiness is best achieved by helping clients clarify their understanding of the good life and then living in accordance with it. For this to be achieved, it must be authentic—it must be based on the client's view of the good life. If one's view of the good life is the one presented to them or imposed upon them by the dominant culture or the psychotherapist without critical reflection, it is not authentic. This has consequences for mental health (see Chapter 7). For Paulo Freire (1968/2018), authentic and liberatory praxis or action requires reflection. From an EH perspective, this ought to be applied to the view of the good life.

In the context of the health care industry, this is problematic. Reflection is not always cost effective in the short term. Often, it requires slowing down the process of therapy. However, although it may not be cost effective in the short term, it may be much more so in the long term because the resultant change is more likely to be authentic, sustained change. This may be why, according to Lambert and Archer's (2006) review of the research, attending therapy for longer is more likely to result in successful, sustained outcomes. Short-term therapies by their nature have to limit the amount of critical reflection and rely upon the therapist's theoretical framework that typically conforms to the dominant

---

[5]In Chapter 2, this competency can be seen in the phenomenological explorations of meaning, as well as other phenomenological explorations.

culture and the implicit values associated with it. This results in an imposition of values. However, happiness derived from conforming to the dominant culture is less likely to be authentic or sustaining.

Once again, what is cost effective—and potentially even therapeutically effective—in the short term may not serve the client's or society's best interest in the long term. Too often, the pressure to be cost effective undermines providing the best available individualized treatments.

An Alternative Approach to Outcome Research

I maintain that a more appropriate approach to outcome research would utilize a variation of participatory action research. In participatory action research, the researchers are collaborators; the participants help formulate the problem, research question, and approach to research (James & Lorenz, 2026). To utilize a similar model with psychotherapy outcome studies, the research would identify a community and approach them about their mental health needs, including the problems within the community and the desired outcomes. From here, the researcher and community would collaboratively discuss an approach to designing a research project on the effectiveness of therapy with this group toward the desired outcome.

The following fictional example may help illustrate. A group of researchers wanted to provide mental health services to a group of community activists and evaluate the effectiveness of the psychotherapy employed. After establishing an initial trusting relationship with the group of community activists, a focus group was set up to discuss the mental health needs of this community and what they perceive as the good life (i.e., the desired outcomes). The results of the focus group indicated that the community activists were not primarily interested in traditional outcomes, such as decreased depression, anxiety, and anger. Instead, their view of the good life included (a) being "creatively maladjusted" (a term coined by Martin Luther King Jr.), (b) recognizing and accepting one's limits, (c) learning to channel anger and hurt as motivation toward changing society and helping members of their community, and (d) achieving collective or community actualization.

After the vision of the good life had been established, the focus group reconvened to review and discuss the results. At this time, consideration was given to common desired psychotherapy outcomes. As these were considered, the group reshaped the outcome of "recognizing one's limits" to also include self-care, which would particularly include culture-specific approaches to self-care. The group also worked to further clarify what it meant to be creatively maladjusted. The focus group retained their rejection of focusing primarily on decreasing depression, anxiety, or anger as appropriate outcomes, noting that this often helped reinforce the status quo and focused too much on individual needs over community needs.

Next, consideration was given as to how to measure the outcomes. Commonplace models, such as outcome measures, were considered and rejected.

The group felt it would be difficult and time consuming to develop these measures, and they did not trust their accuracy. Instead, the focus group preferred to find ways to assess outcomes relationally and within the community.

The next step involved identifying types of psychotherapy that the focus group felt were an appropriate fit or could be an appropriate fit with some modifications. EH therapy was identified as one of the approaches that would be a good fit with some modifications, particularly with adaptations focusing more on collective and community needs and interventions. The focus group learned some about this approach to therapy and offered recommendations for making adaptations to the therapy model for working with community activists. These recommendations were provided to the therapists. Next, the group discussed ways to recruit participants and begin the study.

As the research was completed, the focus group reconvened to review the findings and provide feedback. The feedback helped shape the researchers' interpretation of the results. After this, the researchers wrote up an initial draft of a manuscript. This, too, was presented to the focus group for feedback and modifications before finalizing the manuscript to submit for publication.

An approach to outcome research such as this hypothetical example is more intensive, expensive, and time consuming than current models. A challenge, of course, is that most funding agencies would be resistant to funding a project such as this due to the expense as well as concerns about using a nontraditional approach to research. This challenge says a great deal about the resistance to research models drawing from cultural values and ways of knowing as well as the privileging of mainstream models of science and research (see Yakushko et al., 2016). Funding agencies, too, have a strong preference for the dominant culture's ways of knowing and mainstream values regarding psychotherapy outcomes.

DEMONSTRATING EH THERAPY'S EVIDENCE-BASED FOUNDATIONS

Though EH therapists do not need to fear EBPP, it is important to know how to demonstrate the evidence that supports the therapist's practice. This can be done through the three components of EBPP: best available research evidence; clinical experience and competencies; and client characteristics, culture, and preferences.

In this book, we are advocating that using the best available research is best done through demonstrating the effectiveness of the components of EH therapy and the issues being addressed. When focusing on the specific components, using the best available research entails using the research to improve one's effectiveness with these different components. Each of the chapters in Part II include an overview of the relevant research that can help therapists demonstrate the effectiveness of their approach while also learning to refine their skills related to this component. For example, Vos (Chapter 9) discusses how research can help therapists improve their engagement with clients regarding meaning.

To accomplish demonstrating the effectiveness of components of EH therapy, it is important to have some agreed upon understanding of the problem (formulation of the problem or case formulation) and a treatment plan including goals. EH therapists have often been resistant to adding this structure. There are good reasons for this aversion, as when done poorly, case formulation can limit aspects of psychotherapy. For example, Elkins (2009) noted that it is common for clients to not initially know or reveal their primary reason or reasons for coming to therapy. At times, it may be a general feeling of dis-ease or something they do not yet have adequate words to describe. In other cases, the client may not want to reveal why they are coming to therapy until they have established a good, trusting relationship. This can, at times, take several months to establish, especially for clients who have had bad prior experiences with therapists or the mental health system. Third, as one grows through the process of therapy, new issues may emerge, often either discovered through the therapy process or secondarily resulting from the client's growth. For example, as a client grows and becomes more confident, they may be less willing to continue in unhealthy relationships. This may lead to conflict, grief, and loneliness.

To address these concerns, this book is being developed alongside a second book, *Case Formulation in Existential–Humanistic Therapy* (Hoffman & Cleare-Hoffman, 2025). This approach has been developed to provide a flexible, fluid approach to case formulation and treatment planning that helps clinicians identify particular EH and integrative treatment strategies and interventions to address collaboratively identified challenges and goals.

As the challenges and goals are identified, they are mapped with particular interventions. Some of these interventions, such as presence, may be important for all clients (see Schneider, 2015). However, other interventions may vary depending upon the client, even if valuable for most clients. For example, genuineness and self-disclosure may be more important for clients who struggle with relationships, particularly those who often worry about how others feel about or view them. With clients who struggle with loneliness and isolation primarily due to feeling alienated, empathy may be an important intervention. The skilled therapist, too, may use these differently. For example, at times empathy may be used largely to help understand the client and inform other interventions, whereas with other clients, the direct expression of empathy may be an essential aspect of healing and change.

As therapists clarify challenges and goals, or potentially diagnoses, they then can begin customizing a treatment plan for the clients with specific interventions. To demonstrate research evidence, therapists can then cite or refer to research supporting the different components of therapy being utilized with the particular client. As therapy is fluid, there will likely emerge new issues and goals, which then can be updated in the case formulation and treatment plan. The chapters in Parts II and III of this book are designed to help EH therapists map support for primary interventions. Each of these chapters review the qualitative and quantitative research on these interventions.

The second component of EBPP, therapist experience and competencies, is rooted in generalist competencies, some of which are adapted to be consistent with EH therapy. As these are more global skills to be applied with all clients, this is addressed by Vos in Chapter 2, which focuses on foundational EH therapy competencies. Some of these are highly consistent with generalist therapist competencies with some EH adaptations, whereas others are unique to existential therapy.

The third leg of EBPP is client characteristics, culture, and preferences. Individual client differences regarding characteristics and preferences are naturally part of EH therapy and addressed in the case formulation and treatment planning process. The cultural differences and adaptations require a different approach, which still ought to be a natural, fluid part of EH psychotherapy. However, as EH therapy has struggled with this until recently, each of the chapters in Parts II and III include a section on cultural adaptations. Though it is not possible for these sections to be comprehensive and include all possible adaptations, they lay a foundation for how these strategies can be adapted to be rooted in cultural humility. It is important for therapists to recognize that all therapies contain implicit values, including assumptions about how clients should live. EH therapy, even when striving to be culturally humble, values a particular way of being that includes relational and intrapersonal depth. Most people who read this book likely will align with these values, yet it can be harmful if they are promoted as the right way of being for all individuals.

Through implementing the strategies discussed in this section, EH therapists can demonstrate that they are practicing consistently with EBPP in their work settings, in educational or training programs, and with third party payors.

CONCLUSION

In my over 20 years as a psychologist, I have observed various threats to the freedom to practice EH therapy evolve and fluctuate over time. Early in my career, I was told that if I was willing to use EH therapy with a client presenting with anxiety issues, I should have a complaint filed against me and my license taken away. This astonished me, especially given that Rollo May (1950/1970) wrote one of the first ever psychological books on anxiety: *The Meaning of Anxiety*. This book has been widely read and remains influential. I continued to hear rumors and often concrete evidence of movements in professional psychology that could make it more difficult to practice EH therapy in many settings. Similarly, I heard stories of EH colleagues struggling to convince insurance companies to reimburse them despite a plethora of evidence that supports the benefits of EH therapy.

When teaching at various universities either full time or part time, many of my students who were interested in EH therapy were told by other faculty members that EH therapy was not effective or that there was no evidence that it was effective. At other times, they were told that they could not find a job or pay off student loans if they pursued EH therapy. Yet, in my over 20 years as a faculty member and supervisor, I have had hundreds of students interested in pursuing EH therapy. Despite many of these students not being allowed to focus on EH therapy at their practicum sites and internships, they pursued further developing their rootedness in this approach through seeking training opportunities on their own. I do not know of a single student pursing being an EH therapist who has not been able to find a job or pay off their student loans.

It was these experiences that motivated me to collaborate on writing and editing this book. I want to ensure that students and professionals will retain the right and ability to practice EH therapy. I want clients to be able to pursue EH therapy—or whatever therapy is the right fit for them.

For 20 years, I have advocated that the debate over which therapy is best, most effective, or superior is the wrong debate. This is a distraction that often makes us look foolish to our clients and others outside of the field of psychology. The reality is that psychotherapy in general tends to be effective (Lambert & Archer, 2006; Lutz et al., 2021; Norcross & Wampold, 2019a; Wampold & Imel, 2015), particularly if we are able to establish a good relationship with our clients. It is much easier to establish a good relationship with clients when the modality is a good fit for the client's goals and ways of being. Many clients who have benefited from seeing me for therapy find cognitive behavior therapy simplistic, too rational, limiting, or even oppressive. They have felt unseen, objectified, and devalued by these therapists. Yet, there are clients who have come to me that I have felt would be a better fit for cognitive behavior therapy, EMDR, or other modalities. Although I do not know the result of their experience with the therapists I referred them to, I am confident that these approaches were more likely to benefit these clients.

EH therapists ought to be confident in their approach and the evidence that supports it. This confidence, in fact, can help therapy be more effective (Wampold & Imel, 2015). My hope is that those who read this book find it to be practical and useful, particularly when used with its companion volume, *Case Formulation in Existential–Humanistic Therapy* (Hoffman & Cleare-Hoffman, 2025). Certainly, there are other interventions that could be added to this book, and the research is still developing. A second hope is that this book helps readers develop the skills and resources to build upon it, adding in other interventions and strategies that could be included. This is not intended to be the final statement on practicing EH therapy consistent with EBPP; rather, it is intended to be a starting point that provides a potential path forward to strengthening this foundation. Finally, it is hoped that this book will be useful to researchers interested in filling the gaps in research relevant to EH therapy.

REFERENCES

Ackerman, S. J., Benjamin, L. S., Beutler, L. E., Gelso, C. J., Goldfried, M. R., Hill, C., Lambert, M. J., Norcross, J. C., Orlinsky, D. E., & Rainer, J. (2001). Empirically supported therapy relationships: Conclusions and recommendations of the Division 29

Task Force. *Psychotherapy, 38*(4), 495–497. https://doi.org/10.1037/0033-3204.38. 4.495

Alexander, A. A., Klukoff, H., & Neal, B. (2026). Humanistic and existential approaches to advocacy and activism. In L. Hoffman (Ed.), *APA handbook of humanistic and existential psychology: Vol. 2. Clinical and social applications* (pp. 535–552). American Psychological Association. https://doi.org/10.1037/0000432-026

Anisman, H., Hayley, S., & Kusnecov, A. (2018). *The immune system and mental health.* Academic Press. https://doi.org/10.1016/C2016-0-01000-8

Andrzejewski, A. (2019, June 26). Top U.S. "non-profit" hospitals & CEOs are racking up huge profits. *Forbes.* https://www.forbes.com/sites/adamandrzejewski/2019/06/26/top-u-s-non-profit-hospitals-ceos-are-racking-up-huge-profits/

American Psychiatric Association. (2013). *Diagnostic and statistical manual of mental disorders* (5th ed.). https://doi.org/10.1176/appi.books.9780890425596

American Psychological Association Division 12 Task Force on Promotion and Dissemination of Psychological Procedures. (1995). Training in and dissemination of empirically-validated psychological treatments: Report and recommendations. *The Clinical Psychologist, 48(1).* https://www.div12.org/wp-content/uploads/2017/07/Original-EST-Documents.pdf

American Psychological Association Division 32 Task Force for the Development of Guidelines for the Provision of Humanistic Psychosocial Services. (1997). Guidelines for the provision of humanistic psychosocial services. *The Humanistic Psychologist, 25*(1), 65–107. https://doi.org/10.1080/08873267.1997.9986872

American Psychological Association Division 32 Task Force for the Development of Practice Recommendations for the Provision of Humanistic Psychosocial Services. (2004). Recommended principles and practices for the provision of humanistic psychosocial services: Alternative to mandated practice and treatment guidelines. *The Humanistic Psychologist, 32*(1), 3–75. https://doi.org/10.1080/08873267.2004.9961745

American Psychological Association Presidential Task Force on Evidence-Based Practice. (2006). Evidence-based practice in psychology. *American Psychologist, 61*(4), 271–285. https://doi.org/10.1037/0003-066X.61.4.271

Beasley, D. (2022, August 16). Focus: Newly launched U.S. drugs head toward record-high prices in 2022. *Reuters.* https://www.reuters.com/business/healthcare-pharmaceuticals/newly-launched-us-drugs-head-toward-record-high-prices-2022-2022-08-15/

Beauregard, E. M. (2022). We should all be marching: Why humanistic psychologists should take action toward social justice. *The Humanistic Psychologist, 50*(4), 594–606. https://doi.org/10.1037/hum0000269

Berry Newton, M., & Jackson, T. R. (2026). Integrating multicultural perspectives. In L. Hoffman (Ed.), *APA handbook of humanistic and existential psychology: Vol. 2. Clinical and social applications.* American Psychological Association. https://doi.org/10.1037/0000432-002

Beutler, L. E., & Johannsen, B. E. (2006). Principles of change. In J. C. Norcross, L. E. Beutler, & R. F. Levant (Eds.), *Evidence-based practices in mental health: Debate and dialogue on the fundamental questions* (pp. 226–234). American Psychological Association. https://doi.org/10.1037/11265-000

Cambridge Dictionary. (n.d.). Validate. https://dictionary.cambridge.org/dictionary/english/validate

Carol, L. (2020, January 6). More than a third of U.S. heathcare costs go to bureaucracy. *Reuters.* https://www.reuters.com/article/idUSKBN1Z5260/

Carter, J. A. (2006). Theoretical pluralism and technical eclecticism. In C. D. Goodheart, A. E. Kazdin, & R. J. Sternberg (Eds.), *Evidence-based psychotherapy: Where practice and research meet* (pp. 63–79). American Psychological Association. https://doi.org/10.1037/11423-003

Chávez, T. A., Torres Fernandez, I., Hipolito-Delgado, C. P., & Torres Rivera, E. (2016). Unifying liberation psychology and humanistic values to promote social justice in counseling. *The Journal of Humanistic Counseling*, *53*(3), 166–182. https://doi.org/10.1002/johc.12032

Chigangaidze, R. K., Matanga, A. A., & Katsuro, T. R. (2022). Ubuntu philosophy as a humanistic–existential framework for the fight against the COVID-19 pandemic. *Journal of Humanistic Psychology*, *62*(3), 319–333. https://doi.org/10.1177/00221678211044554

Cleare-Hoffman, H. P., & Hoffman, L. (2017, August 4). *Key influences on the development of existential–humanistic therapy practice* [Poster presentation]. American Psychological Association 125th Annual Convention, Washington, DC, United States.

Cleare-Hoffman, H. P., Hoffman, L., & Wilson, S. S. (2013, July 31–August 4). Existential therapy, culture, and therapist factors in evidence-based practice. In K. Keenan (Chair), *Evidence in support of existential–humanistic psychotherapy: Revitalizing the third force* [Symposium]. American Psychological Association 121st Annual Convention, Honolulu, HI, United States.

Constantino, M. J., Coyne, A. E., Boswell, J. F., Iles, B. R., & Vîslă, A. (2019). Promoting treatment credibility. In J. C. Norcross & M. J. Lambert (Eds.), *Psychotherapy relationships that work: Vol. 1. Evidence-based therapist contributions* (3rd ed., pp. 495–521). Oxford University Press. https://doi.org/10.1093/med-psych/9780190843953.003.0014

Constantino, M. J., Vîslă, A., Coyne, A. E., & Boswell, J. F. (2019). Cultivating positive outcome expectation. In J. C. Norcross & M. J. Lambert (Eds.). *Psychotherapy relationships that work: Vol. 1. Evidence-based therapist contributions* (3rd ed., pp. 461–494). Oxford University Press. https://doi.org/10.1093/med-psych/9780190843953.003.0013

Elkins, D. N. (2009). *Humanistic psychology: A clinical manifesto: A critique of clinical psychology and the need for progressive alternatives.* University of the Rockies Press.

Elkins, D. N. (2015). *The human elements of psychotherapy: A nonmedical model of emotional healing.* American Psychological Association. https://doi.org/10.1037/14751-000

Erman, M., & Wingrove, P. (2023, February 6). Focus: Drug companies face COVID cliff in 2023 as sales set to plummet. *Reuters.* https://www.reuters.com/business/healthcare-pharmaceuticals/drug-companies-face-covid-cliff-2023-sales-set-plummet-2023-02-06/

Finn, S. E., Fischer, C. T., & Handler, L. (Eds.). (2012). *Collaborative/therapeutic assessment: A casebook and guide.* John Wiley & Sons.

Fischer, C. T. (1984). *Individualizing psychological assessment: A collaborative and therapeutic approach.* Routledge.

Frankl, V. E. (1984). *Man's search for meaning: An introduction to logotherapy.* Simon & Schuster. (Original work published 1946)

Freire, E. S. (2006). Randomized controlled clinical trial in psychotherapy research: An epistemological controversy. *Journal of Humanistic Psychology*, *46*(3), 323–335. https://doi.org/10.1177/0022167806286276

Freire, P. (2018). *Pedagogy of the oppressed* (50th anniv. ed.). Bloomsbury Academic. (Original work published in 1968)

Garfield, S. L. (1996). Some problems associated with the "validated" forms of psychotherapy. *Clinical Psychology: Science and Practice*, *3*(3), 218–229. https://doi.org/10.1111/j.1468-2850.1996.tb00073.x

Gelso, C. J., Kivlighan, D. M., Jr., & Markin, R. D. (2019). The real relationship. In J. C. Norcross & M. J. Lambert (Eds.), *Psychotherapy relationships that work: Vol. 1. Evidence-based therapist contributions* (3rd ed., pp. 351–378). Oxford University Press. https://doi.org/10.1093/med-psych/9780190843953.003.0010

Goldfried, M. R. (2007). What has psychotherapy inherited from Carl Rogers? *Psychotherapy*, *44*(3), 249–252. https://doi.org/10.1037/0033-3204.44.3.249

Gupta, N. (2022). Truth, freedom, love, hope, and power: An existential rights paradigm for anti-oppressive psychological praxis. *The Humanistic Psychologist*, *50*(3), 460–475. https://doi.org/10.1037/hum0000274

Hayes, J. A., Gelso, C. J., Kivlighan, M., & Goldberg, S. B. (2019). Managing counter-transference. In J. C. Norcross & M. J. Lambert (Eds.), *Psychotherapy relationships that work: Vol. 1. Evidence-based therapist contributions* (3rd ed., pp. 522–548). Oxford University Press. https://doi.org/10.1093/med-psych/9780190843953.003.0015

Henein, M. Y., Vancheri, S., Longo, G., & Vancheri, F. (2022). The impact of mental stress on cardiovascular health—Part II. *Journal of Clinical Medicine, 11*(15), 4405. https://doi.org/10.3390/jcm11154405

Hoffman, L. (2016). Multiculturalism and humanistic psychology: From neglect to epistemological and ontological diversity. *The Humanistic Psychologist, 44*(1), 56–71. https://doi.org/10.1037/hum0000016

Hoffman, L. (2019). Culture and empathy in humanistic psychology. In L. Hoffman, H. Cleare-Hoffman, N. Granger, Jr., & D. St. John (Eds.), *Humanistic approaches to multiculturalism and diversity: Perspectives on existence and difference* (pp. 103–116). Routledge. https://doi.org/10.4324/9781351133357-9

Hoffman, L. (2024). The possibilities and slippery slope of evidence-based practice in psychology: Why humanistic and existential psychologists must engage the conversation. *The Humanistic Psychologist, 52*(3), 318–324. https://doi.org/10.1037/hum0000347

Hoffman, L., & Bowers, V. (2016, March). *Existential–humanistic therapy and evidence-based practice in psychology: We are on solid ground* [Paper presentation]. Society for Humanistic Psychology 9th Annual Conference, San Francisco, CA, United States.

Hoffman, L., Clark, G., Clark, J., Franklin, M., Henson, A., Smylie, T., & Wilson, S. (2013, August). *Demonstrating existential and humanistic therapy's evidence-based foundation for your practice* [Workshop presentation]. Society for Humanistic Psychology Hospitality Suite at the American Psychological Association 121st Annual Convention, Honolulu, HI, United States.

Hoffman, L., & Cleare-Hoffman, H. P. (2017a, August). *An existential–humanistic approach to case formulation and treatment planning* [Poster presentation]. American Psychological Association 125th Annual Convention, Washington, DC, United States.

Hoffman, L., & Cleare-Hoffman, H. P. (2017b, October). *Existential–humanistic case conceptualization and treatment planning with diverse populations: Ethical considerations and adaptations* [Paper presentation]. International Society for Ethical Psychology and Psychiatry 20th Annual Conference, Denver, CO, United States.

Hoffman, L., & Cleare-Hoffman, H. P. (2025). *Case formulation in existential–humanistic therapy*. American Psychological Association. https://doi.org/10.1037/0000464-000

Hoffman, L., Cleare-Hoffman, H., Granger, N., Jr., & St. John, D. (Eds.). (2019). *Humanistic approaches to multiculturalism and diversity: Perspectives on existence and difference*. Routledge. https://doi.org/10.4324/9781351133357

Hoffman, L., Cleare-Hoffman, H. P., & Jackson, T. (2014). Humanistic psychology and multiculturalism: History, current status, and advancements. In K. J. Schneider, J. F. Pierson, & J. F. T. Bugental (Eds.), *The handbook of humanistic psychology: Theory, research, and practice* (2nd ed., pp. 41–55). Sage.

Hoffman, L., Dias, J., & Soholm, H. C. (2012, August 2–5). Existential–humanistic therapy as a model for evidence-based practice. In S. Rubin (Chair), *Evidence in support of existential–humanistic psychology: Revitalizing the 'third force'* [Symposium]. American Psychological Association 120th Annual Convention, Orlando, FL, United States.

Hoffman, L., Vallejos, L., Cleare-Hoffman, H. P., & Rubin, S. (2015). Emotion, relationship, and meaning as core existential practice: Evidence-based foundations. *Journal of Contemporary Psychotherapy, 45*(1), 11–20. https://doi.org/10.1007/s10879-014-9277-9

Hopkins, J. S. (2023, February 2). Drug prices increase 5.6% as government ramps up pressure to lower costs. *The Wall Street Journal.* https://www.wsj.com/articles/drugmakers-raise-prices-on-nearly-1-000-medicines-but-show-restraint-11675313960

Ingle, M. (2021). Western individualism and psychotherapy: Exploring the edges of ecological being. *Journal of Humanistic Psychology, 61*(6), 925–938. https://doi.org/10.1177/0022167818817181

Ingle, M. (2026). Rethinking individualism, collectivism, and conformity. In L. Hoffman (Ed.), *APA handbook of humanistic and existential psychology: Vol. 1. History, research, philosophy, and theory* (pp. 565–584). American Psychological Association. https://doi.org/10.1037/0000431-024

Jackson, T. (2019). The history of Black psychology and humanistic psychology: Synergetic prospects. In L. Hoffman, H. P. Cleare-Hoffman, N. Granger, Jr., & D. St. John (Eds.), *Humanistic approaches to multiculturalism and diversity: Perspectives on existence and difference* (pp. 29–44). Routledge. https://doi.org/10.4324/9781351133357-4

James, S., & Lorenz, H. (2026). Participatory and relational methodologies: Emergent undercommons, generative refusals, and fugitive movements. In L. Hoffman (Ed.), *APA handbook of humanistic and existential psychology: Vol. 1. History, research, philosophy, and theory.* American Psychological Association. https://doi.org/10.1037/0000431-004

Kamens, S. R., Cosgrove, L., Peters, S. M., Jones, N., Flanagan, E., Longden, E., Schulz, S., Robbins, B. D., Olsen, S., Miller, R., & Lichtenberg, P. (2019). Standards and guidelines for the development of diagnostic nomenclatures and alternatives in mental health research and practice. *Journal of Humanistic Psychology, 59*(3), 401–427. https://doi.org/10.1177/0022167818763862

Kealy, D., & Ogrodniczuk, J. S. (2024). What is the current configuration of evidence-based psychotherapy? Integrating common factors into personalized care. In F. T. L. Leong (Ed.), *APA handbook of psychotherapy: Vol. 2. Evidence-based practice, practice-based evidence, and contextual participant-driven practice* (pp. 153–169). American Psychological Association. https://doi.org/10.1037/0000354-010

Lambert, M. J., & Archer, A. (2006). Research findings on the effects of psychotherapy and their implications for practice. In C. D. Goodheart, A. E. Kazdin, & R. J. Sternberg (Eds.), *Evidence-based psychotherapy: Where practice and research meet* (pp. 111–130). American Psychological Association. https://doi.org/10.1037/11423-005

Lemberger, M. E., & Hutchison, B. (2014). Advocating student-within-environment: A humanistic approach for therapists to animate social justice in the schools. *Journal of Humanistic Psychology, 54*(1), 28–44. https://doi.org/10.1177/0022167812469831

Levant, R. F. (2004). The empirically validated treatment movement: A practitioner/educator perspective. *Clinical Psychology: Science and Practice, 11*(2), 219–224. https://doi.org/10.1093/clipsy.bph075

Levitt, H. M., & Whelton, W. J. (2023). On the need to reconcile cultural and professional power in psychotherapy: Humanistic principles that are foundational for feminist multicultural practice. *The Humanistic Psychologist, 52*(2), 137–162. https://doi.org/10.1037/hum0000327

Lorenz, H., & James, S. (2026). Liberation psychologies and decolonialities: Defecting from environments of domination to build spaces of collective agency, prefigurative politics, and ecological justice. In L. Hoffman (Ed.), *APA handbook of humanistic and existential psychology: Vol. 1. History, research, philosophy, and theory.* American Psychological Association. https://doi.org/10.1037/0000431-028

Lutz, W., Castonguay, L. G., Lambert, M. J., & Barkham, M. (2021). Traditional and new beginnings: Historical and current perspectives on research in psychotherapy and behavioral change. In M. Barkham, W. Lutz, & L. G. Castonguay (Eds.), *Bergin and Garfield's handbook of psychotherapy and behavioral* change (pp. 3–18). John Wiley & Sons.

May, R. (1970). *The meaning of anxiety.* W. W. Norton & Company. (Original work published 1950)

May, R. (1981). *Freedom and destiny.* W. W. Norton & Company.

Mohan, A., Huybrechts, I., & Michels, N. (2022). Psychosocial stress and cancer risk: A narrative review. *European Journal of Cancer Prevention, 31*(6), 585–599. https://doi.org/10.1097/CEJ.0000000000000752

National Council of Schools and Programs of Professional Psychology. (n.d.). *Education model requirements*. https://thencspp.org/training-model/ncspp-educational-model-requirements/

Norcross, J. C. (2001). Purposes, processes, and products of the task force on empirically supported therapy relationships. *Psychotherapy*, *38*(4), 345–356. https://doi.org/10.1037/0033-3204.38.4.345

Norcross, J. C. (2002). *Psychotherapy relationships that work: Therapist contributions and responsiveness to patients*. Oxford University Press.

Norcross, J. C. (2011). *Psychotherapy relationships that work: Evidence-based responsiveness* (2nd ed.). Oxford University Press. https://doi.org/10.1093/acprof:oso/9780199737208.001.0001

Norcross, J. C., & Lambert, M. J. (2006). The therapy relationship. In J. C. Norcross, L. E. Beutler, & R. F. Levant (Eds.), *Evidence-based practices in mental health: Debate and dialogue on the fundamental questions* (pp. 208–218). American Psychological Association. https://doi.org/10.1037/11265-000

Norcross, J. C., & Lambert, M. J. (2019). *Psychotherapy relationships that work: Vol. 1. Evidence-based therapist contributions* (3rd ed). Oxford University Press. https://doi.org/10.1093/med-psych/9780190843953.001.0001

Norcross, J. C., & Wampold, B. E. (2019a). Evidence-based psychotherapy responsiveness: The third task force. In J. C. Norcross & B. E. Wampold (Eds.), *Psychotherapy relationships that work: Vol. 2. Evidence-based therapist responsiveness* (3rd ed., pp. 1–14). Oxford University Press. https://doi.org/10.1093/med-psych/9780190843953.003.0001

Norcross, J. C., & Wampold, B. E. (2019b). *Psychotherapy relationships that work: Vol. 2. Evidence-based therapist responsiveness* (3rd ed.). Oxford University Press. https://doi.org/10.1093/med-psych/9780190843960.001.0001

Pade, H., & Holman, A. (2026). Collaborative assessment. In L. Hoffman (Ed.), *APA handbook of humanistic and existential psychology: Vol. 2. Clinical and social applications* (pp. 49–70). American Psychological Association. https://doi.org/10.1037/0000432-003

Pavlo, A. J. (2026). "A little stand-offish": Existential and humanistic diagnostic perspectives. In L. Hoffman (Ed.), *APA handbook of humanistic and existential psychology: Vol. 1. History, research, philosophy, and theory*. American Psychological Association. https://doi.org/10.1037/0000431-015

Peluso, P. R., & Freund, R. R. (2019). Emotional expression. In J. C. Norcross & M. J. Lambert (Eds.). *Psychotherapy relationships that work: Vol. 1. Evidence-based therapist contributions* (3rd ed., pp. 421–460). Oxford University Press. https://doi.org/10.1093/med-psych/9780190843953.003.0012

Perrin, P. B. (2013). Humanistic psychology's social justice philosophy: Systemically treating the psychosocial and health effects of racism. *Journal of Humanistic Psychology*, *53*(1), 52–69. https://doi.org/10.1177/0022167812447133

Peterson, D. R. (2004). Science, scientism, and professional responsibility. *Clinical Psychology: Science and Practice*, *11*(2), 196–210. https://doi.org/10.1093/clipsy.bph072

Rose, P. R. (2021). *Health, equity, diversity, and inclusion* (2nd ed.). Jones & Bartlett Learning.

Schneider, K. J. (2015). Presence: The core contextual factor of effective psychotherapy. *Existential Analysis*, *2*(2), 304–312.

Shalal, A. (2023, December 14). Biden administration to impose inflation penalties on dozens of drugs. *Reuters*. https://www.reuters.com/business/healthcare-pharmaceuticals/dozens-companies-raised-drug-prices-faster-than-inflation-white-house-says-2023-12-14/

Singal, A. G., Higgins, P. D. R., & Waljee, A. K. (2014). A primer on effectiveness and efficacy trials. *Clinical and Translational Gastroenterology*, *5*(1), e45. https://doi.org/10.1038/ctg.2013.13

Smith, K. R. (2009). Psychotherapy as applied science or moral praxis: The limitations of empirically supported treatment. *Journal of Theoretical and Philosophical Psychology, 29*(1), 34–46. https://doi.org/10.1037/a0015564

Tanenbaum, S. J. (2006). Expanding the terms of the debate: Evidence-based practice and public policy. In C. D. Goodheart, A. E. Kazdin, & R. J. Sternberg (Eds.), *Evidence-based psychotherapy: Where practice and research meet* (pp. 239–259). American Psychological Association. https://doi.org/10.1037/11423-010

Vallejos, L., & Johnson, Z. (2019). Multicultural competencies in humanistic psychology. In L. Hoffman, H. P. Cleare-Hoffman, N. Granger, Jr., & D. St. John (Eds.) *Humanistic approaches to multiculturalism and diversity: Perspectives on existence and difference* (pp. 63–75). Routledge. https://doi.org/10.4324/9781351133357-6

van der Lem, R., van der Wee, N. J. A., van Veen, T., & Zitman, F. G. (2012). Efficacy versus effectiveness: A direct comparison of the outcome of treatment for mild to moderate depression in randomized controlled trials and daily practice. *Psychotherapy and Psychosomatics, 81*(4), 226–234. https://doi.org/10.1159/000330890

Vos, J. (2020). *The economics of meaning in life: From capitalist life syndrome to meaning-oriented economy.* University Professors Press.

Wampold, B. E. (2006). The psychotherapist. In J. C. Norcross, L. E. Beutler, & R. F. Levant (Eds.), *Evidence-based practices in mental health: Debate and dialogue on the fundamental questions* (pp. 200–208). American Psychological Association.

Wampold, B. E., Goodheart, C. D., & Levant, R. F. (2007). Clarification and elaboration on evidence-based practice in psychology. *American Psychologist, 62*(6), 616–618. https://doi.org/10.1037/0003-066X62.6.616

Wampold, B. E., & Imel, Z. E. (2015). *The great psychotherapy debate: The evidence for what makes psychotherapy work* (2nd ed.). Routledge. https://doi.org/10.4324/9780203582015

Washington, H. A. (2008). *Medical apartheid: The dark history of medical experimentation on Black Americans from colonial times to the present.* Vintage.

Whitaker, R. (2011). *The anatomy of an epidemic: Psychiatric drugs and the astonishing rise of mental illness in America.* Crown.

White, D., & Palacios, A. (2020). A culturally responsive existential–phenomenological approach for counseling Black sexual minority youth. *The Journal of Humanistic Counseling, 59*(2), 74–85. https://doi.org/10.1002/johc.12131

World Health Organization. (2019). *International statistical classification of diseases and related health problems* (11th ed.). https://icd.who.int

Yakushko, O., Hoffman, L., Morgan Consoli, M. L., & Lee, G. (2016). On methods, methodologies, and continued colonization of knowledge in the study of "ethnic minorities": Comment on Hall et al. (2016). *American Psychologist, 71*(9), 890–891. https://doi.org/10.1037/amp0000060

Yates, C. (2013). Evidence-based practice: The components, history, and process. *Counseling Outcome Research and Evaluation, 4*(1), 41–54. https://doi.org/10.1177/2150137812472193

2

Existential–Therapeutic Competencies

Joel Vos

Imagine you have been invited to participate in the story of *Alice's Adventures in Wonderland*. Not only have you been asked, but your entire extended family has—even long-lost relatives, your grandparents, and their siblings as well. At some point, Alice's friend, the Dodo bird, suggests doing a bonding activity: a caucus race that has no clearly defined starting places or endpoints. As soon as you start the race, the similarities and dissimilarities between the relatives become clear, as—despite the lack of rules—most relatives run in the same direction and use similar running patterns. Naturally, everyone has their unique strengths and weaknesses, but it becomes clear that you share general directions and competencies. Everyone finishes at the same place, and the Dodo bird concludes that all have won and therefore all deserve prizes.

In the research field of psychological therapies, this is known as the *Dodo bird verdict* or *equivalent therapy effects phenomenon*, as different therapeutic approaches seem to have relatively similar outcomes (Wampold & Imel, 2015). The Dodo bird verdict has sometimes been explained by the observation that different therapeutic approaches have much in common, such as basic therapeutic competencies.

This chapter includes material adapted from "The Existential Therapeutic Competences Framework: Development and Preliminary Validation," by J. Vos, 2021a, *International Journal of Psychotherapy, 25*(1), pp. 9– 51 (https://www.ijp.org.uk/docs/IJP_2021_25_1_Full_Issue.pdf). Copyright 2021 by the European Association of Psychotherapy. Adapted with permission.

https://doi.org/10.1037/0000446-003
The Evidence-Based Foundations of Existential–Humanistic Therapy, L. Hoffman and V. Lac (Editors)

This chapter aims to give an overview of the competencies that the relatives in the family of existential therapies have in common and how these competencies can aid individual therapists in effectively helping clients reach their therapy goals. Focusing on the most effective shared competencies may help existential therapists work most effectually with clients, justify the effectiveness to health insurances and health services, and educate the youngest members of the existential–therapeutic family. Additionally, it may help specific existential approaches, including existential–humanistic (EH) therapy, have a foundation for integrating supported aspects of other existential therapies. This chapter will give an overview of empirical research on existential therapies, as described in detail in several systematic literature reviews and meta-analyses, with a focus on the core competencies of these approaches (J. Vos, 2016a, 2016b, 2017, 2018, 2019, 2021a, 2023b; J. Vos, Cooper, et al., 2015; J. Vos, Craig, & Cooper, 2015; J. Vos & Vitali, 2018).

To give this overview of research-supported existential–therapeutic competencies, this chapter will open with a definition of existential–therapeutic competencies and why identifying these competencies matter. Subsequently, the family tree of existential therapies (ETs) will be described with the philosophical foundations at its roots (ET's grandparents), the common basic existential–therapeutic competencies as its trunk (ET's parents), and unique competencies within specific existential–therapeutic branches (ET's children). See Figure 2.1 for a visual depiction of the family tree.

To understand the common knowledge in ETs (roots and trunks), a brief overview will be provided of the common evidence-based conceptual model and outcomes of ETs. The main part of this chapter will focus on the research evidence for basic existential–therapeutic competencies. The last sections briefly reflect on multicultural considerations, future research, and conclusions.

DEFINING EXISTENTIAL–THERAPEUTIC COMPETENCIES

Since the turn of the millennium, professional bodies worldwide have formulated competencies frameworks for education, training, and the registration and monitoring of practitioner quality (J. Vos, 2021a). For example, in 2006, the American Psychological Association called for establishing and implementing competencies standards throughout the field of psychology across all types of training and professional practice (Campbell et al., 2012; Hope, 2004; Kaslow, 2004; Roberts et al., 2005; Thomas, 2010; J. Vos, 2023a). Example competency frameworks are competency benchmarks (Fouad et al., 2009), the "Competency Assessment Toolkit for Professional Psychology" toolkit (Kaslow et al., 2009), practicum competencies outlines (Hatcher & Lassiter, 2007), and the "Professional Competencies of a European Psychotherapist" core competencies (Young et al., 2013). Several competency frameworks have also been built for specific psychological therapies, such as clinical psychology, cognitive behavior therapy, and psychoanalytic/psychodynamic therapy (University College of

FIGURE 2.1. Conceptual Overview of Existential Therapies

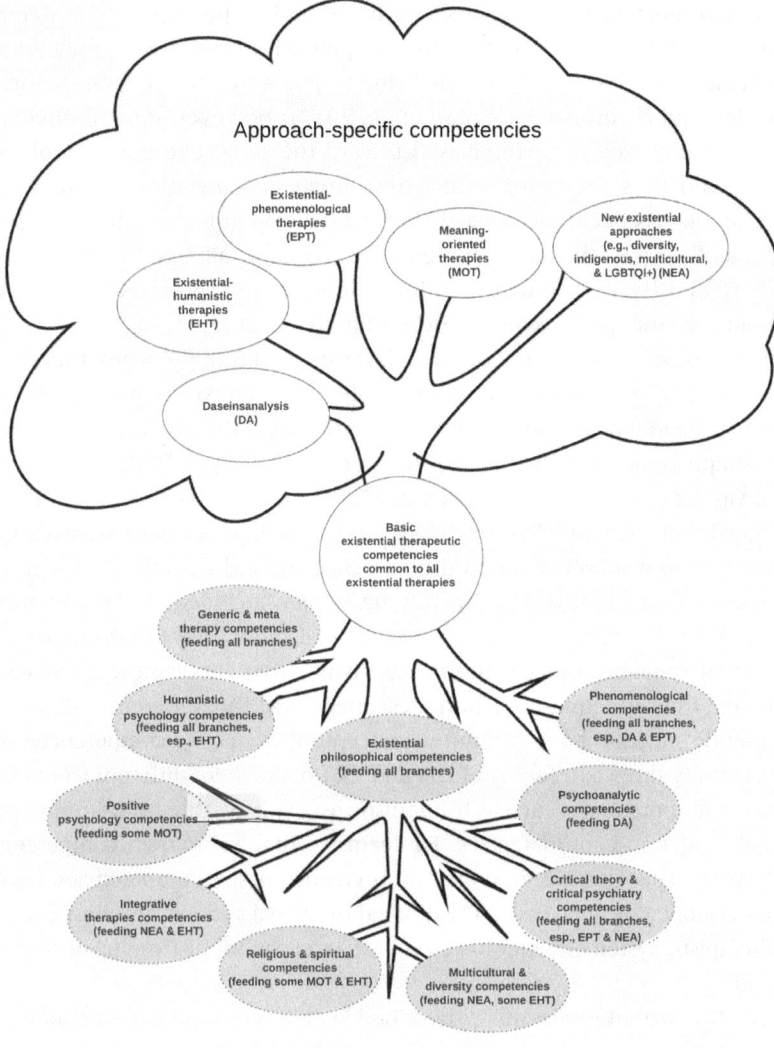

Approach-specific competencies

Existential-phenomenological therapies (EPT)

Meaning-oriented therapies (MOT)

New existential approaches (e.g., diversity, indigenous, multicultural, & LGBTQI+) (NEA)

Existential-humanistic therapies (EHT)

Daseinsanalysis (DA)

Basic existential therapeutic competencies common to all existential therapies

Generic & meta therapy competencies (feeding all branches)

Phenomenological competencies (feeding all branches, esp., DA & EPT)

Humanistic psychology competencies (feeding all branches, esp., EHT)

Existential philosophical competencies (feeding all branches)

Positive psychology competencies (feeding some MOT)

Psychoanalytic competencies (feeding DA)

Integrative therapies competencies (feeding NEA & EHT)

Critical theory & critical psychiatry competencies (feeding all branches, esp., EPT & NEA)

Religious & spiritual competencies (feeding some MOT & EHT)

Multicultural & diversity competencies (feeding NEA, some EHT)

Competencies inspiring existential therapies

London, 2022). One example is the competencies framework for humanistic therapy, which followed previous studies on humanistic competencies (Cain, 2016; Farber, 2010, 2012; Roth, 2015; University College of London, 2022; Vallejos & Johnson, 2019). These frameworks include competences and competencies. Although the terms are often used interchangeably, most psychologists seem to use the term *competence* to refer to an individual's general potential, overall quality, or state of being competent, whereas they seem to use *competencies* (plural of "competency") in regard to specific skills and demonstrable abilities (Stevens, 2013; Whiddett & Hollyforde, 2003). Many of these frameworks have been used in the design of training programs, in the formulation of benchmarks in clinical training and supervision, and in the decision making on which types and competency levels of psychological therapies will be covered by national mental health services and health insurance.

These competencies frameworks are based on best practices and systematic research evidence, so these therapy competencies frameworks may fit the requirements of evidence-based medicine to guarantee the highest quality of education and client care (Hoffman et al., 2012). However, some frameworks have been criticized for being biased toward the subjective opinions of their authors and thus not being sufficiently broad and inclusive (Roth, 2015). Therefore, it has been encouraged that we develop guidelines that represent the broad field (i.e., the basic competencies shared by all, like the trunk in the family tree) as well as show the unique differences of specific schools within the field (i.e., the specific competencies of individual branches).

Even though ETs are some of the oldest therapeutic approaches, there have not been any comprehensive, evidence-based frameworks for ET. Several authors have identified some critical competencies in ET, which seem to reflect their unique position in the field (Hoffman et al., 2015; van Deurzen & Adams, 2016; van Deurzen & Arnold-Baker, 2005; J. Vos, 2017; Wong, 2013). It may be argued that such an ET competencies framework does not exist, as ET may be regarded as a subset of humanistic psychology, and thus these existential–therapeutic competencies may already have been included in the humanistic competencies framework. The next section will show how ET's historical and conceptual roots are indeed intertwined with other therapeutic approaches. However, the subsequent section describes how the different existential–therapeutic branches have a common conceptual model and competencies that seem to unify them as a family of ETs and that make them different from other therapeutic approaches, such as humanistic psychology. Due to its unique conceptual model and competencies, ET seems to require its own competencies framework. This chapter describes the evidence-based competencies framework developed by Joel Vos (2021a) based on global surveys amongst existential therapists, systematic literature reviews, and the input from leaders in the ET field.

Until the turn of the century, there had been a relatively widespread reluctance amongst existential therapists toward identifying key competencies and engaging with quantitative research in general (J. Vos, 2013; J. Vos, Cooper, Correia, & Craig, 2015). This seems to have been caused by a fundamental tendency in existential philosophy to reduce the totality and complexity of phenomena, such as therapeutic practices, to a limited set of operationalized competencies. Of course, any universal model or framework will falter in specific encounters with individual clients, as such models are generalizations across many individuals. Furthermore, postmodernist existential therapists dismiss the modernist idea of identifying an absolute truth (Loewenthal, 2018). It may be argued that, congruent with the thinking of existential philosopher Martin Heidegger (1997), operationalized frameworks are a symptom of how we approach truth in our era (epochè) via calculating thinking (rechnendes Denken) and via explaining psychological phenomena with external instruments and objective observation (erklären) instead of understanding these from within the subjectively lived experience (verstehen; Dilthey, 1895/1996). In contrast, a key value in ET is doing justice to the uniqueness of the lived experiences of each client, therapist, and therapeutic encounter.

Although these critical arguments may be ideologically admirable, seen from an existential–philosophical perspective, they may not be pragmatic and beneficial for the professional status and development of the ET field. Many professional bodies, health care providers, and insurance companies require evidence-based competencies frameworks for training and practice, and thus without such frameworks, they may exclude ET from their smorgasbord of funded treatments. Furthermore, an ET competencies framework may improve the learning efficiency in existential therapy programs and stimulate critical self-reflection and reflexivity in trainees regarding their practices. Thus, we may want to base the ET competencies framework on a pragmatic–phenomenological perspective, which may be described as follows:

> The phenomenon of therapeutic practice may be compared with a multifaceted diamond and a competencies framework is like light cast from one angle, making only one specific facet shine while leaving other facets in the dark. . . . We seem to be needing to cast lights from multiple angles in order to be able to understand the totality of the phenomenon—as seen from a hermeneutic–phenomenological perspective. . . . A light that comes from merely one angle—whatever this angle may be—may not be sufficient to grasp the totality of the phenomenon of the therapeutic encounter. Thus, it may be epistemologically justifiable and clinically pragmatic to develop a competencies framework for ET while we explicitly acknowledge its limitations. Therefore, this study aims to present a competencies framework for ET, which integrates both "bottom-up" and "top-down" perspectives and is based on systematic empirical research. This framework may help—pragmatically—validate, justify, and improve ET training and practices. This framework may, for example, help to translate ET in terms of national occupational standards for mental health care workers. (J. Vos, 2021a, p. 16)

CONTEXTUALIZING EXISTENTIAL-THERAPEUTIC COMPETENCIES

Before we can formulate a common ET competencies framework, we need to understand the similarities and dissimilarities between different ET branches. That is, although there are large overlaps between different ET schools, there may also be some considerable differences (Cooper, 2016; van Deurzen & Arnold-Baker, 2018; van Deurzen et al., 2019). The following sketch of the family tree of ET will be based on a worldwide survey amongst existential therapists by Correia and colleagues (2014, 2016a, 2016b, 2018). Globally, there are 147 existential education and training organizations (Correia et al., 2016b), such as the World Confederation for Existential Therapy, Federation of Existential Therapies Europe, Viktor Frankl Institute, Gesellschaft fur Logotherapie und Existenzanalysis, International Meaning Events & Community, and International Network for Personal Meaning. Authors have categorized these schools into distinct groups, such as Daseinsanalysis, therapies centered around meaning,

EH and existential–integrative therapies, and existential–phenomenological approaches (Cooper, 2016; van Deurzen et al., 2019). However, this classification trend fails to adequately acknowledge the diverse regional schools and unique cultural advancements that exist, particularly in China, Southeast Asia, Africa, and Latin America (Gordon, 1996; Hoffman et al., 2009).

The fundamental aim of Daseinsanalysis is to empower clients to embrace their complete existence and strive for a more authentic way of life (for an overview, see Holzhey-Kunz, 2019). Clients are urged to foster an outlook of "let-it-be-ness" (referred to as Gelassenheit; J. Vos, 2015). Whereas traditional Daseinsanalysts like Binswanger and Boss historically employed a systematic phenomenological approach, contemporary practitioners, exemplified by Holzhey-Kunz, have advanced the approach by integrating it with a myriad of therapeutic skills and placing explicit emphasis on existential themes within client experiences. Daseinsanalysts notably integrate diverse techniques from psychoanalysis, such as free association and dream analysis, into their practice. This integration not only enriches the therapeutic landscape but also underscores the adaptability of Daseinsanalysis in addressing the multifaceted nature of individual experiences, furthering the pursuit of authenticity and holistic well-being.

Meaning-centered therapies, the predominant form of ETs, find frequent application in working with patients confronting chronic or life-threatening illnesses (for overviews, see J. Vos, 2016a, 2016b, 2017). These therapies trace their origins to the establishment of logotherapy (where "logo" signifies "meaning") by Viktor Frankl, succeeded by various meaning-oriented approaches like existential analysis (for an overview, see Längle, 2019); meaning-centered psychotherapy in palliative care (Breitbart, 2016); and evidence-based, meaning-oriented practices (J. Vos, 2016b). Deliberately and methodically addressing inquiries about life's meaning, meaning-centered therapies aim to guide clients toward leading more meaningful and fulfilling lives, embracing life's challenges with an affirmative outlook. Although different meaning-oriented schools employ varied methods, most rely on phenomenological and systematic approaches to help clients unearth their individual perceptions of significance. More recent iterations of meaning-oriented approaches introduce structured, time-limited treatments with systematic steps to unveil the client's unique life meanings, often tailored for specific groups such as cancer patients (Breitbart, 2016; J. Vos, 2017).

EH therapies, prominent primarily in the United States, draw influence from humanistic luminaries like Rollo May and include notable figures such as Bugental and Schneider. These therapies are geared toward guiding clients to attain a heightened sense of presence and a more complete and subjective experience of aliveness (Schneider & Krug, 2010). The pursuit of self-realization is often impeded by unconscious or subconscious anxieties. By aiding clients in confronting and unraveling these barriers (Bugental, 1999), therapists seek to help clients transcend emotions such as guilt, pain, shame, or dread and embrace the entirety of their experiences, including the recognition of their potential and a sense of awe. Therapeutic techniques encompass experiential processing, emotional exploration, self-expression, free association, identification and visualization of emotions, and fostering trust in the capacity to endure negative emotions, often employing strategies and stances as detailed in Parts II and III of this book. Some EH therapists, exemplified by Irvin Yalom (2020), actively encourage clients to surmount their existential defense mechanisms and confront existential realities such as freedom, death, responsibility, and isolation. However, it should be noted that there is disagreement about whether Yalom is an EH therapist or whether his approach represents his own unique existential therapy. Additionally, existential–integrative approaches encompass a spectrum of therapies that amalgamate existential principles with other therapeutic modalities, frequently employing short-term interventions.

The phenomenological–existential therapeutic approaches originated in the United Kingdom, finding inspiration in the works of critical psychiatrist Ronnie Laing and philosopher Hans Cohn and further developed by therapists like Ernesto Spinelli and Emmy van Deurzen. These approaches center on facilitating a nondiagnostic examination of the client's experiences, employing a phenomenological approach with a pronounced focus on the therapeutic alliance. For instance, Spinelli (2005) guides clients in "descriptively clarifying disruptive elements in their worldview, allowing for the relational exploration of their sedimentation and dissociations" (p. 87; see also Spinelli, 1997). Similarly, van Deurzen & Adams (2016) assist clients by employing descriptive–phenomenological inquiries to delve into their experiences and paradoxical emotions within the context of their physical, personal, social, and spiritual spheres. Joel Vos (2017, 2021a) has advocated for the use of more systematic and evidence-based phenomenological approaches in client work to avoid imposing the therapist's agenda, aligning with the principles of the aforementioned influential authors.

In their global survey across existential therapists, Correia and colleagues (2014, 2016a, 2106b, 2018) not only found differences between the four ET branches (existential–humanistic, existential–phenomenological, meaning-oriented, and Daseinsanalysis) but also discovered commonalities. For instance, all existential therapists emphasize the grounding of their practices in existential and phenomenological philosophy, drawing inspiration from humanistic/person-centered approaches, and critical theory/critical psychiatry. Existential therapists commonly employ four interrelated therapeutic competencies: phenomenological skills, relational skills, elucidation of existential themes, and competencies specific to their respective therapeutic schools. It is noteworthy that most existential therapists, as indicated in Correia and colleagues' survey, demonstrate flexibility in not rigidly adhering to a single existential school, instead focusing on commonalities. This observed convergence across theories and practices may suggest that most existential therapists belong to subsequent generations after the inception of ETs, akin to other therapeutic schools. In this conception, the newer generations exhibit a reduced adherence to the unique founders of their school, instead prioritizing commonalities with other approaches and emphasizing therapeutic components supported by empirical research.

The family tree of ET, depicted earlier in Figure 2.1, shows the relationships between ET's underlying philosophies (the roots), its basic general competencies (the trunk), and specific existential approaches (the branches). The five different branches (existential–humanistic, existential–phenomenological, meaning-oriented, Daseinsanalysis, and new existential approaches) share a basic existential–therapeutic conceptual framework and competencies. This shared basic conceptual framework and these competencies have been inspired by existential and phenomenological philosophy as well as humanistic/person-centered approaches and critical theory/critical psychiatry. They also include generic and metatherapy competencies, which all therapeutic approaches (including nonexistential) have in common, as will be elaborated later. Next to these common influences and particularly Heideggerian phenomenology, Daseinsanalysis was also strongly influenced by psychoanalysis. Existential–phenomenological therapies were also strongly influenced by phenomenological philosophy and critical theory/critical psychiatry. Some individual meaning-oriented therapists, such as Paul Wong, have reported influences by positive psychology and religious/spirituality studies, and others, such as Alfried Längle, by phenomenological philosophy. EH therapists have reported influences by other humanistic psychological approaches such as person-centered therapy and, more recently, also by the fields of integrative therapies, multicultural and diversity studies, and religion and spirituality studies.

OVERVIEW OF RESEARCH ON A BASIC EXISTENTIAL–THERAPEUTIC CONCEPTUAL MODEL

The previous section has described how, despite their differences, the different ET branches have much in common. Before we can identify their common basic ET competencies, we need to understand the conceptual model that they have in common. A key competency of any therapeutic school is knowing the main theoretical assumptions that it is based on.

The basic conceptual model of ET consists of multiple components. To be a bona fide therapeutic approach, each component needs to be based on sound research evidence. Bona fide therapies encompass therapeutic practices conducted in good faith, signifying that therapists are professionally trained and dedicated to the therapy through accredited institutions and organizations. Additionally, bona fide therapy necessitates being founded on a robust conceptual framework (Wampold et al., 1997). The conceptual framework of therapies can be deconstructed into various conceptual components, as highlighted in the works of Kazdin (2021) and Joel Vos (2022, 2023a).

> To build a strong conceptual model of a psychological therapy, each component and each of the relationships between the steps need to be supported by strong empirical evidence from quantitative and qualitative research, and by logical reasoning and coherence. If any of these conceptual steps are missing or are not

supported by strong empirical evidence, and/or if the relationship between these steps is illogical or incoherent, it may be concluded that the therapy does not have a strong evidence-based conceptual model, and therefore this therapy may not be *bona fide*. (J. Vos, 2022 p. 65)

In this section, the focus is on delineating the key conceptual components present in ETs and evaluating the extent to which each conceptual component of existential therapy is substantiated by empirical research evidence. These components encompass clinical, etiological, therapeutic, client-oriented, therapist-oriented, relationship-oriented, and competencies-oriented conceptual components. These delineations build upon prior comprehensive reviews on the evidence supporting existential concepts, with forthcoming sections elaborating on research about outcomes and evidence-based therapist competencies (J. Vos, 2019; J. Vos, Cooper, Correia, & Craig, 2015). This chapter highlights a variety of quantitative, qualitative, and mixed methods studies.

Etiological Conceptual Component

The conceptual framework of ETs often originates from a series of ontological assumptions that are inherently unfalsifiable. For example, many existentialists posit that we are thrust into a world characterized by immutable givens such as mortality, freedom, and paradoxes, commonly referred to as "life's givens" or "existential givens." Here, the term "world" serves as a broad descriptor encompassing the entirety of our subjective life and the contextual framework in which we are situated (Heidegger, 1927). In contrast to positivists, phenomenologists assert that we lack direct access to the reality of our world, as our awareness of the world is shaped within our primary subjective phenomenological experiences of daily life. According to existential philosophers like Binswanger (1963) and van Deurzen (2009), individuals can encounter different aspects, domains, or worlds. An empirical review of 109 studies conducted worldwide reveals that individuals notably discern six distinct types of meanings inherent in their experiential flow: materialistic, hedonistic, self-oriented, social, larger, and existential–philosophical meanings (J. Vos, 2023c).

Etiology and Therapeutic Mechanisms of Change

However, as elucidated by philosophers such as Heidegger (1927; J. Vos, 2015, 2021c), individuals in different epochs tend to have a different dominant focus toward different facets of the world. Consequently, within the spectrum of our worldly experiences, we tend to emphasize certain aspects while overlooking others. Phenomenological therapists expound on how individuals often overlay these primary experiences with meaning and interpretations (e.g., Spinelli, 2005; Wrathall, 2010), and as a result, have developed methodologies to delineate this stream of consciousness and differentiate it from secondary interpretations (Smith et al., 2021; J. Vos, 2021b). Thus, a distinction can be made between our unprocessed primary experiences and our subsequent interpreted experiences. For instance, neuropsychological research indicates that consciousness

originates from a primary sense of experiences, even before entering our awareness, which is then subject to our interpretations (Caruso & Flanagan, 2017;
Damasio, 2000). It appears that existential therapists concentrate on aiding clients in opening themselves to their primary flow of experiences and alleviating
emotional barriers or existential defense mechanisms that may impede clients
from fully engaging with the world. Research suggests that when clients are
supported in deepening their experiences and immersing themselves in their
flow—for instance, through focusing techniques (Gendlin, 2003)—they exhibit
enhanced overall well-being (Hendricks, 2002).

Various therapists employ diverse terminology and specific techniques to
assist clients in reconnecting with their primary flow of experiencing the
entirety of the world. In the forthcoming elucidation, the updated stress coping
model proposed by C. L. Park and Folkman (1997) will be utilized; this model
has garnered extensive support from numerous studies, especially in pivotal life
circumstances that explicitly bring existential themes to the forefront. Despite
its robust evidence-based foundation and relevance to existential therapy, this
model and its terminology are infrequently integrated into existential therapy.
The primary appraisal delineates how individuals evaluate a situation: What is
their initial appraisal of the situation? Do they perceive it as a threat or as
benign? Individuals appear to adjust their appraisal of the situation in response
to existential defense mechanisms, or they may endeavor to embrace their
experiences of the situation. For instance, research rooted in terror management theory has furnished substantial evidence of how individuals perceive
and modify their perception of fundamental life givens, such as death awareness or mortality salience (Routledge & Vess, 2018). When individuals are confronted with reminders of their mortality, such as those brought about by the
global COVID-19 situation, these reminders can evoke fear and trigger death
anxiety, which may subsequently be suppressed by altering their perception of
the threat. Studies indicate that existential anxiety heightens the tendency for
individuals to deny the threat posed by COVID-19 (J. Vos, 2021b). Alternatively, individuals may redirect their focus from the threat to something they
find more meaningful, such as their heritage, culture, values, or life's meaning.

In the context of secondary appraisal, individuals are tasked with evaluating
their resources to effectively respond to a given situation. Factors such as
self-efficacy, life experience, and existential competencies often influence an
individual's response to a situation. Viktor Frankl (1946/1985) expounded on
how individuals can alter their internal attitude toward a situation, consequently impacting their well-being. Frankl's focus on finding meaning in life
enabled him to endure the atrocities of being a prisoner in a concentration
camp. In the face of life's boundary situations, individuals can opt to sink to
despair and resignation or distance themselves from the situation by embracing
a leap of faith, transcending the constraints of the situation in both space and
time, thereby cultivating a broader, more authentic, and more meaningful perspective on life (Frankl, 1946/1985; Jaspers, 1925/2013). Although the freedom of will is an unverifiable facet of life (Lukas, 1986), numerous empirical

studies have affirmed the adaptability of individuals in coping with life's experiences (e.g., Zeidner & Endler, 1995). The flexibility in coping styles appears to hold more significance than the reliance on a singular coping strategy to navigate adversity (Kashdan & Rottenberg, 2010).

An illustration of the connection between secondary and tertiary appraisal is evident in the anticipation and protective conduct during the COVID-19 pandemic, which was determined by an individual's sense of self-efficacy, prior encounters with life's uncertainties, and their capacity to endure uncertainties while leading a meaningful life despite life's challenges (J. Vos, 2021b). Tertiary appraisal pertains to the meaning-oriented response that individuals ascribe to a specific situation. Individuals frequently negotiate the significance of a particular situation within the context of their overarching sense of meaning in life (Folkman, 1997; J. Vos, 2011). For instance, a diagnosis of a life-threatening condition can challenge an individual's fundamental assumptions regarding the benevolence of the world, the meaningfulness of life, and the worthiness of the self (Brewin & Holmes, 2003; Janoff-Bulman, 2010). At times, individuals endeavor to uphold these fundamental life assumptions and preserve what holds meaning for them, irrespective of the situation, whereas on other occasions, they may recalibrate their goals and meanings in response to the situation (C. L. Park, 2010; J. Park & Baumeister, 2017). The manner in which individuals experience meaning in demanding situations, such as finding purpose in the face of pain, suffering, and mortality, appears to hinge on several subjective factors. Some existential therapists suppose that clients possess an intrinsic motivation, impetus, or will to find meaning; research indicates that most individuals strive for a meaningful life, although this may not be universally applicable (J. Vos, 2016a, 2018). Moreover, our meaning-oriented coping abilities are contingent on our capacity to lead a meaningful life despite the inherent constraints of the world into which we are thrust, including our mortality, freedom, isolation, and the absence of an absolute true meaning of life bestowed at birth. Consequently, numerous existential therapists have discussed how individuals can hold paradoxes in life, cultivate a sense of tragic optimism, or develop a dual attitude; research suggests that the ability to cultivate a dual attitude can aid in leading a meaningful life while acknowledging life's limitations, which is associated with improved mental well-being (for a review, see J. Vos, 2015, 2018,).

Some of the primary mechanisms of change employed by existential therapists in their work with clients appear to be linked to these appraisal processes. Therapists aid clients in honoring their primary flow of experiencing the world in its entirety by delving into their appraisal processes. This involves enabling individuals to comprehend their situations and lives and scrutinizing how their primary appraisals may be constraining or unproductive. Subsequently, therapists may assist clients in cultivating the resources to formulate an authentic and well-considered response to their situations and life in general (for instance, enhancing well-being and satisfaction when individuals make decisions they deem authentic; Schlegel et al., 2009). Existential therapists also focus on how individuals perceive meaning in life by methodically and explicitly addressing the concept of meaning in life. Research suggests that existential–therapeutic competencies aid clients in these appraisal processes (as elaborated later). Studies indicate that a therapist's personal existential skills, life experience, professional training, and expertise can enhance their therapeutic competencies, subsequently influencing the mechanisms of change that can enhance the clinical components and outcomes in ETs (J. Vos, 2017). Naturally, this provides a broad overview of therapeutic mechanisms, and different existential schools may emphasize varying facets (J. Vos, 2019; J. Vos, Cooper, Correia, & Craig, 2015).

Relational Components

Existential therapists dedicate considerable attention to cultivating a constructive therapeutic relationship, as will be explained later (see also Part II of this volume). Research illustrates how operating at relational depth enhances the therapeutic journey by enabling clients to feel sufficiently secure to delve into their perspectives, resources, and meaning-oriented coping strategies (Norcross & Lambert, 2019). The therapeutic relationship may also provide a platform for experimenting with alternative outlooks and responses.

Clinical Components

Though clients may express concerns about their existential appraisal processes, it is more probable that they seek assistance from an existential therapist due to distinctive existential clinical components. These clinical components stem from etiological mechanisms and can result in outcomes such as psychopathology, diminished quality of life, and physical ailments. For instance, when individuals are confronted with life's fundamental givens and perceive them as threatening, then with inadequate resources and a lack of meaningful coping strategies, they may experience existential moods. Existential moods (referred to by Heidegger as *Grundstimmungen*) are extensively studied affective moods that transcend transient emotions. These moods are not centered on specific objects, such as a fear of dogs, but revolve around profound life concerns such as death, freedom, or responsibility. Existential therapists have identified a wide array of existential moods, with death anxiety and feelings of meaninglessness or meaningfulness being among the most extensively researched (e.g., Brandstätter et al., 2012; Ryff, 1989, 2018; Steger et al., 2006; van Bruggen et al., 2015). These existential moods can manifest explicitly in existential and philosophical inquiries about life, such as the quest for meaning in life; however, many clients seem to grapple with these existential moods in an unconscious manner. These existential moods can underlie other forms of psychopathology and behavior (J. Vos, 2016a, 2016b). Some individuals describe the presence of existential moods and inquiries as an existential crisis, a crisis of meaning in life, an identity crisis, or a spiritual crisis; a crisis may linger before surfacing overtly (J. Vos, 2017). Empirical studies affirm that numerous individuals report experiencing existential moods and questions when they encounter life's fundamental aspects; for instance, most individuals grapple with existential questions following a diagnosis of a chronic or life-threatening illness or during the grieving process after losing a loved one (Henoch & Danielson, 2009; C. L. Park et al., 2008; J. Vos et al., 2016b; Winger et al., 2015). Extensive research indicates that a large majority of the general population actively seeks meaning and that the presence of meaning and meaning-oriented coping styles is moderately to strongly correlated with enhanced quality of life, reduced psychological stress (such as depression and anxiety), and improved physical well-being (Brandstätter et al., 2012; Folkman, 2008; C. L. Park, 2010; Roepke et al., 2014; Ryff et al., 2004; Steger, 2012).

OVERVIEW OF RESEARCH ON GENERAL OUTCOMES OF ETS

As a first indication of which types of ET and which competencies are effective, this section provides an overview of the effects of ET. Similar to other psychological therapies, ET has been developed and validated in multiple stages with different types of studies (e.g. Carroll & Nuro, 2002; Rounsaville et al., 2001). Although various research methodologies may have played an important role in developing and validating ETs, this section will focus only on clinical trials that fulfill the quality criteria of evidence-based medicine.

Joel Vos, Craig, and Cooper (2015) conducted meta-analyses of 21 eligible randomized controlled trials of existential therapy involving 1,792 participants. The inclusion criteria focused on articles in English only. Meaning-oriented therapies ($n = 6$) demonstrated substantial effects on positive meaning in life immediately posttherapy ($d = 0.65$) and at follow-up ($d = 0.57$), with moderate effects on psychopathology ($d = 0.47$) and self-efficacy ($d = 0.48$) at postintervention; however, they did not yield significant effects on self-reported physical well-being ($n = 1$). Supportive–expressive therapy, aligned with the existential therapist Yalom ($n = 5$), exhibited marginal effects at posttreatment and follow-up on psychopathology ($d = 0.20$ and $d = 0.18$, respectively); nevertheless, effects on self-efficacy and self-reported physical well-being were inconclusive ($n = 1$ and $n = 4$, respectively). Notably, there were indications of unreliable data in some publications based on Yalom's approach, as analyses and findings could not be replicated with the same datasets, and clients with substantial negative outcomes had been excluded without disclosure, resulting in publication bias (studies with a high risk of bias were excluded from the meta-analyses). Three studies on existential–integrative therapies (experiential–existential and cognitive–existential therapies) did not yield significant effects. The study samples were diverse, primarily focusing on individuals in challenging life circumstances, such as those with chronic or life-threatening diseases. It is important to note that although the research samples were diverse, they may not fully represent the clinical population, often excluding individuals with complex and comorbid issues. This meta-analysis particularly supported structured interventions incorporating psychoeducation, exercises, and a supportive and relational approach when addressing life's existential aspects, especially in physically ill patients.

To delve deeper into the positive effects of meaning-oriented therapies, Joel Vos and Vitali (2018) conducted a multilingual systematic review and meta-analysis of all clinical trials on meaning-oriented therapies, encompassing 60 trials with a combined population of 3,713. Among these trials, 26 were randomized controlled trials ($n = 1,975$), 15 were nonrandomized controlled trials ($n = 709$), and 19 were nonrandomized noncontrolled trials with pre- and poststudy measurements ($n = 1,029$). The results revealed substantial improvements from pretreatment to immediate posttreatment and follow-up on quality of life ($g = 1.13$, $SE = 0.12$; $g = 0.99$, $SE = 0.20$) and psychological stress ($g = 1.21$, $SE = 0.10$; $g = 0.67$, $SE = 0.20$). Further analyses focusing solely on controlled trials demonstrated that meaning-oriented therapies exhibited large effect sizes compared with control groups, both immediately and at follow-up, on quality of life ($g = 1.02$, $SE = 0.06$; $g = 1.06$, $SE = 0.12$) and psychological stress ($g = 0.94$, $SE = 0.07$, $p < 0.01$; $g = 0.84$, $SE = 0.10$). The researchers observed that immediate effects were more pronounced for general quality of life ($g = 1.37$, $SE = 0.12$) than for meaning in life ($g = 1.18$, $SE = 0.08$), hope and optimism ($g = 0.80$, $SE = 0.13$), self-efficacy ($g = 0.89$, $SE = 0.14$), and social well-being ($g = 0.81$, $SE = 13$). The consistency of these findings was affirmed by the lack of significance of moderators, such as the type of sample, and alternative methods of selecting studies. Furthermore, meta-regression analyses indicated that increases in meaning in life corresponded to decreases in psychological stress ($\beta = -0.56$, $p < 0.001$), validating the existential–therapeutic mechanisms assumed to drive change in clients.

OVERVIEW OF RESEARCH ON BASIC EXISTENTIAL-THERAPEUTIC COMPETENCIES

The preceding sections have presented a comprehensive overview of the various branches in ET and the fundamental conceptual model and outcomes commonly associated with it. This section introduces the evidence-based competencies framework for ETs, developed by Joel Vos in 2021, aimed at validating, justifying, and enhancing the research, training, and practices of existential therapists. The framework was formulated employing strategies akin to those used in other competencies frameworks. Initially, existential–therapeutic competencies were identified in the most frequently cited publications, including the global survey of existential practitioners (Correia et al., 2014, 2016a, 2016b, 2018), a discourse on key features of existential therapy (J. Vos, Craig, & Cooper, 2015), and a discussion following the first World Congress of Existential Therapies concerning the definition of ETs. Each competency was delineated in distinctive and operationalizable terms, resulting in 476 competencies, which were subsequently classified through thematic analysis into 13 groups and 56 subgroups. Each of these 56 subgroups of competencies underwent scrutiny for effectiveness via an exploration of empirical evidence in research studies. Feedback from 12 existential therapists on the final framework was also incorporated. An overview of the findings is illustrated in Figure 2.2, with detailed information available in Joel Vos (2021a).

FIGURE 2.2. Conceptual Overview of Key Assumptions in Existential Therapies

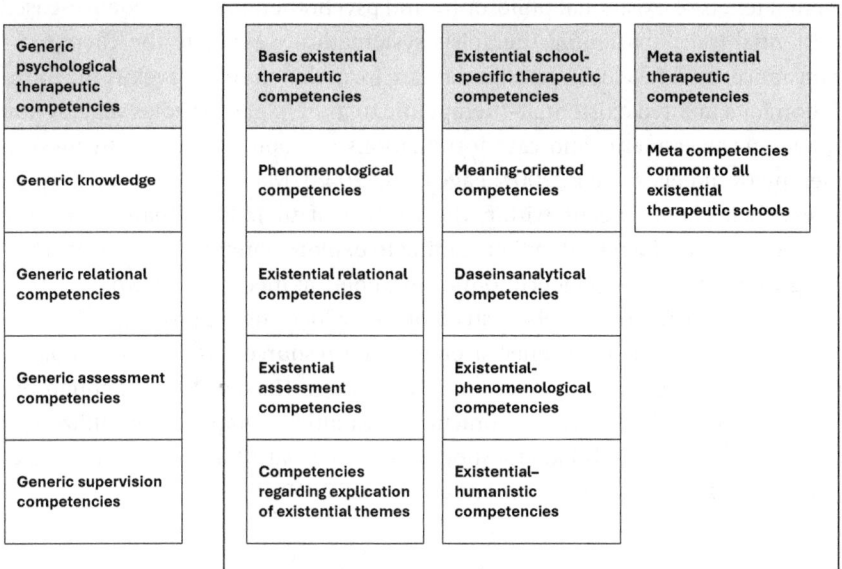

Generic psychological therapeutic competencies	Basic existential therapeutic competencies	Existential school-specific therapeutic competencies	Meta existential therapeutic competencies
Generic knowledge	Phenomenological competencies	Meaning-oriented competencies	Meta competencies common to all existential therapeutic schools
Generic relational competencies	Existential relational competencies	Daseinsanalytical competencies	
Generic assessment competencies	Existential assessment competencies	Existential-phenomenological competencies	
Generic supervision competencies	Competencies regarding explication of existential themes	Existential-humanistic competencies	

Note. Adapted from "The Existential Therapeutic Competences Framework: Development and Preliminary Validation," by J. Vos, 2021a, *International Journal of Psychotherapy, 25*(1), pp. 9–51 (https://www.ijp.org.uk/docs/IJP_2021_25_1_Full_Issue.pdf). Copyright 2021 by the European Association of Psychotherapy. Adapted with permission.

Generic Competencies

Existential therapists utilize a variety of generic competencies that are shared with other therapeutic approaches and have been validated by numerous studies (European Association of Psychotherapy, 2013; Roth, 2015; Young et al., 2013). These encompass generic knowledge, such as understanding mental health issues, familiarity with the specific work environment, adherence to professional standards, and ethical and culturally sensitive conduct. General relational skills involve the ability to establish and sustain a positive therapeutic relationship, as well as the capability to mend any relational disruptions that may arise; research indicates that the therapeutic relationship significantly enhances the effectiveness of therapy (Norcross & Lambert, 2019). Generic assessment skills encompass the well-documented clinical competency to conduct a comprehensive assessment of the client's primary concerns, which are their background, viewpoints, needs, and resources; this assessment serves as the foundation for diagnosis, case formulation, and treatment planning (Roth, 2015). Although less extensively studied, generic supervision skills entail the aptitude to organize and participate in clinical supervision in a constructive manner.

Existential Assessment Competencies

Existential assessment skills center on evaluations aligned with the distinctive clinical, etiological, and therapeutic models of ETs, as delineated earlier. The process of existential assessment often unfolds in a collaborative, relational, and phenomenological manner, encompassing an understanding of the fundamental tenets of existential philosophy and psychotherapies. In evidence-based existential trials, existential therapists systematically evaluate the client's circumstances and develop an existential case formulation that serves as the foundation for a tailored existential–therapeutic treatment plan; studies suggest that systematic assessments and case formulations can bolster the effectiveness of therapy (Kendjelic & Eells, 2007; Page et al., 2008). Many existential therapists assess their clients' needs within the context of their life situation and the broader social and political milieu, aiming to explore potential challenges stemming from structural, socioeconomic, and political inequities (J. Vos, 2020; J. Vos, Roberts, & Davies, 2019). Instead of solely focusing on problems, existential therapists also assess clients' strengths and resources, as a solely problem-focused assessment may inadvertently cause harm (Lukas, 2020). Though not commonly employed in clinical practice, existential therapists may utilize systematic assessment tools like questionnaires, the Goal Attainment Form (Kiresuk et al., 2014), or treatment manuals (J. Vos, 2017).

Phenomenological Competencies

Existential therapists employ phenomenological skills to focus on their clients' subjective experiences and assist them in cultivating deeper self-awareness and insight (J. Vos, Cooper, Correia, & Craig, 2015). Extensive research underscores the benefits of deepening experiential experiences for clients (Elliott et al., 2004). This involves conducting a phenomenological analysis of experiences, with different existential–therapeutic schools employing varied approaches such as philosophical–phenomenological steps (Spinelli, 2005), psychological–phenomenological steps (Längle, 2004), and systematic, pragmatic phenomenological analysis (J. Vos, 2017, 2021c). ETs integrating systematic phenomenological methods alongside other approaches have demonstrated greater effectiveness compared with those lacking a systematic phenomenological approach (J. Vos, Craig, & Cooper, 2015; J. Vos & Vitali, 2018). Additionally, existential therapists possess the ability to foster an attitude of experiential acceptance, aiding clients in embracing and deepening their psychological and existential experiences— instead of denying, overlooking, or rationalizing them—and encouraging immersion in meaningful experiences. For instance, Frankl (1956/2011) advocated for de-reflection, emphasizing the importance of clients immersing themselves in the flow of experiencing rather than being consumed by theoretical reflections (hyper-reflection) and desires (hyper-intention). This also involves phenomenologically exploring hierarchies in clients' experiences, discerning what holds more or less meaning in their encounters; research indicates that this process is often intuitive and unconscious rather than solely cognitive (J. Vos, 2015, 2017, 2020). Many existential therapists adopt a Socratic questioning approach, employing relatively nondirective methods to support clients in self-exploration by asking thought-provoking questions, which has proven to be effective (Britt et al., 2003; Overholser, 2011). Furthermore, existential therapists may utilize specific nonverbal techniques such as focusing, mindfulness, meditation, and guided imagination to help clients explore their experiences, many of which have been supported by research (for overviews, see J. Vos, 2017; see also Elliott et al., 2004; Khoury et al., 2013). Lastly, phenomenological competencies encompass the ability to facilitate clients in actively expressing and articulating emotions (such as making sense of confusing and distressing experiences) and aiding clients in reflecting on and developing emotional meanings.

Relational–Existential Competencies

In ETs, relational competencies assume a pivotal role, aligning with Buber's philosophy that authentic personhood is realized through in-depth encounters between individuals. There is an implicit presumption that clients can deepen their experiences and explicitly engage with existentially profound subjects due to the depth of their therapeutic relationship; correspondingly, existential depth and relational depth may intersect (Golovchanova et al., 2021; J. Vos, 2017). The following competencies are strongly substantiated by a substantial body of research (Norcross & Lambert, 2019; Roth, 2015). These competencies encompass the capacity to navigate the immediate relationship, encompassing both conscious and unconscious processes. For instance, this might be aiding the client in feeling supported and secure enough to articulate challenging experiences and explore them at an existential depth, as well as demonstrating skills to fortify and intensify an authentic, sincere, open, and trustworthy therapeutic relationship. Many existential therapists adopt a person-centered approach, in line with Carl Rogers's (1962) concept of the actualizing tendency: Human development is often viewed as self-directed, and thus therapists are tasked with facilitating this development rather than imposing their own agenda. Existential therapists empathize with the client's life struggles and emphasize that existential challenges are a shared human experience. They acknowledge and unconditionally embrace the significance of existing meanings, religious context, and cultural context. Furthermore, existential therapists commonly aid clients in cultivating ethical and genuine relationships and maintain an ethical stance toward the client and their circumstances.

Competencies About Explicating Existential Themes

Numerous existential therapists, though not all, appear to elucidate existential concepts and provide didactic psychoeducation on topics such as freedom, choice, responsibility, meaning in life, being in the world, mortality, existential anxiety, and the uncertainty of being (J. Vos, 2017; J. Vos, Cooper, Correia, &

Craig, 2015). The explicit exploration and articulation of existential themes often necessitate a delicate equilibrium with the phenomenological and relationally accepting stance, as elucidation should not overshadow the phenomenological and relational processes. Meta-analyses of clinical trials indicate that explicating and systematically delving into existential themes while maintaining the phenomenological and relationally accepting approach can be highly effective for certain clients (J. Vos, Craig, & Cooper, 2015; J. Vos & Vitali, 2018). Similar approaches to explicating and elucidating existential themes can be observed in other therapies, such as schema therapy, acceptance and commitment therapy, and positive psychology (Hayes et al., 2006; Seligman et al., 2005; Sin & Lyubomirsky, 2009; Snyder et al., 2020). These competencies encompass the recognition, articulation, and exploration of existential themes within clients' experiences. Existential therapists can encourage clients to adopt a meaning-oriented coping style to navigate extremely stressful life situations, as cognitive psychological research demonstrates the benefits of meaning-oriented coping (C. L. Park & Folkman, 1997). This entails supporting individuals in finding ways to lead a meaningful and gratifying life while acknowledging life's challenges, adversities, and constraints; this is reminiscent of the Serenity Prayer by existential theologian Martin Niebuhr: "God grant me the serenity to accept the things I cannot change, the courage to change the things I can, and the wisdom to know the difference." Existential therapists delve into clients' paradoxical feelings and ambiguities about life; rather than attempting to resolve these paradoxes or tensions, clients may be encouraged to learn to coexist with these emotions without allowing them to overshadow their daily lives and their ability to lead a meaningful and gratifying life. Existential therapists also pay heed to potential avoidance and denial of existential topics, aiding clients in learning to tolerate existential moods. Extensive studies on terror management theory illustrate how the confrontation with life's ultimate boundaries, such as our mortality, can engender existential anxiety, which individuals may attempt to deny or transform (Routledge & Vess, 2018). Though temporary and partial denial of life's existential themes may offer short-term stress relief or even serve as a source of creativity and productivity, persistent and long-term existential defense mechanisms could lead to reduced life satisfaction and the development of psychopathology (M. S. Vos & De Haes, 2007). Many existential therapists also strive to motivate clients to embrace their responsibility for leading a meaningful life and being authentic with themselves and others, aligning with Sartre's (1943) call to avoid bad faith, or *mauvaise foi*.

School-Specific Existential Competencies

The preceding competencies focused on existential competencies shared by therapists across all existential–therapeutic schools, as evidenced by the research from Correia and colleagues (2014, 2016a, 2016b, 2018). However, each specific school appears to have slightly different conceptual models and competencies. The majority of empirical research pertains to meaning-specific competencies in meaning-oriented therapies. For instance, an overview of the commonalities among treatment manuals of meaning-oriented therapies reveals specific evidence-based, meaning-oriented competencies, including providing meaning-centered didactics, emphasizing long-term meaning over short-term gratification and pleasure, and uncovering the potential benefits of this focus, among others (J. Vos, 2016a, 2017). Additionally, EH therapies appear to diverge from other ET branches in several aspects. These therapies seem to place greater emphasis in their conceptual theories on the topics of freedom and embodied presence, likely influenced by their strong roots in humanistic and person-centered psychology. Presence encompasses research-supported competencies such as focusing on experiences in the present, evoking the authentic, vitalizing, and confronting self-protections. Moreover, many EH therapists appear to more frequently and explicitly seek integration with other nonexistential therapeutic approaches, while other ET branches also often employ research-supported metacompetencies, such as tailoring the therapeutic approach to the unique client in their individual situation. Although meta-analyses do not demonstrate significant effects for existential–integrative therapies, this may be attributed to the limited number of studies (J. Vos, Craig, & Cooper, 2015), and there are some positive indications for the effectiveness of integrative and pluralistic therapies (Cooper & Dryden, 2015; Zarbo et al., 2016).

Metacompetencies

Metacompetencies encompass the skills that therapists utilize to tailor the therapy to the unique needs of each client in every individual moment. These competencies are prevalent across all therapeutic modalities and have garnered substantial empirical support (Young et al., 2013); however, they seem to assume a more explicit role in ETs (e.g., Cooper, 2016). Metacommunication involves customizing therapy objectives and techniques to the client's needs, abilities, and preferences. It also encompasses therapeutic flexibility, which entails the capacity to respond to a client's specific needs at any given moment, such as navigating change, challenging circumstances, trauma, and crises. Existential therapists employ metacommunication and shared decision making to collaboratively formulate therapy objectives that hold significance for the client, as well as techniques that align with their abilities and inclinations (Campbell et al., 2012; Mearns & Cooper, 2017). They may solicit explicit feedback from clients about the therapy and utilize this input to enhance their practices. Although existential therapists are capable of adhering to the principles of their therapy approach, they can integrate alternative therapeutic mechanisms to meet the client's needs when necessary, which appears to enhance therapeutic effectiveness (Roth, 2015).

Lastly, critical self-reflection and reflexivity play a significant role in existential therapy, influenced by the hermeneutic turn in phenomenology. Self-reflection involves introspection on one's own existential and psychological growth (e.g., through personal therapy), whereas reflexivity denotes "bending back upon oneself" etymologically, signifying a form of critical self-reflection on the intersubjective dynamics among the therapist, client, and social-professional-socioeconomic context. The training of existential therapists often integrates numerous self-reflective and reflexive exercises, although this approach has been criticized for not consistently being systematic, potentially leading to self-affirming bias and narcissistic self-indulgence (J. Vos, 2022c, 2023a). Figure 2.3 gives an overview of all possible levels of self-reflection and reflexivity, with different types of relationships indicated by Roman numerals, Arabic numerals, and letters. A label with a prime symbol indicates a relationship between one level and another. Each label doesn't necessarily correlate to a specific concept—rather, they reflect a range of possible types of possible relationships within a level. Numbers I–III describe the mutual relationships between clients, the client's concerns, and their social context; for example, a client talks about their depression (I) which may be influenced by the cultural norms and taboos about depression (II) and their underprivileged, marginalized social position (III). Numbers 1–6 describe the client's higher level influences on these relationships; for example, a client's personality may influence how they talk about their depression (1) and their depressive state may

FIGURE 2.3. Overview of Existential-Therapeutic Competencies

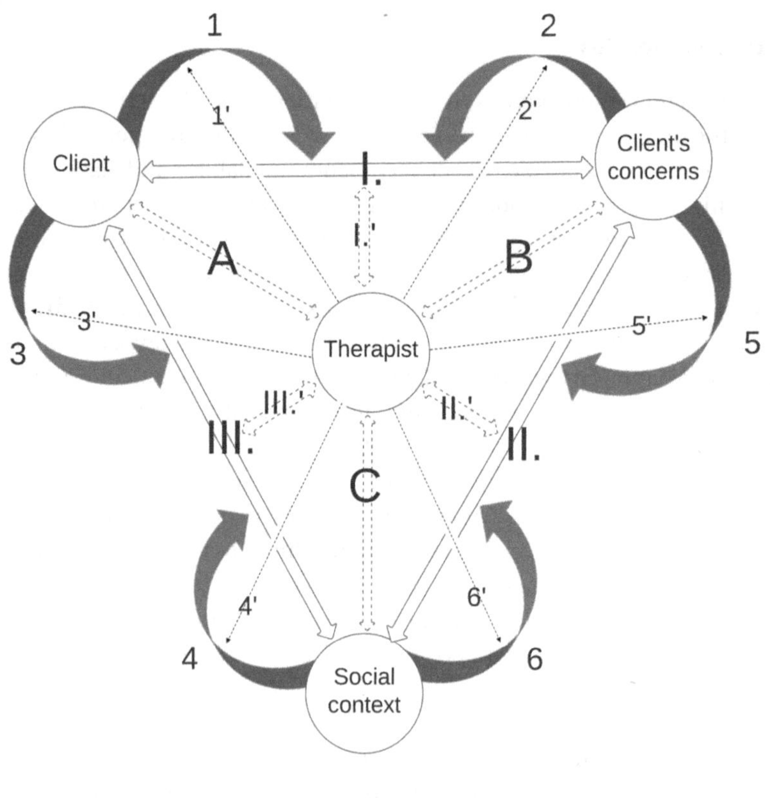

Note. From *Doing Research in Psychological Therapies: A Step-by-Step Guide*, by J. Vos, 2023, Sage. Copyright 2023 by Joel Vos. Reprinted with permission.

influence how they talk about depression, such as feeling more negative about its prognosis (2). The therapist assesses, perceives, and possibly intervenes with the client, their concerns, and social context (A–C), the relationships between the client, concerns, and social context (I'–III'), and the client's higher level influences (1'–6'). For example, the therapist may not merely assess the client's symptoms (B) but also who they are in general as a person and their personality, values, norms, and life history (A) and their social context (C). The therapist may reflect on how the client's social position may have influenced the client in general (III') and their experience and expression of depressive symptoms (II'). The therapist is aware of how the client's symptoms may not be reduced to a simple, single diagnosis, as their experiences and expression of depression may be influenced by the client's unique personality, values, norms, life history (1') and depression (2'). See further details in Joel Vos (2023a) and find self-reflective questions for each relationship in the figure online (https:// joelvos.com/doingresearch/).

MULTICULTURAL CONSIDERATIONS AND FUTURE RESEARCH NEEDS

Since the turn of the millennium, many critiques have been emerging about the dominance of Western White male perspectives in ETs and how many existential ideas have already existed in non-Western cultures and religions long before modern existential philosophy emerged in continental Europe (Gordon, 1996; Hoffman et al., 2009). For example, almost all cited studies in this chapter are based on research in White, higher-educated, cisgender people in Western countries. This lack of diversity seems common to all research on psychological therapies. There have been some initiatives to examine and publish on existential topics in diverse populations, although much more research is needed (Hoffman et al., 2009; Hoffman et al., 2019). Unfortunately, it seems too early to conclude what conceptual models and competencies this existential literature on diversity has in common. Several studies have seemed to compare multicultural conceptual models and competencies with the existing four ET schools, particularly with the branch of EH therapies. However, it seems important not to impose any pre-existing conceptual models and competency frameworks of ET onto these diverse conceptual models and frameworks. It may be hypothesized that, over time, a fifth branch of new existential approaches has been emerging, which seems to have basic conceptual models and competencies in common but also may have unique components regarding ETs with diverse, indigenous, multicultural, and LGBTQI+ communities. A related point of attention for future research regarding the experiences and existential treatment of individuals who are confronted with a lack of privileges—such as due to belonging to an ethnic or socioeconomic minority group, structural injustice, moral injustice, and complex posttraumatic stress disorder). For example, there is much research on the applicability of terror management theory on many psychological topics, including racism, nationalism, and extremist responses to

COVID-19, and researchers are investigating how terror management theory could be used to prevent structural injustice, such as racism and homophobia (J. Vos, 2020).

Although all components of the basic conceptual model and basic competencies of ET have been supported by some empirical literature, these findings should be validated by more studies with rigorous methodologies and experimental designs. More research is needed on the unique conceptual components and competencies of specific ET branches. For example, more research is necessary on integrative–existential therapies, and more in general into what conceptual assumptions and competencies ET has in common with other therapeutic approaches, such as cognitive behavior therapies. For example, it could be that a topic such as meaning can be addressed effectively in different approaches. Research on integration with neuroscience and biomedical sciences is still in its infancy but shows promising findings (Caruos & Flanagan, 2017; Ryff et al., 2004). Furthermore, more research is needed on ET in the general population, as research has disproportionately focused on individuals in boundary situations in life, such as psychotrauma or severe physical illness; for example, research is needed into the competencies and effectiveness of brief existential–therapeutic counseling in general and primary mental health care settings (for a study indicating promising findings, see Rayner & Vitali, 2016).

Finally, it seems important to defend the field of ET from disproportionate commercial influences that may bias or overly simplify research, training, and practices, as it seems that existential psychological ideas have been misrepresented—possibly deliberately—by some business coaches, human resource managers, and positive psychologists (Kaufman, 2021; J. Vos, 2020). Therefore, it seems important to use benchmarks, such as the basic conceptual model and competency framework in this chapter, for clinical training, clinical supervision, and practice in mental health care settings.

CONCLUSION

A substantial body of empirical literature provides support for the conceptual model, competencies, and outcomes of ETs, suggesting that overall, ETs are bona fide therapeutic approaches. Meaning-oriented therapies, in particular, have demonstrated strong evidence of reducing psychological stress and enhancing quality of life, with effect sizes comparable to other humanistic therapies (Cain, 2016; Elliott, 2002; J. Vos & van Rijn, 2022) and psychological therapies such as cognitive behavior therapy (Goodheart et al., 2006; J. Vos, 2023a), a phenomenon often referred to as the *equivalent therapy effects phenomenon* or the *Dodo bird verdict* (Wampold & Imel, 2015). Consequently, the key consideration for individual therapists is not which existential–therapeutic branch is universally superior, but rather which therapeutic interventions are most effective for specific individuals (cf. Roth & Fonagy, 2006). Although ETs appear to benefit a broad spectrum of clients, they have been most extensively studied in individuals facing pivotal life situations, such as those grappling with psychological traumas, death (J. Vos, 2018), grief (Neimeyer, 2012), chronic or life-threatening physical illnesses (J. Vos, 2016b), and the impact of COVID-19 (J. Vos, 2021b).

This review of empirical research on ETs underscores the potential for therapists to leverage existential–therapeutic knowledge and competencies, emphasizing evidence-based concepts and competencies outlined in this chapter. The framework of existential–therapeutic competencies can serve to refine and structure the curriculum of existential psychotherapy training programs, providing a foundation for training and development. Given the substantial effect sizes observed in clinical trials, as well as the evidence-based conceptual model and accredited ET training institutions, it is advisable for health insurance and service organizations to consider funding existential therapies. Moreover, health insurance companies, commissioners, and service organizations can utilize the evidence-based competencies framework to define and monitor appropriate competence levels among existential therapists. Similarly, professional bodies can adopt this framework as a benchmark for the required competencies in accrediting training programs and registering individual therapists, thereby contributing to the formulation of training, trade, and professional employment standards.

REFERENCES

Binswanger, L. (1963). *Being-in-the-world: Selected papers of Ludwig Binswanger*. Basic Books.

Brandstätter, M., Baumann, U., Borasio, G. D., & Fegg, M. J. (2012). Systematic review of meaning in life assessment instruments. *Psycho-Oncology, 21*(10), 1034–1052. https://doi.org/10.1002/pon.2113

Breitbart, W. S. (Ed.). (2016). *Meaning-centered psychotherapy in the cancer setting: Finding meaning and hope in the face of suffering*. Oxford University Press.

Brewin, C. R., & Holmes, E. A. (2003). Psychological theories of posttraumatic stress disorder. *Clinical Psychology Review, 23*(3), 339–376. https://doi.org/10.1016/S0272-7358(03)00033-3

Britt, E., Blampied, N. M., & Hudson, S. M. (2003). Motivational interviewing: A review. *Australian Psychologist, 38*(3), 193–201. https://doi.org/10.1080/00050060310001707207

Bugental, J. F. (1999). *Psychotherapy isn't what you think: Bringing the psychotherapeutic engagement into the living moment*. Zeig Tucker & Theisen Publishers.

Cain, D. J., Keenan, K., & Rubin, S. (Eds.). (2016). *Humanistic psychotherapies: Handbook of research and practice* (2nd ed.). American Psychological Association. https://doi.org/10.1037/14775-000

Campbell, L., Fouad, N., Grus, C., Hatcher, R., Leahy, K., & McCutcheon, S. (2012, July). *A practical guidebook for the competency benchmarks*. American Psychological Association. https://www.apa.org/ed/graduate/guide-benchmarks.pdf

Carroll, K. M., & Nuro, K. F. (2002). One size cannot fit all: A stage model for psychotherapy manual development. *Clinical Psychology: Science and Practice, 9*(4), 396–406. https://doi.org/10.1093/clipsy.9.4.396

Caruso, G., & Flanagan, O. (Eds.). (2017). *Neuroexistentialism: Meaning, morals, and purpose in the age of neuroscience*. Oxford University Press.

Cooper, M. (2016). *Existential therapies*. Sage.

Cooper, M., & Dryden, W. (Eds.). (2015). *The handbook of pluralistic counselling and psychotherapy*. Sage.

Correia, E. A., Cooper, M., & Berdondini, L. (2014). The worldwide distribution and characteristics of existential counsellors and psychotherapists. *Existential Analysis, 25*(2), 321–337.

Correia, E. A., Cooper, M., & Berdondini, L. (2016a). Existential psychotherapy: An international survey of the key authors and texts influencing practice. In S. E. Schulenberg (Ed.), *Clarifying and furthering existential psychotherapy* (pp. 5–17). Springer. https://doi.org/10.1007/978-3-319-31086-2_2

Correia, E. A., Cooper, M., & Berdondini, L. (2016b). Existential therapy institutions worldwide: An update of data and the extensive list. *Existential Analysis, 27*(1), 155–200.

Correia, E. A., Cooper, M., Berdondini, L., & Correia, K. (2018). Existential psychotherapies: Similarities and differences among the main branches. *Journal of Humanistic Psychology, 58*(2), 119–143. https://doi.org/10.1177/0022167816653223

Damasio, A. (2000). *The feeling of what happens: Body and emotion in the making of consciousness*. Vintage.

Dilthey, W. (1996). *Wilhelm Dilthey: Selected works: Vol. 4. Hermeneutics and the study of history* (R. A. Makkreel & F. Rodi, Eds.). Princeton University Press. (Original work published 1895)

Elliott, R. (2002). The effectiveness of humanistic therapies: A meta-analysis. In D. J. Cain (Ed.), *Humanistic psychotherapies: Handbook of research and practice* (pp. 57–81). American Psychological Association. https://doi.org/10.1037/10439-002

Elliott, R. K., Greenberg, L. S., Lietaer, G., & Lambert, M. J. (2004). Research on experiential psychotherapies. In M. J. Lambert (Ed.), *Bergin and Garfield's handbook of psychotherapy and behavior change* (5th ed., pp. 493–539). John Wiley & Sons.

European Association of Psychotherapy. (2013). *The core competencies of a European psychotherapist*. https://www.psychotherapy-competency.eu/Documents/Revised_Core_Competencies_Feb_2013.pdf

Farber, E. W. (2010). Humanistic–existential psychotherapy competencies and the supervisory process. *Psychotherapy, 47*(1), 28–34. https://doi.org/10.1037/a0018847

Farber, E. W. (2012). Supervising humanistic–existential psychotherapy: Needs, possibilities. *Journal of Contemporary Psychotherapy, 42*(3), 173–182. https://doi.org/10.1007/s10879-011-9197-x

Folkman, S. (1997). Positive psychological states and coping with severe stress. *Social Science & Medicine, 45*(8), 1207–1221.

Folkman, S. (2008). The case for positive emotions in the stress process. *Anxiety, Stress & Coping, 21*(1), 3–14. https://doi.org/10.1080/10615800701740457

Fouad, N. A., Grus, C. L., Hatcher, R. L., Kaslow, N. J., Hutchings, P. S., Madson, M. B., & Crossman, R. E. (2009). Competency benchmarks: A model for understanding and measuring competence in professional psychology across training levels. *Training and Education in Professional Psychology, 3*(4, Suppl.), S5–S26. https://doi.org/10.1037/a0015832

Frankl, V. E. (1985). *Man's search for meaning*. Simon and Schuster. (Original work published 1946)

Frankl, V. E. (2011). *The unheard cry for meaning*. Simon and Schuster. (Original work published 1956)

Gendlin, E. T. (2003). *Focusing: How to gain direct access to your body's knowledge* (25th anniv. ed.). Random House.

Golovchanova, N., Dezutter, J., & Vanhooren, S. (2021). Meaning profiles and the perception of the working alliance at the start of outpatient person-centered, experiential, and existential psychotherapies. *Journal of Clinical Psychology, 77*(3), 770–781. https://doi.org/10.1002/jclp.23057

Goodheart, C. D., Kazdin, A. E., & Sternberg, R. J. (Eds.). (2006). *Evidence-based psycho-therapy: Where practice and research meet.* American Psychological Association. https://doi.org/10.1037/11423-000

Gordon, L. (Ed.). (1996). *Existence in Black: An anthology of Black existential philosophy.* Routledge.

Hatcher, R. L., & Lassiter, K. D. (2007). Initial training in professional psychology: The practicum competencies outline. *Training and Education in Professional Psychology, 1*(1), 49–63. https://doi.org/10.1037/1931-3918.1.1.49

Hayes, S. C., Luoma, J. B., Bond, F. W., Masuda, A., & Lillis, J. (2006). Acceptance and commitment therapy: Model, processes and outcomes. *Behaviour Research and Therapy, 44*(1), 1–25. https://doi.org/10.1016/j.brat.2005.06.006

Heidegger, M. (1927). *Sein und zeit* [Being and time]. Klostermann.

Heidegger, M. (1997). *Der satz vom grund* [The principle of reason]. Klostermann.

Hendricks, M. N. (2002). Focusing-oriented/experiential psychotherapy. In D. J. Cain (Ed.), *Humanistic psychotherapies: Handbook of research and practice* (pp. 221–251). American Psychological Association. https://doi.org/10.1037/10439-007

Henoch, I., & Danielson, E. (2009). Existential concerns among patients with cancer and interventions to meet them: An integrative literature review. *Psycho-Oncology, 18*(3), 225–236. https://doi.org/10.1002/pon.1424

Hoffman, L., Cleare-Hoffman, H., Granger, N., Jr., & St. John, D. (Eds.). (2019). *Humanistic approaches to multiculturalism and diversity: Perspectives on existence and difference.* Routledge. https://doi.org/10.4324/9781351133357

Hoffman, L., Dias, J., & Soholm, H. C. (2012, August 2–5). Existential–humanistic therapy as a model for evidence-based practice. In *Evidence in support of existential–humanistic psychology: Revitalizing the 'third force'* [Symposium]. American Psychological Association 120th Annual Convention, Orlando, FL, United States.

Hoffman, L., Vallejos, L., Cleare-Hoffman, H. P., & Rubin, S. (2015). Emotion, relationship, and meaning as core existential practice: Evidence-based foundations. *Journal of Contemporary Psychotherapy, 45*(1), 11–20. https://doi.org/10.1007/s10879-014-9277-9

Hoffman, L., Yang, M. E., Kaklauskas, F. J., & Chan, A. E. (Eds.). (2009). *Existential psychology East–West.* University of the Rockies Press.

Holzhey-Kunz, A. (2019). Daseinsanalysis—An ontological approach to psychic suffering based on the philosophy of Martin Heidegger. In E. Deurzen, E. Craig, A. Längle, K. J. Schneider, D. Tantam, and S. Plock (Eds.), *The Wiley world handbook of existential therapy* (pp. 55–67). John Wiley & Sons. https://doi.org/10.1002/9781119167198

Hope, R. (2004). *The ten essential shared capabilities—A framework for the whole of the mental health workforce.* National Institute for Mental Health England and the Sainsbury Centre for Mental Health Joint Workforce Support Unit.

Janoff-Bulman, R. (2010). *Shattered assumptions: Towards a new psychology of trauma.* Simon and Schuster.

Jaspers, K. (2013). *Psychologie der weltanschauungen* [Psychology of worldviews]. Springer-Verlag. (Original work published 1925)

Kashdan, T. B., & Rottenberg, J. (2010). Psychological flexibility as a fundamental aspect of health. *Clinical Psychology Review, 30*(7), 865–878. https://doi.org/10.1016/j.cpr.2010.03.001

Kaslow, N. J. (2004). Competencies in professional psychology. *American Psychologist, 59*(8), 774–781. https://doi.org/10.1037/0003-066X.59.8.774

Kaslow, N. J., Grus, C. L., Campbell, L. F., Fouad, N. A., Hatcher, R. L., & Rodolf, E. R. (2009). Competency assessment toolkit for professional psychology. *Training and Education in Professional Psychology, 3*(4, Suppl), S27–S45. https://doi.org/10.1037/a0015833

Kaufman, S. B. (2021). *Transcend: The new science of self-actualization.* Penguin.

Kazdin, A. E. (2021). *Research design in clinical psychology.* Cambridge University Press. https://doi.org/10.1017/9781108993647

Kendjelic, E. M., & Eells, T. D. (2007). Generic psychotherapy case formulation training improves formulation quality. *Psychotherapy, 44*(1), 66–77. https://doi.org/10.1037/0033-3204.44.1.66

Khoury, B., Lecomte, T., Fortin, G., Masse, M., Therien, P., Bouchard, V., Chapleau, M. A., Paquin, K., & Hofmann, S. G. (2013). Mindfulness-based therapy: A comprehensive meta-analysis. *Clinical Psychology Review, 33*(6), 763–771. https://doi.org/10.1016/j.cpr.2013.05.005

Kiresuk, T. J., Smith, A., & Cardillo, J. E. (Eds.). (2014). *Goal attainment scaling: Applications, theory, and measurement.* Psychology Press. https://doi.org/10.4324/9781315801933

Längle, A. (2004). The search for meaning in life and the existential fundamental motivations. *International Journal of Existential Positive Psychology, 1*(1), 1–10.

Längle, A. (2019). The history of logotherapy and existential analysis. In E. Deurzen, E. Craig, A. Längle, K. J. Schneider, D. Tantam, and S. Plock (Eds.), *The Wiley world handbook of existential therapy* (pp. 309–323). John Wiley & Sons. https://doi.org/10.1002/9781119167198

Loewenthal, D. (2018). *Post-existentialism and the psychological therapies: Towards a therapy without foundations.* Routledge. https://doi.org/10.4324/9780429478420

Lukas, E. (2020). *Logotherapy: Principles and methods.* Elisabeth-Lukas-Archiv GmBH.

Lukas, E. S. (1986). *Meaning in suffering: Comfort in crisis through logotherapy.* Institute of Logotherapy Press.

Mearns, D., & Cooper, M. (2017). *Working at relational depth in counselling and psychotherapy* (2nd ed.). Sage.

Neimeyer, R. A. (Ed.). (2012). *Techniques in grief therapy: Creative practices for counseling the bereaved.* Taylor & Francis Group. https://doi.org/10.4324/9780203152683

Norcross, J. C., & Lambert, M. J. (Eds.). (2019). *Psychotherapy relationships that work: Vol. 1. Evidence-based therapist contributions* (3rd ed.). Oxford University Press. https://doi.org/10.1093/med-psych/9780190843953.001.0001

Overholser, J. C. (2011). Collaborative empiricism, guided discovery, and the Socratic method: Core processes for effective cognitive therapy. *Clinical Psychology: Science and Practice, 18*(1), 62–66. https://doi.org/10.1111/j.1468-2850.2011.01235.x

Page, A. C., Stritzke, W. G., & Mclean, N. J. (2008). Toward science-informed supervision of clinical case formulation: A training model and supervision method. *Australian Psychologist, 43*(2), 88–95. https://doi.org/10.1080/00050060801994156

Park, C. L. (2010). Making sense of the meaning literature: An integrative review of meaning making and its effects on adjustment to stressful life events. *Psychological Bulletin, 136*(2), 257–301. https://doi.org/10.1037/a0018301

Park, C. L., Edmondson, D., Fenster, J. R., & Blank, T. O. (2008). Meaning making and psychological adjustment following cancer: The mediating roles of growth, life meaning, and restored just-world beliefs. *Journal of Consulting and Clinical Psychology, 76*(5), 863–875. https://doi.org/10.1037/a0013348

Park, C. L., & Folkman, S. (1997). Meaning in the context of stress and coping. *Review of General Psychology, 1*(2), 115–144. https://doi.org/10.1037/1089-2680.1.2.115

Park, J., & Baumeister, R. F. (2017). Meaning in life and adjustment to daily stressors. *The Journal of Positive Psychology, 12*(4), 333–341. https://doi.org/10.1080/17439760.2016.1209542

Rayner, M., & Vitali, D. (2016). Short-term existential psychotherapy in primary care: A quantitative report. *Journal of Humanistic Psychology, 56*(4), 357–372. https://doi.org/10.1177/0022167815569884

Roberts, M. C., Borden, K. A., Christiansen, M. D., & Lopez, S. J. (2005). Fostering a culture shift: Assessment of competence in the education and careers of professional psychologists. *Professional Psychology: Research and Practice, 36*(4), 355–361. https://doi.org/10.1037/0735-7028.36.4.355

Roepke, A. M., Jayawickreme, E., & Riffle, O. M. (2014). Meaning and health: A systematic review. *Applied Research in Quality of Life, 9*(4), 1055–1079. https://doi.org/10.1007/s11482-013-9288-9

Rogers, C. R. (1962). Toward becoming a fully functioning person. In A. W. Combs (Ed.), *Perceiving, behaving, becoming: A new focus for education* (pp. 21–33). National Education Association. https://doi.org/10.1037/14325-003

Roth, A., & Fonagy, P. (2006). *What works for whom? A critical review of psychotherapy research* (2nd ed.). Guilford Press.

Roth, A. D. (2015). Are competence frameworks fit for practice? Examining the validity of competence frameworks for CBT, psychodynamic, and humanistic therapies. *Psychotherapy Research, 25*(4), 460–472. https://doi.org/10.1080/10503307.2014.906763

Rounsaville, B. J., Carroll, K. M., & Onken, L. S. (2001). A stage model of behavioral therapies research: Getting started and moving on from stage I. *Clinical Psychology: Science and Practice, 8*(2), 133–142. https://doi.org/10.1093/clipsy.8.2.133

Routledge, C., & Vess, M. (Eds.). (2018). *Handbook of terror management theory*. Academic Press.

Ryff, C. D. (1989). Happiness is everything, or is it? Explorations on the meaning of psychological well-being. *Journal of Personality and Social Psychology, 57*(6), 1069–1081. https://doi.org/10.1037/0022-3514.57.6.1069

Ryff, C. D. (2018, October). Eudaimonic well-being: Highlights from 25 years of inquiry. In K. Shigemasu, S. Kuwano, T. Sato, & T. Matsuzawa (Eds.), *Diversity in harmony: Insights from psychology—Proceedings of the 31st International Congress of Psychology* (pp. 375–395). John Wiley & Sons.

Ryff, C. D., Singer, B. H., & Love, G. D. (2004). Positive health: Connecting well-being with biology. *Philosophical Transactions of the Royal Society of London. Series B, Biological Sciences, 359*(1449), 1383–1394. https://doi.org/10.1098/rstb.2004.1521

Sartre, J. P. (1943). *Being and nothingness: An essay in phenomenological ontology*. Routledge.

Schlegel, R. J., Hicks, J. A., Arndt, J., & King, L. A. (2009). Thine own self: True self-concept accessibility and meaning in life. *Journal of Personality and Social Psychology, 96*(2), 473–490. https://doi.org/10.1037/a0014060

Schneider, K. J., & Krug, O. T. (2010). *Existential–humanistic therapy*. American Psychological Association. https://doi.org/10.1037/12050-000

Seligman, M. E., Steen, T. A., Park, N., & Peterson, C. (2005). Positive psychology progress: Empirical validation of interventions. *American Psychologist, 60*(5), 410–421. https://doi.org/10.1037/0003-066X.60.5.410

Sin, N. L., & Lyubomirsky, S. (2009). Enhancing well-being and alleviating depressive symptoms with positive psychology interventions: A practice-friendly meta-analysis. *Journal of Clinical Psychology, 65*(5), 467–487. https://doi.org/10.1002/jclp.20593

Smith, J. A., Flowers, P., & Larkin, M. (2021). *Interpretative phenomenological analysis: Theory, method and research* (2nd ed.). Sage.

Snyder, C. R., Lopez, S. J., Edwards, L. M., & Marques, S. C. (Eds.). (2020). *The Oxford handbook of positive psychology* (3rd ed.). Oxford University Press.

Spinelli, E. (1997). *Tales of un-knowing: Therapeutic encounters from an existential perspective*. New York University Press.

Spinelli, E. (2005). *The interpreted world: An introduction to phenomenological psychology*. Sage.

Steger, M. F. (2012). Making meaning in life. *Psychological Inquiry, 23*(4), 381–385. https://doi.org/10.1080/1047840X.2012.720832

Steger, M. F., Frazier, P., Oishi, S., & Kaler, M. (2006). The meaning in life questionnaire: Assessing the presence of and search for meaning in life. *Journal of Counseling Psychology, 53*(1), 80–93. https://doi.org/10.1037/0022-0167.53.1.80

Stevens, G. W. (2013). A critical review of the science and practice of competency modelling. *Human Resource Development Review, 12*(1), 86–107. https://doi.org/10.1177/1534484312456690

Thomas, J. C. (2010). *Handbook of clinical psychology competencies*. Springer.

University College of London. (2022, November 25). *Competence frameworks*. The UCL Division of Psychology and Language Sciences. https://www.ucl.ac.uk/pals/research/clinical-educational-and-health-psychology/research-groups/competence-frameworks

Vallejos, L., & Johnson, Z. (2019). Multicultural competencies in humanistic psychology. In L. Hoffman, H. Cleare-Hoffman, N. Granger Jr., & D. St. John (Eds.), *Humanistic approaches to multiculturalism and diversity: Perspectives on existence and difference* (pp. 63–75). Routledge. https://doi.org/10.4324/9781351133357-6

van Bruggen, V., Vos, J., Westerhof, G., Bohlmeijer, E., & Glas, G. (2015). Systematic review of existential anxiety instruments. *Journal of Humanistic Psychology, 55*(2), 173–201. https://doi.org/10.1177/0022167814542048

van Deurzen, E. (2009). *Everyday mysteries: A handbook of existential psychotherapy*. Routledge.

van Deurzen, E., & Adams, M. (2016). *Skills in existential counselling & psychotherapy* (2nd ed.). Sage.

van Deurzen, E., & Arnold-Baker, C. (Eds.). (2005). *Existential perspectives on human issues: A handbook for therapeutic practice*. Macmillan.

van Deurzen, E., & Arnold-Baker, C. (2018). *Existential therapy: Distinctive features*. Routledge.

van Deurzen, E., Craig, E., Längle, A., Schneider, K. J., Tantam, D., & du Plock, S. (Eds.). (2019). *The Wiley world handbook of existential therapy*. John Wiley & Sons. https://doi.org/10.1002/9781119167198

Vos, J. (2011). *Opening the psychological black box in genetic counseling* [Doctoral thesis, Leiden University].

Vos, J. (2013). Quantitative research and existential therapies: Hard science versus hard words. *Hermeneutic Circular, 24*(2), 22–24.

Vos, J. (2015). Meaning and existential givens in the lives of cancer patients: A philosophical perspective on psycho-oncology. *Palliative & Supportive Care, 13*(4), 885–900. https://doi.org/10.1017/S1478951514000790

Vos, J. (2016a). Working with meaning in life in mental health care: A systematic literature review of the practices and effectiveness of meaning-centred therapies. In P. Russo-Netzer, S. E. Schulenberg, & A. Batthyany (Eds.), *Clinical perspectives on meaning: Positive and existential psychotherapy* (pp. 59–87). Springer. https://doi.org/10.1007/978-3-319-41397-6_4

Vos, J. (2016b). Working with meaning in life in physical health care. In P. Russo-Netzer, S. E. Schulenberg, & A. Batthyany (Eds.), *Clinical perspectives on meaning: Positive and existential psychotherapy* (pp. 59–87). Springer. https://doi.org/10.1007/978-3-319-41397-6_4

Vos, J. (2017). *Meaning in life: An evidence-based handbook for practitioners*. Macmillan.

Vos, J. (2018). Death in existential psychotherapies: A critical review. In R. E. Menzies, R. G. Menzies, & L. Iverach (Eds.), *Curing the dread of death: Theory, research and practice* (pp. 145–160). Australian Academic Press.

Vos, J. (2019). A review of research on existential–phenomenological therapies. In E. van Deurzen, E. Craig, A. Längle, K. J. Schneider, D. Tantam, & S. du Plock (Eds.), *The Wiley world handbook of existential therapy* (pp. 592–614). John Wiley & Sons. https://doi.org/10.1002/9781119167198.ch37

Vos, J. (2020). *The economics of meaning in life: From capitalist life syndrome to meaning-oriented economy*. University Professors Press.

Vos, J. (2021a). The existential therapeutic competences framework: Development and preliminary validation. *International Journal of Psychotherapy, 25*(1), 9–51. https://www.ijp.org.uk/docs/IJP_2021_25_1_Full_Issue.pdf

Vos, J. (2021b). *The psychology of COVID-19: Building resilience for future pandemics.* Sage.

Vos, J. (2021c). Systematic pragmatic phenomenological analysis: Step-wise guidance for mixed methods research. *Counselling & Psychotherapy Research, 21*(1), 77–97. https://doi.org/10.1002/capr.12366

Vos, J. (2022). Meaning in life across cultures and times: An evidence-based overview. In A. Chan (Ed.), *Meaning in life* (pp. 21–40). Atlantis Press.

Vos, J. (2023a). *Doing research in psychological therapies: A handbook and step-by-step guide.* Sage.

Vos, J. (2023b). Existential psychological therapies: An overview of empirical research. *Pratiques Psychologiques, 29*(4), 211–229. https://doi.org/10.1016/j.prps.2023.06.001

Vos, J. (2023c). The meaning sextet: A systematic literature review and further validation of a universal typology of meaning in Life. *Journal of Constructivist Psychology, 36*(2), 204–231. https://doi.org/10.1080/10720537.2022.2068709

Vos, J., Cooper, M., Correia, E., & Craig, M. (2015). Existential therapies: A review of their scientific foundations and efficacy. *Existential Analysis, 26*(1), 49–69.

Vos, J., Craig, M., & Cooper, M. (2015). Existential therapies: A meta-analysis of their effects on psychological outcomes. *Journal of Consulting and Clinical Psychology, 83*(1), 115–128. https://doi.org/10.1037/a0037167

Vos, J., Roberts, R., & Davies, J. (2019). *Mental health in crisis.* Sage.

Vos, J., & van Rijn, B. (2022). The effectiveness of transactional analysis treatments and their predictors: A systematic literature review and explorative meta-analysis. *Journal of Humanistic Psychology.* Advance online publication. https://doi.org/10.1177/00221678221117111

Vos, J., & Vitali, D. (2018). The effects of psychological meaning-centered therapies on quality of life and psychological stress: A metaanalysis. *Palliative & Supportive Care, 16*(5), 608–632. https://doi.org/10.1017/S1478951517000931

Vos, M. S., & De Haes, J. C. J. M. (2007). Denial in cancer patients, an explorative review. *Psycho-Oncology, 16*(1), 12–25. https://doi.org/10.1002/pon.1051

Wampold, B. E., & Imel, Z. E. (2015). *The great psychotherapy debate: The evidence for what makes psychotherapy work.* Routledge. https://doi.org/10.4324/9780203582015

Wampold, B. E., Mondin, G. W., Moody, M., Stich, F., Benson, K., & Ahn, H. N. (1997). A meta-analysis of outcome studies comparing bona fide psychotherapies: Empirically, "all must have prizes." *Psychological Bulletin, 122*(3), 203–215. https://doi.org/10.1037/0033-2909.122.3.203

Whiddett, S., & Hollyforde, S. (2003). *A practical guide to competencies: How to enhance individual and organisational performance.* Chartered Institute of Personnel and Development.

Winger, J. G., Adams, R. N., & Mosher, C. E. (2015). Relations of meaning in life and sense of coherence to distress in cancer patients: A meta-analysis. *Psycho-Oncology, 25*(1), 2–10. https://doi.org/10.1002/pon.3798

Wong, P. T. P. (Ed.). (2013). *The human quest for meaning: Theories, research, and applications.* Routledge. https://doi.org/10.4324/9780203146286

Wrathall, M. A. (2010). *Heidegger and unconcealment: Truth, language, and history.* Cambridge University Press. https://doi.org/10.1017/CBO9780511777974

Yalom, I. D. (2020). *Existential psychotherapy.* Basic Books.

Young, C., Szyszkowitz, T., Oudijk, R., Schultess, P., & Stabingis, A. (2013). The EAP Project to Establish the Professional Competencies of a European Psychotherapist. *International Journal of Psychotherapy, 17*(2), 40–58.

Zarbo, C., Tasca, G. A., Cattafi, F., & Compare, A. (2016). Integrative psychotherapy works. *Frontiers in psychology, 6*, 2021.

Zeidner, M., & Endler, N. S. (Eds.). (1995). *Handbook of coping: Theory, research, applications.* John Wiley & Sons.

3

Research on Existential–Humanistic Psychotherapy

Andrew M. Bland

This chapter surveys both qualitative and quantitative research published since 2010 to supplement and follow up on extant reviews of research on existential–humanistic (EH) and allied therapies (Angus et al., 2015; Cain et al., 2016; Cooper et al., 2010b; Di Malta et al., 2024; Elliott et al., 2021; Hoffman, 2019b; Hoffman, Vallejos, et al., 2015; Schneider & Krug, 2017, 2020; Scholl et al., 2014; Vos, 2019). It heeds Vos's (2019) call for epistemological and methodological pluralism to provide support for EH therapy. Moreover, it serves to further dispel the false narrative that no evidence exists for EH therapy's effectiveness (Cooper et al., 2010c), especially in a zeitgeist characterized by precarious movement in the direction of therapeutic monoculture (Cooper et al., 2010c; Leichsenring et al., 2018).

The chapter begins with a brief overview of EH therapy, as well as the closely related humanistic–experiential (HE) therapies. Next, qualitative and quantitative research on the effectiveness of the general relational principles of EH therapy is reviewed, along with that of HE therapies—which Hoffman, Vallejos, and colleagues (2015) and Schneider and Krug (2017, 2020) identified as principal empirical support for EH therapy. This is further expanded upon in many of the subsequent chapters in this volume. Included here is a summary of common factors research as well as investigations of specific factors that are central in EH therapy. Then, given the numerous theoretical, philosophical, and practical similarities between EH and HE therapies—person-centered therapy (PCT),

Thanks to my graduate assistant, Hannah Standish, for helping with library research. Also, thanks to Dr. Kand McQueen for providing consultation on this chapter.

https://doi.org/10.1037/0000446-004
The Evidence-Based Foundations of Existential–Humanistic Therapy, L. Hoffman and V. Lac (Editors)

process–experiential and emotion-focused therapies (PE/EFTs), and gestalt therapy—research pertaining to the utility and therapeutic outcomes of those therapies with specific populations and presenting concerns is outlined in order to provide further empirical support for EH by proxy. Thereafter, a similar approach is employed with existential–phenomenological (EP) therapy. Finally, recommendations for future research are proposed.

When available, meta-analysis and -synthesis articles have been selected and reviewed first. Those are followed by additional empirical studies that were not included in the aforementioned literature reviews or extant meta-analyses and -syntheses. Also, note that (a) case studies based on fictitious or composite clients have been omitted in order to preserve the chapter's empirical focus and (b) occasionally, qualitative studies are briefly mentioned at the conclusion of some sections pertaining more specifically to quantitative research in order to maintain the thematic flow of the text.

OVERVIEW OF EH THERAPY

EH therapy is a "deeply relational" (Scholl et al., 2014, p. 219), collaborative (i.e., "acting with clients, not on them" [Scholl et al., 2014, p. 221]), phenomenologically oriented approach intended to "set people free" by addressing their problems as the "outward signs of unused inner possibilities" (May, 1981, pp. 19–20; see also Schneider, 2019a).[1] That is, EH therapists employ the therapeutic relationship as a platform for helping clients see and act upon their ability to make choices within the natural, cultural, and self-imposed limits of living and to accept life's paradoxes without engaging in denial of either their freedom or constraints (Schneider, 2008). Predicated on therapeutic and conceptual principles articulated by Bugental (1978, 1987), Krug (2019a, 2019b; Schneider & Krug, 2017, 2020), May (1983; Schneider & May, 1995), Schneider (2008, 2019b; Schneider & Krug, 2017, 2020), and Yalom (1980), EH therapy promotes increased self-reflection and "individuals' ability to venture into unfamiliar territory and respond more spontaneously and adaptively in the face of challenges" (Scholl et al., 2014, p. 228).

To facilitate this exploration, first, EH therapists place a premium on the "potentially curative" (Elliott et al., 2021, p. 1) value of *healing through meeting* (Friedman, as cited in Schneider & Krug, 2020) by way of "authentic but boundaried" therapeutic relationships (Elliott et al., 2021, p. 1). Second, with the therapist as a "process expert" (Scholl et al., 2014, p. 222), EH therapy aims to help clients (a) become more present to themselves and others, (b) experience the ways they both mobilize and block themselves from fuller presence, (c) take responsibility for how they have constructed their current lives, and

---

[1] Portions of this section have been adapted from "The Humanistic Perspective," by A. M. Bland and E. M. DeRobertis, in V. Zeigler-Hill and T. K. Shackelford (Eds.), *Encyclopedia of Personality and Individual Differences* (pp. 2061–2079), 2020, Springer (https://doi.org/10.1007/978-3-319-28099-8_1484-2). Copyright 2020 by Springer Nature Switzerland AG. Adapted with permission.

(d) choose or actualize ways of being based on facing (vs. avoiding) *existential givens* and *boundary situations* (Greening, 1992; Jaspers, 1970; Yalom, 1980; see also Cooper, 2017; Hoffman, 2019b) as well as cultivating meaning and awe (Hoffman, 2019b; Schneider & Krug, 2017). Third, EH conceptualization is holistic and nonreductive (i.e., "[opening] up possibilities instead of restricting ways [clients] can be understood" [Hoffman, 2019b, p. 9]), and EH therapy serves to promote integration both within clients and with their lived world and the cosmos (Schneider & Krug, 2020).

Further, clients are understood to be experts on both their own experience and potentials within themselves in relation to multiple intersecting ecological and cultural contexts (Bland & DeRobertis, 2020; Jackson, 2019; Vallejos & Johnson, 2019; see also Schneider & Krug, 2020). EH therapists value both the content and the process of client experiencing and create relational conditions for clients to forge their identities and senses of control, responsibility, and teleological purpose out of their contextually situated lived experience (Cooper, 2017; Schneider & Krug, 2020). Thus, clients are granted an active and autonomous role in the therapy process, with therapists respecting clients' freedom and potential to make choices, set goals, and even fail (Rogers, as cited in Scholl et al., 2014) as they use the therapeutic experience to both construe and construct meaning in their lives.

Needs have been identified for the individualistic aspects of EH theorizing to be augmented by and situated amongst other ways of knowing (Hoffman, Cleare-Hoffman, et al., 2019; Jackson, 2019; Vallejos & Johnson, 2019), and for EH principles like freedom (Hoffman, Cleare-Hoffman, et al., 2015) and empathy (Hoffman, 2019a) to be broadened insofar as they are conceptualized differently internationally and in cultural contexts different from those in which EH therapy was originally developed (Hoffman, Jackson, et al., 2019). This has contributed to adaptations of EH theorizing through multicultural lenses that acknowledge parallel constructs and principles while preserving and respecting the integrity of the variations (Hoffman, Cleare-Hoffman, & Jackson, 2015; Hoffman, Cleare-Hoffman, et al., 2019; Hoffman, Yang, Kaklauskas, et al., 2019; Hoffman, Yang, Mansilla, et al., 2019; van Deurzen et al., 2019). Meanwhile, Hannush (2007) conceptualizes culture as the form by which existential givens are collectively negotiated as a means of guiding its members. DeRobertis and Bland (2020) provide phenomenological evidence using an international sample that supports EH theorizing on the trajectory by which people approach others who are different: first as a threat and then from a place of empathy and openness to the other. According to this perspective, this transformation occurs through a process of cross-cultural learning by which new meanings emerge from the interpersonal exchange and compartmentalized, intellectualized understandings of the other become outmoded.

Contemporary EH therapy has two vectors: a more experiential approach and an existential analytic approach (Cooper, 2017). Despite some subtle nuances, these vectors share much in common with other allied therapies that will be explored in this chapter: (a) for the experiential vector, HE therapies including Rogerian PCT (a forerunner to EH therapy) as well as contemporary "neo-humanistic" (Elliott & Greenberg, 2007, p. 1) PE/EFT[2] and (b) for the analytic vector, EP therapy (see Vos, 2019). The existential–integrative (EI) approach (see Schneider, 2008) also has been developed as a "bona fide off-spring" of EH therapy (Schneider, 2019a, p. 231) and also is represented in this chapter. As described by Angus and colleagues (2015; see also Elliott et al., 2021; Hoffman, 2019b; Scholl et al., 2014), all of these models emphasize several evidence-based principles of therapeutic practice:

- By entering empathetically into clients' subjective experience—deemed an essential aspect of their humanity—therapists offer clients a new, emotionally validating interpersonal experience (a *corrective experience*; see Bland, 2014; see also Chapter 6 of this volume on working with emotions).

- Tacit experiencing is an important guide to the conscious adaptive experience. An attuned, supportive therapeutic relationship serves to help clients develop comfort looking inward and, therefore, to render emotional pain more bearable.

- Therapists' responses and interventions are intended to stimulate and deepen the process of clients' immediate experiencing and ongoing awareness throughout the course of therapy. This includes clients' perceiving, sensing, feeling, thinking, and striving.

- Emphasis is given to clients' integrative, formative tendencies toward not only survival but also growth, agency, and the creation of meaning through symbolization. The collaborative nature of the therapeutic relationship is key to the unfolding process of therapy and to clients disclosing narratives or personal stories that further develop and maintain a shared understanding and trust.

- Clients are seen as unique individuals with complex arrays of emotions, behaviors, stories, and capacities that can, at times, be viewed as representative of a particular clinical diagnostic category but never reduced to one. As an alternative to viewing clients through the lens of pathology or deficits, their concerns are approached from the stance of thwarted potential and truncated development. In addition, therapists emphasize and affirm how clients' strengths can be employed to address challenges.

The chapters in this volume further delineate evidence-based aspects of EH practice.

Rather than focus solely on *first-order change* (i.e., symptom reduction and adjustment) that offers temporary relief to clients but runs the risk of leaving

---

[2]It is important to note that HE therapies mainly parallel the aspects of EH therapy that are centered around potential (as noted in the May quotation in the Overview of EH Therapy section), as well as experiencing, self-determination, growth, authenticity, and presence (as discussed further in the Research on Specific HE Therapeutic Outcomes section). More broadly, EH therapy also focuses on freedom within limitations that is experienced and responded to along a constrictive–expansive continuum (Schneider, 2008, 2019a), as well as on existential givens that are assumed to be universal but also are nonprescriptive (Hoffman, Serlin, et al., 2019).

underlying problems relatively unaddressed and prone to eventual return (May, as cited in Schneider et al., 2009), EH therapists emphasize transformative *second-order change* processes, also known as *existential liberation* (Schneider & Krug, 2017). Second-order change involves a deep restructuring of self that results in long-term, core-level shifts in and expansions of clients' perspectives of their presenting concerns, their world, and themselves (for a review of theoretical and empirical literature on this topic, see Bland, 2013). EH therapists rely less on prescriptive techniques that uphold their role as expert and, instead, employ their presence and reflexive capacities as instruments for understanding and reflecting the client's unique patterns of lived experience.

EH therapists attend to clients' narratives, metaphors, nonverbal behaviors, responses to feedback, and other interaction patterns to help clients explore how these may point toward formative histories that contribute to defensive interpersonal or behavior patterns in an effort to uphold a false sense of self. Therapists' presence serves to "reflect back aspects that are evident but unnoticed" and, "in effect, hold a mirror up to the client" (Schneider & Krug, 2017, pp. 4, 44; see also Chapter 5 of this volume) to guide understanding of how the client is both presently living and willing to live (Schneider, 2019a). Accordingly, clients' resistance to growth becomes exposed and challenged to promote *disidentification*—that is, surrendering the need to defend their current position, having confused it for their greater self-identity. Rather than cling to past knowledge and expectations of themselves, others, and situations, clients become better able to realize and act on a sense of presence and capacity for meaning making in all their experience and appreciation of their situatedness in time. The therapeutic relationship offers a safe space in which clients may consider their underactualized potential and limitations in a way that stimulates neural plasticity and therefore new learning. When the process goes well, clients "reclaim and re-own their lives" (Schneider & Krug, 2017, p. 3), developing a worldview and behavior that authentically and responsibly expresses their core values.

The therapeutic encounter presents clients with the choice between (a) becoming consumed by suffering to the point that they attempt to evade it (i.e., engaging in *experiential avoidance*) and thereby generate even more suffering for themselves or others and (b) accepting the aspects of their lives over which they have no control and committing their attention and energy to those which they do (i.e., resiliently suffering well). This sense of *intentionality* (May, 1969; Schneider & Krug, 2017, 2020) enables a person to set goals and self-determinedly move forward instead of become mired in the face of adversity as they deal with the daimonic using self-awareness, integrity, and creativity (Hoffman, 2019b). Accordingly, EH (and especially EI) therapists may also incorporate, amongst other strategies, role play, rehearsal, visualization, problem solving, and mindfulness-based techniques to help clients try out new experiences and behaviors in the interest of incorporating and maintaining them outside the therapy relationship (Cooper, 2017; Schneider, 2019a; Schneider & Krug, 2017; Scholl et al., 2014; see also Part III of this volume). EH therapy has been successfully integrated with cognitive behavior therapy (CBT) and family systems therapy (Shumaker, 2017) as well as narrative therapy (Richert, 2010).

Under- and Misrepresentation of EH Therapy in Textbooks

In a content analysis of 21 introductory psychology textbooks, Henry (2017) notes that EH and HE therapies were represented almost entirely by PCT. Rogers's (1957, 1959) facilitative conditions for change were found to be misconstrued as abilities instead of attitudes. Worse, Rogers's nondirective qualities were characterized as "highly passive," as exemplified by one textbook author who rhetorically inquired what therapists actually do during sessions (Henry, 2017, p. 286).[3] Moreover, although gestalt therapy was also mentioned in over a third of the textbooks, it was exclusively Perls's version without consideration of its contemporary iterations (e.g., Lac, 2016, 2017 as well as PE/EFT). In the meantime, 80% of the books omitted existential therapies altogether, and only one book discussed human science (i.e., qualitative) research methods—a principal means of providing empirical support for existential therapies (Vos, 2019)—and did so in a dismissive manner at that.

At the level of graduate training, Prochaska and Norcross's (2018) *Systems of Psychotherapy* textbook does include chapters on existential, PCT, and experiential therapies. However, they are presented in separate chapters with EH and EI therapy (a) mentioned only briefly and (b) "interchangeably" merged with EP therapy (p. 93) without acknowledging their subtle differences (see Cooper, 2017; van Deurzen et al., 2019). More importantly, though the research cited to support experiential therapy is generally more favorable, much of the research selected by the authors to represent existential therapy and PCT tends to include older studies or those involving variant models that employ only isolated fragments of EH theorizing. Not surprisingly, these studies fail to offer support for those therapies. This overlooks evidence to the contrary from studies that are newer and that maintain a greater degree of fidelity to the original models. As Elliott and Freire (2010) observe, if EH and HE therapists "let others define our reality by studying watered-down versions of what we do, we are going to be in trouble" (p. 12).

Existing Reviews of EH and Related Therapies

As an antidote to this predicament, during the 2010s, critical reviews of empirical research supporting EH and allied therapies have been published (Angus et al., 2015; Cain et al., 2016; Cooper et al., 2010b; Elliott et al., 2021; Hoffman, 2019b; Hoffman, Vallejos, et al., 2015; Scholl et al., 2014; Schneider & Krug, 2017, 2020; Vos, 2019). In particular, these authors have focused on 21st-century research in

---

[3]This problematically conflates PCT—and, with that, EH therapy—with supportive/nondirective therapy that will be discussed later in this chapter and which researchers have found to be ineffective. In contrast, with its emphases on promoting openness to immediate emotional and cognitive experiencing, a "shift from incongruence to congruence," and a "change in [one's] manner of relating" as well as in their "relationship to [their] problems" (Rogers, 1961/1995, p. 157, emphasis added), PCT qualifies as a legitimate psychotherapy, described by Wampold (2007) as entailing "understanding the [client's] explanation (i.e., [their] folk psychology) and modifying it to be more adaptive" (p. 863).

an effort to render it "inappropriate for academicians and policymakers to consider these treatments ineffective or inferior" (Lambert et al., 2016, p. 59). Moreover, Elkins (2016) summarized classic research findings on relational healing (including Rogers's seminal research on PCT; Rogers, 1961/1995) as well as contemporary research on attachment and relational neuroscience to make the case that the human element is the most potent determinant of psychotherapy effectiveness because it draws on humans' evolutionarily derived ability to heal emotionally via social means. This chapter surveys research published since 2010 to supplement and follow up on these extant reviews—which primarily, though not exclusively, cover studies from before 2010 and up to 2015.

REVIEW OF QUALITATIVE RESEARCH ON EH THERAPY

Qualitative methodologies have long been favored by EH psychologists for their phenomenological, holistic, narratively based, and tentative (e.g., hypothesis-generating as an alternative to hypothesis-testing; Charon & Marcus, 2017) stance (Timulak & Creaner, 2010; see also Bland & DeRobertis, 2020). Qualitative methodologies are particularly conducive to (a) understanding clients' internal experiencing from their frame of reference and (b) identifying contextual factors to inform therapists' decision making and enhance their responsiveness and intentionality (Levitt, 2016). Taken together, these contributions lend themselves to better understandings of "the experience of change [that] consists of a qualitative shift into a whole new way of seeing the world" (Rousmaniere et al., 2020, p. 569).

Case Studies

Case studies produced by EH psychologists have been valuable not only for establishing effectiveness but also for theory building (Elliott et al., 2021). Adding to EH therapy's "enduring lineage" (Schneider & Krug, 2020, p. 282) of "some of the most eloquent case studies in the professional literature" (Schneider & Krug, 2017, p. 101), Krug and colleagues (2019), Schneider and Krug (2017, 2020), and Shumaker (2017) provide case histories and vignettes to illustrate EH therapists' responsiveness to clients' feelings, experiences, and protective patterns via a process orientation, as well as successful integration of EH principles with psychodynamic and CBT approaches.

Gordon and colleagues (2021) demonstrate how EH therapy illuminates therapists' ability to help clients with preexisting medical conditions reflect on the unanticipated changes and anxieties ignited by the COVID-19 pandemic while simultaneously reinforcing the potential to live with greater purpose and intention. Case illustrations depict the practical import of EH therapy as being its ability to help clients reevaluate their values and priorities, engage in life review and cultivate presence, integrate mindfulness and meaning in life, redefine meaning in life and priorities, and enhance their strengths and find resilience.

Further, Himelstein (2011) provides case illustrations to demonstrate the effectiveness of EH therapy for incarcerated adolescents. The EH emphases on self-awareness (vs. change as a necessity), authentic human encounters, exploration of resistance, and exploration of the client's relationship with death were found to resonate with that population. Next, Thompson (2012) discusses how an addiction treatment center's shift from a behavioral model to a meaning-centered EI approach was conducive to a more positive environment that resulted in a drop in attrition as well as elimination of behavioral problems. Moreover, Lac (2017) explores the effectiveness of EI equine-assisted therapy for helping an adolescent girl with anorexia develop a sense of safety and increased presence that alleviated her constricted way of being in the world and enabled her to feel a greater sense of significance.

Finally, Ribeiro studies therapeutic collaboration during the emergence of *reconceptualization innovative moments* (i.e., exceptions to and/or contrasts with problematic self-narratives in session; Ribeiro et al., 2018) as well as the effectiveness of PCT (Ribeiro et al., 2014), narrative therapy (Ribeiro, Braga, et al., 2016), and PE/EFT (Ribeiro, Cunha, et al., 2016) for depression. Taken together, Ribeiro's findings suggest the importance of (a) therapists' sensitivity to clients' Vygotskian zones of proximal development and responsiveness to clients' moment-to-moment experiencing and growth within the bounds of their readiness for change and (b) therapists balancing supportive and challenging interventions as clients move into areas of unfamiliarity and healthy risk taking.

Empirical Support for General Relational Principles

As noted, research on the fundamental relational principles that undergird HE therapies also provides empirical support for the effectiveness of EH therapy by proxy. Timulak and Creaner (2010) conduct a metasynthesis of qualitative investigations into outcomes of PCT and PE/EFT. The metasynthesis is based on eight studies—all from 1990 to 2009, as well as one 1950s study—involving a total of 108 clients (including two couples). Elliott and colleagues (2021) follow with an updated metasynthesis of an additional nine studies with 71 more clients that yields largely consistent findings. They maintain the general thematic structure from the 2010 metasynthesis but also consolidate some subthemes and fine-tune the wording to emphasize newly understood nuances of experiences involving the self and interpersonal changes. Taken together, these findings reflect EH's focus on promoting clients' ability to be present to—and stand in awe of—life's paradoxes (Schneider & Krug, 2020). First, in the domain of appreciating experiences of self, EH therapy's focus rests upon clients'

- smoother and healthier emotional experiencing (e.g., becoming more hopeful or optimistic and energetic while also more stable, calmer, and at peace; enhancing emotional openness as well as expression and regulation);

- self-acceptance of vulnerability: (a) appreciating vulnerability (e.g., experiencing openness to and transparently showing a greater range of emotion) and (b) strengthening self-compassion and self-acceptance, and valuing self (e.g., improving self-esteem, practicing self-care, engaging internal support);

- mastery and resilience of problematic experiences: (a) cultivating resilience (e.g., restructuring and transcending pain); (b) feeling empowered (e.g., improving confidence, coping, decisiveness, ability to take action, assertiveness); and (c) mastering symptoms; and

- enjoyment of changes in life circumstances.

Second, in the domain of appreciating one's experience of self in relation to others, EH therapy prioritizes clients'

- feeling supported (e.g., deepening interpersonal relations, building a greater support network) and

- being different or healthier in interpersonal encounters (e.g., increasing openness or tolerance, establishing relational priorities).

Third, in the domain of changed view of self and others, EH therapy promotes clients'

- self-insight and self-awareness (e.g., developing meaning, authenticity, self-understanding) and

- changed view of others (e.g., perspective taking in interpersonal encounters, accepting imperfections).

In addition, Elliott and colleagues' (2021) metasynthesis examines clients' perspectives on the helpful aspects of HE therapies. Themes include (a) clients feeling understood, listened to, and validated by the therapist; (b) clients and therapists coconstructing new awareness and meaning regarding clients' experience; (c) clients attending to their own needs in session and thereby feeling free and empowered; (d) clients expressing vulnerability, processing painful emotional experiences, and accessing adaptive ones; and (e) clients arriving at a new awareness and recognition of their own agency in experiences such as self-criticism. Unhelpful aspects reported by some clients include experiencing continuing symptoms, finding experiential work overwhelming, and encountering misunderstandings in the therapeutic relationship.[4]

---

[4]This finding seems attributable in part to EH therapy's eudaimonic or chaironic instead of hedonic focus (Bland & DeRobertis, 2020; Hoffman, 2019) as well as to its likelihood to increase emotional arousal (Pos et al., 2017). Indeed, Brintzinger and colleagues (2021) find that only clients with an underregulated style of emotional processing benefited from mindfulness—a core ingredient of EH psychology and psychotherapy since its beginning (Bland & DeRobertis, 2020)—to reduce depressive symptoms, whereas therapeutic success actually was hindered for clients with an over- or well-regulated style of emotional processing. As Schneider and Krug (2017) acknowledge, EH therapy is not for everyone: "Clients who seek short-term, symptom-reducing therapy probably will not appreciate" its depth-oriented approach (p. 104). This implies the need for EH therapists to be competent in multiple therapeutic modalities reflecting a breadth of theoretical orientations in order to honor and suit clients' preferences.

Further, Elliott and colleagues identify how the studies in their metasynthesis have begot more precision in descriptions of (a) productive therapy processes (e.g., self-reflection on broader meanings spurred by shifts from descriptions of external events to internal experiences), (b) spiraling movement between action and reflection in the development of new narratives, (c) assimilation of problematic or painful client experiences, (d) favorable outcomes from client emotional expression grounded in autobiographical memories and accompanied by deeper levels of experiencing, and (e) the need to provide clients opportunities for growth via the healthy tension between therapist responses that are supportive and following (e.g., providing safety and openness) and those that are challenging and process guiding. Taken together, these findings support the position that successful therapy involves movement "from an undifferentiated, global, symptomatic distress; through underlying core painful feelings of shame, fear, and/or loneliness; to unmet needs; and eventually to a response to those unmet needs in the form of self-compassion and/or boundary-setting healthy anger" (Elliott et al., 2021, p. 29).

REVIEW OF QUANTITATIVE RESEARCH ON EH THERAPY

During the last decade, researchers have heeded Cooper and colleagues' (2010a) call for outcome studies involving HE—and with that, EH—therapies that employ symptom-based measures, a focus on specific presenting conditions, more clearly defined practices of seasoned therapists, and follow-up data. In addition, researchers have furnished both randomized controlled trial (RCT) studies that can be included in meta-analyses in order "to fully impact on policy" (p. 244), as well as process–outcome research to identify specific factors that make the therapies unique and to study specific means of conveying relational conditions that serve as a vehicle for meaningful change.

Common Factors

Since the 1990s, researchers including Wampold (see Duncan, 2015; Elkins, 2019; Wampold & Imel, 2015) and Norcross (see Norcross & Lambert, 2019) have conducted meta-analyses of therapy research studies to identify therapeutic factors to which effective therapy can be attributed, irrespective of theoretical orientation. Their findings have shown that common factors—including goal consensus/collaboration, empathy, alliance, positive regard/affirmation, therapist variables, congruence/genuineness, cultural adaptation of evidence-based treatments, and expectations—have been shown to be the most salient agents of change. Notably, these researchers had not set out to bolster EH therapy. However, their findings are "a major vindication of [EH therapy's] emphasis on the importance of the human and relational elements of psychotherapy" (Elkins, 2019, p. 5). In particular, the common factors findings lend support to Rogers's (1957, 1959) three facilitative conditions for meaningful change (i.e., unconditional positive regard, accurate empathetic understanding of the client's internal frame of reference, and congruence/genuineness). Indeed, employment of Rogers's facilitative conditions has been shown to beget small and small to moderate effects in therapy outcome (empathy: $r = 0.28$ [Elliott et al., 2018]; positive regard: $g = 0.28$ [Farber et al., 2018]; congruence/genuineness: $r = 0.23$ [Kolden et al., 2018]). Moreover, Bayliss-Conway and colleagues (2021) note that therapeutic relationships incrementally increase clients' authenticity over the course of 10 sessions. Also, therapists' long-term (12 months posttherapy) effectiveness has been found to be at least partially an artifact of their facilitative interpersonal skills (Anderson et al., 2016).

It is important to note that this should not be construed as saying that EH therapy holds a monopoly on effective therapy. Rather, "the common factors perspective transcends the 'battle of the brands'" (Elkins, 2019, p. 4; see also Goldman, 2019; Norcross & Lambert, 2019). Indeed, CBT, psychodynamic therapy, and PCT have been shown to yield comparable pre–post outcomes (Stiles et al., 2008). Similarly, as discussed further later, Stephenson and Hale (2020) find that CBT and EP therapy yield comparable effectiveness. Moreover, Flückiger and colleagues' (2018) meta-analysis of 295 studies involving over 30,000 clients suggests a small to moderate effect of therapeutic alliance upon outcome across theoretical orientations in both face-to-face ($r = 0.278$) and teletherapy ($r = 0.275$) formats. Likewise, Leibert and Dunne-Bryant (2015) find that the therapeutic alliance ($\beta = 0.35$) plus an additional common factor, client expectancy, most significantly predicts therapy outcome. Interestingly, client expectations about outcome tend to hinder therapeutic success ($\beta = -0.28$); this seems to reflect EH and HE therapies' focus on promoting openness to experience as an alternative to symptom reduction alone. Further, Bartholomew and colleagues (2021) note that, after controlling for client level of distress as well as for number of sessions, when clients' perceptions of the working alliance with their therapist increased, their positive affect also increased ($\beta = 0.20$).

Per the report of the Third Interdivisional American Psychological Association Task Force on Evidence-Based Relationships and Responsiveness, therapeutic relationships account for client improvement (or lack thereof) as much as, and probably more than, the particular treatment method (Norcross & Lambert, 2019). In light of these findings, the task force concludes their review of multiple meta-analyses by proposing that psychotherapy relationships (a) should be promoted by therapist qualities and behaviors that are explicitly addressed in practice and treatment guidelines (otherwise, evidence-based treatments may be "seriously incomplete and potentially misleading" [p. 631]); (b) enhance treatment effectiveness when they are adapted to specific client characteristics, including transdiagnostic ones, in addition to diagnosis; and (c) act in concert with treatment methods, client characteristics, and helper qualities to determine and form a comprehensive understanding of effectiveness.

Additional characteristics of EH therapy that were discussed in the introduction to this chapter, such as corrective experiences and second-order change, also have been treated as common factors by Castonguay and Hill (2012) and Fraser and Solovey (2007), respectively. Further, Bland (2013, 2014, 2019) satisfies Cooper and colleagues' (2010a) and Elliott and colleagues' (2021) recommendations for more case studies to shed additional light on these processes.

Specific Factors

Fulfilling Cooper and colleagues' (2010a) and Raffagnino's (2019) calls for research into more specific factors associated with EH and HE therapies, both quantitative and qualitative investigations have been conducted on additional EH and HE therapies constructs and principles beyond Rogers' facilitative conditions. These include presence (Geller & Greenberg, 2022; see also Bland, 2013, and Chapter 5 of this volume); self-disclosure (Hill et al., 2018; Pinto-Coelho et al., 2018; see also Chapter 13 of this volume); immediacy (closely related to the EH strategy of invoking the actual; Hill et al., 2018, 2020); human flourishing (Fosha & Thoma, 2020); relational savoring (i.e., helping clients recognize and benefit from moments of positive connection; Borelli et al., 2020); the real relationship (i.e., authenticity between therapist and client; Gelso et al., 2018; Gelso & Silberberg, 2016; see also Chapter 12 of this volume); mutuality (Cornelius-White et al., 2018); therapists' hope for their clients (Bartholomew et al., 2019); and confronting existential givens (Bland, 2021; Frediani et al., 2023). In addition, Fisher and colleagues (2020) find that clients' capacity to negotiate between conflicted self-states and the ability to experience and process emotions work synergistically to predict symptomatic improvement. Also, meta-analyses have shown that symptom improvement can be predicted by client experiencing in session ($r = -0.19$; Pascual-Leone & Yeryomenko, 2017) as well as by therapists' ($d = 0.56$) and clients' ($d = 0.85$) emotional expression (Peluso & Freund, 2018). Using Cohen's (1988) guidelines, these are moderate and large effects, respectively.

Finally, providing support for the meaning making component of EH therapy (Schneider & Krug, 2020; see also Chapter 10 of this volume), Vos's (2016a) meta-analyses show that meaning-centered therapies spur improvements in clients' existential, psychological, physical, and general well-being when compared not only to baseline measurement but also to other modalities (such as acceptance and commitment therapy) that do not include a meaning component. Moreover, incorporating a meaning-centered perspective in CBT for chronic pain has been found to significantly lower pain-related disability compared with traditional CBT alone, especially for clientele with a spiritual orientation (Gebler & Maercker, 2014). Further, chronically ill patients can use meaning to deal with and transcend the limitations of their disease, with "the goal of helping patients to live a meaningful life despite their disease at its center" (Vos, 2016b, p. 183). Likewise, existential interventions have been found to improve existential well-being, quality of life, hope, and self-efficacy in cancer patients that can serve as a protective factor against depression, demoralization, and desire for death (Bauereiß et al., 2018). Similarly, meaning-centered group therapy has been found to promote long-term positive effects on positive interpersonal relations and sense of personal growth in cancer survivors (Holtmaat et al., 2020); increase psychological and physical well-being; improve satisfaction with life and retirement; and also reduce depressive symptoms, hopelessness, loneliness, and suicidal ideation in men confronting existential givens as they transition into late adulthood (Heisel et al., 2019).

RESEARCH ON SPECIFIC HE THERAPEUTIC OUTCOMES

As noted, EH therapy shares much in common with HE therapies, particularly PE/EFT (which are treated as synonymous in this chapter insofar as EFT evolved out of PE therapy; Goldman, 2019). Both EH and PE/EFT have mutual roots in the therapeutic approaches of PCT, gestalt therapy, Gendlinian focusing, and existential therapy (Elliott & Greenberg, 2007; Goldman, 2019). They share foundational values and assumptions that experience is central, people are greater than the sum of their parts and are capable of self-determination, a growth tendency exists, and therapists need to be authentic and present with their clients (Elliott & Greenberg, 2007; see also Greenberg et al., 1996).

Moreover, like EH, the PE/EFT therapist is an "expert on process" (Greenberg et al., 1996, p. 23) who strives to foster clients' immediate experiencing, presence/authenticity, agency, wholeness (which arises out of dialectic creative tension), pluralism/diversity (i.e., equality and empowerment), and growth (i.e., increasing differentiation and adaptive flexibility). This is done via (a) empathetic attunement (e.g., entering and tracking clients' immediate and evolving experiencing), (b) therapeutic bond (e.g., communicating empathy, caring, and presence to the client), (c) task collaboration (e.g., mutual goal setting, engaging the client as an active participant in therapy), (d) experiential processing (e.g., helping clients work in different ways at different times), (e) task completion (e.g., resolving key therapeutic foci over time), and (f) self-development (e.g., fostering client responsibility and empowerment; Elliott & Greenberg, 2007; see also Greenberg et al., 1996). Importantly, a key point of divergence from EH therapy is PE/EFT's being comparably more directive in guiding the client toward engaging in particular affective information-processing and meaning-making strategies (see Greenberg et al., 1996). On the other hand, both aim to promote clients' ownership of emotions and other denied aspects of self, changes outside of therapy, and interpersonal impacts (Greenberg et al., 1996; Scholl et al., 2014).

Elliott and Freire (2010) summarize and critically review six meta-analyses of HE therapies, particularly PCT and PE/EFT, that were conducted between 1980 and 2008. Their overall conclusions are outlined here and are supplemented with statistics from Elliott and colleagues' (2021) replication meta-analysis of 91 additional studies from 2009 to 2018 on the effectiveness of HE therapies—including EH/EI therapy—for a broader range of clinical populations and cultural backgrounds. The results were found to be generally consistent with the previous research:

- HE therapies produce large effects ($g = 0.73$) when comparing clients' reported frequency, duration, and intensity of symptoms pre- and post-therapy.

- Clients reported that these therapeutic benefits were maintained during follow-up assessment both within a year ($ES_w = 0.88$) and over a year ($ES_w = 0.92$) after termination.

- Clients who received HE therapies showed large gains relative to clients who received no therapy ($ES_w = 0.88$).

- HE therapies are clinically and statistically equivalent to other therapies ($ES_w = -0.08$).

- Broadly, HE therapies may be trivially less effective than CBT ($ES_w = -0.26$). However, when supportive–nondirective therapies ("diluted, non–bona fide versions of PCT" [Elliott et al., 2021, p. 9]) were removed, the effect size raised to −0.15. Elliott and colleagues attributed these findings to negative researcher allegiance (to CBT) as well as to studies involving particularly complex client issues for which HE therapies may not be as well-suited.

- HE therapies have been found to be as or more effective than other therapies (like CBT) for addressing relationship and interpersonal problems, chronic health problems, eating difficulties, and psychotic conditions. For anxiety and depression, evidence was mixed—but again, the scales may have been tipped in favor of CBT due to allegiance effects.

Further, Marren and colleagues' (2022) metasynthesis of 11 qualitative studies on clients' experience of the helpful versus unhelpful aspects of PE/EFT showed comparable outcomes as those identified by Elliott and colleagues (2021), as summarized earlier.

Effectiveness Research on PCT, PE/EFT, and Gestalt Therapy

During the last decade, researchers have satisfied Elliott and Freire's (2010) recommendation for effectiveness research to be conducted on PCT for depression (Watson & Pos, 2017) and chronic health problems (Epstein et al., 2018; Lynass & Gillon, 2017); PCT and PE/EFT therapies for generalized anxiety (Elliott, 2013; Timulak, 2018; Timulak et al., 2022; Watson et al., 2017) and social anxiety (Elliott & Shahar, 2017; MacLeod & Elliott, 2014); PE/EFT for eating disorders (Compare & Tasca, 2016; Hibbs et al., 2020; Wnuk et al., 2015); and psychological contact for psychosis (García-Mieres et al., 2019) and dementia (Chenoweth et al., 2019; Kim & Park, 2017). Additional areas researched during the last decade include

- PCT for addressing intrapersonal differentiation (i.e., fragmentation) in psychosis (García-Mieres et al., 2019);

- PE/EFT for facilitating identity integration and resolution of grief in third culture kids (Davis et al., 2015), addressing fear of cancer reoccurrence (Almeida et al., 2022), and working with autism (Robinson, 2020; Robinson & Elliott, 2017);

- humanistic–integrative therapy (van Rijn & Wild, 2013) and PE/EFT (Pos et al., 2017), including couples therapy (Wittenborn et al., 2019), for depression;

- HE therapies for child anxiety (Nuding, 2013), trauma (Khayyat-Abuaita et al., 2019; see also Serlin et al., 2019), depression (Petrei & Gemescu, 2020), and incarcerated offenders of intimate partner violence (Pascual-Leone et al., 2011);

- humanistic school-based counseling (Cooper et al., 2010; Pearce et al., 2017); and

- HE-oriented, social–emotional and mindfulness-based interventions for promoting self-awareness, improved emotional reactivity, and present centeredness in early childhood educators (Palacios & Lemberger-Truelove, 2019).

Further, Di Malta and colleagues (2024) summarize research findings related to the effectiveness of PCT (including person-centered arts therapies) for working with a variety of populations including children and adolescents, couples and families, and older adults as well as concerns involving grief, trauma, and addiction. Qualitative studies have brought increased attention to the role of developmental processes and narrative expression for enhanced emotion regulation in PE/EFT (Angus et al., 2015). Also, Timulak and Keogh (2022) published a clinical guide (which includes interview transcriptions) that demonstrates the integration of PE/EFT with a transdiagnostic framework to guide clients' transformation of emotional pain.

Traditional gestalt experiential interventions also have been investigated. Raffagnino's (2019) systematic review of 11 studies on gestalt therapy conducted since the mid-2000s suggested its effectiveness for promoting clients' reflection on their life narrative, confidence in interpersonal participation, and ability to overcome experiential avoidance and enhance presence and self-compassion. Illustrations of the effectiveness of chairwork for promoting emotional experiencing, expression, and enactment in session have been provided by Kellogg and Garcia Torres (2021). Also, Lac (2016) showcased the effectiveness of gestalt-oriented equine therapy for providing a supportive developmental environment that fosters children's self-direction of their own growth and learning through a phenomenological and embodied experience of playing. Finally, gestalt-oriented pastoral care in both individual and especially group formats has been found to decrease anxiety, depression, and trauma symptoms and spiritual distress (Thomas et al., 2022).

RESEARCH ON EXISTENTIAL-PHENOMENOLOGICAL THERAPY

Steeped in the tradition of Heidegger, Husserl, Buber, Boss, Binswanger, and Laing (see Cooper, 2017), EP therapy (see Spinelli, 2015; van Deurzen, 2019;

van Deurzen & Adams, 2016), also known as the British school, emphasizes "a descriptive, non-diagnostic exploration of clients' lives and experiences" that promotes *unknowing*—"an openness and receptivity to what which emerges in the therapeutic encounter in all its novelty, mystery, and otherness" (Cooper, 2017, pp. 135, 156). EP therapy shares in common with EH therapy (a) a client-centered focus on the therapeutic relationship (Stephenson & Hale, 2020; Vos, 2019) and close alignment with the common factors (Alegria et al., 2016) and (b) a focus on clients' "attempts to evade [existential] reality" that are "the primary fount of [their] psychological difficulties" via sedimentations in worldview (Cooper, 2017, p. 141). The therapist's role is to help clients develop a deeper understanding of the physical, social, personal/psychological, and spiritual dimensions across or along which they are pulled to "identify their core values: [what] they think [is] worth living or dying for" (p. 147).

EP therapists employ relational and intersubjective processes and a "genuinely engaged posture" to convey a sense of interest in clients' subjective experiencing to promote analysis of clients' personal existential meaning as emerging in contradictory tensions and paradoxes as well as choice and responsibility for their life path (Alegria et al., 2016, p. 87; see also van Deurzen, 2019). Also, like EH therapy, EP therapy "focuses on challenges in everyday life, breaking down our self-deception . . . that life can be challenge-free, and instead accepting life as it comes and realizing our freedom" (Vos, 2019, p. 599).

Explored in relation to clients' life context, EP therapists tend to understand symptoms as, in some cases, healthy responses (Wharne, 2021), and in other contexts, normal responses to an abnormal situation (Jackson, 2019; Vallejos & Johnson, 2019). They employ the phenomenological methods of bracketing (i.e., setting aside biases and assumptions), description (i.e., exploration, challenge, clarification), and horizontalization (i.e., treating all phenomena as equal). These methods are focused on what emerges in the here-and-now and are grounded in descriptive exploration of what it means to be a human being capable of language and reflection, which provides the capacity for freedom, responsibility, and choice as to how to live one's life (Stephenson & Hale, 2020).

As with PCT and PE/EFT, researchers have noted that EP therapy's effectiveness is contingent upon an active therapist who not only helps clients develop a deeper understanding of their core values and beliefs but also challenges the contradictions in their narratives (Alegria et al., 2016; Bauereiß et al., 2018). This is consistent with Wampold's (2007) suggestion that legitimate therapies involve clients acquiring a "new, more adaptive explanation" (p. 862) in conjunction with empirical findings that "laypersons want things to 'happen' in their therapy" (Cooper et al., 2019, p. 213) and, as aforementioned, supportive/nondirective therapy is ineffectual (Elliott et al., 2021; Vos, Cooper, et al., 2015).

Quantitative Research

Notably, quantitative research on EP therapy has been limited. This is attributable in part to its theoretical incompatibility with the positivistic assumptions of the medical paradigm that focuses on objective explanations at the expense of understanding individuals' subjective lived experience (Vos, 2019)—and, with that, its aforementioned outcomes not aligning with the typical outcome measures used in conventional effectiveness research. On the other hand, Stephenson and Hale (2020) conducted a quantitative analysis that compared EP therapy with CBT for treating patients in a National Health Service (NHS) secondary care setting in the United Kingdom. They observed that both therapies resulted in a comparable amount of change—from severe to moderate distress and with a quarter of participants having moved from a clinical to a nonclinical population. These findings contribute to the feasibility of EP therapy being included among therapies that further provide empirical support for EH therapy by proxy. Accordingly, they also "open up the possibility of a real choice for NHS patients, in line with NHS directives" (p. 448).

Also, Vos (Vos, Cooper, et al., 2015; Vos, Craig, et al., 2015) performs a systematic literature review and meta-analysis of 15 studies (including RCTs) involving EP therapy for 1,792 clients facing *boundary situations* including health crises. EP therapies were found to spur moderate to large effects ($d = 0.64$) in terms of clients' ability to experience meaning in life, as well as moderate increases in self-efficacy and moderate decreases in psychopathology.

Moreover, Daei Jafari and colleagues (2020) study the effectiveness of EH therapy with Iranian couples. They find that an EP-oriented psychoeducational modality promotes relationships characterized by greater search for meaning (e.g., partners committed to cooperation and responsibility in the face of relational tension) as well as intimacy, respect, mutual understanding, and compatible expectations and common goals between partners.

Case Studies

Rayner and colleagues (2017) demonstrate the effectiveness of EP therapy for helping a depressed, middle-aged, adult female client align her possibilities for a future self (i.e., a realistic view of where she might be in 5 years) with her ideal self in a way that integrates EP principles with NHS standards of practice to "achieve a 'both/and' stance" (p. 66).

Vanhooren and colleagues (2018) study the outcomes of an existential–experiential intervention for promoting posttraumatic growth in an incarcerated female client in her thirties. They note improved self-care and awareness of her finiteness and vulnerability (i.e., the physical dimension), appreciation for individual differences while incarcerated and more authentic relationships after release (i.e., the social dimension), shifts in self-knowledge and self-concept that allows both positive and negative self-experiences (i.e., the physical/psychological dimension), and steps toward a more meaningful life (i.e., the spiritual dimension). Taken together, developing alternatives to existential alienation or isolation and to destructive behavior as a means of meeting the client's needs for intimacy, contact, and meaning "gave her important keys to desist from crime" (p. 161).

Case reports also have explored (a) the themes of waiting and the experience of despair that arose during existential therapy with a midthirties woman who anticipated heart transplantation following a heart attack (Schulz, 2015); (b) the role of existential therapy for helping clients accept death, which resulted in decreased death anxiety and recurring dreams involving death (Akbari, 2019); and (c) the role of EP therapy for helping a gay man in his forties overcome self-condemnation in light of his religious background (van Deurzen & Arnold-Baker, 2019).

Integrative and Brief Therapy Models

The effectiveness of EP therapy also has been supported by quantitative investigations of integrative and brief therapy models that employ existential theorizing and practice assumptions. For example, Cooper and colleagues (2015) find that clients in pluralistic therapy for depression—an integrative approach that employs phenomenological bracketing of therapists' assumptions about therapeutic method and outcome as well as focuses on experienced needs and client preferences (Vos, 2019)—report reduced anxiety and depression and greater attainment of personal goals, as well as having found both the relational and the technical dimensions of therapy helpful. Similarly, VITA (Latin for "life"), an existential, short-term, dynamic group modality, has been found to improve symptom distress and relational problems for clients with treatment-resistant depression—both during the course of treatment and at one year follow-up, when employment was likely to be higher and medication use to be lower (Stålsett et al., 2012). Further, short-term therapy that incorporates existential experimentation (proactive and creative engagement with clients with their personal difficulties) has been shown to reduce depressive and anxiety symptoms, perceived distress, and need for psychological services in primary care settings (Rayner & Vitali, 2016, 2018).

CONCLUSION

The literature summarized in this chapter clearly supports the position that EH and allied therapies are "empirically supported by multiple lines of scientific evidence"—which include both "'gold standard' RCTs" and qualitative inquiries (Elliott et al., 2021, p. 42). In addition to symptom reduction, EH therapy's focus on second-order change via healing relationships, working with emotions and experience, and meaning making (Hoffman, Vallejos, et al., 2015) promotes outcomes that involve a more complex identity, greater authenticity/congruence, increased levels of self-directedness, self-compassion, and perspective taking (Scholl et al., 2014). However, despite the consistency of the evidence, EH therapy has not found its way into mainstream treatment guidelines in either the United States or the United Kingdom. Among other factors, this seems attributable to a rise of conservative cultural and political ideologies

(Elkins, 2009), to infiltration of interest groups onto committees that review evidence (Elliott et al., 2021), and to a focus on outcomes at the expense of process as well as the disconnect between research outcomes and clinical outcomes (Scholl et al., 2014). Accordingly, to help promote the effectiveness of EH therapy, both lists of evidence-based treatments (Angus et al., 2015; Elliott & Freire, 2010) and textbooks (see Henry, 2017) should be updated to better account for the research presented in this chapter.

Stamoulos and colleagues (2016) note that although the majority of therapists continue to regard the therapeutic alliance and therapist empathy as salient predictors of successful therapy outcome, on the whole, they view factors such as unconditional positive regard, clients' hope for recovery, and clients' emotional expression more neutrally. This seems attributable to EH and related therapies having become underemphasized, if not dismissed, in clinical training in the face of therapeutic monoculture, as aforementioned. Importantly, therapists' undervaluing of these qualities comes despite the abundance of research evidence supporting their relevance. To illustrate, meta-analyses have shown that positive regard is a "demonstrably effective" element of the therapy relationship (Norcross & Lambert, 2019, p. 632), and clients' emotional expression has been found to have a large effect ($d = 0.85$) upon therapy outcome (Peluso & Freund, 2018). Further, the value of therapeutic presence was implied in Abargil and Tishby's (2021) research, which concluded that "therapists should pay attention to their feelings in the course of treatment" and be cautious about becoming stuck in specific emotions when clients are not progressing (p. 13).

Recommendations

First and foremost, to complement research pertaining to the experiential vector of EH therapy, more quantitative research that directly assesses the effectiveness of EH/EI and EP therapies without relying on common factors or evidence by proxy from other models is recommended to enhance the empirical canon for the analytic vector. Such research could serve as an opportunity to build bridges between EH/EI and EP modalities and other therapies and to strengthen the foundation of existing evidence reviewed in this chapter in order to prevent them from becoming atrophied in the current evidence-based practice era. Equally, given that symptom reduction is not necessarily a principal goal of EH/EI and EP therapies,[5] "it is very important to develop and validate measures that can identify the kind of changes that [EH] therapy would be hypothesized to bring about" (Cooper et al., 2010a, p. 246). Instruments pertaining to EH-oriented therapeutic and outcome constructs (see Freire & Grafanaki,

---

[5]EH therapists typically view many of the goals of mainstream therapy (e.g., symptom reduction, decreased sadness, increased happiness) as byproducts of a well-lived life. Thus, even though symptom reduction is not a direct goal of therapy, it is often a side effect (Elkins, 2009; see also Bland, 2013).

2010; Kaufman, 2020; Watson & Watson, 2010) also should be reviewed and potentially employed in future studies.[6]

Second, given the "theoretical, practical, and political barriers" faced by those who have attempted to conduct research on EH therapy in conjunction with the increasing legitimization of qualitative inquiry in psychology (Schneider & Krug, 2020, p. 282), as aforementioned, further qualitative studies can better capture EH/EI and EP therapies in their relational as well as philosophical depth. In particular, though quantitative research on symptom reduction has suggested that therapies are equivalent in their effectiveness, qualitative methods may reveal "greater effectiveness of therapies that emphasize client growth and transformation" (Elkins, 2019, p. 7). Accordingly, further research that defines and describes transformative phenomena experienced by clients is recommended to supplement extant literature on clients' experiences of second-order change (e.g., Murray, 2002). This would serve as a relevant antidote to the ubiquity of reductionistic thinking and brief therapy models in health care at the expense of continuity (Mauksch & Fogarty, 2018). Further, EH therapy is well-suited to heed Hammer's (2019) call for both qualitative and quantitative research that examines additional factors like "compassion, hospitality, wisdom, and serenity and the ways these soulful qualities of the therapist enhance and deepen the therapeutic encounter" and, thus, enhance therapy outcome (p. 143).

Third, Elliott and colleagues (2021) call for research to compare more versus less process-guiding HE therapies. Doing so could help clarify and contribute to closing the theory–practice gap regarding the role of directiveness in effective therapy as well as stimulate further theory development in EH/EI therapy and PE/EFT circles. In addition, given the between-study variability in effects between HE therapies and other therapies, Elliott and colleagues also recommend more thorough examination of possible moderators of comparative outcome effects.

Fourth, Tarsha (2016) suggests that compulsive engagement in social media is a contemporary supplement to the maladaptive defenses against existential isolation identified by Yalom (1980). Accordingly, EH therapy has promise to be effective for both preventing and treating social media–induced anxiety (fear of missing out) in adolescents—especially as they have grappled with isolation and loneliness both during the COVID-19 pandemic and in a hypertechnologized era (Twenge, 2017). Research that both reflects and guides the development of therapeutic strategies in this area seems warranted.

Fifth, to help make EH therapy more palatable in a multicultural, global society, additional research on its effectiveness not only with a variety of client

---

[6]Moreover, with respect to the centrality of the therapeutic relationship in EH/EI and EP therapies, Duncan and colleagues' (2018) *Partners for Change Outcome Management System* offers measurement of (a) holistic second-order change to complement existing measures of symptom reduction, (b) global functioning, and (c) therapy experience. In addition, Levitt's *Client Experiences of Therapy Scale* (Levitt et al., 2019) provides a tool for assessing the quality of in-session therapy based within the experiences of clients and what they value.

populations and presenting concerns but also from a range of cultural–contextual backgrounds is recommended. Researchers continuing to integrate "the cultural and social aspects of the client in a more explicit and direct manner" (Hoffman, Vallejos, et al., 2015, p. 14) should help overcome criticisms of EH therapy as overly individualistic (Prochaska & Norcross, 2018; see also Hoffman, Cleare-Hoffman, et al., 2019; Jackson, 2019; Vallejos & Johnson, 2019). Also, empirical explorations of international variations of EH therapy, like Zhi Mian therapy (see Dueck & Wei, 2019; Hoffman, 2019b; Hoffman, Jackson, et al., 2019; Wang, 2019), are suggested.

Finally, bringing this chapter full circle, given the centrality of therapists' presence in EH therapy, especially as a means of both modeling and nurturing clients' own sense of presence (Schneider & Krug, 2017, 2020), Angus and colleagues (2015) and Geller and Greenberg (2022) identify the development of the helper-as-person as an area ripe for exploration. Bland (2018) offers one such pedagogical/supervision strategy, and further inquiry into multiple facets of the development of the helper-as-person within clinical training is recommended.

REFERENCES

Abargil, M., & Tishby, O. (2021). Fluctuations in therapist emotions and their relation to treatment processes and outcomes. *Journal of Psychotherapy Integration*, *31*(1), 1–18. https://doi.org/10.1037/int0000205

Akbari, M. (2019). How dreams help us to accept death: A case study. *International Journal of Dream Research*, *12*(2), 72–76.

Alegria, S., Carvalho, I., Sousa, D., Correia, E. A., Fonseca, J., Pires, B. S., & Fernandes, S. (2016). Process and outcome research in existential psychotherapy. *Existential Analysis*, *27*(1), 78–92.

Almeida, S. N., Elliott, R., Silva, E. R., & Sales, C. M. D. (2022). Emotion-focused therapy for fear of cancer recurrence: A hospital-based exploratory outcome study. *Psychotherapy*, *59*(2), 261–270. https://doi.org/10.1037/pst0000389

Anderson, T., McClintock, A. S., Himawan, L., Song, X., & Patterson, C. L. (2016). A prospective study of therapist facilitative interpersonal skills as a predictor of treatment outcome. *Journal of Consulting and Clinical Psychology*, *84*(1), 57–66. https://doi.org/10.1037/ccp0000060

Angus, L., Watson, J. C., Elliott, R., Schneider, K., & Timulak, L. (2015). Humanistic psychotherapy research 1990–2015: From methodological innovation to evidence-supported treatment outcomes and beyond. *Psychotherapy Research*, *25*(3), 330–347. https://doi.org/10.1080/10503307.2014.989290

Bartholomew, T. T., Gundel, B. E., Li, H., Joy, E. E., Kang, E., & Scheel, M. J. (2019). The meaning of therapists' hope for their clients: A phenomenological study. *Journal of Counseling Psychology*, *66*(4), 496–507. https://doi.org/10.1037/cou0000328

Bartholomew, T. T., Kang, E., Joy, E. E., Robbins, K. A., & Maldonado-Aguiñiga, S. (2021). Clients' perceptions of the working alliance as a predictor of increases in positive affect. *Journal of Psychotherapy Integration*, *32*(3), 310–325. https://doi.org/10.1037/int0000265

Bauereiß, N., Obermaier, S., Özünal, S. E., & Baumeister, H. (2018). Effects of existential interventions on spiritual, psychological, and physical well-being in adult patients with cancer: Systematic review and meta-analysis of randomized controlled trials. *Psycho-Oncology*, *27*(11), 2531–2545. https://doi.org/10.1002/pon.4829

Bayliss-Conway, C., Price, S., Murphy, D., & Joseph, S. (2021). Client-centred therapeutic relationship conditions and authenticity: A prospective study. *British Journal of Guidance & Counselling, 49*(5), 637–647. https://doi.org/10.1080/03069885.2020.1755952

Bland, A. M. (2013). A vision of holistic counseling: Applying humanistic-existential principles in the therapeutic relationship. *Journal of Holistic Psychology, 2*(1), 277–282.

Bland, A. M. (2014). Corrective experiences in corrections counseling. *Journal of Theoretical and Philosophical Criminology, 6*(1), 46–74. https://www.jtpcrim.org/Jan-2014/Article-2-Andrew-Bland.pdf

Bland, A. M. (2018). Facilitating and assessing personal growth in helper development using Hart's (2014) *Four Virtues. The Humanistic Psychologist, 46*(1), 6–29. https://doi.org/10.1037/hum0000078

Bland, A. M. (2019). The personal hero technique: A therapeutic strategy that promotes self-transformation and interdependence. *Journal of Humanistic Psychology, 59*(4), 634–657. https://doi.org/10.1177/0022167818763207

Bland, A. M. (2021). The existential obituary writing technique for emerging adults: Thematic and content analyses. *The Humanistic Psychologist, 49*(3), 435–458. https://doi.org/10.1037/hum0000176

Bland, A. M., & DeRobertis, E. M. (2020). Humanistic perspective. In V. Zeigler-Hill & T. K. Shackelford (Eds.), *Encyclopedia of personality and individual differences* (pp. 2061–2079). Springer. https://doi.org/10.1007/978-3-319-24612-3_1484

Borelli, J. L., Smiley, P. A., Kerr, M. L., Hong, K., Hecht, H. K., Blackard, M. B., Falasiri, E., Cervantes, B. R., & Bond, D. K. (2020). Relational savoring: An attachment-based approach to promoting interpersonal flourishing. *Psychotherapy, 57*(3), 340–351. https://doi.org/10.1037/pst0000284

Brintzinger, M., Tschacher, W., Endtner, K., Bachmann, K., Reicherts, M., Znoj, H., & Pfammatter, M. (2021). Patients' style of emotional processing moderates the impact of common factors in psychotherapy. *Psychotherapy, 58*(4), 472–484. https://doi.org/10.1037/pst0000370

Bugental, J. F. T. (1978). *Psychotherapy and process: The fundamentals of an existential–humanistic approach.* McGraw-Hill.

Bugental, J. F. T. (1987). *The art of the psychotherapist.* W. W. Norton & Company.

Cain, D. J., Keenan, K., & Rubin, S. (Eds.). (2016). *Humanistic psychotherapies: Handbook of research of research and practice* (2nd ed.). American Psychological Association. https://doi.org/10.1037/14775-000

Castonguay, L. G., & Hill, C. E. (Eds.). (2012). *Transformation in psychotherapy: Corrective experiences across cognitive behavioral, humanistic, and psychodynamic approaches.* American Psychological Association. https://doi.org/10.1037/13747-000

Charon, R., & Marcus, E. R. (2017). A narrative transformation of health and healthcare. In R. Charon, S. DasGupta, N. Hermann, C. Irvine, E. R. Marcus, E. R. Colón, D. Spencer, & M. Spiegel (Eds.), *The principles and practice of narrative medicine* (pp. 271–291). Oxford University Press. https://doi.org/10.1093/med/9780199360192.003.0013

Chenoweth, L., Stein-Parbury, J., Lapkin, S., Wang, A., Liu, Z., & Williams, A. (2019). Effects of person-centered care at the organisational-level for people with dementia. A systematic review. *PLoS One, 14*(2), e0212686. https://doi.org/10.1371/journal.pone.0212686

Cohen, J. (1988). *Statistical power analysis for the behavioral sciences* (2nd ed.). Erlbaum.

Compare, A., & Tasca, G. A. (2016). The rate and shape of change in binge eating episodes and weight: An effectiveness trial of emotionally focused group therapy for binge-eating disorder. *Clinical Psychology & Psychotherapy, 23*(1), 24–34. https://doi.org/10.1002/cpp.1932

Cooper, M. (2017). *Existential therapies* (2nd ed.). Sage.

Cooper, M., Norcross, J. C., Raymond-Barker, B., & Hogan, T. P. (2019). Psychotherapy preferences of laypersons and mental health professionals: Whose therapy is it? *Psychotherapy, 56*(2), 205–216. https://doi.org/10.1037/pst0000226

Cooper, M., Rowland, N., McArthur, K., Pattison, S., Cromarty, K., & Richards, K. (2010). Randomised controlled trial of school-based humanistic counselling for emotional distress in young people: Feasibility study and preliminary indications of efficacy. *Child and Adolescent Psychiatry and Mental Health, 4*(1), 12. https://doi.org/10.1186/1753-2000-4-12

Cooper, M., Watson, J. C., & Hölldampf, D. (2010a). Key priorities for research in the person-centered and experiential field: "If not now, when?" In M. Cooper, J. C. Watson, & D. Hölldampf (Eds.), *Person-centered and experiential therapies work: A review of the research on counseling, psychotherapy, and related practices* (pp. 240–251). PCCS.

Cooper, M., Watson, J. C., & Hölldampf, D. (Eds.). (2010b). *Person-centered and experiential therapies work: A review of the research on counseling, psychotherapy, and related practices.* PCCS.

Cooper, M., Watson, J. C., & Hölldampf, D. (2010c). Preface. In M. Cooper, J. C. Watson, & D. Hölldampf (Eds.), *Person-centered and experiential therapies work: A review of the research on counseling, psychotherapy, and related practices* (pp. i–iii). PCCS.

Cooper, M., Wild, C., van Rijn, B., Ward, T., McLeod, J., Cassar, S., Antoniou, P., Michael, C., Michalitsi, M., & Sreenath, S. (2015). Pluralistic therapy for depression: Acceptability, outcomes and helpful aspects in a multisite study. *Counselling Psychology Review, 30*(1), 6–20. https://doi.org/10.53841/bpscpr.2015.30.1.6

Cornelius-White, J. H. D., Kanamori, Y., Murphy, D., & Tickle, E. (2018). Mutuality in psychotherapy: A meta-analysis and meta-synthesis. *Journal of Psychotherapy Integration, 28*(4), 489–504. https://doi.org/10.1037/int0000134

Daei Jafari, M. R., Aghaei, A., & Rashidi Rad, M. (2020). Existential humanistic therapy with couples and its effect on meaning of life and love attitudes. *The American Journal of Family Therapy, 48*(5), 530–545. https://doi.org/10.1080/01926187.2020.1770142

Davis, P. S., Edwards, K. J., & Watson, T. S. (2015). Using process-experiential/emotion-focused therapy techniques for identity integration and resolution of grief among third culture kids. *The Journal of Humanistic Counseling, 54*(3), 170–186. https://doi.org/10.1002/johc.12010

DeRobertis, E. M., & Bland, A. M. (2020). From personal threat to cross-cultural learning: An eidetic investigation. *Journal of Phenomenological Psychology, 51*(1), 1–15. https://doi.org/10.1163/15691624-12341368

Di Malta, G., Cooper, M., O'Hara, M., Gololob, Y., & Stephen, S. (Eds.). (2024). *The handbook of person-centered psychotherapy and counseling* (3rd ed.). Bloomsbury.

Dueck, A., & Wei, G. Q. (2019). The indigenous psychology of Lu Xun and Xuefu Wang. In L. Hoffman, M. Yang, M. Mansilla, J. Dias, M. Moats, & T. Claypool (Eds.), *Existential psychology East–West* (Vol. 2, pp. 17–46). University Professors Press.

Duncan, B. L. (2015). The person of the therapist: One therapist's journey to relationship. In K. J. Schneider, J. F. Pierson, & J. F. T. Bugental (Eds.), *The handbook of humanistic psychology: Theory, research, and practice* (pp. 457–472). Sage. https://doi.org/10.4135/9781483387864.n37

Duncan, B. L., Sparks, J. A., & Timimi, S. (2018). Beyond critique: The partners for change outcome management system as an alternative paradigm to psychiatric diagnosis. *Journal of Humanistic Psychology, 58*(1), 7–29. https://doi.org/10.1177/0022167817719975

Elkins, D. N. (2009). *Humanistic psychology: A clinical manifesto.* University of the Rockies Press.

Elkins, D. N. (2016). *The human elements of psychotherapy: A nonmedical model of emotional healing.* American Psychological Association. https://doi.org/10.1037/14751-000

Elkins, D. N. (2019). Common factors: What are they and what do they mean for humanistic psychology? *Journal of Humanistic Psychology, 62*(1), 21–30. https://doi.org/10.1177/0022167819858533

Elliott, R. (2013). Person-centered/experiential psychotherapy for anxiety difficulties: Theory, research and practice. *Person-Centered and Experiential Psychotherapies, 12*(1), 16–32. https://doi.org/10.1080/14779757.2013.767750

Elliott, R., Bohart, A. C., Watson, J. C., & Murphy, D. (2018). Therapist empathy and client outcome: An updated meta-analysis. *Psychotherapy, 55*(4), 399–410. https://doi.org/10.1037/pst0000175

Elliott, R., & Freire, E. (2010). The effectiveness of person-centered and experiential therapies: A review of the meta-analyses. In M. Cooper, J. C. Watson, & D. Hölldampf (Eds.), *Person-centered and experiential therapies work: A review of the research on counseling, psychotherapy, and related practices* (pp. 1–15). PCCS.

Elliott, R., & Greenberg, L. S. (2007). The essence of process-experiential/emotion-focused therapy. *American Journal of Psychotherapy, 61*(3), 241–254. https://doi.org/10.1176/appi.psychotherapy.2007.61.3.241

Elliott, R., & Shahar, B. (2017). Emotion-focused therapy for social anxiety (EFT-SA). *Person-Centered and Experiential Psychotherapies, 16*(2), 140–158. https://doi.org/10.1080/14779757.2017.1330701

Elliott, R., Watson, J. C., Timulak, L., & Sharbanee, J. (2021). Research on humanistic-experiential psychotherapies: Updated review. In M. Barkham, W. Lutz, & L. Castonguay (Eds.), *Bergin and Garfield's handbook of psychotherapy and behavior change* (50th anniv. ed., pp. 421–468). John Wiley & Sons.

Epstein, A. S., O'Reilly, E. M., Shuk, E., Romano, D., Li, Y., Breitbart, W., & Volandes, A. E. (2018). A randomized trial of acceptability and effects of values-based advance care planning in outpatient oncology: Person-centered oncologic care and choices. *Journal of Pain and Symptom Management, 56*(2), 169–177.e1. https://doi.org/10.1016/j.jpainsymman.2018.04.009

Farber, B. A., Suzuki, J. Y., & Lynch, D. A. (2018). Positive regard and psychotherapy outcome: A meta-analytic review. *Psychotherapy, 55*(4), 411–423. https://doi.org/10.1037/pst0000171

Fisher, H., HaCohen, N., Shimshi, S., Rand-Lakritz, S., Shapira, K., & Tuval-Mashiach, R. (2020). Ability to move between self-states and emotional experiencing and processing as predictors of symptomatic change. *Psychology and Psychotherapy, 93*(4), 723–738. https://doi.org/10.1111/papt.12256

Flückiger, C., Del Re, A. C., Wampold, B. E., & Horvath, A. O. (2018). The alliance in adult psychotherapy: A meta-analytic synthesis. *Psychotherapy, 55*(4), 316–340. https://doi.org/10.1037/pst0000172

Fosha, D., & Thoma, N. (2020). Metatherapeutic processing supports the emergence of flourishing in psychotherapy. *Psychotherapy, 57*(3), 323–339. https://doi.org/10.1037/pst0000289

Fraser, J. S., & Solovey, A. D. (2007). *Second-order change in psychotherapy: The golden thread that unifies effective treatments.* American Psychological Association. https://doi.org/10.1037/11499-000

Frediani, G., Krieckemans, L., Seijnaeve, A., & Vanhooren, S. (2023). Engaging with the client's existential concerns: The impact on therapists and counselors. *Person-Centered and Experiential Psychotherapies, 22*(3), 283–302. https://doi.org/10.1080/14779757.2022.2133000

Freire, E., & Grafanaki, S. (2010). Measuring the relationship conditions in person-centered and experiential psychotherapies: Past, present, and future. In M. Cooper, J. C. Watson, & D. Hölldampf (Eds.), *Person-centered and experiential therapies work: A review of the research on counseling, psychotherapy, and related practices* (pp. 188–214). PCCS.

García-Mieres, H., Niño-Robles, N., Ochoa, S., & Feixas, G. (2019). Exploring identity and personal meanings in psychosis using the repertory grid technique: A systematic review. *Clinical Psychology & Psychotherapy, 26*(6), 717–733. https://doi.org/10.1002/cpp.2394

Gebler, F. A., & Maercker, A. (2014). Effects of including an existential perspective in a cognitive-behavioral group program for chronic pain: A clinical trial with 6 months follow-up. *The Humanistic Psychologist, 42*(2), 155–171. https://doi.org/10.1080/08873267.2013.865188

Geller, S. M., & Greenberg, L. S. (2022). *Therapeutic presence: A mindful approach to effective therapy* (2nd ed.). American Psychological Association. https://doi.org/10.1037/13485-000

Gelso, C. J., Kivlighan, D. M., Jr., & Markin, R. D. (2018). The real relationship and its role in psychotherapy outcome: A meta-analysis. *Psychotherapy, 55*(4), 434–444. https://doi.org/10.1037/pst0000183

Gelso, C. J., & Silberberg, A. (2016). Strengthening the real relationship: What is a psychotherapist to do? *Practice Innovations, 1*(3), 154–163. https://doi.org/10.1037/pri0000024

Goldman, R. N. (2019). History and overview of emotion-focused therapy. In L. S. Greenberg & R. N. Goldman (Eds.), *Clinical handbook of emotion-focused therapy* (pp. 3–35). American Psychological Association. https://doi.org/10.1037/0000112-001

Gordon, R. M., Dahan, J. F., Wolfson, J. B., Fults, E., Lee, Y. S. C., Smith-Wexler, L., Liberta, T. A., & McGiffin, J. N. (2021). Existential–humanistic and relational psychotherapy during COVID-19 with patients with preexisting medical conditions. *Journal of Humanistic Psychology, 61*(4), 470–492. https://doi.org/10.1177/0022167820973890

Greenberg, L. S., Rice, L. N., & Elliott, R. (1996). *Facilitating emotional change: The moment-by-moment process.* Guilford Press.

Greening, T. (1992). Existential challenges and responses. *The Humanistic Psychologist, 20*(1), 111–115. https://doi.org/10.1080/08873267.1992.9986784

Hammer, D. (2019). Cultivating soulfulness in psychotherapy. *Spirituality in Clinical Practice, 6*(2), 139–143. https://doi.org/10.1037/scp0000173

Hannush, M. J. (2007). An existential-dialectical-phenomenological approach to understanding cultural tilts: Implications for multicultural research and practice. *Journal of Phenomenological Psychology, 38*(1), 7–23. https://doi.org/10.1163/156916207X190229

Heisel, M. J., Moore, S. L., Flett, G. L., Norman, R. M. G., Links, P. S., Eynan, R., O'Rourke, N., Sarma, S., Fairlie, P., Wilson, K., Farrell, B., Grunau, M., Olson, R., & Conn, D. (2019). Meaning-centered men's groups: Initial findings of an intervention to enhance resiliency and reduce suicide risk in men facing retirement. *Clinical Gerontologist: The Journal of Aging and Mental Health.* https://doi.org/10.1080/07317115.2019.1666443

Henry, C. D. (2017). Humanistic psychology and introductory textbooks: A 21st-century reassessment. *The Humanistic Psychologist, 45*(3), 281–294. https://doi.org/10.1037/hum0000056

Hibbs, R., Pugh, M., & Fox, J. R. E. (2020). Applying emotion-focused therapy to work with the "anorexic voice" within anorexia nervosa: A brief intervention. *Journal of Psychotherapy Integration, 31*(4), 327–347. https://doi.org/10.1037/int0000252

Hill, C. E., Kivlighan, D. M., III, Rousmaniere, T., Kivlighan, D. M., Jr., Gerstenblith, J. A., & Hillman, J. W. (2020). Deliberate practice for the skill of immediacy: A multiple case study of doctoral student therapists and clients. *Psychotherapy, 57*(4), 587–597. https://doi.org/10.1037/pst0000247

Hill, C. E., Knox, S., & Pinto-Coelho, K. G. (2018). Therapist self-disclosure and immediacy: A qualitative meta-analysis. *Psychotherapy, 55*(4), 445–460. https://doi.org/10.1037/pst0000182

Himelstein, S. (2011). Engaging the moment with incarcerated youth: An existential–humanistic approach. *The Humanistic Psychologist, 39*(3), 206–221. https://doi.org/10.1080/08873267.2011.592436

Hoffman, L. (2019a). Culture and empathy in humanistic psychology. In L. Hoffman, H. Cleare-Hoffman, N. Granger, Jr., & D. St. John (Eds.), *Humanistic approaches to multiculturalism and diversity: Perspectives on existence and difference* (pp. 103–116). Routledge. https://doi.org/10.4324/9781351133357-9

Hoffman, L. (2019b). Introduction to existential-humanistic psychology in a cross-cultural context. In L. Hoffman, M. Yang, F. J. Kaklauskas, A. Chan, & M. Mansilla (Eds.), *Existential psychology East–West* (Vol. 1, Rev. ed., pp. 1–72). University Professors Press.

Hoffman, L., Cleare-Hoffman, H., Granger, N., Jr., & St. John, D. (2019). Introduction. In L. Hoffman, H. Cleare-Hoffman, N. Granger, Jr., & D. St. John (Eds.), *Humanistic approaches to multiculturalism and diversity: Perspectives on existence and difference* (pp. 3–14). Routledge. https://doi.org/10.4324/9781351133357-1

Hoffman, L., Cleare-Hoffman, H., & Jackson, T. (2015). Humanistic psychology and multiculturalism: History, current status, and advancements. In K. J. Schneider, J. F. Pierson, & J. F. T. Bugental (Eds.), *The handbook of humanistic psychology: Theory, research, and practice* (pp. 41–55). Sage. https://doi.org/10.4135/9781483387864.n4

Hoffman, L., Jackson, T., Mendelowitz, E., Wang, X., Yang, M., Bradford, K., & Schneider, K. J. (2019). Challenges and new developments in existential–humanistic and existential–integrative therapy. In E. van Deurzen, E. Craig, A. Längle, K. J. Schneider, D. Tantam, & S. du Plock (Eds.), *The Wiley world handbook of existential therapy* (pp. 290–303). Wiley Blackwell. https://doi.org/10.1002/9781119167198.ch18

Hoffman, L., Serlin, I. A., & Rubin, S. (2019). The history of existential–humanistic and existential–integrative therapy. In E. van Deurzen, E. Craig, A. Längle, K. J. Schneider, D. Tantam, & S. du Plock (Eds.), *The Wiley world handbook of existential therapy* (pp. 235–246). Wiley Blackwell. https://doi.org/10.1002/9781119167198.ch13

Hoffman, L., Vallejos, L., Cleare-Hoffman, H. P., & Rubin, S. (2015). Emotion, relationship, and meaning as core existential practice: Evidence-based foundations. *Journal of Contemporary Psychotherapy, 45*(1), 11–20. https://doi.org/10.1007/s10879-014-9277-9

Hoffman, L., Yang, M., Kaklauskas, F. J., Chan, A., & Mansilla, M. (Eds.). (2019). *Existential psychology East–West* (Vol. 1, Rev. ed.). University Professors Press.

Hoffman, L., Yang, M., Mansilla, M., Dias, J., Moats, M., & Claypool, T. (Eds.). (2019). *Existential psychology East–West* (Vol. 2). University Professors Press.

Holtmaat, K., van der Spek, N., Lissenberg-Witte, B., Breitbart, W., Cuijpers, P., & Verdonck-de Leeuw, I. (2020). Long-term efficacy of meaning-centered group psychotherapy for cancer survivors: 2-Year follow-up results of a randomized controlled trial. *Psycho-Oncology, 29*(4), 711–718. https://doi.org/10.1002/pon.5323

Jackson, T. (2019). The history of Black psychology and humanistic psychology. In L. Hoffman, H. Cleare-Hoffman, N. Granger, Jr., & D. St. John (Eds.), *Humanistic approaches to multiculturalism and diversity: Perspectives on existence and difference* (pp. 29–44). Routledge. https://doi.org/10.4324/9781351133357-4

Jaspers, K. (1970). *Philosophy* (E. B. Ashton, Trans.; Vol. 2.). University of Chicago Press.

Kaufman, S. B. (2020). *Transcend: The new science of self-actualization*. Tarcher-Perigee.

Kellogg, S., & Garcia Torres, A. (2021). Toward a chairwork psychotherapy: Using the four dialogues for healing and transformation. *Practice Innovations, 6*(3), 171–180. https://doi.org/10.1037/pri0000149

Khayyat-Abuaita, U., Paivio, S., Pascual-Leone, A., & Harrington, S. (2019). Emotional processing of trauma narratives is a predictor of outcome in emotion-focused therapy for complex trauma. *Psychotherapy, 56*(4), 526–536. https://doi.org/10.1037/pst0000238

Kim, S. K., & Park, M. (2017). Effectiveness of person-centered care on people with dementia: A systematic review and meta-analysis. *Clinical Interventions in Aging, 12*, 381–397. https://doi.org/10.2147/CIA.S117637

Kolden, G. G., Wang, C.-C., Austin, S. B., Chang, Y., & Klein, M. H. (2018). Congruence/genuineness: A meta-analysis. *Psychotherapy, 55*(4), 424–433. https://doi.org/10.1037/pst0000162

Krug, O. T. (2019a). Existential–humanistic and existential–integrative therapy: Method and practice. In E. van Deurzen, E. Craig, A. Längle, K. J. Schneider, D. Tantam, & S. du Plock (Eds.), *The Wiley world handbook of existential therapy* (pp. 257–266). Wiley Blackwell. https://doi.org/10.1002/9781119167198.ch15

Krug, O. T. (2019b, August 11). *Existential, humanistic, and experiential therapies in historical perspective*. Krug Counseling. https://www.krugcounseling.com/post/existential-humanistic-and-experiential-therapies-in-historical-perspective

Krug, O. T., Granger, N., Yalom, I., & Schneider, K. J. (2019). Case illustrations of existential–humanistic and existential–integrative therapy. In E. van Deurzen, E. Craig, A. Längle, K. J. Schneider, D. Tantam, & S. du Plock (Eds.), *The Wiley world handbook of existential therapy* (pp. 267–281). Wiley Blackwell. https://doi.org/10.1002/9781119167198.ch16

Lac, V. (2016). Horsing around: Gestalt equine psychotherapy as humanistic play therapy. *Journal of Humanistic Psychology, 56*(2), 194–209. https://doi.org/10.1177/0022167814562424

Lac, V. (2017). Amy's story: An existential–integrative equine-facilitated psychotherapy approach to anorexia nervosa. *Journal of Humanistic Psychology, 57*(3), 301–312. https://doi.org/10.1177/0022167815627900

Lambert, M. J., Fidalgo, L. G., & Greaves, M. R. (2016). Effective humanistic psychotherapy processes and their outcomes. In D. J. Cain, K. Keenan, & S. Rubin (Eds.), *Humanistic psychotherapies: Handbook of research and practice* (2nd ed., pp. 49–79). American Psychological Association. https://doi.org/10.1037/14775-003

Leibert, T. W., & Dunne-Bryant, A. (2015). Do common factors account for counseling outcome? *Journal of Counseling and Development, 93*(2), 225–235. https://doi.org/10.1002/j.1556-6676.2015.00198.x

Leichsenring, F., Abbass, A., Hilsenroth, M. J., Luyten, P., Munder, T., Rabung, S., & Steinert, C. (2018). "Gold standards," plurality and monocultures: The need for diversity in psychotherapy. *Frontiers in Psychiatry, 9*, 159. https://doi.org/10.3389/fpsyt.2018.00159

Levitt, H. M. (2016). Qualitative research and humanistic psychotherapy. In D. J. Cain, K. Keenan, & S. Rubin (Eds.), *Humanistic psychotherapies: Handbook of research and practice* (2nd ed., pp. 81–113). American Psychological Association. https://doi.org/10.1037/14775-004

Levitt, H. M., Morrill, Z., Grabowski, L., & Minami, T. (2019, August 8). *Going beyond symptoms and measuring psychotherapy outcomes as clients experiencing it: The Clients' Experiences in Therapy Scale (CETS)* [Paper presentation]. Division 32 Hospitality Suite at the American Psychological Association 127th Annual Convention, Chicago, IL, United States.

Lynass, R., & Gillon, E. (2017). A thematic analysis of the experience of person-centred counselling for clients with multiple sclerosis: A pilot study. *Counselling Psychology Review, 32*(4), 49–57. https://doi.org/10.53841/bpscpr.2017.32.4.49

MacLeod, R., & Elliott, R. (2014). Nondirective person-centered therapy for social anxiety: A hermeneutic single-case efficacy design study of a good outcome case. *Person-Centered and Experiential Psychotherapies, 13*(4), 294–311. https://doi.org/10.1080/14779757.2014.910133

Marren, C., Mikoška, P., O'Brien, S., & Timulak, L. (2022). A qualitative meta-analysis of the clients' experiences of emotion-focused therapy. *Clinical Psychology & Psychotherapy, 29*(5), 1611–1625. https://doi.org/10.1002/cpp.2745

Mauksch, L., & Fogarty, C. T. (2018). Behavioral health integration and the risks of reductionism. *Families, Systems & Health, 36*(1), 1–3. https://doi.org/10.1037/fsh0000346

May, R. (1969). *Love and will*. W. W. Norton & Company.

May, R. (1981). *Freedom and destiny*. W. W. Norton & Company.

May, R. (1983). *The discovery of being: Writings in existential psychology*. W. W. Norton & Company.

Murray, R. (2002). The phenomenon of psychotherapeutic change: Second-order change in one's experience of self. *Journal of Contemporary Psychotherapy, 32*(2/3), 167–177. https://doi.org/10.1023/A:1020592926010

Norcross, J. C., & Lambert, M. J. (2019). What works in the psychotherapy relationship: Results, conclusions, and practices. In J. C. Norcross & M. J. Lambert (Eds.),

Psychotherapy relationships that work: Vol. 1. Evidence-based therapist contributions (3rd ed., pp. 631–646). Oxford University Press. https://doi.org/10.1093/med-psych/9780190843953.003.0018

Nuding, D. (2013). Anxiety in childhood—Person-centered perspectives. *Person-Centered and Experiential Psychotherapies, 12*(1), 33–45. https://doi.org/10.1080/14779757.2013.767746

Palacios, A. F., & Lemberger-Truelove, M. E. (2019). A counselor-delivered mindfulness and social–emotional learning intervention for early childhood educators. *The Journal of Humanistic Counseling, 58*(3), 184–203. https://doi.org/10.1002/johc.12119

Pascual-Leone, A., Bierman, R., Arnold, R., & Stasiak, E. (2011). Emotion-focused therapy for incarcerated offenders of intimate partner violence: A 3-year outcome using a new whole-sample matching method. *Psychotherapy Research, 21*(3), 331–347. https://doi.org/10.1080/10503307.2011.572092

Pascual-Leone, A., & Yeryomenko, N. (2017). The client "experiencing" scale as a predictor of treatment outcomes: A meta-analysis on psychotherapy process. *Psychotherapy Research, 27*(6), 653–665. https://doi.org/10.1080/10503307.2016.1152409

Pearce, P., Sewell, R., Cooper, M., Osman, S., Fugard, A. J. B., & Pybis, J. (2017). Effectiveness of school-based humanistic counselling for psychological distress in young people: Pilot randomized controlled trial with follow-up in an ethnically diverse sample. *Psychology and Psychotherapy, 90*(2), 138–155. https://doi.org/10.1111/papt.12102

Peluso, P. R., & Freund, R. R. (2018). Therapist and client emotional expression and psychotherapy outcomes: A meta-analysis. *Psychotherapy, 55*(4), 461–472. https://doi.org/10.1037/pst0000165

Petrei, L. M., & Gemescu, M. M. (2020). Humanistic experiential psychotherapy for depression: A case study. *Journal of Experiential Psychotherapy, 23*(2), 56–65.

Pinto-Coelho, K. G., Hill, C. E., Kearney, M. S., Sarno, E. L., Sauber, E. S., Baker, S. M., Brady, J., Ireland, G. W., Hoffman, M. A., Spangler, P. T., & Thompson, B. J. (2018). When in doubt, sit quietly: A qualitative investigation of experienced therapists' perceptions of self-disclosure. *Journal of Counseling Psychology, 65*(4), 440–452. https://doi.org/10.1037/cou0000288

Pos, A. E., Paolone, D. A., Smith, C. E., & Warwar, S. H. (2017). How does client expressed emotional arousal relate to outcome in experiential therapy for depression? *Person-Centered and Experiential Psychotherapies, 16*(2), 173–190. https://doi.org/10.1080/14779757.2017.1323666

Prochaska, J. O., & Norcross, J. C. (2018). *Systems of psychotherapy: A transtheoretical analysis* (9th ed.). Oxford University Press.

Raffagnino, R. (2019). Gestalt therapy effectiveness: A systematic review of empirical evidence. *Open Journal of Social Sciences, 7*(6), 66–83. https://doi.org/10.4236/jss.2019.76005

Rayner, M., Kauntze, C., & Sayers, L. (2017). Existential experimentation: From being and doing to an approach that addresses the theme of 'insider and outsider.' *Existential Analysis, 28*(1), 66–81.

Rayner, M., & Vitali, D. (2016). Short-term existential psychotherapy in primary care: A quantitative report. *Journal of Humanistic Psychology, 56*(4), 357–372. https://doi.org/10.1177/0022167815569884

Rayner, M., & Vitali, D. (2018). Existential experimentation: Structure and principles for a short-term psychological therapy. *Journal of Humanistic Psychology, 58*(2), 194–213. https://doi.org/10.1177/0022167816655925

Ribeiro, A. P., Braga, C., Stiles, W. B., Teixeira, P., Gonçalves, M. M., & Ribeiro, E. (2016). Therapist interventions and client ambivalence in two cases of narrative therapy for depression. *Psychotherapy Research, 26*(6), 681–693. https://doi.org/10.1080/10503307.2016.1197439

Ribeiro, E., Cunha, C., Teixeira, A. S., Stiles, W. B., Pires, N., Santos, B., Basto, I., & Salgado, J. (2016). Therapeutic collaboration and the assimilation of problematic experiences in emotion-focused therapy for depression: Comparison of two cases. *Psychotherapy Research*, *26*(6), 665–680. https://doi.org/10.1080/10503307.2016. 1208853

Ribeiro, E., Fernandes, C., Santos, B., Ribeiro, A., Coutinho, J., Angus, L., & Greenberg, L. (2014). The development of therapeutic collaboration in a good outcome case of person-centered therapy. *Person-Centered and Experiential Psychotherapies*, *13*(2), 150–168. https://doi.org/10.1080/14779757.2014.893250

Ribeiro, E., Gonçalves, M., & Santos, B. (2018). How reconceptualization of the self is negotiated in psychotherapy: An exploratory study of the therapeutic collaboration. *Journal of Humanistic Psychology*, *62*(5), 718–747. https://doi.org/10.1177/0022167818 792123

Richert, A. J. (2010). *Integrating existential and narrative therapy*. Duquesne University Press.

Robinson, A. (2020). Enhancing empathy in emotion-focused group therapy for adolescents with autism spectrum disorder: A case conceptualization model for interpersonal rupture and repair. *Journal of Contemporary Psychotherapy*, *50*(2), 133–142. https://doi.org/10.1007/s10879-019-09443-6

Robinson, A., & Elliott, R. (2017). Emotion-focused therapy for clients with autistic process. *Person-Centered and Experiential Psychotherapies*, *16*(3), 215–235. https://doi.org/ 10.1080/14779757.2017.1330700

Rogers, C. R. (1957). The necessary and sufficient conditions of therapeutic personality change. *Journal of Consulting Psychology*, *21*(2), 95–103. https://doi.org/10.1037/ h0045357

Rogers, C. R. (1959). A theory of therapy, personality, and interpersonal relationships, as developed in the client-centered framework. In S. Koch (Ed.), *Psychology: A study of a science: Vol. 3. Formulations of the person and the social context* (pp. 184–256). McGraw-Hill.

Rogers, C. R. (1995). *On becoming a person: A therapist's view of psychotherapy*. Houghton-Mifflin. (Original work published 1961)

Rousmaniere, T., Wright, C. V., Boswell, J., Constantino, M. J., Castonguay, L., McLeod, J., Pedulla, D., & Nordal, K. (2020). Keeping psychologists in the driver's seat: Four perspectives on quality improvement and clinical data registries. *Psychotherapy*, *57*(4), 562–573. https://doi.org/10.1037/pst0000227

Schneider, K. J. (Ed.). (2008). *Existential–integrative psychotherapy: Guideposts to the core of practice*. Routledge.

Schneider, K. J. (2019a). Existential–humanistic and existential–integrative therapy. In E. van Deurzen, E. Craig, A. Längle, K. J. Schneider, D. Tantam, & S. du Plock (Eds.), *The Wiley world handbook of existential therapy* (pp. 231–233). Wiley Blackwell. https:// doi.org/10.1002/9781119167198.part3

Schneider, K. J. (2019b). Existential–humanistic and existential–integrative therapy: Philosophy and theory. In E. van Deurzen, E. Craig, A. Längle, K. J. Schneider, D. Tantam, & S. du Plock (Eds.), *The Wiley world handbook of existential therapy* (pp. 247–256). Wiley Blackwell. https://doi.org/10.1002/9781119167198.ch14

Schneider, K. J., Galvin, J., & Serlin, I. (2009). Rollo May on existential psychotherapy. *Journal of Humanistic Psychology*, *49*(4), 419–434. https://doi.org/10.1177/0022167809340241

Schneider, K. J., & Krug, O. T. (2017). *Existential–humanistic therapy* (2nd ed.). American Psychological Association. https://doi.org/10.1037/0000042-000

Schneider, K. J., & Krug, O. T. (2020). Existential–humanistic psychotherapies. In S. B. Messer & N. J. Kaslow (Eds.), *Essential psychotherapies: Theory and practice* (4th ed., pp. 257–293). Guilford Press.

Schneider, K. J., & May, R. (1995). *The psychology of existence: An integrative, clinical perspective*. McGraw-Hill.

Scholl, M. B., Ray, D. C., & Brady-Amoon, P. (2014). Humanistic counseling process, outcomes, and research. *The Journal of Humanistic Counseling*, *53*(3), 218–239. https:// doi.org/10.1002/j.2161-1939.2014.00058.x

Schulz, C. (2015). Existential psychotherapy with a person who lives with a left ventricular assist device and awaits heart transplantation: A case report. *Journal of Humanistic Psychology, 55*(4), 429–473. https://doi.org/10.1177/0022167814539192

Serlin, I. A., Krippner, S., & Rockefeller, K. (Eds.). (2019). *Integrated care for the traumatized: A whole-person approach.* Rowman & Littlefield.

Shumaker, D. (2017). *Existential–integrative approaches to treating adolescents.* Palgrave Macmillan/Springer Nature. https://doi.org/10.1057/978-1-349-95211-3

Spinelli, E. (2015). *Practicing existential therapy* (2nd ed.). Sage.

Stålsett, G., Gude, T., Rønnestad, M. H., & Monsen, J. T. (2012). Existential dynamic therapy ("VITA") for treatment-resistant depression with Cluster C disorder: Matched comparison to treatment as usual. *Psychotherapy Research, 22*(5), 579–591. https://doi.org/10.1080/10503307.2012.692214

Stamoulos, C., Trepanier, L., Bourkas, S., Bradley, S., Stelmaszczyk, K., Schwartzman, D., & Drapeau, M. (2016). Psychologists' perceptions of the importance of common factors in psychotherapy for successful treatment outcomes. *Journal of Psychotherapy Integration, 26*(3), 300–317. https://doi.org/10.1037/a0040426

Stephenson, L., & Hale, B. (2020). An exploration into effectiveness of existential–phenomenological therapy as a U.K. NHS psychological treatment intervention. *Journal of Humanistic Psychology, 60*(3), 436–453. https://doi.org/10.1177/0022167817719178

Stiles, W. B., Barkham, M., Mellor-Clark, J., & Connell, J. (2008). Effectiveness of cognitive-behavioural, person-centred, and psychodynamic therapies in UK primary-care routine practice: Replication in a larger sample. *Psychological Medicine, 38*(5), 677–688. https://doi.org/10.1017/S0033291707001511

Tarsha, A. A. (2016). The role of existential therapy in the prevention of social media–driven anxiety. *Existential Analysis, 27*(2), 382–388.

Thomas, M., Crabtree, M., Janvier, D., Craner, W., Zechner, M., & Bussian, L. B. (2022). Bridging religion and spirituality with gestalt psychotherapy to improve clinical symptoms: Preliminary findings using gestalt pastoral care. *Psychotherapy, 59*(3), 400–404. https://doi.org/10.1037/pst0000425

Thompson, G. (2012). A meaning-centered therapy for addictions. *International Journal of Mental Health and Addiction, 10*(3), 428–440. https://doi.org/10.1007/s11469-011-9367-9

Timulak, L. (2018). Humanistic–experiential therapies in the treatment of generalized anxiety: A perspective. *Counselling & Psychotherapy Research, 18*(3), 233–236. https://doi.org/10.1002/capr.12172

Timulak, L., & Creaner, M. (2010). Qualitative meta-analysis of outcome of person-centered and experiential psychotherapies. In M. Cooper, J. C. Watson, & D. Hölldampf (Eds.), *Person-centered and experiential therapies work: A review of the research on counseling, psychotherapy, and related practices* (pp. 65–90). PCCS.

Timulak, L., & Keogh, D. (2022). *Transdiagnostic emotion-focused therapy: A clinical guide for transforming emotional pain.* American Psychological Association. https://doi.org/10.1037/0000253-000

Timulak, L., Keogh, D., Chigwedere, C., Wilson, C., Ward, F., Hevey, D., Griffin, P., Jacobs, L., Hughes, S., Vaughan, C., Beckham, K., & Mahon, S. (2022). A comparison of emotion-focused therapy and cognitive-behavioral therapy in the treatment of generalized anxiety disorder: Results of a feasibility randomized controlled trial. *Psychotherapy, 59*(1), 84–95. https://doi.org/10.1037/pst0000427

Twenge, J. M. (2017, September). Have smartphones destroyed an entire generation? *The Atlantic.* https://www.theatlantic.com/magazine/archive/2017/09/has-the-smartphone-destroyed-a-generation/534198/

Vallejos, L., & Johnson, Z. (2019). Multicultural competencies in humanistic psychology. In L. Hoffman, H. Cleare-Hoffman, N. Granger, Jr., & D. St. John (Eds.), *Humanistic approaches to multiculturalism and diversity: Perspectives on existence and difference* (pp. 63–75). Routledge. https://doi.org/10.4324/9781351133357-6

van Deurzen, E. (2019). Existential–phenomenological therapy. In E. van Deurzen, E. Craig, A. Längle, K. J. Schneider, D. Tantam, & S. du Plock (Eds.), *The Wiley world handbook of existential therapy* (pp. 127–131). Wiley Blackwell. https://doi.org/10.1002/9781119167198.part2

van Deurzen, E., & Adams, M. (2016). *Skills in existential counselling and psychotherapy* (2nd ed.). Sage.

van Deurzen, E., & Arnold-Baker, C. (2019). Existential–phenomenological therapy illustration: Rahim's dilemma. In E. van Deurzen, E. Craig, A. Längle, K. J. Schneider, D. Tantam, & S. du Plock (Eds.), *The Wiley world handbook of existential therapy* (pp. 181–197). Wiley Blackwell. https://doi.org/10.1002/9781119167198.ch10

van Deurzen, E., Craig, E., Längle, A., Schneider, K. J., Tantam, D., & du Plock, S. (Eds.). (2019). *The Wiley world handbook of existential therapy*. Wiley Blackwell. https://doi.org/10.1002/9781119167198

Vanhooren, S., Leijssen, M., & Dezutter, J. (2018). Posttraumatic growth during incarceration: A case study from an experiential–existential perspective. *Journal of Humanistic Psychology, 58*(2), 144–167. https://doi.org/10.1177/0022167815621647

van Rijn, B., & Wild, C. (2013). Humanistic and integrative therapies for anxiety and depression: Practice-based evaluation of transactional analysis, gestalt, and integrative psychotherapies and person-centered counseling. *Transactional Analysis Journal, 43*(2), 150–163. https://doi.org/10.1177/0362153713499545

Vos, J. (2016a). Working with meaning in life in chronic or life-threatening disease: A review of its relevance and the effectiveness of meaning-centered therapies. In P. Russo-Netzer, S. E. Schulenberg, & A. Batthyany (Eds.), *Clinical perspectives on meaning: Positive and existential psychotherapy* (pp. 171–200). Springer. https://doi.org/10.1007/978-3-319-41397-6_9

Vos, J. (2016b). Working with meaning in life in mental health care: A systematic literature review of the practices and effectiveness of meaning-centered therapies. In P. Russo-Netzer, S. E. Schulenberg, & A. Batthyany (Eds.), *Clinical perspectives on meaning: Positive and existential psychotherapy* (pp. 59–87). Springer. https://doi.org/10.1007/978-3-319-41397-6_4

Vos, J. (2019). A review of research on existential-phenomenological therapies. In E. van Deurzen, E. Craig, A. Längle, K. J. Schneider, D. Tantam, & S. du Plock (Eds.), *The Wiley world handbook of existential therapy* (pp. 592–614). Wiley Blackwell. https://doi.org/10.1002/9781119167198.ch37

Vos, J., Cooper, M., Correia, E., & Craig, M. (2015). Existential therapies: A review of their scientific foundations and efficacy. *Existential Analysis, 26*(1), 49–69.

Vos, J., Craig, M., & Cooper, M. (2015). Existential therapies: A meta-analysis of their effects on psychological outcomes. *Journal of Consulting and Clinical Psychology, 83*(1), 115–128. https://doi.org/10.1037/a0037167

Wampold, B. E. (2007). Psychotherapy: The humanistic (and effective) treatment. *American Psychologist, 62*(8), 857–873. https://doi.org/10.1037/0003-066X.62.8.857

Wampold, B. E., & Imel, Z. E. (2015). *The great psychotherapy debate: The evidence for what makes psychotherapy work* (2nd ed.). Routledge. https://doi.org/10.4324/9780203582015

Wang, X. (2019). The symbol of the iron house: From survivalism to existentialism. In L. Hoffman, M. Yang, M. Mansilla, J. Dias, M. Moats, & T. Claypool (Eds.), *Existential psychology East–West* (Vol. 2. pp. 3–15). University Professors Press.

Watson, J. C., & Pos, A. E. (2017). Humanistic and experiential perspectives. In R. J. DeRubeis & D. R. Strunk (Eds.), *The Oxford handbook of mood disorders* (pp. 459–468). Oxford University Press.

Watson, J. C., Saedi Chekan, S., & McMullen, E. (2017). Emotion-focused psychotherapy for GAD: Individual case comparison of a good and poor outcome case. *Person-Centered and Experiential Psychotherapies, 16*(2), 118–139. https://doi.org/10.1080/14779757.2017.1330707

Watson, J. C., & Watson, N. (2010). Operationalizing incongruence: Measures of self-discrepancy and affect regulation. In M. Cooper, J. C. Watson, & D. Hölldampf (Eds.), *Person-centered and experiential therapies work: A review of the research on counseling, psychotherapy, and related practices* (pp. 164–187). PCCS.

Wharne, S. (2021). How is distress understood in existential philosophies and can phenomenological therapeutic practices be "evidence-based"? *Theory & Psychology, 31*(2), 273–289. https://doi.org/10.1177/0959354320964586

Wittenborn, A. K., Liu, T., Ridenour, T. A., Lachmar, E. M., Mitchell, E. A., & Seedall, R. B. (2019). Randomized controlled trial of emotionally focused couple therapy compared to treatment as usual for depression: Outcomes and mechanisms of change. *Journal of Marital and Family Therapy, 45*(3), 395–409. https://doi.org/10.1111/jmft.12350

Wnuk, S. M., Greenberg, L., & Dolhanty, J. (2015). Emotion-focused group therapy for women with symptoms of bulimia nervosa. *Eating Disorders, 23*(3), 253–261. https://doi.org/10.1080/10640266.2014.964612

Yalom, I. (1980). *Existential psychotherapy.* Basic Books.

II

EVIDENCE-BASED FOUNDATIONS OF EXISTENTIAL–HUMANISTIC STANCES

4

Therapeutic Presence in Existential–Humanistic Psychotherapy

Orah T. Krug, Chris Bradshaw, Juanita Ratner, and Almudena Sánchez-Mazarro

Existential–humanistic (EH) therapy is a relational and experiential therapy focusing on the actual, lived experiences of both client and therapist as they exist in the therapeutic encounter. Lived experience includes the immediate, cognitive, affective, kinesthetic, and profound aspects of an experience. Within a safe and collaborative therapeutic relationship, EH therapy aims to (a) help clients become more present to themselves and others, (b) assist clients in identifying ways they block themselves from fuller presence, (c) challenge clients to assume responsibility for designing their present lives, and (d) encourage clients to choose more expanded ways of being in their daily lives (Schneider & Krug, 2010, 2017).

To accomplish this, EH therapists cultivate presence to the *here-and-now*. This phrase, utilized by Fritz Perls, is integral in gestalt therapy (Perls, 1947) as well as foundational to the interpersonal approach of Irvin Yalom (Yalom, 1980, 2002). In EH therapy, the "here" refers to the therapy room and the "now" refers to inter- and intrapersonal processes actual in the present moment. These processes expand awareness, healing, and change.

Waking up and truly experiencing life now, presently and actively, has the potential to bring about an inner evolution and to improve one's life (Bugental, 1978). Bugental believed that (a) humans are rarely fully present, (b) presence is essential for living a meaningful and engaged life, and (c) becoming present is a fundamental task of humanity. May (1983) posits that presence is the ability to pause in the face of what life throws at us and to choose a response with our whole organism (i.e., mind, body, emotions, and spirit). In his conception, this constitutes true freedom.

https://doi.org/10.1037/0000446-005

The Evidence-Based Foundations of Existential–Humanistic Therapy, L. Hoffman and V. Lac (Editors)

Much has been written about the challenges to being fully present in modern life and in therapy itself (Bugental, 1978; Geller & Greenberg, 2022; Hayes & Vinca, 2017). EH therapy sees presence, though it may express itself differently in different cultural contexts, as a birthright of human beings (Bugental, 1978; May, 1983; Ratner, 2017). Consequently, the cultivation of therapeutic presence is understood as the foundation and primary aim of EH therapy (Schneider & Krug, 2017; Schneider & May, 1995). Being fully present in a relationship promotes mental, emotional, neurobiological, and physiological health within us and within the people around us, and it may be at the core of what makes psychotherapy effective (Geller, 2017; Geller & Greenberg, 2022; Geller & Porges, 2014; Schneider, 2015b; Schneider & Krug, 2017; Siegel, 2007, 2011, 2018).

DEFINING PRESENCE

Presence can only be provisionally defined and is defined differently by various theorists and clinicians within EH psychology and in other systems of psychology (Geller & Greenberg, 2022; Hoffman, 2019). A general linguistic, general psychotherapeutic, and EH definition of presence is offered. The Latin root of presence is *prae* ("before") and *esse* ("to be") creating a word that literally means "to be before." Merriam-Webster's dictionary defines presence as "existence" or "being there" (Merriam-Webster, n.d.). Another aspect of presence refers to an individual's demeanor, stance, or bearing. Therapeutic presence may involve the following process: the therapist being grounded in and aware of their physical experience in session (i.e., body existence); "immersed in what is poignant in the moment within the client" and in the therapeutic relationship (i.e., emotion/heart existence); experiencing expanded mental perception (i.e., mind existence); and being fully "with and for the client" (i.e., service-oriented/spiritual coexistence; Geller & Greenberg, 2022, p. 12).

Schneider (2015b) defines therapeutic presence from an EH perspective as "a complex mix of appreciative openness, concerted engagement, support, and expressiveness, and it both holds and illuminates that which is palpably significant within the client and between client and therapist" (p. 305). Presence involves safety (holding) while simultaneously mirroring (illuminating) and exploring what is physically, emotionally, imaginatively, and intuitively (or palpably) felt as vital and alive in the present moment within the client, within the therapist, and between client and therapist.

CONTEXTUALIZING PRESENCE IN AN EH CONTEXT

EH therapists cultivate presence and invite their clients to do the same so that a copresence exists between client and therapist (Bugental, 1999; Cooper, 2005; Geller & Greenberg, 2002; Krug, 2009, 2017; Schneider & Krug, 2010,

2017). EH therapists turn the therapeutic soil, adding the life-affirming nutri-ents of acceptance, empathy, attunement, and appropriate responsiveness. Therapists cannot make a client heal or change any more than farmers can make their crops grow.

The cultivation of presence is both the ground for a genuine encounter and a method for effecting transformational change. By "ground" here we mean the foundation and basis, but with connotations of the earth and the life-giving soil. The ground includes EH therapists' intention to create a safe and intimate therapeutic relationship whereby the client can find their own authentic ground. Within this relationship clients can face and reflect on disavowed ways of being and coping, past wounds, and attitudes about self and others; clients also learn to work with and trust differences both within themselves and toward the world. EH therapy sees presence as the existential connection with the ground of a person's being (May, 1983; Ratner, 2015). In a collectivist cul-ture, this ground may be more communal, and in an individualist culture, more individual. EH therapy emphasizes the client's self-discovery and the therapist coming humbly from a place of not knowing and is thus open to where the client leads in terms of rediscovering their own presence (Bugental, 1999; Schneider & Krug, 2017).

The method of presence expands experiential awareness of clients' personal worlds. Personal world or context refers to self or other and world constructs and their functional yet constrictive protections. Protections (often *unregarded* by the client) are constructed to cope with painful, overwhelming, or frighten-ing beliefs and feelings regarding self or others and the world as well as with traumatic experiences and other alienating or stressful life experiences such as being the object of racism, violence, or abandonment.

To paraphrase Irvin Yalom (1980), nothing takes precedence over the health and well-being of the therapeutic relationship. Yalom describes the interper-sonal field as the in-between space. Cultivating presence to the *in-between* brings the client's attention to the therapeutic relationship with comments and questions like "I feel farther away from you right now. Do you notice if you feel distant?"; "How was that to tell me?"; or "You seem to not like what I just said to you." This relational focus creates a sense of genuineness, openness, and trust. Krug's extensive training with Bugental and Yalom shaped her perspec-tive that EH therapists are more effective when they cultivate presence to both the subjective processes within the therapist and within the client (i.e., the intrapersonal processes) and the interpersonal process between client and ther-apist (Krug, 2009, 2019, 2021a, 2021b; Krug & Piwowarski, 2019; Krug & Schneider, 2016; Schneider & Krug, 2010, 2017).

The phrase *self and world constructs* refers to how the client implicitly under-stands and manifests their own nature and relationship to the world through behaviors and attitudes. They are subjective because they are self-created. For example, a client believes that they are damaged, that others will shun them, and that the world is cold and unloving. In order to function, the client dis-avows awareness of these beliefs and related pain by constructing a protective life stance such as being a people pleaser or a people avoider. Protective life stances are actual but often unregarded by the individual (Bugental 1999). That is, these protective life stances (sometimes referred to as defense mechanisms or maladaptive coping strategies in other approaches) often show up in the room with the therapist and certainly manifest in moments of the client's life. However, these are often seemingly unnoticed by the client, or noticed and not recognized for what they in fact are.

An individual's self and world constructs express themselves in the present moment through bodily gestures, vocal tones, dreams, and behavior patterns and not so much through words spoken. For this reason, EH therapists focus more on illuminating implicit processes than on addressing objective content through being present. The relationship between implicit process and objective content is like the relationship between the music of a song and the words of a song. The music conveys the tone and the mood, often at a deeper level than the words themselves. Consequently, EH therapists ask themselves, "How is my client telling me their story? Is their voice flat and unemotional or filled with trembling emotion? What am I feeling as I sit with my client (e.g., do I want to move toward or away from them)?"

In presence, EH therapists may attend to how the client occupies personal space—with confidence and ease or with hesitation and constraint. They may comment on a client's relational ways of being, such as "You seem to not like what I just said." Or they may simply attend to how clients relate to them—in engaged, open or detached, or aloof ways.

Illustrations of Cultivating Presence

The following vignette illustrates how Orah Krug cultivated presence to her client, Mary's,[1] unfolding, implicit process. This was Krug's first session with Mary. She began by telling Krug about her breakup with her boyfriend. She told Krug he wanted more intimacy but felt that she was hard to get close to and didn't seem to need him. After a year together, he decided to end the relationship. Mary cried as she told Krug more about what happened. Krug listened but noticed that her attention was drawn to how Mary was holding on to a shredded tissue and not taking another, even though there was a whole box of tissues next to her. Krug decided to trust her focus on Mary's tissue behavior.

KRUG: I notice you haven't taken another tissue even though yours is shredded from your tears.

MARY: [pausing and looking up at Krug with dawning awareness] I never ask or reach for help. I always make do.

---

[1]Mary is a fictional composite of several clients.

This vignette illustrates how a therapist's focus on what is most alive in the moment can lead to a deepening of the process. Krug has learned to trust that what is most alive in her client is almost always a reflection of something meaningful to them. By cultivating presence to Mary's tissue behavior, Krug discovered and felt a self-created protective stance, namely "I always make do." Mary's protective stance was what Bugental (1999) described as actual but unregarded. In other words, Mary always making do was a real and visible way of being (i.e., actual), but one that was out of her conscious awareness. EH therapists are trained to cultivate presence to a client's implicit process—to bring awareness to unregarded ways of being.

Cultivating personal and relational presence often allows clients to feel the pain of a wound, as they are no longer numbed by the protective pattern. The belief about self finds expression for Mary: "I've never felt worthy of being cared for—I'm damaged, that's why I don't reach out to you." By supporting clients to experientially embody their self-restrictive protections in the safety of the present therapeutic relationship, clients can face and accept the givens of existence and their core decisions and wounds that may have been avoided, denied, or repressed. Responsibility is assumed for constructing the protective pattern, along with a newfound sense of agency and choice. The deepest roots of trauma cannot be talked about or explained away; they must be discovered, felt, and lived through (Krug, 2019; Krug & Schneider, 2016; Krug et al., 2019; Schneider & Krug, 2010, 2017).

RESEARCH SUPPORT

Presence is a difficult concept to directly research, in part because it is an abstract concept and understood differently by different therapists (Geller & Greenberg, 2022; see also Geller & Greenberg, 2002, 2010). A deep presence is an inner experience with esoteric and noetic nuances that must be experienced—words can only point to it. Additionally, presence may have some overlap at times with other constructs, such as warmth, empathy, and genuineness (Geller & Greenberg, 2022; see also Geller et al., 2010). In this section, we review the quantitative and qualitative research literature on presence.

Leading therapy outcome researcher Bruce Wampold (2008), in a review of Kirk Schneider's edited book *Existential–Integrative Psychotherapy*, writes: "I have no doubt that EI [existential–integrative] approaches would satisfy any criteria used to label other psychological treatments as scientific" (p. 5). He continues, "It could be . . . that an understanding of the principles of existential therapy is needed by all therapists, as it adds a perspective that might, as Schneider contends, form the basis of all effective treatments" (p. 6).

Effective psychotherapy is better explained by certain common, contextual, or atmospheric factors that carry across the major therapeutic approaches when they are effective as opposed to by the specific techniques and concepts particular to each unique approach (Wampold & Imel, 2015). Schneider (2015b) proposes that many of these factors are existential–humanistic in nature and that therapist presence may be the center of the wheel of the common factors (see Figure 4.1).

Carl Rogers (1957) wrote that therapists need to offer certain conditions in the therapy room in order to create the growth-promoting environment where clients can accept themselves, become congruent, harness their strengths, and grow. Rogers referred to these as therapist-offered conditions (TOCs): congruence, unconditional positive regard, and empathy. Later in his career, Rogers wrote about the healing power of being fully present with clients (Rogers, 1979, 1980). In an interview published after his death (Baldwin, 2000), Rogers discusses that presence may be one of the primary goals of therapy. Therapeutic presence may be either a fourth TOC in therapy, or a precursor that makes the other TOCs possible or more effective (Baldwin, 2000; Cain, 2010; Geller et al., 2010).

In a study of clients' perceptions of their existentially oriented therapists, Schneider (1985) reports that although techniques were important to long-term success, the personal involvement of the therapist (their genuineness, support, and understanding) was by far the most critical factor identified. Such involvement inspired clients to become more self-aligned and to experience themselves as increasingly "secure, valued and valuable, expressive, realistic, and

FIGURE 4.1. Presence May Be the Hub of the Common Factors Wheel

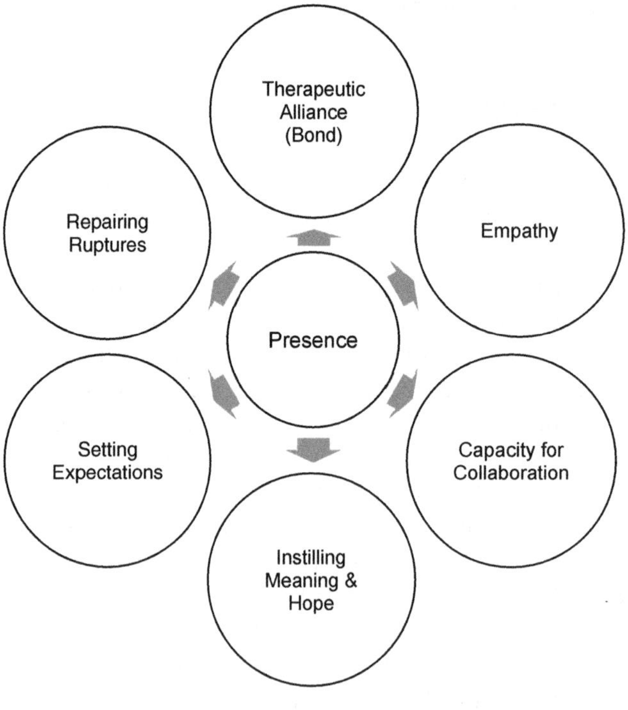

Note. Adapted from *The Client Experience of Therapeutic Presence* [Doctoral dissertation], by C. C. Bradshaw, 2024, ProQuest Dissertations & Theses (https://www.proquest.com/openview/ae61cbded2a853da0167a5b4cd86dc41/1?cbl=18750&diss=y&loginDisplay=true&pq-origsite=gscholar). Copyright 2024 by Christopher C. Bradshaw. Adapted with permission.

optimistic" (p. iii; for a comprehensive review of these and other EH therapeutic investigations see also Angus et al., 2015; Elliot, 2002; Rennie, 2002; Walsh & McElewain, 2002; Watson & Bohart, 2015). Additional studies show that presence can be considered as the foundation for creating the conditions needed for a strong therapeutic alliance and empathy (Dunn et al., 2013; Geller, 2017; Geller & Greenberg, 2022; Geller et al., 2010; Geller & Porges, 2014).

Quantitative Research

Quantitative studies may find it difficult to embrace the deep complexity of the process and ground of presence. These studies are often based on the idea that a client and the therapist themselves can evaluate the therapist's presence during the session as more or less present. This is worth deep questioning and reflection. Therapist's presence cannot be reduced to what the client or therapist might perceive (Bernhardt et al., 2020). Although often presence creates a sense of safety and allows for empathy and warmth, it also may be uncomfortable (Geller & Greenberg, 2022; Schneider, 2015a, 2015b; Schneider & Krug, 2017). Not only this, but EH therapists being attuned to the discomfort of presence can at times be therapeutic in relational work.

At the same time, presence as measured by client and therapist may be impactful. Shari Geller and Leslie Greenberg engaged seminal qualitative, quantitative, and theoretical work on presence (Geller & Greenberg, 2022; see also Geller & Greenberg, 2002, 2010). Geller and colleagues (2010) developed the Therapist Presence Inventory (TPI), with versions to be self-administered postsession by therapists regarding their own presence (TPI-T) and by clients regarding their therapist's presence in session (TPI-C; Geller & Greenberg, 2010). Their research utilizes factor analysis and finds the TPIs to be reliable and valid. Further, they set out to determine if increased therapist presence, as measured by the TPIs, improved in-session alliance (as measured by the Working Alliance Inventory), the therapeutic relationship (as measured by the Relationship Inventory), and outcomes in the form of insight and behavior change (as measured by the Client Task Specific Measure—Revised). Results are in favor of client perception of increased therapist presence correlating with positive session outcomes (Geller et al., 2010). The research shows that "therapists' presence is related to their experience of the therapeutic relationship, and that clients' perception of therapist presence relates to session outcome and the therapeutic alliance" (Geller et al., 2010, p. 608). Also, therapist rated presence predicts clients' perception of their therapists' empathy, congruence, and unconditional regard.

Results further indicate that client-centered (CC) therapy, a humanistic approach, and processing experiential (PE) therapy, an approach with similarities to EH therapy, yield higher ratings of therapist presence both from clients in the TPI-C and from therapists themselves in the TPI-T as compared with cognitive behavior therapy (CBT). Geller's research further shows that presence is related to the TOCs proposed by Rogers (i.e., empathy, congruence, and positive regard). Presence may be a fourth TOC or an especially adaptable TOC that helps the others function more effectively (Geller & Greenberg, 2022; Geller et al., 2010). Results show that clients found the therapists who utilized the CC and PE approaches to be higher in the TOCs than were the CBT therapists. However, regardless of the type of therapy utilized, clients reported greater positive change when presence was rated higher. This suggests that, regardless of the method of therapy utilized, increased presence will likely improve outcome and connects back to the idea that presence might be related to the common factors.

This study aimed to create a measure for presence, test the reliability and validity of this measure, and explore the possible connection between presence and good outcomes in therapy. In their work related to the construction of the TPI measures, the authors consulted therapists who emphasize presence in their practices (Geller & Greenberg, 2010). Demographically, these therapists are discussed in terms of gender (male or female identifying). In measuring the effectiveness of the TPIs and of presence therapeutically, the authors collected client participant data on age, gender identification (male or female identifying), race, marital status, and education level. Regarding these demographic variables, Geller and colleagues (2010) did not find any statistically significant differences between these groups concerning any of the outcomes measured. This could suggest that presence, and the lack of presence, apply as significant in therapy across these demographics represented. It could also be argued that good therapists attune to and adjust to the client according to cultural presentations, and their presence manifests accordingly.

Additional cultural contexts that might influence an individual participant or therapist and that may influence the process and experience of presence in session are not considered, such as (but not limited to) sexual orientation, additional gender identities, the presence of experienced disability or other ability, immigration status, and socioeconomic status. A total of 114 participants (39 identifying as men, 75 identifying as women) ages 21–65 years old were drawn from two Canadian universities in two randomized controlled trials and met criteria for the diagnosis for major depression. Significantly, 89.5% of participants identified as White, 7.9% identified as Asian, and 2.6% Hispanic. There were no participants of Black or African descent, no participants of Indigenous descent, and no other races or ethnicities were identified. The therapists (21 female, 4 male) in this study included four licensed doctoral-level psychologists; two PhD clinical psychologists not yet licensed; and 19 advanced doctoral students. Eight therapists utilized CBT, four utilized PE therapy, and 13 utilized PE and CC therapy. From a multicultural perspective, it is noteworthy that we are not aware of the race of the therapists.

This study contributes much to our understanding of presence and is an important piece of literature; however, the demographic data highlights a gap in the literature. More remains to be done in terms of understanding the role that cultures and intersectionality may play in the experience and process of presence. Additional research explores connections with presence and empathy, the need to prepare for presence to produce good outcomes, session quality, the therapeutic alliance, and other factors and outcomes in therapy. Presence was found to be a predictor for therapeutic alliance and successful session outcomes across emotion-focused therapy, CBT, and person-centered therapy (Geller et al., 2010) and clients' symptom reduction (Hayes & Vinca, 2017). Hayes and Vinca (2017) found that a therapist's presence perceived by the client was correlated to the therapist's empathy perceived by the client.

Mindfulness and Presence

Presence is fundamental in creating a therapeutic environment of trust and safety at the neurobiological and nervous system levels (Geller & Porges, 2014). Largely through a calm, alert, warm, and safe presence, therapists help clients to tolerate difficult emotion and distress in an adaptive way. It also has been advanced that therapy helps to a degree that enhances neuroplasticity (Cozolino, 2017).

Mindfulness meditation cultivates presence such that presence becomes more consistently practiced by humans—an example of neuroplasticity (Farb et al., 2013; Geller, 2017; Lazar et al., 2005; Siegel, 2011). However, psychotherapeutic presence is, of course, not synonymous with mindfulness meditation (Geller & Greenberg, 2022; Schneider, 2015b). Mindfulness meditation, a potentially presence-generating practice, strengthens and thickens parts of the brain involved in attention, focus, and awareness of body senses (Lazar et al., 2005). All forms of meditation may engage the insular cortex region of the brain, which is involved in "monitoring of body states, empathy, and metacognition" (Geller, 2017, p. 49). Relatedly, EH therapists use their own embodied experience to model and encourage a fuller presence in the client (Bugental, 1978; Schneider & Krug, 2017; Schneider & May, 1995;). Awareness of embodied experience bears some similarity to aspects of mindfulness (see also Chapter 14 of this volume). However, EH therapists have been doing this before mindfulness became popular in psychotherapy (Bugental, 1978; May, 1975)

Electroencephalography, functional magnetic resonance imaging, and positron emission tomography scans show that meditation mostly stimulates the rest- and digest-oriented parasympathetic nervous system but has some arousal of the sympathetic fight–flight system, allowing for a skillful balance of peace and engagement (Geller & Greenberg, 2022). This parallels the recommended neurobiology of therapy involving overall safety with a healthy amount of challenge-oriented stress (Cozolino, 2017).

Polyvagal Theory: Safety Through Presence

Polyvagal theory discusses the process of neuroception, the neurological process by which human beings instinctively evaluate safety and risk in relationships through responding to signals such as facial expression, tone of voice, body posture, and emotional expression (Dana, 2018). People respond to threat by nervous system states commonly referred to as fight, flight, freeze, fawn, and faint. The *self-protections* referred to in EH therapy (Schneider & Krug,

2017)—designed largely unconsciously to protect the client from the present moment and yet paradoxically cutting them off from deeper meaning—through the lens of polyvagal theory would likely be rooted in one of these listed nervous system states or combinations of them.

Nonverbal communication of therapeutic presence—such as a well-calibrated tone of voice, a receptive and attentive body posture, and a centered yet emotionally warm and expressive face—may help facilitate clients' neuroception of safety. This helps clients feel safe enough to process in a directly experiential way, often even with difficult or even traumatic material (Geller & Greenberg, 2022; Geller & Porges, 2014; Porges & Dana, 2018), facilitating healing and the sense of freedom to build self-efficacy within a neurological context as well as a psychotherapeutic one.

It should be noted, however, that, similar to presence, it is the experience and perception of the client regarding safety that matters, not the therapist's perception of themselves. That is, it is important for EH therapists to understand that feeling present or feeling that we are holding a safe space may not mean the client feels this way. To call back to Schneider's definition of presence, there is an engagement element with what is felt as vital within the client. Further, as the work of Menakem (2017) shows, in multicultural situations with clients from marginalized groups, the experience of suffering from systemic racism that some clients have experienced may create an embodied reaction resulting in not feeling safe in therapy in general with any therapist, especially White therapists. Clients from marginalized groups may experience automatic self-protective nervous system states of fight, flight, freeze, fawn, and faint simply by being in the room with a therapist from a nonmarginalized group. A mature EH therapist sensitive to their own context and to what is present in the room generally would be alert to this phenomenon and allow it to inform how they express presence and attune to what might be significant within the client who may have suffered from systemic racism.

Presence in the therapist tends to invoke presence in the client (Bugental, 1978; May, 1983: Ratner, 2015), whether or not it is perceived as such. While on the one hand it is the client's perception of therapist presence that matters in terms of quantitatively measured outcomes (Geller et al., 2010), on the other hand a client also may not recognize when a therapist is present or may even be highly uncomfortable with presence in the therapist and in themselves (Geller & Greenberg, 2022).

Schneider (2015a) writes about levels of experiential liberation: physiological, environmental, cognitive, psychosexual, interpersonal, and experiential (i.e., the immediate, affective, kinesthetic, and profound). In EH therapy, the experiential level of presence and liberation is the deepest and, often, most demanding level. Cultural and intersectionality issues can present and be worked with at every level of liberation and presence. EH therapists monitor a client's readiness, willingness, and capacity for full experiential presence and modulate their expression of presence accordingly, factoring in the balance of safety and growth (Schneider, 2015a; Schneider & Krug, 2017; Schneider &

May, 1995). In EH therapy, the therapist invites the client into a fuller presence and may in turn vivify for a client how they block their own presence, or, selectively, confront how this client blocks their presence and limits their growth and access to a meaningful life. An alert and sensitive presence on the part of the therapist may recognize discomfort in the client and intuitively judge how to respond: to hold space; to ask, "How are we doing?"; and, when appropriate, to normalize the client's response. As will be discussed later, multicultural and intersectionality issues come into play in terms of the EH therapist modulating how presence is expressed. In summary, EH presence aims to first create a sense of safety and acceptance, but it does not hold that safety is sufficient for healing and change. As previously stated, presence both holds (safety) and illuminates constrictive protective patterns and invites engagement with disavowed parts to heal painful wounds and bring about lasting change. There are special considerations related to multiculturalism, cultural humility, and awareness of the legacy of systemic racism that need to be engaged with when seeking to be an effectively present therapist with clients from marginalized groups.

Interpersonal Neurobiology: Integration Through Presence

The field of interpersonal neurobiology, as written about by Siegel and others, may offer insights into aspects of the positive effects and processes of presence and its importance in therapy. According to Siegel (2017), physical and psychological health starts with a process of *integration*, which in turn starts through therapeutic presence. Through presence we may integrate attention, awareness, intention, and the rational and later developed areas of the brain with the earlier developed and more emotionally reactive regions. Synaptic connections strengthen through presence, and, for example, rational cognition synergizes in an adaptive way with emotional feeling or the body senses harmonizing with thinking and emotions. This facilitates an individual to be present in their own life cognitively, emotionally, and palpably in their senses. Thus, it can help with the all-too-common issue of one's emotions overriding their rationality, leading one to ignore warning signs from the body and which wreaks havoc in one's life, or a person's thinking being cut off from what their bodies tell them, which can cause them to think themselves into physical ailments.

Integration, thus, refers to working well together or harmonizing, a bidirectional influencing of disparate parts to the positive holistic generation of resilience, empathy, compassion, flexibility, attunement, morality, and health (Siegel, 2011). This enables a discerning and more fully human state to be more conducive to authentic choice and the ability to better embody one's potential. Presence can help us be more open and attuned in our relationships (Siegel, 2018). Presence also enhances our ability to attune to what is going on within ourselves, which is the basis for being able to empathize with others (Siegel, 2007). Further, being in a state of presence may help improve our health in the cardiovascular, chromosomal, inflammation response, stress response, and immune function areas (Siegel, 2011).

Qualitative Research

Qualitative research shows the importance of presence and offers nuanced descriptions of how presence might function in therapy as well as what it may demand of the therapist. Several studies interview therapists about their experiences with presence. Fraelich (1989) engages a hermeneutic study interviewing six therapists about presence and settles on 14 elements representing the therapist's relationship with presence. These elements refer to presence as spontaneous, involving being fully in the moment, a sense of openness on the part of the therapist, a sense in the therapist of freshly registering raw experience real-time as it comes, an element of intentional service and bracketing of self-concerns, a deep interest in the client, authenticity in the therapist, deep engagement with the client's subjective world, a palpably strong relationship, unconditional positive regard, and other elements.

Geller and Greenberg (2002), in the qualitative study that would lead to their later quantitative work resulting in the creation of the TPI (Geller & Greenberg, 2010), engage in interviews with therapists who have either written about presence or who consider presence an important element in their work. The study collects data on experience level and modalities utilized by therapist participants, but not any demographic data such as race, age, or gender identification. It is not noted in the study whether or not these therapists identified as multicultural or as emphasizing a multicultural approach to therapy.

Geller and Greenberg (2010) include therapists from a range of approaches: CBT, person-centered therapy, and PE therapy. Therapists were interviewed about presence, its importance, and its role in effective therapy. It is worth touching on a few of the items in the TPI scales, as they align with EH practice. The client version (TPI-C) consists of questions on a Likert scale ranging from 0 to 7. Here are two such examples: "My therapist was fully there in the moment with me" and "My therapist's responses were really in tune with what I was experiencing in the moment." The therapist version consists of 21 questions, also on a 0 to 7 scale, exploring the process, experience, and absence of presence, many of which align with EH practice. The following are two examples from the TPI-T: "I was aware of my own internal flow of experiencing" and "I felt fully immersed in my client's experience and yet still centered within myself."

Other literature warns against reducing presence down to a list of elements or traits and reminds us that presence is a process taking place in dynamic relationships (Schneider, 2015b; see also Geller & Greenberg, 2022; Phelon, 2001, 2004). This aligns with EH theory and core stances (Schneider, 2015b; Schneider & Krug, 2017). Phelon (2001, 2004) engages a rich qualitative study of presence, utilizing a range of methods: hermeneutic text work, observing therapists who reported experiencing presence when they themselves were in therapy, and interviews of therapists. Phelon concludes that presence is a fundamental process and not reducible to a list of traits or characteristics. Phelon further notes that therapists' ongoing "commitment to personal growth" and "spiritual practice and belief" is integrated into their therapy practice, and the therapists' level of personal "inner awareness" tends to be involved in the lives of highly present therapists (Phelon, 2001, p. iii). Inner awareness includes, among other elements, an attunement to the therapist's own emotions and physical sensations in session. Having a spiritual practice is not a requirement per Phelon's findings. The key is finding a way of talking about and practicing inner awareness and integrating that inner awareness practice into the therapy work.

Marie-Miller (2016), exploring how therapist training programs might look at presence, completed a dissertation employing a transcendental phenomenological inquiry into counseling students' development of therapeutic presence through their counselor education program. Three findings from this study align with the manner in which therapists receive training in EH through organizations such as the Existential–Humanistic Institute (see Krug & Schneider 2016): counselors-in-training "benefit from self-awareness activities"; "education pertaining to client encounters can help to develop therapeutic presence"; and certain "personal characteristics" of counselors affect their level of therapeutic presence (Marie-Miller, 2016, p. iii). The study also looks at different concepts of presence and the characteristics counselors might need to acquire to develop presence from within different theoretical approaches to counseling. For example, "personal characteristics" discussed by Marie-Miller include the EH values of acceptance, unconditional positive regard, empathy, and genuineness. Similarly, a qualitative literature review of 14 studies in the nursing literature, resulting in a metasynthesis of presence, finds presence to be a process engaged interpersonally and marked by elements such as openness, sensitivity, intimacy, vulnerability and the ability to adapt to diverse contexts (Finfgeld-Connett, 2006).

The question of how therapists can grow in their experiential practice of presence and in their conceptual understanding of presence is something that needs to be researched more, and yet there is a body of literature on this (Geller, 2017; Geller & Greenberg, 2022; Pierson et al., 2015; Schneider, 2015b; Schneider & Krug, 2016, 2017; Schneider & May, 1995). The level of professional maturity and self-awareness of the therapist is also, of course, relevant to the way they manifest presence and relate to the client. A good therapist is committed to a lifetime of personal growth, doing their own inner work, becoming increasingly aware, and increasingly mastering the art of therapy.

Research has looked at possible connections between therapeutic presence and depth in psychotherapy. This research aligns with the writings of Rollo May (1983), Bugental (1987, 1989), and other seminal existential, humanistic, and EH theorists and practitioners where presence is seen as the essential precursor to depth in therapy. EH writers and clinicians have written about and discussed depth in therapy in terms of depth of connection in the therapeutic relationship and working with deep underlying issues that may be hidden from conscious awareness—such as the givens of existence or ultimate human concerns as written about by Yalom (1980) and Schneider (2015a)—as well as depth of change, growth, and experiential transformation in the client and therapist. Depth also refers to working at a level below conceptual construct, in the actual immediacy of experience (Schneider & Krug, 2017). This is felt by EH therapists to be fundamental to the possibility of change within the deeper dimensions of the person and significant in the development of will, choice, self-efficacy, and transformation of traumatic experience.

Cooper (2005) engages a person-centered, phenomenological interview study of eight therapists from the person-centered tradition about their experience encountering their clients in relational depth. Therapists reported enhanced experiences of empathy, acceptance, receptivity, immersion, clarity, and awareness. During moments of relational depth, the interviewed therapists reported that their clients were transparent, addressing important issues in therapy and returning the therapist's level of attunement. Cooper acknowledges parallels and synergies between this research and research on presence and flow. He offers the definition that relational depth refers to cultivating a copresence in therapy.

Colosimo and Pos (2015) complete a task-analysis study to create an observational measure for determining how presence relates to other processes and outcomes in therapy. The authors identify four main ways, each accompanied by behaviors, that therapists show presence: "being-here, being-now, being-open, and being with and for the client" (p. 100). Additional qualitative work explores presence as an important element in therapy and touches on presence as an embodied experience and as essential for helping the client develop the capacity for choice. Bohart and Tallman (1999) and Rennie (1994) have demonstrated the value of such existential concepts as presence and the expansion of the capacity for choice in effective facilitation. Presence becomes the ground, or foundation, for the therapist during the encounter and it needs to be embodied (Geller & Greenberg, 2022; Krug, 2021)

Presence is featured strongly in case studies. As written in Schneider and Krug (2017), "existential psychotherapy has produced some of the most eloquent case studies in the professional literature (e.g., Binswanger, 1958; Boss, 1963; Bugental, 1976; May, 1983; Schneider & May, 1995; Spinelli, 1997; van Duerzen, 2015; Yalom, 1989)" (p. 101). Bugental (1976) has vividly elucidated his personal struggles—thoughts, feelings, and even kinesthetic reactions—in his depictions of his work with clients; Yalom (1989) has explicated the liveliness and even humor of profoundly present therapeutic rapport.

Other studies show the importance of presence in trauma-focused psychotherapy. Cameron (2019) explores the utilization of humanistic approaches to presence in the treatment of trauma. The article stresses that, in traumatized clients, classic EH ideas such as the need to encounter our freedom and limitation, constrictions and expansion, play heavily. Presence is the primary way to work effectively with clients struggling in these polarities, helping clients be able to consciously experience their contradictions, come to understand them, and develop greater discernment and agency. It has been written that trauma often robs us of the ability to feel safe in the present moment (Dana, 2018; Levine,

1997). This aligns with EH theory that presence helps with timing in therapy, and that it is essential that therapists not become rigidly attached to technique (May, 1983; Schneider & May, 1995). An emphasis is placed on interpersonal and intrapersonal awareness, through presence, and the notion that this awareness is how authentic exchange happens between client and therapist, fostering, ultimately, trauma healing. An EH theoretical position that bears repeating is the following: Often, the deepest roots of trauma cannot be talked about or explained away; they must be discovered, felt, and lived through (Krug 2019, Krug & Schneider 2016; Krug et al., 2019; Schneider & Krug, 2010, 2017).

Studies have explored presence in teletherapy, especially during the COVID-19 pandemic. Rathenau and colleagues (2021) write that therapists quickly had to look hard at how they cultivate therapeutic relationships given the sudden and extreme challenges presented by having to switch entirely to telehealth at the height of the pandemic. Presence is a precursor to a healthy therapeutic relationship, including in the online space. Careful attention is paid to how presence can help reduce therapist burnout, especially when working exclusively online. The study shows that therapists' attitudes about providing therapy online and their perceived difficulties in working online affect their ability to be present under those circumstances. The authors propose that strengthening therapist presence online would improve their attitudes and experiences as online therapists, and possibly vice versa.

MULTICULTURAL CONSIDERATIONS

Because presence in EH therapy is about holding and illuminating what is significant in the therapy room and an individual cannot be fully understood or related to outside of their cultural contexts, then cultural considerations are important in presence. Hoffman and colleagues (2019), writing about how humanistic psychology can work to better fulfill its multicultural promise and improve its attunement to diversity, argue that an even broader contextualist view of the individual is necessary. That is, an individual (both client and therapist) and their behavior can be even more fully understood within their cultural and intersectional contexts and the cultural and intersectional contexts that they bring together when they meet.

In EH therapy, a therapist needs to be aware of their own context from the perspective of intersectionality (Crenshaw, 1989; Federman, 2020; Hayes, 2015; Krug & Schneider, 2016; Vallejos & Johnson, 2019), including the idea that one has various cultural identities and areas of advantage and disadvantage that interrelate in the person's experience and self-identity. Ongoing work with this as well as continuing self-education around diversity issues form a foundation from which an EH therapist can be better attuned to the role of context in the therapeutic session.

One of many examples of how this is often creatively approached in the training of EH therapists is illustrated by an exercise Krug has used in the

Existential–Humanistic Institute training retreats. Krug has participants make a context bag with note cards delineating all the aspects they can be aware of concerning their context, both multicultural and personally historical. After a discussion, participants are to bring the bag to all the remaining gatherings within the retreat and sit on it to emphasize to themselves that they are never without their context. The multicultural context will affect the experience of presence in most situations, likely for both the therapist and client. Marginalized clients, for example, may be suspicious of the therapist's presence (particularly if the therapist is White and of a different socioeconomic strata) and may not feel safe enough to move toward a copresence or relational depth until trust has been established. Even then, there may remain some caution. Marginalized therapists may also feel unsafe at times in session with clients from nonmarginalized groups, or within clinical settings where the majority of therapists are from nonmarginalized groups.

Understanding the implications of presence in a multicultural context points to the need for EH therapists to explore their cultural biases related to individualism, or the assumption that one can work with a pure and total presence that is not impacted by issues of culture and intersectionality (Hoffman, 2019; Vallejos & Johnson, 2019). Presence may not equate experientially with safety within a one-on-one therapy session between, for example, a White male therapist and a client of color. What the therapist perceives as safe may be quite different than what the client perceives as safe, especially in this context of individual therapy. A worthy goal, in these cases, may involve moving toward safer spaces and recognizing that total relational safety may be unrealistic due to cultural factors. Cultural factors aside, moving toward safer spaces is a worthy (and a more realistic) goal for all therapists. Realistically, pure and total presence is not possible and moreover does not equate to total relational safety. Awareness of this on the part of the therapist can help the client experience the environment, paradoxically, as safer.

As EH therapy is a relational therapy, the experience of, for example, a White EH therapist and a client who is a person of color feeling unsettled in the presence of the therapist can, potentially, become material for healing. This type of discomfort, even if encountered and worked with by the EH therapist from a place of presence, does not always result in greater healing, but it is possible. The EH therapist can consider attuned ways of addressing cultural differences with appropriate relational check-ins. These check-ins may initially involve the therapist checking in with themselves about how their cultural biases are influencing the session, along with the other impressions the therapist includes in their awareness. Vallejos and Johnson (2019) write that failure to acknowledge cultural differences in session between the therapist and client can obstruct positive outcomes and harm the therapeutic relationship.

In cultures that are hierarchical or less emotionally expressive, some aspects of a given therapist's typical approach with presence may not feel safe or okay at first, or maybe not ever. For example, a middle-aged, White, American, male EH therapist from an upper-middle socioeconomic status may inadvertently assume that the following are excellent examples of demonstrating intrapersonal and interpersonal safety and presence: monitoring his own anxiety and regulating himself to become calmer in demeanor, using a soft voice, making steady eye contact, smiling, and encouraging the assertive expression of emotion in the client when he notices the client seems repressed or hesitant. However, a given cultural experience in the client may find this invasive, offensive, suspicious, smug, or excessively anxiety-provoking. A given cultural experience in the client may feel that a more assertive, upbeat, declarative, and physically stern posture may connote more of a subjective feeling of presence. A relational check-in, such as, "How are we doing?" followed by an exploration of the client's experience in therapy, allows the therapist to better understand the client's experience and recalibrate, if necessary, their posture, attitude, and interventions.

Our experience working with clients from a wide range of demographics (including race, region of the United States, socioeconomic status, sexual orientation, gender identification and expression, personality features, mental health diagnoses, abilities, age, and indigenous heritage) in diverse settings (such as outpatient, inpatient, Medicaid-funded, private pay, court-mandated, voluntary, and educational settings) is that presence is one of the core stances in therapy that applies readily across a spectrum of human interactions and cultural contexts. Yet, in a true existential dialectic, presence is modulated with sensitivity to how cultures manifest in the moment within the client, within the therapist, within the setting of therapy and surrounding settings, and within the relationship. That is, it seems that presence applies in any cultural context—it is a question of how presence is expressed and perhaps the expectations one places on presence.

The definition of presence given by Schneider (2015b) is quite apt here. First, Schneider refers to presence as a complex mix of various elements, including expressiveness, engagement, and support. Indeed, the reason this definition is abstract and there are not always clear procedures for presence (e.g., sitting up straight, steady eye contact, even breathing) is precisely because what support means to one client may be very different from how support is experienced by other clients. The expressiveness element, for example, can be modulated based on intersectionality issues, including consideration of eye contact, voice volume, vocal tone, frequency of questions, degree of formality, and other factors. These are all important questions, often with cultural influences, about how presence actually will manifest in a multicultural setting.

Yalom (2002) and May (1983) suggest that we create a new therapy for every client. EH therapists are trained to tailor the therapy to the unique needs of every client (Krug & Schneider 2016). Thus, an element of presence, paradoxically, is questioning one's own manifestation of presence based on, among many factors, intersectionality and cultural concerns and responsibilities. It is important to note that there is often a dialectic between therapists adjusting their presence and expressiveness to the client, on the one hand, and, on the other hand, providing a useful counterpoint to the client, or even creating some tension with the client or simply noting what is present in the moment but unregarded. A fundamental stance in EH therapy is mirroring (Schneider & Krug, 2017). This involves holding a mirror up to the client in terms of their strengths and desires as well as ways they block themselves from presence and a fully engaged, meaningful life. In a given client case, it could be that it is the therapist's differences in presence and expressiveness that provides a point of contrast and helps the client to see themselves. An example of how this might play out involves differences in culture related to age and temperament. An older Black male therapist with a calm demeanor and a younger Black male client who feels restless and on edge may experience differences in certain elements in culture, yet the therapist may be able to mirror the client back to him in useful ways. Therapy is complex like human beings are complex. EH emphasizes not having ready-made procedures and rigid techniques for this reason (Schneider & Krug, 2017).

Hoffman (2019) writes that presence may be important in the development of empathy, which is shown to be important in effective psychotherapy in general and EH therapy in particular (Schneider & Krug, 2017; Wampold & Imel, 2015). However, presence and empathy in multicultural contexts can be especially challenging due, in part, to different conceptualizations across cultures experientially and in terms of what it means to be an individual or part of a community, and what constitutes a healthy sense of self, among other differences (Hoffman, 2019). Hoffman recommends that, in order for therapists to be able to cultivate a presence and an empathy that is appropriate multiculturally, therapists must do "one's own work pertaining to cultural biases, developing knowledge about cultural differences, and engaging with narratives and the arts relevant to cultural differences and intersectionality" (p. 114).

Krug and Schneider hold that a stance of essential humility (i.e., of not knowing) opens the therapist to the uniquely personal world of the client, helping them set aside their own preconceptions so they may enter their client's world with curiosity and empathy (Krug & Schneider 2016; Schneider & Krug 2017). Cultural humility is also an essential stance and attitude for EH therapists to foster deep within themselves (Vallejos & Johnson, 2019). Cultural humility is necessary for therapeutic presence to have value within a multicultural context. In years past, the humanistic approach (and in fact the entire field of psychology) had been dominated by White, male, Eurocentric, and individualistic perspectives. Over the years, this has begun changing. The tent has expanded and now the field of psychology in general and the humanistic approach in particular includes more individuals reflecting a broader spectrum of genders, races, religions, cultures, and perspectives. Vallejos and Johnson (2019) write that EH therapists must challenge themselves to first become aware of their cultural biases and to become knowledgeable, in a deep way, about other cultures while maintaining humility (as one cannot become fully competent in another's culture and must remain open to individual nuances and experiences of their cultures).

EH has the framework to align with cultural humility. Due to EH's humanistic roots and emphasis on presence, EH holds that the client is the expert in their experience and that therapists must actively seek to engage with and be present with the client experience (Schneider & Krug, 2017). Presence itself is potentially a practice of humility—of opening to what is palpably significant, regardless of whether or not it fits in with our agendas and biases, while knowing and holding, in true dynamic and paradoxical existential fashion, the fact that we cannot fully rise above our agendas and biases. The key, perhaps, is for the therapist to know enough—to have done their own cultural work of identifying and questioning their biases and researching other cultures—to stop and humbly assess the interplay of culture in session.

CASE EXAMPLE

We will present one hypothetical case of how these ideas might play out in an EH therapy session. Suppose the client is a gay Black man and the therapist is a White heterosexual woman. As the therapeutic relationship progresses it becomes clear that, although the client is bringing issues that seem, to the White female EH therapist, influenced by cultural factors and experiences he has had as a gay Black man, he is not initially presenting them in that multicultural context. Adding humility and needed complexity, the therapist is aware she might be projecting on him from her own contexts. It is rather his own experience that he focuses on. The implicit meanings he takes from experience can be highlighted as they are expressed. The therapist can be sensitive to both his cultures as influences and his beliefs about how he just is, separate from his cultures. The therapist might draw attention to how he manifests his own perceptions of himself and only obliquely refer to issues around gay male culture or racial questions with which he is struggling. By pointing to such instances, drawing attention to what may be present and at play but unrecognized, the therapist can help illustrate for him the interplay and significance of his own experience—that he attended a prestigious university, or that he is an educated professional seeking meaningful relationships in the gay culture, and so on. Coming to perceive the implicit meanings he has made of various formative experiences (e.g., those of family, education, past relationships) can support him to find new meanings, leading to a confident self-construct and thus even more efficacy in professional and personal settings.

As therapy unfolds, the therapist became aware of generalized stereotypes she projected onto this client from his initial presentation in their early sessions. As trust grew in their working relationship, she found she was able to use that awareness in moments where it was useful for the client to understand mannerisms or protections he had adopted to protect from experiencing others projecting similar preconceptions onto him. As therapy progressed, by honoring these experiences in a sacred way, it became safer for the client to explore microaggressions he had experienced and how they had become part of his self and world construct, sort through the meanings he had made, and continue to embody and empower his authentic self more and more. Further, the therapist sought to understand any of her biases around what constitutes a healthy self, healthy relationships, and healthy self-expression. She sought literature and consultation around working with Black males and yet remained humble and perhaps could engage relational check-ins about how cultural differences may be influencing the session from the client's perspective.

EH therapists must continue working to cultivate presence to their own context and that of their client; educate themselves about cultural diversity and microaggressions; operate from a place of cultural humility and a sincere wish to live with more freedom, presence, and autonomy; and attend closely to the nuances of the relationship in the present moment. If we do this, continued growth in multicultural work and service is possible. The unique intersectionality of cultural identities and experiences each client brings will be attended to in presence as the client processes in direct experience.

FUTURE RESEARCH

Geller and colleagues (2010) did not investigate how specifically EH therapists fared in terms of outcomes related to presence but did include similar approaches, such as CC therapy (humanistic) and PE therapy (similar to EH therapy). This study needs to be replicated to focus on EH therapy directly. Additional quantitative and qualitative studies on presence and therapy outcomes need to be engaged and should include EH therapy in the approaches utilized by therapists in the studies.

In Geller and Greenberg (2002), the question of how presence manifested and impacted therapy was put to therapists, not to clients. Since EH therapy holds that the expertise is within the client, it makes sense to conduct formal studies about presence where clients are considered the experts. Geller and Greenberg (2010) essentially showed that it is client perception of therapist presence that matters in terms of outcomes, not the therapist perception of their own presence. It could be that our understanding of what presence is, and what it might mean to clients, has not been finely tuned enough to know how to evaluate clients' experience of presence.

Bradshaw (2024) explored the client experience of therapeutic presence through a mixed-methods research design. This included use of the TPIs, descriptive statistics, reflexive thematic analysis, audio-recorded semistructured interviews with clients, and affective and embodied follow-up questions to help determine the participant's emotional and physical experience in moments they found their therapist fully present or less present. Further, in keeping with EH practices of humility and intrapersonal awareness, Bradshaw kept a reflexive journal questioning his decisions, biases (including cultural), and experiences while conducting the research and analysis.

Bradshaw discovered eight themes for the client experience of therapeutic presence: safety, connection, feeling deeply seen and heard, respect, feeling supportively challenged, being accepted, feeling empowered, and good timing. The study included cisgender and transgender male and female individuals. Of note was that the transgender clients reported having experienced past therapists as un-present to the client's cultural needs related to gender, whereas their current highly present therapists expressed present attunement to their cultural needs. Bradshaw found three themes for the client experience of a lack of therapeutic presence with past therapists: disconnection, disrespect, and lack of safety.

Geller and Greenberg (2022) assess that some clients may not be ready for a fuller presence in therapy. This aligns with Schneider (2015a) discussing that existential therapists need to assess, in real time and on an ongoing basis, a client's readiness, capacity, and willingness for the deep experiential work of full presence. This, of course, does not mean that therapists don't need to be present, aware both internally and externally, and attuned and adaptive. Research should be done into assessing client readiness for a fuller experiential and relational presence and perhaps on signs that a client is not ready or willing for a deeper exploration of their experience. For instance, clients with traumatic experience may need their defensive stance and behavior. Schneider and Krug (2017) echo Bugental's respect for defenses as serving an important purpose for the client. Understanding defenses as protections, they advocate for a collaborative exploration of the protection's function and usefulness. As clients engage with their protections, especially as they manifest in the therapy room, they typically experience their protections as both useful and constrictive.

EH therapists recognize the important function self-protections serve and the vulnerability and possible retriggering that might occur should those protections be too early challenged or undermined. Moving slowly and checking in during sessions cultivates therapeutic collaboration that helps to mitigate retriggering. And yet, triggering does happen. Working through such breeches is an important aspect of the work, allowing clients to experience and explore their triggers and therapists to explore theirs. What follows may be a stronger and a more intimate connection. However, if repair isn't possible, then a mutually agreed upon ending and referral out is needed. Even though this is a failed outcome, it remains a failed collaborative outcome through a process of presence, care, and sensitivity.

The influence of culture in shaping the client and therapist experience of presence is an area where further research is needed. How experiences of presence manifest may vary depending on cultural contexts, personality type within cultural contexts (e.g., degrees of introversion or extroversion, agreeableness or disagreeableness, emotional and facial expression), and related intersectional factors such as areas of disadvantage or advantage, gender, sexuality. Indeed, Geller and Greenberg (2022) discuss this as a possible reason for the disconnect in their quantitative study (Geller et al., 2010) between therapist and client perception of therapist presence is related to cultural factors and perceptions.

Longitudinal studies on the client and the therapist's experience of therapeutic presence in session over time, and its development over time, is also warranted. It has been proposed that therapeutic presence is the hub of the common factors wheel (Schneider, 2015b), and research has shown that the therapeutic relationship is the most important factor early in treatment in predicting longer term outcomes (Wampold, 2018; Wampold & Imel, 2015). It has been proposed that presence is essential throughout the therapeutic process, from start to finish (Geller & Greenberg, 2022; Schneider & Krug, 2017). Studying presence early in treatment, and its effect and development over longer periods of time, is needed. It is particularly important, as practicing EH clinicians, to see more mixed-methods research, incorporating, for example, the TPI and other EH-aligned outcome scales and measures with qualitative methods such as thematic analysis, heuristic inquiry, case study, and others. Bradshaw (2024) identified themes for the client experience of therapeutic presence and lack of therapeutic presence. These themes will need to be tested and explored further to test their validity in different cultural contexts and over longer courses of therapy as the relationship with the therapist develops.

CONCLUSION

EH therapists use the cultivation of presence to be the foundation, method, and goal of therapy. A reclaiming of one's life is the goal: efficacy, awareness, and authentic responses rather than a life determined and limited by defensive postures in relation to the personal and social environments the person has experienced. This cannot be achieved until one knows what has been disowned. This type of change is in the core of one's being, it is whole-bodied and transformative. Presence involves aspects of awareness, acceptance, availability, cultural humility, awareness of intersectionality, and attuned expressiveness in both therapist and client. It affords an experience of one's being (May, 1983; May et. al, 1958). If one can work to be truly present with another human being, then a genuine encounter may occur in which disowned protective patterns and wounds can be faced, dissolved, or managed. New and more functional patterns can emerge. This whole-bodied transformation can even, at times, lead clients to notably new attitudes toward life in general, an attitude of humility and wonder or a sense of adventure that can fruitfully be termed "awe-inspiring" (Krug, 2017, 2019; Krug & Schneider, 2016; Schneider, 2023; Schneider & Krug, 2010, 2017, 2020). A person can find and enliven a fluid center that can remain intact within the vicissitudes of life's experience (Schneider, 2023).

Presence has been shown to facilitate health at the levels of subjective psychological experience, the nervous system, and neurobiologically. Through presence, a skillful integration or harmonizing may occur resulting in greater empathy, flexibility, attunement, and well-being. Although quantitative outcome studies are not abundant yet, they do show promising results linking therapeutic presence with improved behavior change and insight, empathy, therapeutic relationship, and other key factors, processes, and outcomes in therapy. Qualitative studies indicate presence is an important factor in good therapy and add rich detail to our knowledge of the characteristics, demands, and functions of presence in therapy. Theory, case study, and the lived experience of therapists and clients have a long and rich history exploring the essential nature of presence in healing relationships.

REFERENCES

Angus, L. E., Watson, J. C., Elliott, R., Schneider, K., & Timulak, L. (2015). *The handbook of narrative psychotherapy: Practice, theory, and research*. Sage.

Baldwin, M. (2000). Interview with Carl Rogers on the use of the self in therapy. In S. Geller & L. Greenberg (Eds.), *Therapeutic presence: A mindful approach to psychotherapy* (pp. 39–40). American Psychological Association.

Bernhardt, I. S., Nissen-Lie, H. A., & Råbu, M. (2020). The embodied listener: A dyadic case study of how therapist and patient reflect on the significance of therapist's personal presence for the therapeutic change process. *Psychotherapy Research, 30*(4), 417–432. https://doi.org/10.1080/10503307.2020.1808728

Binswanger, L. (1958). The case of Ellen West. In R. May, E. Angel, & H. F. Ellenberger (Eds.), *Existence: A new dimension in psychiatry and psychology* (pp. 237–364). Basic Books.

Bohart, A. C., & Tallman, K. (1999). *How clients make therapy work: The process of active self-healing*. American Psychological Association. https://doi.org/10.1037/10323-000

Boss, M. (1963). *Psychoanalysis and daseinsanalysis* (L. B. Lefebre, Trans.). Basic Books.

Bradshaw, C. C. (2024). *The client experience of therapeutic presence* (Publication No. 31770698) [Doctoral dissertation, Saybrook University]. ProQuest Dissertations & Theses. https://www.proquest.com/openview/ae61cbded2a853da0167a5b4cd86dc41/1?cbl=18750&diss=y&pq-origsite=gscholar

Bugental, J. F. T. (1976). *The search for existential identity: Patient–therapist dialogues*. Jossey-Bass.

Bugental, J. F. T. (1978). *Psychotherapy and process: The fundamentals of an existential-humanistic approach*. Addison-Wesley

Bugental, J. F. T. (1987). *The art of the psychotherapist: How to develop the skills that take psychotherapy beyond science*. W. W. Norton & Company.

Bugental, J. F. T. (1989). *Psychotherapy isn't what you think: Bringing the psychotherapeutic engagement into the living moment*. Zeig, Tucker & Theisen.

Bugental, J. F. T. (1999). *Psychotherapy isn't what you think*. Zeig.

Cain, D. J. (2010). *Person-centered psychotherapies*. American Psychological Association. https://doi.org/10.1037/17330-000

Cameron, A. (2019). Trauma-focused presence. *Journal of Humanistic Psychology, 64*(5), 813–841. https://doi.org/10.1177/0022167819880653

Colosimo, K. A., & Pos, A. E. (2015). A rational model of expressed therapeutic presence. *Journal of Psychotherapy Integration, 25*(2), 100–114. https://doi.org/10.1037/a0038879

Cooper, M. (2005). Therapists' experiences of relational depth: A qualitative interview study. *Counselling & Psychotherapy Research, 5*(2), 87–95. https://doi.org/10.1080/17441690500211130

Cozolino, L. (2017). *The neuroscience of psychotherapy* (3rd ed.). W. W. Norton & Company.

Crenshaw, K. (1989). Demarginalizing the intersection of race and sex: A Black feminist critique of antidiscrimination doctrine, feminist theory and antiracist politics. *University of Chicago Legal Forum, 1989*(1), 139–167.

Dana, D. (2018). *The polyvagal theory in therapy: Engaging the rhythm of regulation.* W. W. Norton & Company.

Dunn, R., Callahan, J. L., Swift, J. K., & Ivanovic, M. (2013). Presence as the foundation for empathy: A therapeutic relationship necessity. *Psychotherapy, 50*(3), 3–8.

Elliott, R. (2002). Hermeneutic single-case efficacy design. *Psychotherapy Research, 12*(1), 1–20. https://doi.org/10.1080/713869614

Farb, N. A. S., Segal, Z. V., & Anderson, A. K. (2013). Mindfulness meditation training alters cortical representations of interoceptive attention. *Social Cognitive and Affective Neuroscience, 8*(1), 15–26. https://doi.org/10.1093/scan/nss066

Federman, D. (2020). Existential intersectionality: The impact of social context on existential therapy. *Journal of Humanistic Psychology, 60*(5), 622–639.

Finfgeld-Connett, D. (2006). Meta-synthesis of presence in nursing. *Journal of Advanced Nursing, 55*(6), 708–714. https://doi.org/10.1111/j.1365-2648.2006.03961.x

Fraelich, C. B. (1989). *A phenomenological investigation of the psychotherapist's experience of presence* [Doctoral dissertation, The Union for Experimenting Colleges and Universities]. ProQuest One Academic.

Geller, S. M. (2017). *A practical guide to cultivating therapeutic presence.* American Psychological Association. https://doi.org/10.1037/0000025-000

Geller, S. M., & Greenberg, L. S. (2002). Therapeutic presence: Therapists' experience of presence in the psychotherapeutic encounter. *Person-Centered and Experiential Psychotherapies, 1*(1–2), 71–86. https://doi.org/10.1080/14779757.2002.9688279

Geller, S. M., & Greenberg, L. S. (2010). *Therapeutic Presence Inventories (TPI)—Client and therapist versions.* https://www.sharigeller.ca/_images/pdfs/Therapeutic_Presence_Inventory_Therapist_copyright.pdf

Geller, S. M., & Greenberg, L. S. (2022). *Therapeutic presence: A mindful approach to effective therapeutic relationships.* American Psychological Association. https://doi.org/10.1037/13485-000

Geller, S. M., Greenberg, L. S., & Watson, J. C. (2010). Therapist and client perceptions of therapeutic presence: The development of a measure. *Psychotherapy Research, 20*(5), 599–610. https://doi.org/10.1080/10503307.2010.495957

Geller, S. M., & Porges, S. W. (2014). Therapeutic presence: Neurophysiological mechanisms mediating feeling safe in therapeutic relationships. *Journal of Psychotherapy Integration, 24*(3), 178–192. https://doi.org/10.1037/a0037511

Hayes, J. A., & Vinca, M. (2017). Therapist presence, absence, and extraordinary presence. In L. G. Castonguay & C. E. Hill (Eds.), *How and why are some therapists better than others? Understanding therapist effects* (pp. 85–99). American Psychological Association. https://doi.org/10.1037/0000034-006

Hayes, P. A. (2015). *Addressing cultural complexities in practice: Assessment, diagnosis, and therapy* (2nd ed.). American Psychological Association. https://doi.org/10.1037/11650-000

Hoffman, L. (2019). Culture and empathy in humanistic psychology. In L. Hoffman, H. Cleare-Hoffman, N. Granger Jr., & D. St. John (Eds.), *Humanistic approaches to multiculturalism and diversity: Perspectives on existence and difference* (pp. 103–116). Routledge. https://doi.org/10.4324/9781351133357-9

Hoffman, L., Cleare-Hoffman, H., Granger, N., Jr., & St. John, D. (Eds.). (2019). *Humanistic approaches to multiculturalism and diversity: Perspectives on existence and difference.* Routledge. https://doi.org/10.4324/9781351133357

Krug, O. T. (2009). James Bugental and Irvin Yalom: Two masters of existential therapy cultivate presence in the therapeutic encounter. *Journal of Humanistic Psychology, 49*(3), 329–354. https://doi.org/10.1177/0022167809334001

Krug, O. T. (2017). Existential, humanistic, and experiential therapies in historical per-spective. In A. J. Consoli, L. E. Beutler, & B. Bongar (Eds.), *Comprehensive textbook of psychotherapy: Theory and practice* (2nd ed., pp. 91–105) Oxford University Press.

Krug, O. T. (2019). Existential-humanistic and existential-integrative therapy: Method and practice. In E. van Deurzen, E. Craig, A. Längle, K. J. Schneider, D. Tantum, & S. du Plock (Eds.), *The Wiley world handbook of existential therapy* (pp. 257–266). John Wiley & Sons. https://doi.org/10.1002/9781119167198.ch15

Krug, O. T. (2021, Spring). *Existential meaning making: The heart of therapeutic change* [Workshop]. *California Psychological Association Quarterly.*

Krug, O. T., Granger, N., Yalom, I., & Schneider, K. J. (2019). Case illustrations of exis-tential–humanistic and existential–integrative therapy. In E. van Deurzen, E. Craig, A. Längle, K. J. Schneider, D. Tantum, & S. du Plock (Eds.), *The Wiley world handbook of existential therapy* (pp. 267–281). John Wiley & Sons. https://doi.org/10.1002/9781119167198.ch16

Krug, O. T., & Piwowarski, T. (2019). Ethical issues in existential–humanistic psycho-therapy. In M. Trachsel, J. Gaab, N. Biller-Andorno, S. Tekin, & J. Z. Sadler (Eds.), *Oxford handbook of psychotherapy ethics* (pp. 562–578). Oxford University Press. https://doi.org/10.1093/oxfordhb/9780198817338.013.46

Krug, O. T., & Schneider, K. J. (2016). *Supervision essentials for existential–humanistic ther-apy.* American Psychological Association. https://doi.org/10.1037/14951-000

Lazar, S. W., Kerr, C. E., Wasserman, R. H., Gray, J. R., Greve, D. N., Treadway, M. T., McGarvey, M., Quinn, B. T., Dusek, J. A., Benson, H., Rauch, S. L., Moore, C. I., & Fischl, B. (2005). Meditation experience is associated with increased cortical thick-ness. *NeuroReport, 16*(17), 1893–1897. https://doi.org/10.1097/01.wnr.0000186598.66243.19

Levine, P. A. (1997). *Waking the tiger: Healing trauma—The innate capacity to transform over-whelming experiences.* North Atlantic Books.

Marie-Miller, J. (2016). *Development of therapeutic presence in mental health counselors* [Doc-toral dissertation, University of Phoenix]. https://www.researchgate.net/publication/322602766_Dissertation_development_of_therapeutic_presence_in_mental_health_counselors

May, R. (1975). *The courage to create.* W. W. Norton & Company.

May, R. (1983). *The discovery of being.* W. W. Norton & Company.

May, R., Angel, E., & Ellenberger, H. (Eds.). (1958). *Existence: A new dimension in psychiatry and psychology.* Basic Books. https://doi.org/10.1037/11321-000

Menakem, R. (2017). *My grandmother's hands: Radicalized trauma and the pathway to mend-ing our hearts and bodies.* Central Recovery Press.

Merriam-Webster. (n.d.). Presence. In *Merriam-Webster.com dictionary.* Retrieved January 28, 2024, from https://www.merriam-webster.com/dictionary/presence

Perls, F. (1947). *Ego hunger and aggression.* The Gestalt Journal Press.

Phelon, C. R. (2001). *Healing presence: An intuitive inquiry into the presence of the psychothera-pist* [Doctoral dissertation, Institute of Transpersonal Psychology). ProQuest One Academic.

Phelon, C. R. (2004). Healing presence in the psychotherapist. *The Humanistic Psychologist, 32*(4), 342–356. https://doi.org/10.1080/08873267.2004.9961759

Pierson, J. F., Krug, O. T., Sharp, J. G., & Piwowarski, T. (2015). Cultivating therapeutic artistry: Model existential–humanistic training programs. In K. J. Schneider, J. F. Pier-son, & J. F. T. Bugental (Eds.), *The handbook of humanistic psychology: Leading edges in theory, practice, and research* (2nd ed., pp. 631–652). Sage. https://doi.org/10.4135/9781483387864.n50

Porges, S. W., & Dana, D. (2018). *Clinical applications of the polyvagal theory: The emergence of polyvagal-informed therapies.* W. W. Norton & Company.

Rathenau, S., Sousa, D., Vaz, A., & Geller, S. (2021). The effect of attitudes toward online therapy and the difficulties in online therapeutic presence. *Journal of Psychotherapy Integration, 32*(1), 19–33. https://doi.org/10.1037/int0000266

Ratner, J. (2015). Rollo May and the search for being: Implications of May's thought for contemporary existential–humanistic psychotherapy. *Journal of Humanistic Psychology, 59*(2), 252–268. https://doi.org/10.1177/0022167815613880

Ratner, J. (2017). *Presence, being, initiation: Understanding and teaching presence, the lineage and legacy of James Bugental.* https://ehinstitute.org/wp-content/uploads/2021/04/JRatner_Presence_Being_Initiation_Bugental_Legacy_Lineage_2017.pdf

Rennie, D. L. (2002). Experiencing psychotherapy: Grounded theory studies. In D. J. Cain & J. Seeman (Eds.), *Humanistic psychotherapies: Handbook of research and practice* (pp. 117–144). American Psychological Association. https://doi.org/10.1037/10439-005

Rennie, D. L. (1994). Clients' deference in psychotherapy. *Journal of Counseling Psychology, 41*(4), 427–437. https://doi.org/10.1037/0022-0167.41.4.427

Rogers, C. R. (1957). The necessary and sufficient conditions of therapeutic personality change. *Journal of Consulting Psychology, 21*(2), 95–103. https://doi.org/10.1037/h0045357

Rogers, C. R. (1979). *The foundations of the person-centered approach.* University of California Press.

Rogers, C. R. (1980). *A way of being.* Mariner Books.

Schneider, K. J. (1985). *The paradoxical self: Toward an understanding of existential meaning therapy* [Doctoral dissertation, Saybrook University].

Schneider, K. J. (2015a). *Existential–integrative psychotherapy: Guideposts to the core of practice.* Routledge.

Schneider, K. J. (2015b). Presence: The core contextual factor in effective psychotherapy. *Existential Analysis, 2*(2), 304–312.

Schneider, K. J. (2023). *Life-enhancing anxiety: Key to a sane world.* University Professors Press.

Schneider, K. J., & Krug, O. T. (2010). *Existential–humanistic therapy.* American Psychological Association. https://doi.org/10.1037/12050-000

Schneider, K. J., & Krug, O. T. (2016). *Supervision essentials for existential–humanistic therapy.* American Psychological Association.

Schneider, K. J., & Krug, O. T. (2017). *Existential–humanistic therapy* (2nd ed.). American Psychological Association. https://doi.org/10.1037/0000042-000

Schneider, K. J., & Krug, O. T. (2020). Existential–humanistic psychotherapies. In S. Messer & N. Kaslow (Eds.), *Essential psychotherapies: Theory and practice* (4th ed., pp. 257–293). Guilford Press.

Schneider, K. J., & May, R. (1995). *The psychology of existence: An integrative, clinical perspective.* McGraw-Hill.

Siegel, D. J. (2007). *The mindful brain: Reflection and attunement in the cultivation of well-being.* W. W. Norton & Company.

Siegel, D. J. (2011). *Mindsight: The new science of personal transformation.* Bantam.

Siegel, D. J. (2017). Foreword. In S. M. Geller, *A practical guide to therapeutic presence* (pp. ix–xi). American Psychological Association.

Siegel, D. J. (2018). *Aware: The science and practice of presence.* TarcherPerigee.

Spinelli, E. (1997). *Tales of un-knowing: Therapeutic encounters from an existential perspective.* Open University Press.

Vallejos, L., & Johnson, Z. (2019). Multicultural competencies in humanistic psychology. In L. Hoffman, H. Cleare-Hoffman, N. Granger, Jr., & D. St. John (Eds.), *Humanistic approaches to multiculturalism and diversity: Perspectives on existence and difference* (pp. 63–76). Routledge. https://doi.org/10.4324/9781351133357-6

van Deurzen, E. (2015). *Existential psychotherapy and counselling in practice* (3rd ed.). Sage.

Walsh, R. A., & McElwain, B. (2002). Existential and humanistic approaches to therapy. In J. C. Norcross (Ed.), *Psychotherapy relationships that work* (pp. 235–253). Oxford University Press.

Wampold, B. E. (2008). Existential–integrative psychotherapy: Coming of age [Review of the book *Existential–Integrative Psychotherapy: Guideposts to the Core of Practice,* by K. J. Schneider, Ed.]. *PsycCritiques, 53*(3). https://doi.org/10.1037/a0011070

Wampold, B. E., & Imel, Z. I. (2015). *The great psychotherapy debate: The evidence for what makes psychotherapy work* (2nd ed.). Routledge. https://doi.org/10.4324/9780203582015

Wampold, B. E. (2018). *The basics of psychotherapy: An introduction to theory and practice* (2nd ed.). American Psychological Association. https://doi.org/10.1037/0000117-000

Watson, J. C., & Bohart, A. C. (2015). Humanistic–experiential psychotherapy. In N. Kazantzis, M. A. Reinecke, & A. Freeman (Eds.), *Cognitive and behavioral therapies* (pp. 202–216). Guilford Press.

Yalom, I. (1980). *Existential psychotherapy.* Basic Books.

Yalom, I. (1989). *Love's executioner and other tales of psychotherapy.* Basic Books.

Yalom, I. (2002). *The gift of therapy.* HarperCollins.

5

Empathy in Existential–Humanistic Psychotherapy

Arthur C. Bohart, Jerrold Lee Shapiro, and Gayle Byock

In this chapter, we explore the role of empathy in existential–humanistic (EH) psychotherapy, outline how it is supposed to function, and review both quantitative and qualitative research. We consider how the construct of empathy is situated in a multicultural framework and conclude with suggestions for future research.

THE CONCEPT OF EMPATHY

Bohart and Greenberg (1997) note that empathy is a complex, multidimensional construct. For them, empathy involves at least the following four dimensions: (a) a cognitive or understanding component; (b) an experiential component; (c) an action component, specifically in the form of communication; and (d) a way of being together in relationship. Elliott and colleagues (2018) focus on cognitive and affective aspects of empathy. In social and developmental psychology, the characteristic focus is on empathy as either perceiving the feelings and emotions of others or, sometimes in addition, sharing somewhat the same emotion that another person is experiencing (Bohart & Greenberg, 1997; Feshbach, 1997).

This tendency to define empathy as primarily focusing on feelings and emotions is also found in the field of psychotherapy (e.g., Brems, 2000). However, Bohart and Greenberg (1997) note that for many psychotherapists, the focus is actually more on cognitive aspects—that is, viewing the world as others see the

https://doi.org/10.1037/0000446-006
The Evidence-Based Foundations of Existential–Humanistic Therapy, L. Hoffman and V. Lac (Editors)

world. Several studies have found that the therapeutic responses of Carl Rogers, despite the notion that what he did was reflect feelings, were more directed to the meaning/cognitive aspects of the client's experience and communications than to emotional aspects (Bohart & Greenberg, 1997). Rogers (1986) emphasized *empathic understanding*, and Bohart (2021) has argued that empathy, at least from a person-centered perspective, should be thought of more in terms of a manner of knowing, in particular what Belenky and colleagues (1986) have called *connected knowing* as opposed to *separate knowing*.

Therapeutic empathy is not primarily feeling the same feeling. Greenberg and Rushanski-Rosenberg (2002), using an interpersonal process recall procedure in which therapists reviewed recordings of empathy episodes, conclude that therapists do not necessarily feel the same feeling as their clients. However, empathy cannot be understood as a primarily cold intellectual understanding either. It involves striving to get a sense of the essence of what and how a person is feeling, thinking, and experiencing their world. Most importantly, at core, it is an attempt to engage with the client—to meet them, so to speak.

For current purposes, we operationalize the construct of empathy as a process of trying to understand the other person, and that includes understanding both the window through which they see their world (Yalom, 2001) and how they are emotionally responding to it. Understanding is not strictly cognitive. Understanding includes an emotional and experiential grasp of the other person's intent and history as well as what they are experiencing. It includes entering into and sharing their experience, as we shall see in the next section, or coexperiencing. At a practical, practicing, experiential level, the cognitive–affective split is a false dichotomy. It is neither cool, intellectual perspective taking, nor emotional immersion. Rather, it is a kind of grasping of the other's experience.

Empathy and Mutuality

There is evidence that empathy is coconstructed (MacFarlane et al., 2017). Jordan (1997), Murphy and Cramer (2014), and Elliott and colleagues (2018) all argue that empathy is not one way. Empathy is coconstructed through dialogue between therapist and client. Therapists may initiate empathic conversation, but clients promote empathy by listening to therapists, empathically understanding where therapists are coming from, and cocreating a dialogue and climate in therapy. Each partner is trying to attune to the meanings of the other, and the therapist takes their lead from an empathic, understanding response from the client.

One approach to therapy of particular relevance to this chapter is \relational cultural therapy (RCT). It emphasizes the ideas of mutuality and cultural sensitivity. Jordan (1997) clarifies RCT as an approach to mutuality: "When empathy and concern flow both ways, there is an intense affirmation of the self and paradoxically a transcendence of the self, a sense of self as part of a larger relational unit" (Jordan & Surrey, 1986, p. 1; 1997, p. 347). The goal of RCT is to transform patterns of power and control into empathy and mutual respect (Jordan, 1997, pp. 346–347). As a client develops "accurate empathy" for the therapist, this transformation generalizes to other relationships, and integration of empathy for the self, other, and relationship occurs (Jordan, 1997, p. 349).

Jordan (2000) illustrates that an understanding of process—seeing content in context—ties together the power of mutual empathy in the therapeutic relationship with the notion of healing in connection. She underscores the impact of isolation as a form of human suffering and immobilization that prevents reconnection after disconnection. Thus, healing from isolation occurs in relationship with others. The obstacle to connection is the therapeutic goal of separateness, self-autonomy, self-sufficiency, and independence. "Context and community are paid lip service, but rarely seen as primary" (p. 1006). Empathic connection that embraces a client's embedded context thus serves as an antidote for isolation that in turn enhances the therapeutic relationship.

As previously noted, Bohart (2021) has suggested that empathy be thought of as connected knowing. The search for connected knowing is at the foundation of RCT first put forward in Jean Baker Miller's (1976/1986) book *Toward a New Psychology of Women*. Her focus was on women and other historically marginalized groups who are affected by the domination–subordination roles that American culture supports. In 1991, Miller wrote,

> Modern American theorists of early psychological development and, indeed, of the entire life span, from Erik Erikson (1950) to Daniel Levinson (1978), tend to see all of development as a process of separating oneself out from the matrix of others—'Becoming one's own man [sic]'—in Levinson's words. Development of the self presumably is attained via a series of painful crises, by which the individual accomplishes a sequence of allegedly essential separations from others, thereby achieving an inner sense of separated individuation. (p. 11)

More recently, Banks (2015) suggested quite a different paradigm that builds on Miller's emphasis of relation rather than focus on isolated self and states that relational cultural theory "doesn't imagine people as defined by boundaries; it sees relationships as more like a magician's linking rings. The rings are a set, but they are not stuck in a rigid configuration" (p. 12).

If the therapy relationship is primarily aimed at a client's individuation and internal change, it focuses on increasing an individual's unique personal control over their experiences. Such an approach seems to regard a client's cultural and societal environment as both external and immutable in therapy. This denies the internalization of sociocultural aspects of being and is counter to the development of mutual empathy, more full understanding, and even to some extent, the therapeutic alliance. To be fully empathic, the client's relationship to the external is a significant component of self-knowledge.

From this perspective, empathy becomes a way of being in therapy. At its most basic level, it is connection, understanding the other person is making a union with them in order to facilitate most accurately and effectively to intervene with them and help them.

A Working Definition of Empathy

Bohart and Greenberg (1997) have comprehensively reviewed the history of the concept of empathy, and we will not replicate that here. Briefly, however, Wispé (1987) argued that it was the humanistic psychotherapist Carl Rogers who made the concept of empathy popular in the United States. Most people would probably agree with Rogers's definition of empathy:

> The therapist's sensitive ability and willingness to understand the client's thoughts, feelings and struggles from the client's point of view. [It is] this ability to see completely through the client's eyes, to adopt his [sic] frame of reference . . . . It means entering the private perceptual world of the other . . . . [It is] being sensitive, moment by moment, to the changing felt meanings which flow in this other person. It means sensing meanings of which he or she [sic] is scarcely aware. (Rogers, 1980, p. 85, 142)

Rogers (1959) added that empathy had to have an as-if quality; that is, that therapists were not to immerse themselves so much in the experience of the other that they came to lose themselves. Nor were they ever to forget that their experience of the other is not the truth about the other's experience, but that it is as if the therapist were the other. In this regard, the therapist must keep personally centered while also being in the other's shoes, trying to see things through the other's eyes. That is, they focus on the process of how the other sees and experiences things, not how the therapist would if they were in the other's position. This suggests a kind of dual awareness of one's own experience and that of the other (Shlien, 1997).

How one defines empathy in part determines how empathy is assumed to play a role in therapy. For current purposes, we are adopting Rogers's definition that empathy is a set of concepts and actions that share in common the perspective that somehow the therapist is trying to see, feel, or experience the world from the point of view of the client. The key part, then, is that of projecting oneself into the experience of another person, and, metaphorically, walking in their shoes. However, as we have already seen and will see discussed further in the next section, the EH concept of empathy goes beyond the focus of sharing the experience of the other.

CONTEXTUALIZING EMPATHY IN AN EH CONTEXT

Although empathy is an essential component in all relationship-based therapies, none more so than phenomenologically based existential psychotherapy, the term itself is curiously absent in the vast majority of books on existential psychotherapy. For example, the word "empathy" doesn't appear in the indexes of texts by Bugental (1976, 1987), May (1969), Schneider (2008), Schneider and Krug (2017), Shapiro (2016), Spinelli (1997), or Yalom (1980). The closely related variable "presence" is also strangely absent from these indexes.

There are many possible explanations for this absence, but the most likely is that empathy is so ubiquitous and such a core component of all relationship therapy work that it mirrors David Foster Wallace's timeless notion about fish having no awareness of water. Because empathy in existential therapy is so essential, it isn't easy to delineate. There is something ineffable in defining and separating out empathy and presence as an embodied process in existential psychotherapy (Shapiro, 2016).

There may in fact be a subtle difference in the ways existential therapists conceive of empathy. Empathy within existential work is empathy not only for the person, but for the process in which individuals are engaged together (Shapiro, 2016). It is that full cognitive, affective, and spiritual connection that is unmistakable in the moment; it is a transcendent experience akin to Buber's (1970) I–thou moments that alter both individuals. When this is translated into therapy, there is empathy not only for the "thou" but also for the phenomenological "us" that is temporarily created by the intimate interaction. O'Hara (1984) has said that empathy is not only getting inside the skin of the other but also getting inside the skin of the relationship.

Observing this phenomenon that encompasses each individual, the intimate combination of the two, and the nature of the interaction itself requires understanding the subtle differences between a therapist personally experiencing anxiety and reflecting that of the client. Normative empathic responses to a client's description of affect might include statements such as "You are feeling really scared" or "You are feeling very sad." The existential therapist might instead reflect, "It's really scary" or tearfully express, "That feels really sad" in the moment.

From an existential perspective, there are certain universal human conditions that create significant levels of (existential) anxiety: mortality, isolation, freedom versus responsibility, and meaninglessness (i.e., Yalom, 1980). These anxieties are all parts of being alive and conscious. When a client expresses any of these (e.g., a fear of mortality), therapists can meet that anxiety with their own personal anxieties about life ending and share the emotion. This must be done within a client's personal, cultural, gendered experience (Shapiro, 2021). When this occurs, the possibility arises for what Bugental (1999) describes as *life-changing therapy*. It is something that goes far beyond symptom amelioration, although that may occur as well. Thus, for an existential therapist, one way of expressing empathy is through empathically attuned self-disclosure of the immediate process. In short, self-disclosure of facts of the therapist's life is less germane than the therapist's phenomenological experience of the interaction in real time.

Many authors have used musical terms to try to describe the intimate therapy interaction (i.e., Bohart & Rosenbaum, 1995; Bugental, 1987; Shapiro, 2016, 2021; van Deurzen, 2002). They all describe a special resonance and harmony between the client and therapist. Like individual musical instruments played alone are somewhat transformed when combined with others, such as in an orchestra, the resultant music is more than the sum of the two parts.

There is something new and creative between the individual instruments. Instead of focusing on the you-and-me interaction, it includes a newly created (if only momentarily) "us." The therapeutic focus is less on either person, but instead on awareness of what is occurring in the here-and-now interaction. Van Deurzen (2010) describes that resonance as "this ability to tune into the human dimension of a person's troubles and to figuratively let the vibrations of it set off a similar sound in oneself" (p. 257).

One of the ways that such resonance and harmony can be achieved within this framework is the therapist joining with the clients' manner of representing the sensory and internal input of their experience. This is often done by adopting the argot, images, and style in which a client processes their experiences at both conscious and unconscious levels. Close listening to a client will inform the therapist of their idioms, language, style, primary representational system (Bandler & Grinder, 1975), and, even more so, the metaphors of the client. In doing so, the likelihood of connecting at both conscious and unconscious levels is increased.

For example, in speaking with a client who continually used sports metaphors to question how they could possibly know the right way to connect more deeply with significant others in their life, including the therapist, the therapist opined aloud, "It's like the knowledge that the ball is going in the hoop by the way it feels as you let it go—you don't even have to look. What can we do now that allows for the same 'right' feeling?" Once that occurs in a session, the likelihood of transfer of learning from the therapy session to daily life is enhanced.

In another example, a Star Wars fan who was constantly "trying and failing" at his job, was asked, "What would Yoda say about that?" As a slight grin appeared on his face, he quoted, "Do or do not. There is no try!" The therapist replied, "So what would doing be like in here?" To both of their slight surprise, the client responded, "I would stop trying to impress you and tell you how much I fear being a total failure." That led to some very fruitful discussions of the difference between doing the right thing instead of trying to do things right, both in therapy and in his life.

A final example expresses the fear of death by a 45-year-old woman. A professor of history at a local university, she specialized in Greek and Roman mythology. When she came into therapy, she was contemplating an affair that she acknowledged would threaten her marriage and family life with their three children. Yet, she was enticed by her fantasy of what it would be like with this stranger with whom she was having a texting relationship. She came to therapy saying, "Convince me to do it. My friends all tell me not to meet him or text back!" As the therapy progressed, she expressed, "This could be my last chance before I get old and die." She continually obsessed about the "decision to continue her texting relationship, or more." Despite the therapist's exploration of her upset balance of freedom and security, she continued to be stuck.

In almost every session, she used a number of metaphors about ancient Greek myths. In the fourth session, she mentioned, almost as an aside, that she was struggling to complete a paper for presentation on the relevance of Homer's

Odyssey for later attributions of characteristics to Roman gods. Joining her, the therapist asked if she saw herself as one of the sirens or Ulysses. She answered immediately, "Ulysses of course," and then laughed. She asked, "Why would you ask me that? What does it have to do with my dilemma?"

The therapist responded, "I had the sense of what it would be like to be so tempted by the siren's call that I'd tie myself to the mast to avoid madness and drowning. Ulysses handled a dilemma one way. Is there a viable alternative for you?"

She said in an almost trance-like state, "You know what I was listening to on the way over here? You probably don't know it. Tom Paxton—I can't help but wonder where I'm bound."

Entering into her metaphor, the therapist noted, "The last stanza is 'Nail your shoes to the kitchen floor, lace 'em up and bar the door / Thank the stars for the roof that's over you.'"

"I know that's right," she said, "but where am I going to find the excitement in life?"

"That sounds like a very interesting question for us to explore," the therapist said. "What are you feeling now?"

She responded, in a way that seemed to surprise herself, "I'm feeling pretty excited!" This led directly into how she wanted to live with her death anxiety.

In that example, the therapist joined the client in her academic cognitive framework, shared her images and metaphors, and accompanied her in what Erickson (1980, 2009) calls a "mutual trance state." Instead of trying to convince her to make either decision, the therapist reflected what she was relating from a shared mythical and musical framework. This empathy included each person and also their interactional "we."

Is the Interaction Truly Mutual?

What do we know about client empathy or shared empathy? Summarizing the extant literature, de Wied and colleagues (2020) conclude that the research is fairly silent on that matter. We know a lot about therapist empathy and outcome, but what do we know about changes in client empathy? In contrast to hundreds of studies on development of therapist empathy, there are precious few on changes in client empathy and virtually none on the correlation between the two or on relational empathy (i.e., the empathy of the "us"). Jordan (2004) includes "movement toward mutuality and mutual empathy (caring and learning flows both ways), where empathy expands for both self and other as the first of six elements of relational competence" (p. 15). Do those existential, shared I–thou encounters increase the clients' empathy as well? Are both parties, indeed, changed by the interaction?

From a logical perspective, empathy seems positively related to altruism. Thus, any increases in client empathy could also increase their experience of altruism. Batson (2016) makes a connection between empathy and altruism: "In both earlier philosophical writing and more recent psychological work, the most frequently mentioned possible source of altruistic motivation is an other-oriented emotional reaction to seeing another in need" (p. 2). Shapiro and colleagues (2019) expand the salience of altruism, arguing that the experience of altruism is incompatible with low self-esteem, anxiety, and depression, common reasons clients seek therapy. Thus, development of client empathy seems valuable as a component of existential psychotherapy. The dearth of studies on the correlation between empathy and altruism make this a heuristic supposition at this time. In addition, the lack of reported research on the impact of, and changes in, mutual empathy is a major deficit in evidence in the prevailing understanding of existential empathy.

RESEARCH

Our focus in this brief research review is on the efficacy of empathy in promoting therapeutic change. There are a few comprehensive research reviews on empathy in psychotherapy available (e.g., Elliott et al., 2018; Watson, 2016). We will briefly summarize results from Elliott and colleagues' (2018) review, adding selected findings of interest. We have divided this review into two sections: quantitative and qualitative findings. In the quantitative section, we will primarily focus on the relationship of empathy to psychotherapy outcome. In the qualitative section we explore clients' experiences of empathy and its benefits.

Quantitative Research Findings

The topic of measures of empathy is complex. We do not have space to go into this here; we simply observe that there are multiple measures. Elliott and colleagues (2018) break them down into four categories: measures from the client's perspective, measures from the therapist's perspective, so-called objective ratings made by third-party observers, and measures of so-called empathic accuracy. Personality trait measures of empathy (e.g., Baron-Cohen, 2011; Davis, 1983) exist but have not been used extensively in psychotherapy research.

These different measures of empathy do not necessarily correlate highly with one another (Bohart & Greenberg, 1997). Of these different classes of measures, Elliott and colleagues' meta-analysis (2018) finds that clients' perceptions of their therapists' empathy are better predictors of outcome than are therapists' perceptions or those of third-party observer ratings. There were only a few studies on empathic accuracy measures and personality trait measures, and these were not found to be useful.

Elliott and colleagues' (2018) review is the third in a series of comprehensive meta-analyses of research on the relationship of empathy to outcome in psychotherapy. These reviews were commissioned as part of a repeating project headed by John Norcross and originally instigated when he was president of

Division 29 (Society for the Advancement of Psychotherapy) of the American Psychological Association. The project goal was to document the evidence on empirical support for the impact of therapeutic relationships on psychotherapy outcome. Empathy was one of the components studied, and based on these extensive studies, it has been designated as an empirically supported relationship component (Norcross, 2002, 2011; Norcross & Lambert, 2018).

In one meta-analysis, Elliott and colleagues (2018) analyzed the results of 82 studies of 6,138 clients. Clients were seen for an average of 25 sessions. The relationship of empathy to outcome was studied at both the effects level (290 different measurements of effects in 82 studies), and at the study level (82 studies). The following variables were considered: number of sessions; treatment setting; experience level of therapists; therapists' theoretical orientation; types of problems; and various aspects of measurement, such as when measurements were taken, types of measures, and so on. These data were analyzed in various ways, but the best estimate of the relationship of empathy to outcome was the study-level random effects weighted r of 0.28, 95% CI [0.23–0.33]. This equated to a moderate effect size of $d = 0.58$. This means that empathy accounted for about 9% of the variance in outcome, which is approximately equivalent to the variance accounted for by the therapeutic alliance in general (Flückiger et al., 2018) and is higher than the variance accounted for by specific treatment methods in Wampold & Imel's (2015) estimate of $d = 0.20$ for intervention effects.

Elliott and colleagues (2018) did not break the results down by specific approaches to psychotherapy. However, they did look at classes of therapies. Humanistic–experiential (HE) therapies was one of the classes. This included person-centered therapy, emotion-focused therapy, existential therapy, Gestalt therapy, and other humanistic approaches. The two most studied approaches have been person-centered therapy and emotion-focused therapy. While both of these are commonly included within the rubric EH approaches, they are not identical to existential therapy. Emotion-focused therapy (originally called process–experiential therapy), however, is a mixture of person-centered relationship principles and Gestalt therapy procedures, among other things (see Greenberg et al., 1993). According to one Gestalt therapist, Gestalt therapy can be defined as "existential therapy with a technology" (Robert Resnick, personal communication, September 1968). Thus, the results of the analysis of HE therapies are pertinent to existential therapies, although not directly applicable.

With that caveat in mind, of particular interest to this chapter is finding the effects of empathy in the HE and psychodynamic therapies and comparing them with the cognitive behavior therapies. Theoretically, for both HE and psychodynamic therapies, empathy is seen as having a curative component. It does not merely provide support for other therapist interventions; it is itself a healing component. Furthermore, it is emphasized as more central to the therapeutic process in HE therapies than for cognitive behavior therapies. Therefore, one might expect that it would play a larger role in outcome for HE and psychodynamic therapies than it does in cognitive behavior therapies. However, for the third time (Elliott et al., 2018; the two previous meta-analyses [i.e., Elliott et al., 2011, and Bohart et al., 2002] found the same thing), the relationship of empathy to outcome was stronger in cognitive behavior therapy than it was in the HE and psychodynamic therapies. In order, the correlations between empathy and outcome for the three major groupings were cognitive behavior therapy at $r = 0.30$, HE therapies at $r = 0.24$ and psychodynamic therapy at $r = 0.21$. The correlation for HE therapies of $r = 0.24$ equates to an effect size of $d = 0.49$, a moderate or medium effect size. Thus, it can be argued that empathy plays an important role in HE therapies, although not quite as important a role as it appears to play in cognitive behavior therapy.

We shall briefly mention some of the other findings (for a more comprehensive review, see Elliott et al., 2018). First, it is important to know that there was significant heterogeneity in the results, indicating a wide range of difference in studies in terms of finding a relationship between empathy and outcome, with some studies finding high correlations while others found low or minimal correlations. These varied somewhat as a function of the type of measures used to measure both empathy and outcome. This also suggests that further research and analyses are needed to understand what variables, other than the ones we have mentioned, moderate the relationship between empathy and outcome.

Finally, we mention the results for which client populations' empathy is more or less useful. Elliott and colleagues (2018) did not break these findings down by therapeutic approach, so the HE therapies were mixed in with both cognitive behavior and psychodynamic approaches. The largest empathy outcome association was for depressed or anxious clients, severely distressed or chronic incarcerated populations, and clients with mixed or unspecified problems. Smaller effects were found for clients who engaged in self-damaging activities (e.g., substance misuse) and those with mild, normal, or physical problems.

Aside from the meta-analysis, we want to mention some specific findings. There is evidence that empathy facilitates emotional reprocessing (Greenberg & Paivio, 1997). It is associated with raising levels of productive experiencing (Klein & Mathieu-Coughlan, 1986; Rice & Saperia, 1984). Bohart (2021) has argued that empathy facilitates clients' thinking in more wise ways, and Sachse (1990a, 1990b) found evidence that empathy facilitates productive client thinking. There is also evidence that empathy increases the likelihood of clients seeking treatment. In particular, Chafetz and colleagues (1962, 1964) found that a single empathic counseling session significantly increased the odds of patients with alcohol problems being willing to enter therapy. Additionally, that single session increased their odds of staying in treatment. Finally, empathy has been found to reduce the chances of clients dropping out of therapy prematurely (Altmann, 1973; Landfield, 1971).

Three Research Examples
This section details three research examples of the relationship between therapist empathy and outcome. The first is a study by William R. Miller and colleagues (1980) on the treatment of alcoholism. This study was one of the factors

that led Miller and Rollnick to develop motivational interviewing (W. R. Miller & Rollnick, 2012). Although motivational interviewing is not specifically an EH therapy, it shares many characteristics with client-centered therapy and existential therapy. In particular, a major focus is on client resistance, and empathy is a key tool for dealing with that. Miller and colleagues (1980) studied a cognitive behavior treatment for problem drinking. The empathy of the therapists involved in the study was rated by observers, based both on how the therapists were performing in therapy as well as what they said in supervision sessions. The ratings were done before the outcome of therapy was known. The authors found a significant 0.82 correlation between the therapists' empathy and positive outcome in terms of a reduction in drinking. Although the relationship was somewhat weaker at follow-up, it was still statistically significant. The relationship of empathy to outcome was stronger than the relationship of the cognitive behavior interventions to outcome.

Emotion-focused therapy utilizes both a philosophy and a number of interventions that are directly relevant to EH psychotherapies. Watson and colleagues (2020) studied depressed clients who received 16 weeks of either cognitive behavior therapy or emotion-focused therapy. The authors found that the empathy of the therapist predicted positive changes in depression. This appeared to work through empathy's impact on changes in clients' affect regulation, which in turn was related to clients' positive changes in depressive symptomatology.

Finally, Watson and colleagues (2014) studied clients who received either cognitive behavior therapy or emotion-focused therapy for their depression. They found that the clients' ratings of their therapists' empathy were correlated with changes in the clients' attachment styles. Clients became more self-accepting and less insecure. These changes were associated with reductions in their feelings of depression.

Client Empathy and Mutuality in Psychotherapy

A unique emphasis of EH psychotherapy is its emphasis on the interrelationship of therapist and client empathy and the idea that we need to look at the therapist–client relationship as a whole, rather than simply looking at therapist empathy for the client. It has been argued that mutuality is a salient factor in psychotherapy outcomes (Cornelius-White et al., 2018). Elliott and colleagues (2018) conclude, from their overview of the research, that

> empathy is not only something that is "provided" by the therapist as if it were a medication, but is a cocreated experience between a therapist trying to understand the client and a client trying to communicate with the therapist and be understood. (p. 406)

In one study, Murphy and Cramer (2014) found that when there was mutuality in how therapists and clients perceived one another—that is, when clients saw their therapists as empathic, and when therapists saw these same clients as high in empathy—this mutuality was associated with better therapeutic outcome in both HE and cognitive behavior therapies. Looking at the topic of mutuality more generally, Murphy and Cramer (2014) reviewed evidence that shows that mutuality is associated with greater levels of positive therapeutic change (such as with lower levels of bulimic symptoms) and fewer symptoms of depression. Cornelius-White and colleagues (2018) did a meta-analysis on studies that measured mutuality in therapy. Empathy was a significant variable in their analysis. They reported large effect sizes in relationship to session quality and other therapeutic variables.

Qualitative Studies

There are by now a massive number of studies on clients' experiences in therapy (see Fuertes, 2022). Cullari (2001) published a review of studies until 2001, including one of his own. Consistently across studies, one of the top variables that clients reported as being important fell into the category of empathic listening and understanding. For example, Cullari found that the single most common thing clients wanted in the ideal therapist was that the therapist be a good listener. Howe (1993) summarized his findings on what clients wanted in terms of three themes: accept me, understand me, and talk with me.

Levitt and colleagues (2016) did a qualitative meta-analysis of client experiences in therapy. They concluded that the overarching core category found was "Being Known and Cared for Supports Clients' Ability to Agentically Recognize Obstructive Experiential Patterns and Address Unmet Vulnerable Needs." Similarly, one of the subclusters they found was "Caring, Understanding, and Accepting Therapists Allow Clients to Internalize Positive Messages and Enter the Change Process of Developing Self-Awareness." Two lower level subclusters also had to do with empathy: "Category 2.2: Being deeply understood and accepted helps clients engage in self-reflection nondefensively and increase their self-awareness" and "Category 2.4: Feeling unheard, misunderstood, or unappreciated challenges the alliance and requires discussions of differences."

In two other qualitative meta-analyses or metasyntheses of client experiences, Timulak (2007) found that in a study of seven qualitative studies on clients' reports of helpful processes in therapy, acceptance and understanding of the client by the therapist was one of the major helpful elements. Similarly, Timulak (2010) investigated 41 studies on significant moments in psychotherapy. Feeling understood and reassured was one of the major findings. By contrast, one of the major problematic events was when clients felt misunderstood by their therapists. Finally, McElvaney and Timulak (2013) did a meta-analysis of studies on insight events in therapy. Therapist empathic responding was one process that appeared to facilitate client insight.

In terms of specific research projects, Myers (2000, 2003; Myers & White, 2010) conducted three linked qualitative studies. Myers studies the experience of five female psychotherapy clients who had participated in a humanistic, empathy-based therapy for at least 20 sessions. Clients were interviewed after therapy had ended. Clients were selected because they had had a good relationship with their therapist as well as because they were articulate about their experiences. All clients interviewed reported being listened to as an essential element of their relationship with their therapists. Feeling empathically listened to was associated with an increased sense of personal agency, a redefined sense of self, a renewed sense of being-in-the world, increased self-acceptance, and increased self-empathy. A 10 year follow-up showed that these positive changes had persisted and clients continued to attribute them to being empathically understood by their therapists.

MacFarlane and colleagues (2017) interviewed nine clients about their experiences of empathy in psychotherapy. The nine clients were seen by eight therapists. The researchers explore three features of the empathic experience: clients' phenomenological experience of empathy, clients' interpretations of the psychotherapists' empathic communication, and clients' perceptions of the utility (e.g., benefits and consequences) of empathy. These clients participated in an interpersonal process recall (Elliott, 1986) procedure where they reviewed videotapes of their sessions. Three types of empathy were discovered from the qualitative analysis. The first was clients' perceptions of therapists' cognitive empathy. This category included a complex combination of therapist attentiveness, asking pertinent questions, reflections, and trying to see things from the client's perspective. Emotional empathy was a second theme. This consisted of clients' perceptions of therapists' emotional attunement. The third category was client empathy, which consisted of clients' attunement to the therapist.

The researchers also discovered two categories of benefits from empathy. The first had to do with how empathy facilitated the therapy process. This included impacts on things like the pacing of the session, facilitating openness, helping overcome demographic differences between therapist and client, facilitating trust, and facilitating openness. The second category had to do with benefits to the client, such as an improvement in self-understanding, having corrective experiences, and feeling better.

In sum, qualitative research strongly supports the proposition that clients view feeling understood, known, listened to, and empathically related to by their therapists as helpful. Furthermore, specifically in relationship to the EH view of empathy, there is some evidence that client empathy also plays a role in therapy.

MULTICULTURAL CONSIDERATIONS

Psychotherapy in general is defined as the science of individual differences. From this perspective, each therapeutic interaction is unique to the individuals in relationship. Indeed, existential therapists would also posit that each moment within each session may provide a unique fleeting moment in time in which empathy may occur. Nonetheless, it is important to understand some general trends that reflect individuals' cultural (broadly defined) backgrounds. Crosscultural counseling and psychotherapy adopting from the fields of cultural anthropology and linguistics offers two potentially contrasting levels of analysis in understanding cultural norms and experiences: emic and etic (Pedersen et al., 1981).

Simply put, emic analyses begin with the unique different culture of interest, and etic comprehension is based initially on similarities across all human beings. In exploring a central variable like empathy in psychotherapy, both considerations are germane. Accurate empathy requires being with the client as a fellow human being with universal concerns and also understanding as best as possible the culturally centric demands and motivations that are crucial to the client's unique self.

In addition, although we know that intragroup differences within a culture, ethnicity, or gender, for example, are greater than intergroup differences, the individual client in our presence is uniquely influenced by both. This is particularly relevant to empathy. In order to be effectively empathic, therapists must be attuned to the intricate intersectionality of real-world clients. Their gender, culture, and even generational issues greatly influence who they are.

What empathy means to a first-generation immigrant from an East Asian culture and what it means to their third-generation grandchild are likely to be quite distinctly different. Similarly, empathy from a male therapist with a female client may also be far different. Equally important are the unique qualities of a person from within a distinct cultural, gender, and generational frame. Thus, a *sansei* (third-generation) immigrant from Japan will share some common experiences with other third-generation Japanese immigrants and with all third-generation immigrants. However, they will also be different from those with whom they share a cohort.

The assumption that a client may be pigeonholed in reference to their ethnicity, ancestors, or sex can lead to significant ruptures in the therapeutic encounter. Indeed, mistakes in culturally sensitive therapeutic empathy may come when there is assumed similarity because of shared characteristics. Just because both the client and therapist identify as Methodist and Californian does not mean that those similarities will lead to automatic empathy. An assumption that it naturally does is more hubris than empathy. In short, placing the construct of accurate empathy into a cultural context is quite complex and insufficiently studied from a combined emic and etic framework.

Several authors have made crucial inroads into better placing empathy into a cultural framework. Some focus on emic considerations and other on etic. For example, one question involves whether people from collective cultures exhibit more empathy (i.e., Pedersen et al., 1981). Answers to this question come from various perspectives including the significance of political, value, and socioeconomic influences. For example, in his commencement address at Northwestern University on June 16th, 2006, then–future president of the United States Barack Obama avers,

> We live in a culture that discourages empathy. A culture that too often tells us our principle [*sic*] goal in life is to be rich, thin, young, famous, safe, and entertained. A culture where those in power too often encourage these selfish impulses. (Northwestern University, 2008)

Obama continues on to say that self-centeredness is rife among the American people and argues that this empathy deficit is a result of a very American, culturally sanctioned quest for individualistic goals of self-enhancement rather than the collective good.

Taking the importance of political sensitivity to the psychotherapeutic realm, Peter Schmid (2015) argues that "psychotherapy is politics or it isn't psycho-therapy" (p. 230). According to Schmid, people are inextricably connected to their physical and social environments. Problems are therefore not simply due to internal psychological factors; social factors must not be neglected. If a client has no place to live or does not have enough food, this will affect their psycho-logical functioning. Thus, focusing solely on internal psychological work alone is an exercise in futility. Empathy, therefore, must include a sensitivity to the client's social–ecological context and its effect on them.

Empathy Through a Multicultural Lens

As indicated earlier, we define culture broadly, including differences in ances-try, race, ethnicity, gender identities, spirituality, and power. We also construe it to mean differences in experience across different identities that may have an impact on the therapist–client relationship, including various forms of societal oppression that may affect the client's daily existence. Therapists need to be keenly aware of the intersectionality that defines each client's personality.

From an EH perspective, therapy at heart is what Carl Rogers has described as a meeting of persons (Cissna & Anderson, 1994), as we have previously mentioned. Taking culture into account, we can reconstrue therapy as a place where true dialogue between cultures and diverse experiences can meet. Sha-piro and Patterson (2020), in their focus on couples therapy, argue that because of differences in families of origin, all relationships contain crosscultural char-acteristics. Similarly, Pedersen (1977; 1991) states that all therapy is multicul-tural, and Bohart and Rosenbaum (1995) say that therapy is a "meeting of persons and of cultures." This implies that therapeutic empathy is not merely therapist empathy for the client, nor therapist and client empathy for one another, nor even getting inside the skin of the relationship (to paraphrase O'Hara, 1984). It needs to be getting inside the skin of the therapist–client rela-tionship embedded in all the larger cultural forces that are impacting on each of them as well as on their relationship together.

Various writers have supported this position (Hoffman, 2019). For example, Pedersen and colleagues (1981, 2008) have argued that inclusive cultural empathy implies that therapists need to pay attention to the cultural factors that are part of an individual's identity. Similarly, Comas-Diaz (2016) defines *cultural empathy* as "a process of perspective taking by using a cultural and con-textual framework as a guide for understanding the client from outside" (p. 163). In keeping with this, Hoffman (2019) notes that

> empathy must take into account individual subjective experience as well as the recognition that the person is part of a larger whole that entails other relation-ships . . . . This . . . allows for empathy that recognizes and embraces others who may maintain a different conception of the self not consistent with more ego-centric Western views. (p. 109)

Further, Elliott and colleagues (2018) note,

> It is important for therapists working with diverse populations to be empathic with their clients' specific circumstances, as well as the complexities inherent in their social and political locations (Fuertes et al., 2006). This in-depth understanding includes sensitivity to race, socioeconomic status, gender, sex, religion, and sociopolitical forces such as oppression and perceived microaggressions. Competent therapists working with diverse populations display high levels of not just rapport and communicative attunement to clients in session but also person empathy that embeds understanding of the client's social identities and the possible impact of societal discrimination. (p. 405)

Therefore, as Fuertes and colleagues (2007) have observed, there may be diversity-related aspects of empathy that are not captured with general measures of empathy. In terms of being sensitive, Grzanka and colleagues (2017) point out that therapists need to be aware of how their theories may interfere with their sensitivity to the power and oppression implicit in clients' intersectional identities. They also suggest that therapists should understand how their work is influenced by issues of privilege and oppression and how these factors affect their clients' lives. Being sensitive as well as showing empathic understanding, emotional support, and nonjudgment may be particularly important in facilitating participation in therapy for clients from diverse backgrounds (Gillispie et al., 2005).

Fitting in with this, for the relational–cultural approach to therapy that we have previously mentioned, relational competence emphasizes that power held by one party (the therapist) must be addressed by "creating good connection rather than exercising power over others as the path of growth" (Jordan, 2004, p. 15). Power over becomes power with (Jordan, 2004). Power differentials, isolation, and shame are obstacles to relational empathy; rather, "relational competence occurs within a context of wishing to empower others and appreciating the life-giving nature of community building, of treating strength with others rather than in isolation" (Jordan, 2004, p 15).

Therapist, Know Thyself

Therapists need to be cautious in assuming the accuracy of their empathy across cultures. There are several essential implications of this. First, it implies the salience of *therapist self-awareness*. The more therapists are aware of their own embedded and implicit cultural assumptions about the nature of the individual, cognition, and emotion and their roles in everyday life, the more able therapists will be in empathically entering into productive I–thou moments with their clients. This self-knowledge includes cultural norms and standards about a wide variety of values, the nature of time, how to approach problems, and some sense of their own personal triggers. For instance, O'Hara (1996) shows how Carl Rogers's implicit Western masculine assumptions subtly influenced his work with a woman client.

Second, this emphasizes the importance for the therapist of continual *empathic checking*. There is no way that we can be completely aware of our implicit cultural assumptions. That means we need to continually and carefully listen and check our understanding. Third, it means that we must be open to allowing the client to teach us about their experience of their culture. They are, in fact, the expert here about how their culture translates to them personally. This has the added benefit of equalizing the relationship between therapist and client, something that research has shown clients prize (Bohart & Tallman, 2022).

Equalizing the therapy relationship is a laudable goal. However, there are aspects of the professional relationship that implicitly say to the client that the therapist is in a power position. In many cases, they are paying the therapist, meeting at the therapist's office, waiting in their waiting room, and so on. Additionally, clients themselves, especially clients from some cultures, may have been socialized to believe that the therapist is the boss (although this may not be true in some cases where a therapist who is a person of color may be working with a White client). Nonetheless, therapists, through their sensitive listening as well as their genuine attempt to understand the client and meet them, can equalize this power dynamic, at least to some degree.

Fourth, our discussion about multiculturalism implies that the more we know about different cultures, the better. As Hoffman (2019) notes,

> although it is not realistic for therapists to have knowledge about all cultures, particularly when considering the intersectionality of various cultures or aspects of identity that often exist within individuals, being familiar with a range of cultural variations . . . helps a therapist improve their ability to recognize difference otherwise hidden. (p. 110)

We would add that the wider the variety of cultures therapists meet with openness and willingness to learn (two crucial components of empathy), the greater flexibility there is in adjusting to clients, whether or not they come from a particular previously encountered culture. The combination of knowledge and cultural humility enhance the ability of the therapist to listen to the individual client without mechanistically applying cultural stereotypes.

EH Therapies and Diversity

Because EH psychotherapies focus on universal challenges or givens encountered that all people must face, they can offer a particular opportunity to address the challenges of working with people from many cultures. These approaches especially value working with the unique individual and understanding their phenomenological experience of the world (which is infused with their cultural place in the world), rather than applying diagnostic and other stereotypes to them. Such approaches have the following characteristics:

- They place emphasis on continual therapist self-awareness.

- They underscore the necessity of meeting each particular client in the here-and-now, enhancing I–thou dialogue, with the therapists and clients building a common ground of understanding and coexperiencing.

- EH theories emphasize certain basics of human experience. They hypothesize that there are universal anxieties that humans inevitably encounter, regardless of culture of origin. These include anxiety around mortality, isolation, finding and creating meaning in life, and facing freedom and the attendant responsibility. Each client can be best understood by their responses to these personal challenges within the cultural frame in which they live and function (Shapiro, 2016; Yalom, 1980).

In this way, EH therapies can be culturally inclusive when practiced with appropriate cultural awareness and humility. They provide an antidote to what Obama refers to as a cultural deficit, reducing isolation, tribalism, and lack of human connection (Northwestern University, 2008).

Research on Empathy and Cultural Diversity

Here we look at the limited research on empathy with clients from diverse cultural backgrounds. It should be noted that this research is not specifically on EH therapy. Looking more broadly at the relationship of therapist performance to client outcome with respect to multicultural diversity, there is evidence that therapists' multicultural competence and multicultural sensitivity is positively correlated with outcome. Norcross and Wampold (2018) report an effect size of 0.50 (a medium effect size) between outcome and therapists adapting their therapy approaches and procedures to clients' cultural backgrounds. In their review of the literature, Tao and colleagues (2015) report that therapists' multicultural competency correlates positively with building a positive therapeutic alliance as rated by clients, the impact of sessions on them, and client satisfaction. They found less evidence on the relationship of multicultural competence and outcome, but what they did find was in a positive direction. Tao and colleagues (2015) conducted a meta-analysis of all the studies relating multicultural competence to the previous factors as well as other therapeutic factors. They find a high correlation between multicultural competence and process measures ($r = 0.75$) and a moderate correlation with outcome ($r = 0.29$).

Because the results reported by Norcross and Wampold (2018) and Tao and colleagues (2015) support the importance of multicultural competency, which includes a sensitivity to clients' cultural backgrounds, we can expect that therapist empathy likely contributes to therapists' ability to be multiculturally sensitive. This inference is buttressed by the fact that Fuertes and colleagues (2006) find a strong correlation between clients' perception of their therapists' multicultural competence and their therapists' empathy ($r = 0.81$). We should note, however, that there is more to multicultural competency than empathy (Fuertes et al., 2006).

There is little research that looks specifically at empathy with clients from different cultural groups in psychotherapy and its effects on psychotherapy outcome. One study by Fuertes and colleagues (2006) examines the relationships among therapists' empathy, the working alliance, multicultural competence, and client satisfaction. The therapists were 34 Americans of European descent and 17 from historically marginalized groups. Of the clients, 39 were from historically marginalized groups and 12 were European American. The authors reported no significant differences in results depending on how therapists and clients were matched. The authors found a significant correlation between clients' ratings of their therapists' empathy and their satisfaction with therapy ($r = 0.83$). Another study by Gillispie and colleagues (2005) finds that African American clients' satisfaction with the mental health services they were receiving was positively correlated with their therapists' empathy. Of the 11 therapists studied, six were of European-descended American backgrounds, and five were from historically marginalized groups. Staff empathy also correlated positively to clients' intent to pursue aftercare.

We mention one last finding, although it is not directly a test of empathy and therapeutic outcome. Hettema and colleagues (2005) report on a meta-analysis of evidence for the effectiveness of motivational interviewing (MI). The meta-analysis found that the effect size of MI with client samples predominantly made up of persons of color was three times as large as with other client samples ($d = 0.79$ vs. $d = 0.26$). The therapists were predominantly not persons of color. Empathy is at the core of MI, but it is not the only component. Thus, this is suggestive but inconclusive.

There are few studies that have looked at other diversity variables, such as those of clients' socioeconomic status, religion, gender, intersectionality, or degree of oppression and their relationship to therapist empathy and to therapeutic outcome. In one research project, Woodin and colleagues (2012) study the usefulness of MI to reduce violent abusive behavior in couples. It was found that a greater empathic reflection-to-question ratio from the therapist was correlated with a reduction in aggression for both men and women. There was a nonsignificant trend for global therapist empathy to predict a reduction in aggression for women.

Overall, these studies are informative and have construct validity with EH theories. However, there is much more to be discerned about the relationship of empathy and culture. In particular, it should be considered that most, though not all, of the research has been conducted by individuals from Western culture. It is possible that this has impacted some of the focus on empathy research. More research is needed on how cultural variables may complicate empathic communications between therapists and clients as well.

FUTURE RESEARCH NEEDS

Elliott and colleagues (2018) have noted that it is time to move beyond research that correlates measures of empathy with therapeutic outcomes. Previous research analyses have composited measures of empathy and related them to composites of outcome measures. Now, more sensitive research is needed. It is essential to explore more differentiated questions that deal with both the definition of empathy and its measurement. We need to more intensively study what empathy actually is.

We need more rigorous studies of how empathy per se functions as a curative factor across multiple forms of psychotherapy and, specifically, how it works and what it means within an intersectional context. In so doing, we need to do more fine-grained analyses looking at considerations such as intersectionality. We also should consider the experiences of therapists themselves with marginalization and oppression. In order to do this, we must use a mix of research methods. Some of these involve research that is based on the inductive process of EH therapy. Such studies could presumably explore the manner in which empathy develops within and between sessions as well as the effect of varying forms and levels of empathy.

Much of psychotherapy research, particularly that of outcome studies, is a deductive process. Researchers begin with a theory, develop hypotheses, and use observations to reject the null hypothesis. Existential psychotherapy and measures of variables like van Deurzen's *copathy* are primarily inductive, beginning with observations and developing phenomenological theories from there (Shapiro, 2016).

The challenge is to be able to evaluate—in some reliable manner—therapist empathy, client empathy, shifts in the unconscious combined entity state that reflects the "us" interconnection, and how those shifts affect the overall therapeutic encounter and results. This is particularly the province of qualitative research. However, both qualitative and quantitative methods are needed.

One approach might involve simultaneous physiological recordings of the therapist and client in real time during sessions and an exploration of how those measures affect therapeutic outcome. Such ongoing measures of client and therapist could also be used to understand the mutual empathy in the relationship (i.e., the "we") of empathy in therapy. Another approach involves the use of interpersonal process recall (Elliott, 1986). Both therapists, as well as clients, could be interviewed by culturally sensitive interviewers shortly after therapy, while clients listen to recordings of sessions, in order to get the clients' take on issues like therapist empathy, therapist sensitivity to diverse issues, egalitarianism, and the like.

Finally, there are a trio of adjudicatory methods for studying change in single cases that allow for the more fine-grained analyses we are calling for. These methods—the research jury (Bohart et al., 2021), the hermeneutic single-case efficacy design (Elliott et al., 2009), and the panel of psychological inquiry method of case study research (R. B. Miller et al. 2021)—rely upon intensive study of a rich case record by a jury of evaluators who then draw conclusions as to whether a given client changed or not, and if so, how therapy contributed. Studies done so far have demonstrated that the change process in therapy is more complex than how things appear from randomized controlled clinical trials.

Expansive research is particularly important in EH therapy modalities because the role empathy plays in these therapies is more complex than the role of empathy in some other therapies.

CONCLUSION

Empathy is currently considered an empirically supported relationship characteristic. Because it plays an important role in EH therapy, the research we have summarized therefore provides empirical support for the practice of EH therapy. At the same time, further research is needed to explore a more differentiated view of the role of empathy in EH therapy.

REFERENCES

Altmann, H. A. (1973). Effects of empathy, warmth, and genuineness in the initial counseling interview. *Counselor Education and Supervision, 12*(3), 225–228. https://doi.org/10.1002/j.1556-6978.1973.tb01555.x

Bandler, R., & Grinder, J. (1975). *The structure of magic: A book about language and therapy.* Science and Behavior Books.

Banks, A. (2015). *Wired to connect: The surprising link between brain science and strong, healthy relationships.* Penguin Random House.

Baron-Cohen, S. (2011). *The science of evil: On empathy and the origins of cruelty.* Basic Books.

Batson, C. D. (2016). Empathy and altruism. In K. W. Brown & M. R. Leary (Eds.), *The Oxford handbook of hypo-egoic phenomena* (pp. 161–174). Oxford University Press. https://doi.org/10.1093/oxfordhb/9780199328079.013.11

Belenky, M. F., Clinchy, B. M., Goldberger, N. R., & Tarule, J. (1986). *Women's ways of knowing: The development of self, voice, and mind.* Basic Books.

Bohart, A., & Rosenbaum, R. (1995). The dance of empathy: Empathy, diversity, and technical eclecticism. *The Person-Centered Journal, 2,* 5–29.

Bohart, A. C. (2021). *The art of Bohart: Person-centred therapy and the enhancement of human possibility.* PCCS Books.

Bohart, A. C., & Greenberg, L. S. (1997). Introduction. In A. C. Bohart & L. S. Greenberg (Eds.), *Empathy reconsidered: New directions in psychotherapy* (pp. 3–31). American Psychological Association. https://doi.org/10.1037/10226-018

Bohart, A. C., Shenefiel, L., & Alejandro, M. (2021). What can we learn about therapeutic change from case history data? The research jury method with the couple case of "Carl" and "Sandra." *Pragmatic Case Studies in Psychotherapy, 17*(2), 210–234. https://doi.org/10.14713/pcsp.v17i2.2096

Bohart, A. C., & Tallman, K. (2022). Client expertise: The active client in psychotherapy. In J. N. Fuertes (Ed.), *The other side of psychotherapy: Understanding clients' experiences and contributions in treatment* (pp. 13–43). American Psychological Association. https://doi.org/10.1037/0000303-002

Bordin, E. S. (1979). The generalizability of the psychoanalytic concept of working alliance. *Psychotherapy, 16*(3), 252–260. https://doi.org/10.1037/h0085885

Brems, C. (2000). *Basic skills in psychotherapy and counseling.* Wadsworth/Thomson.

Buber, M. (1970). *I and thou* (W. Kaufmann, Trans.). Scrivener. (Original work published 1937)

Bugental, J. F. T. (1976). *The search for existential identity: Patient-therapist dialogue in humanistic psychotherapy.* Jossey-Bass.

Bugental, J. F. T. (1987). *The art of the psychotherapist.* W. W. Norton & Company.

Bugental, J. F. T. (1999). *Psychotherapy isn't what you think.* Zeig, Tucker & Company.

Chafetz, M. E., Blane, H. T., Abram, H. S., Clark, E., Golner, J. H., Hastie, E. L., & McCourt, W. F. (1964). Establishing treatment relations with alcoholics: A supplementary report. *Journal of Nervous and Mental Disease, 138*(4), 390–393. https://doi.org/10.1097/00005053-196404000-00010

Chafetz, M. E., Blane, H. T., Abram, H. S., Golner, J., Hastie, E. L., McCourt, W. F., Clark, E., & Meyers, W. (1962). Establishing treatment relations with alcoholics. *Journal of Nervous and Mental Disease, 134*(5), 395–409. https://doi.org/10.1097/00005053-196205000-00001

Chui, H., & Liu, F. (2021). Emotional experience of psychotherapists: A latent profile analysis. *Psychotherapy, 58*(3), 401–413. https://doi.org/10.1037/pst0000379

Cissna, K. N., & Anderson, R. (1994). The 1957 Martin Buber–Carl Rogers dialogue, as dialogue. *Journal of Humanistic Psychology, 34*(1), 11–45. https://doi.org/10.1177/00221678940341003

Comas-Diaz, L. (2016). Multicultural therapy. In H. S. Friedman (Ed.), *Encyclopedia of mental health* (2nd ed., pp. 163–168). Academic Press. https://doi.org/10.1016/B978-0-12-397045-9.00184-1

Cornelius-White, J. H. D., Kanamori, Y., Murphy, D., & Tickle, E. (2018). Mutuality in psychotherapy: A meta-analysis and meta-synthesis. *Journal of Psychotherapy Integration, 28*(4), 489–504. https://doi.org/10.1037/int0000134

Cullari, S. (2001). *Counseling and psychotherapy*. Allyn & Bacon.

Davis, M. (1983). Measuring individual differences in empathy: Evidence for a multidimensional approach. *Journal of Personality and Social Psychology, 44*(1), 113–126. https://doi.org/10.1037/0022-3514.44.1.113

de Wied, M., van der Graaff, J., de Rooij, G., Scheepers, F., Hoekstra, P. J., Branje, S., & van de Schoot, R. (2020). The role of client empathy in treatment outcome in a sample of adolescents referred to forensic youth psychiatric services. *Children and Youth Services Review, 118*, 105301. https://doi.org/10.1016/j.childyouth.2020.105301

Elliott, R. (1986). Interpersonal process recall (IPR) as a psychotherapy process research method. In L. S. Greenberg & W. M. Pinsof (Eds.), *The psychotherapeutic process: A research handbook* (pp. 503–528). Guilford Press.

Elliott, R., Bohart, A. C., Watson, J. C., & Murphy, D. (2018). Therapist empathy and client outcome: An updated meta-analysis. *Psychotherapy, 55*(4), 399–410. https://doi.org/10.1037/pst0000175

Elliott, R., Partyka, R., Alperin, R., Dobrenski, R., Wagner, J., Messer, S. B., Watson, J. C., & Castonguay, L. G. (2009). An adjudicated hermeneutic single-case efficacy design study of experiential therapy for panic/phobia. *Psychotherapy Research, 19*(4–5), 543–557. https://doi.org/10.1080/10503300902905947

Erickson, M. H. (1980). *The collected papers of Milton H. Erickson* (E. L. Rossi, Ed.). Irvington Publishers.

Erickson, M. H. (2009). Naturalistic techniques of hypnosis. *The American Journal of Clinical Hypnosis, 51*(4), 333–340. (Original work published 1958)

Feshbach, N. D. (1997). Empathy: The formative years—Implications for clinical practice. In A. C. Bohart & L. S. Greenberg (Eds.), *Empathy reconsidered: New directions in psychotherapy* (pp. 33–59). American Psychological Association. https://doi.org/10.1037/10226-001

Flückiger, C., Del Re, A. C., Wampold, B. E., & Horvath, A. O. (2018). The alliance in adult psychotherapy: A meta-analytic synthesis. *Psychotherapy, 55*(4), 316–340. https://doi.org/10.1037/pst0000172

Fuertes, J. N. (Ed.). (2022). *The other side of psychotherapy: Understanding clients' experiences and contributions in treatment*. American Psychological Association. https://doi.org/10.1037/0000303-000

Fuertes, J. N., Mislowack, A., Brown, S., Gur-Arie, S., Wilkinson, S., & Gelso, C. J. (2007). Correlates of the real relationship in psychotherapy: A study of dyads. *Psychotherapy Research, 17*, 423–430.

Fuertes, J. N., Stracuzzi, T. I., Bennett, J., Scheinholtz, J., Mislowack, A., Hersh, M., & Cheng, D. (2006). Therapist multicultural competency: A study of therapy dyads. *Psychotherapy, 43*(4), 480–490. https://doi.org/10.1037/0033-3204.43.4.480

Gillispie, R., Williams, E., & Gillispie, C. (2005). Hospitalized African American mental health consumers: Some antecedents to service satisfaction and intent to comply with aftercare. *American Journal of Orthopsychiatry, 75*(2), 254–261. https://doi.org/10.1037/0002-9432.75.2.254

Greenberg, L. S., & Paivio, S. C. (1997). *Working with emotions in psychotherapy.* Guilford Press.

Greenberg, L. S., Rice, L. N., & Elliott, R. (1993). *Facilitating emotional change: The moment-by-moment process.* Guilford Press.

Greenberg, L. S., & Rushanski-Rosenberg, R. (2002). Therapists' experience of empathy. In J. C. Watson, R. N. Goldman, & M. S. Warner (Eds.), *Client-centered and experiential psychotherapy in the 21st century: Advances in theory, research and practice* (pp. 204–220). PCCS Books.

Grzanka, P. R., Santos, C. E., & Moradi, B. (2017). Intersectionality research in counseling psychology. *Journal of Counseling Psychology, 64*(5), 453–457. https://doi.org/10.1037/cou0000237

Hettema, J., Steele, J., & Miller, W. R. (2005). Motivational interviewing. *Annual Review of Clinical Psychology, 1*(1), 91–111. https://doi.org/10.1146/annurev.clinpsy.1.102803.143833

Hoffman, L. (2019). Culture and empathy in humanistic psychology. In L. Hoffman, H. Cleare-Hoffman, N. Granger, Jr., & D. St. John (Eds.), *Humanistic approaches to multiculturalism and diversity: Perspectives on existence and difference* (pp. 103–116). Routledge. https://doi.org/10.4324/9781351133357-9

Howe, D. (1993). *On being a client.* Sage.

Jordan, J. V. (1997). Relational development through mutual empathy. In A. C. Bohart & L. S. Greenberg (Eds.), *Empathy reconsidered: New directions in psychotherapy* (pp. 343–353). American Psychological Association. https://doi.org/10.1037/10226-015

Jordan, J. V. (2000). The role of mutual empathy in relational/cultural therapy. *Journal of Clinical Psychology, 56*(8), 1005–1016. https://doi.org/10.1002/1097-4679(200008)56:8<1005::AID-JCLP2>3.0.CO;2-L

Jordan, J. V. (2004). Toward competence and connection. In J. V. Jordan, M. Walker, & L. M. Hartling (Eds.), *The complexity of connection: Writings from the Stone Center's Jean Baker Miller Training Institute* (pp. 11–27). Guilford Press.

Jordan, J. V., & Surrey, J. L. (1986). The self-in-relation: Empathy and the mother-daughter relationship. In T. Bernay & D. Cantor (Eds.), *The Psychology of Today's Woman* (pp. 81–104). Routledge.

Klein, M. H., & Mathieu-Coughlan, P. (1986). Measures of client and therapist vocal quality. In L. S. Greenberg & W. M. Pinsof (Eds.), *The psychotherapeutic process: A research handbook* (pp. 21–72). Guilford Press.

Landfield, A. W. (1971). *Personal construct systems in psychotherapy.* Rand McNally.

Levinson, D. (1978). *The seasons of a man's life.* Alfred A. Knopf.

Levitt, H. M., Pomerville, A., & Surace, F. I. (2016). A qualitative meta-analysis examining clients' experiences of psychotherapy: A new agenda. *Psychological Bulletin, 142*(8), 801–830. https://doi.org/10.1037/bul0000057

MacFarlane, P., Anderson, T., & McClintock, A. S. (2017). Empathy from the client's perspective: A grounded theory analysis. *Psychotherapy Research, 27*(2), 227–238. https://doi.org/10.1080/10503307.2015.1090038

May, R. (1969). *Love and will.* W. W. Norton & Company.

McElvaney, J., & Timulak, L. (2013). Clients' experience of therapy and its outcomes in 'good' and 'poor' outcome psychological therapy in a primary care setting: An exploratory study. *Counselling & Psychotherapy Research, 13*(4), 246–253. https://doi.org/10.1080/14733145.2012.761258

Miller, J. B. (1986). *Toward a new psychology of women.* Beacon Press. (Original work published 1976)

Miller, J. B. (1991). The development of women's sense of self. In J. V. Jordan, A. G. Kaplan, J. B. Miller, I. P. Stiver, & J. L. Surrey (Eds.), *Women's growth in connection: Writings from the Stone Center* (pp. 11–26). Guilford Press.

Miller, R. B., Ashley, B., Mount, K., Tuepker, S., Powell, T., O'Leary, D., Fouts, M., Allshouse, K., Rusczek, J., Hennebarrows, K., & Dombroski, A. (2021). Further developments in the Panel of Psychological Inquiry Method of case study research: The case of "Ronan." *Pragmatic Case Studies in Psychotherapy, 17*(2), 129–209. https://doi.org/10.14713/pcsp.v17i2.2095

Miller, W. R., & Rollnick, S. (2012). *Motivational interviewing: Helping people change* (3rd ed.). Guilford Press.

Miller, W. R., Taylor, C. A., & West, J. (1980). Focused versus broad-spectrum behavior therapy for problem drinkers. *Journal of Consulting and Clinical Psychology, 48*(5), 590–601. https://doi.org/10.1037/0022-006X.48.5.590

Murphy, D., & Cramer, D. (2014). Mutuality of Rogers's therapeutic conditions and treatment progress in the first three psychotherapy sessions. *Psychotherapy Research, 24*(6), 651–661. https://doi.org/10.1080/10503307.2013.874051

Myers, S. (2000). Empathic listening: Reports on the experience of being heard. *Journal of Humanistic Psychology, 40*(2), 148–173. https://doi.org/10.1177/0022167800402004

Myers, S. (2003). Relational healing: To be understood and to understand. *Journal of Humanistic Psychology, 43*(1), 86–104. https://doi.org/10.1177/0022167802238815

Myers, S., & White, C. M. (2010). The abiding nature of empathic connections: A 10-year follow-up study. *Journal of Humanistic Psychology, 50*(1), 77–95. https://doi.org/10.1177/0022167809337475

Norcross, J. C. (Ed.). (2002). *Psychotherapy relationships that work.* Oxford University Press.

Norcross, J. C. (Ed.). (2011). *Psychotherapy relationships that work: Evidence-based responsiveness* (2nd ed.). Oxford University Press. https://doi.org/10.1093/acprof:oso/9780199737208.001.0001

Norcross, J. C., & Lambert, M. J. (2018). Psychotherapy relationships that work III. *Psychotherapy, 55*(4), 303–315. https://doi.org/10.1037/pst0000193

Norcross, J. C., & Wampold, B. E. (2018). A new therapy for each patient: Evidence-based relationships and responsiveness. *Journal of Clinical Psychology, 74*(11), 1889–1906. https://doi.org/10.1002/jclp.22678

Northwestern University. (2008, July 15). *2006 Northwestern Commencement—Sen. Barack Obama* [Video]. Youtube. https://www.youtube.com/watch?v=2MhMRYQ9Ez8

O'Hara, M. M. (1984). Person-centered gestalt: Towards a holistic synthesis. In R. F. Levant & J. M. Shlien (Eds.), *Client-centered therapy and the person-centered approach: New directions in theory, research and practice* (pp. 203–221). Praeger.

O'Hara, M. M. (1996). Rogers and Sylvia: A feminist analysis. In B. A. Farber, D. C. Brink, & P. M. Raskin (Eds). *The psychotherapy of Carl Rogers: Cases and commentary* (pp. 284–300). Guilford Press.

Pedersen, P. B. (1977). The triad model of cross-cultural counselor training. *The Personnel and Guidance Journal, 56*(2), 94–100. https://doi.org/10.1002/j.2164-4918.1977.tb04491.x

Pedersen, P. B. (1991). Multiculturalism as a generic approach to counseling. *Journal of Counseling & Development, 70*(1), 6–12. https://doi.org/10.1002/j.1556-6676.1991.tb01555.x

Pedersen, P. B., Crethar, H. C., & Carlson, J. (2008). *Inclusive cultural empathy: Making relationships central in counseling and psychotherapy.* American Psychological Association. https://doi.org/10.1037/11707-000

Pedersen, P. B., Draguns, J. G., Lonner, W. J., & Trimble, J. E. (1981). *Counseling across cultures* (Rev. ed.). University of Hawaii Press.

Rice, L. N., & Saperia, E. P. (1984). Task analysis of the resolution of problematic reactions. In L. N. Rice & L. S. Greenberg (Eds.), *Patterns of change: Intensive analysis of psychotherapy process* (pp. 67–123). Guilford Press.

Rogers, C. R. (1959). A theory of therapy, personality and interpersonal relationships, as developed in the client-centered framework. In S. Koch (Ed.), *Psychology: A study of science: Vol. 3. Formulations of the person and the social context* (pp. 184–256). McGraw-Hill.

Rogers, C. R. (1980). *A way of being*. Houghton Mifflin.

Rogers, C. R. (1986). Reflection of feelings. *Person-Centered Review, 1(4)*, 375–377.

Sachse, R. (1990a). Concrete interventions are crucial: The influence of the therapist's processing proposals on the client's interpersonal exploration in client-centered therapy. In G. Lietaer, J. Rombauts, & R. Van Balen (Eds.), *Client-centered and experiential psychotherapy in the nineties* (pp. 295–308). Leuven University Press.

Sachse, R. (1990b). The influence of therapist process proposals on the explication process of the client. *Person-Centered Review, 5(3)*, 321–344.

Schmid, P. F. (2015). Person and society: Toward a person-centered sociotherapy. *Person-Centered and Experiential Psychotherapies, 14(3)*, 217–235. https://doi.org/10.1080/14779757.2015.1062795

Schneider, K. J. (Ed.). (2008). *Existential–integrative psychotherapy: Guideposts to the core of practice*. Routledge.

Schneider, K. J., & Krug, O. T. (2017). *Existential–humanistic therapy* (2nd ed.). American Psychological Association. https://doi.org/10.1037/0000042-000

Shapiro, J. L. (2016). *Pragmatic existential counseling and psychotherapy: Intimacy, intuition and the search for meaning*. Sage. https://doi.org/10.4135/9781483397535

Shapiro, J. L. (2021, June 12). *An existential approach to anxiety and to COVID-19 and its sequelae* [Presentation]. Society for the Exploration of Psychotherapy Integration 37th Annual Meeting.

Shapiro, J. L., & Patterson, T. (2020). *Real world couple counseling and psychotherapy*. Cognella Academic Press.

Shapiro, J. L., Peltz, L. S., & Bernadett-Shapiro, S. T. (2019). *Basics of group counseling and psychotherapy: An introductory guide*. Cognella Academic Press.

Shlien, J. (1997). Empathy in psychotherapy: A vital mechanism? Yes. Therapist's conceit? All too often. By itself enough? No. In A. C. Bohart & L. S. Greenberg (Eds.), *Empathy reconsidered: New directions in psychotherapy* (pp. 63–80). American Psychological Association. https://doi.org/10.1037/10226-002

Spinelli, E. (1997). *Tales of un-knowing: Eight stories of existential therapy*. New York University Press.

Tao, K. W., Owen, J., Pace, B. T., & Imel, Z. E. (2015). A meta-analysis of multicultural competencies and psychotherapy process and outcome. *Journal of Counseling Psychology, 62(3)*, 337–350. https://doi.org/10.1037/cou0000086

Timulak, L. (2007). Identifying core categories of client-identified impact of helpful events in psychotherapy: A qualitative meta-analysis. *Psychotherapy Research, 17(3)*, 305–320. https://doi.org/10.1080/10503300600608116

Timulak, L. (2010). Significant events in psychotherapy: An update of research findings. *Psychology and Psychotherapy: Theory, Research and Practice, 83(4)*, 421–447. https://doi.org/10.1348/147608310X499404

van Deurzen, E. (2002). *Existential counselling and psychotherapy in practice*. Sage.

van Deurzen, E. (2010). *Everyday mysteries: A handbook of existential psychotherapy* (2nd ed.). Routledge.

Wampold, B. E., & Imel, Z. E. (2015). *The great psychotherapy debate: The evidence for what makes psychotherapy work*. Routledge. https://doi.org/10.4324/9780203582015

Watson, J. C. (2016). The role of empathy in psychotherapy: Theory, research, and practice. In D. J. Cain, K. Kennan, & S. Rubin (Eds.), *Humanistic psychotherapies: Handbook of research and practice* (2nd ed., pp. 115–145). American Psychological Association. https://doi.org/10.1037/14775-005

Watson, J. C., McMullen, E. J., Rodrigues, A., & Prosser, M. C. (2020). Examining the role of therapists' empathy and clients' attachment styles on changes in clients' affect regulation and outcome in the treatment of depression. *Psychotherapy Research, 30*(6), 693–705. https://doi.org/10.1080/10503307.2019.1658912

Watson, J. C., Steckley, P. L., & McMullen, E. J. (2014). The role of empathy in promoting change. *Psychotherapy Research, 24*(3), 286–298. https://doi.org/10.1080/10503307.2013.802823

Wispé, L. (1987). History of the concept of empathy. In N. Eisenberg & J. Strayer (Eds.), *Empathy and development* (pp. 17–37). Cambridge University Press.

Woodin, E. M., Sotskova, A., & O'Leary, K. D. (2012). Do motivational interviewing behaviors predict reductions in partner aggression for men and women? *Behaviour Research and Therapy, 50*(1), 79–84. https://doi.org/10.1016/j.brat.2011.11.001

Yalom, I. D. (1980). *Existential psychotherapy.* Basic Books.

Yalom, I. D. (2001). *The gift of therapy.* Harper Collins.

6

Working With Emotions in Existential–Humanistic Psychotherapy

Brittany Varisco and Louis Hoffman

Emotion is a central focus of psychotherapy, and successful emotional processing has repeatedly been associated with positive treatment outcomes and change across therapeutic modalities (Whelton, 2004). Existential and phenomenological perspectives have sought to more deeply understand the experiential, subjective, lived experience of feelings across a variety of contexts from everyday emotional experiences to mood disorders, depression, and psychosis (Bortolan, 2017; Ghaemi, 2006; Heavey et al., 2012; Vodušek et al., 2014). The controversy surrounding the definition, understanding, and place of emotion is as long as the history of the field itself. Furthermore, there has historically been a lack of research surrounding specific change processes, therapeutic factors, and therapist and client characteristics that contribute to working with emotions. In this chapter, we begin with a brief generalist overview of emotion before detailing an existential–humanistic (EH) understanding of emotion. In considering research on emotion, we focus on qualitative and quantitative research that supports the EH approach to emotion in psychotherapy. As the understanding, expression, and valuing of emotion is strongly influenced by culture, we next give consideration to multicultural perspectives before concluding with consideration of future research needs.

https://doi.org/10.1037/0000446-007
The Evidence-Based Foundations of Existential–Humanistic Therapy, L. Hoffman and V. Lac (Editors)

UNDERSTANDING EMOTIONS IN PSYCHOTHERAPY

Emphasis on emotions and emotional processing gained momentum in the early 2000s and onward, and the bulk of the existing research comes from the career-long pursuits of Greenberg and colleagues' work in emotion-focused therapy (EFT), an integrative, neo-humanistic, experiential approach that synthesizes aspects of person-centered therapy, Gestalt therapy, experiential therapy, and existential therapy alongside modern cognitive, attachment, interpersonal, psychodynamic, and narrative theories (Greenberg, 2017). EFT has endeavored to distinguish core processes and principles for working with emotions across therapeutic modalities and believes the therapeutic relationship to be critically important for facilitating and holding emotional transformation. Through this lens, emotions are believed to be innately adaptive as well as the means and measure of one's engagement in the world (Whelton, 2004). Emotions provide information about our existential needs and are evolutionarily essential to our survival by organizing our experiences and motivating us to take purposeful action (Pascual-Leone et al., 2016). In essence, emotions should not be viewed as problematic aspects of the human experience to be controlled or eradicated but instead should be faced, experienced, explored, and processed to gain information, create meaning, and motivate adaptive and productive action (Greenberg & Pascual-Leone, 2006; Pos & Greenberg, 2007; Pos et al., 2009). Although this is one of many definitions, it points to the complexity of emotions and emotional processing and highlights the nuanced relationships between physiology, lived experience, cognition, and behavior.

Emotional processing therefore requires both the visceral, somatic experience of emotion as well as cognitive evaluation and meaning making (Teasdale, 1999; Whelton, 2004) in the pursuit of helping clients identify, experience, express, explore, make sense of, and flexibly respond to their emotions (Greenberg, 2002, as cited in Pos et al., 2009). Dysfunction and distress are believed to arise from the experience of emotions rather than the emotions themselves, such as a lack of emotional awareness, unproductive emotional responses (born from unprocessed affect, trauma, secondary emotions, and undifferentiated emotions), emotion dysregulation (over- and underregulated emotions), and difficulty in developing adaptive narratives and meaning from emotional experiences (Greenberg et al., 2019).

In much of Western culture, emotions are often viewed as something to be controlled, suppressed, or eradicated (Hoffman, 2019). Furthermore, there is an implicit assumption that uncomfortable or painful emotions, such as anxiety, sadness, and anger, are bad, whereas pleasant emotions, such as happiness, are good. This has impacted the norms about emotions and emotional expression, which deeply influenced the field of psychology and psychiatry, especially through the development of the various versions of the *Diagnostic and Statistical Manual of Mental Disorders* (5th ed.; American Psychiatric Association, 2013) and the *International Statistical Classification of Diseases and Related Health Problems* (11th ed; World Health Organization, 2019*)*. Henretty and colleagues (2008) pose a criticism of Western psychology's subscription to diagnoses and the *Diagnostic and Statistical Manual of Mental Disorders*, as they believe it to perpetuate the pathologization and stigmatization of emotional experiences that may be especially pronounced when approaching the expression, experience, and meaning of emotions of diverse cultures.

CONTEXTUALIZING EMOTIONS IN AN EH CONTEXT

Hoffman and colleagues (2015) view working with emotion as a core aspect of EH therapy. Yet the emphasis on emotions is not always agreed upon. Bugental (1987) likens emotions in therapy to blood in surgery, stating, "Both are inevitable as the work goes forward; both importantly serve a cleansing function and foster healing; both must be respected and dealt with by the professional; and neither is the point of the procedure" (p. 113). He believes increasing awareness of one's existence, powers, choices, and limits to be the purpose of therapy, guided and accompanied by strong and painful feelings. For many EH psychologists, emotions are embedded within the broader idea of embodiment, or one's lived experience, and are a central component of depth therapy.

Rollo May (1950/1977), the primary originator of EH therapy, writes extensively about anxiety, which he views as ontological. In other words, anxiety is embedded in the human condition and arises from the threat of nonexistence and the need to fulfill one's potential. Its presence is a marked sign of inner conflict that seeks to convey information and impart lessons. May as well as Kierkegaard (1844/1944, 1844/1976) describe *healthy anxiety* as life enhancing in its ability to move a person toward actualization, adaptivity, and creativity, whereas *unhealthy anxiety* is life constricting in its sacrifice of freedom, movement away from potential, and stagnation. Their belief is that unhealthy anxiety stems from the inability to face, move through, and process ontological anxiety and that this understanding of healthy and unhealthy experiences can be more broadly applied to all emotions. In stating that emotions are ontological, one is maintaining that emotions are a normal part of the human condition and that all emotions, at their core, are healthy. As discussed by May and Kierkegaard, this is not to say that all emotional experiences are healthy. The way individuals respond and relate to their emotions—including repression, suppression, avoidance, denial, and impulsive acting based upon strong feelings—can be problematic (Hoffman, 2019). Similarly, Diamond's (1996) expansion of May's work with the daimonic speaks to the natural tendency of emotions that have both constructive and destructive potentials and are considered to be neither inherently good nor inherently evil. It is when these tendencies and emotions are denied, avoided, and repressed that they can become problematic, distressing, and all consuming.

Hoffman (2019) maintains that, from an EH perspective, emotions can be understood as a way of knowing. As such, instead of managing, controlling, or repressing emotions, it behooves the individual to listen to them. However, at times, emotions may become intense enough to overwhelm the client, making it difficult to listen to the wisdom the emotion has to offer. When this occurs, it may be necessary to help clients develop emotional management skills that build confidence in regulating emotions and improve the ability to withstand uncomfortable and painful affect (Hoffman, 2020). If these emotions cannot be managed relationally or through the client's current coping mechanisms, EH therapists utilize somatic interventions, mindfulness, or integrative approaches (e.g., polyvagal exercises) to sufficiently regulate emotions in order to begin working with them in therapy.

In therapy, EH therapists work with emotion in a variety of ways. Bugental (1987) describes a process of moving in and out of emotion, warning against the strategy of focusing solely on the arousal as he acknowledges the idiosyncratic differences between clients' capacities to experience and express emotion. He highlights the need to attend to not only what is stated but also how it is said, and he posits that the use of more or less attention to client affectivity facilitates and modulates the emotional flow. For Bugental, curiosity is also foundational. Moving in and out of emotion with curiosity allows clients to experience and learn from their emotions, as well as gain distance from the emotion to engage in meaning making. He also believes in the importance of making explicit that which is manifest but implicit. This may be done through reflection, attunement, and well-timed phrasing, which means helping clients express and articulate their inner subjective experiences. Bugental's emphasis on emotion and nervous system regulation in therapy was ahead of his time, and echoes of his work can be found in prominent theories today such as Schore's (1994) regulation theory and Porges's (2011) polyvagal theory.

Schneider (2008; Schneider & Krug, 2017) discusses therapeutic stances that are foundational to EH therapy, including invoking the actual and vivifying self-protections (i.e., resistance), which serve as invitations for clients to engage with their inner emotional world. Invoking the actual invites the client to connect with a fuller presence or embodiment, including emotions. Similarly, vivifying self-protections works to intensify their experience of self-protection, which generally entails an emotional component. Schneider also utilizes what he refers to as *embodied meditation* that involves meditative strategies to encourage clients to engage with what is palpably present. An important aspect of his existential–integrative model of therapy is its ability to adapt EH practices in a variety of settings, across clinical presentations, and among diverse populations (Schneider, 2008). The utility of this approach is of importance when considering unique client capacities for emotional awareness, expression, and regulation, especially when more structured and skill-based interventions are necessary alongside or prior to depth worth.

The concept of presence is foundational to working with emotions (see Chapter 5 of this volume). The development of therapeutic presence creates a space that invites emotions into the therapy room. Yalom (1980, 1989) discusses the therapist's disclosure, particularly here-and-now disclosure, which can be understood as an aspect of presence. Through the client's own embodiment and sharing of aspects of their emotional experience, clients are able to witness and experience the value of emotional disclosure and move into their own emotional experience and expression.

QUANTITATIVE RESEARCH

Building on the original principles and processes for working with emotion (Greenberg & Pascual-Leone, 2006), Pascual-Leone and colleagues (2016) adapted the categories for humanistic–experiential therapies. Each of these processes will be explored in our review of existing research and are believed to be necessary, though not individually sufficient, for successful work with emotions and, ultimately, transformation: (a) emotional awareness and engagement, (b) arousal and expression or enactment, (c) regulation and self-soothing, and (d) reflection and meaning making. The process of emotional transformation will be discussed more thoroughly in the review of qualitative research. The message we hope to convey is that working with emotions is dynamic and nuanced, involves multiple interrelated and overlapping processes, relies on a strong therapeutic relationship impacted by therapist characteristics, and is unique to the features and capacity of each client.

Emotional Awareness and Engagement

Emotional awareness is a cognitive skill demonstrated by the ability to both recognize and describe bodily felt emotions in oneself and in others, which precedes and is differentiated from emotional expression. Lane and colleagues' (1990) early work serves as the foundation for the development of the five levels of emotional awareness of increasing complexity that progress from awareness of bodily sensations and urges to naming emotions to feeling multiple differentiated emotions and developing empathy (Levels of Emotional Awareness Scale; Lane et al., 1990, 2022). Difficulties with emotional awareness— and arguably other emotional processes, such as depth of experiencing, emotional arousal, and emotion regulation—are believed to stem from skill deficits (i.e., developmental disruptions) and self-protective mechanisms (i.e., suppression, avoidance, and repression; Lane et al., 2022). This aligns with EH psychology's belief that emotional distress arises from a lack of emotional awareness and the inability to approach and move through painful emotions (Kierkegaard, 1844/1944, 1844/1976; May 1950/1977) as well as that the avoidance and suppression of emotional experiences can result in all-consuming distress (i.e., the daimonic; Diamond, 1996).

Emotional awareness has been shown to correlate positively with self-restraint and impulse control, and it is believed to be essential for emotion regulation (Lane et al., 2022). In a summary of research, Lane and colleagues (2022) explore the role of enhanced emotional awareness in promoting change across cognitive behavior, emotion-focused and experiential, and psychodynamic

therapies. All three approaches deemed the enhancement of emotional awareness to be necessary but not sufficient by itself for therapeutic change and shared
a mutual belief that until painful emotions are attended to, they will influence
thoughts, emotions, and behaviors outside of one's awareness. These findings
highlight emotional awareness as a gateway for depth work and the embodiment of emotions, which aligns with interventions used in EH therapy.

Thompson and colleagues (2011) investigate the relationship between emotional awareness and intensity of emotional experience in a nonclinical sample
of adults utilizing negative and positive affect measures derived from the Positive Affect Negative Affect Scale (D. Watson et al., 1988), Ekman's basic emotions (Ekman et al., 1972), and the Trait Meta-Mood Scale (Salovey et al.,
1995). Over the course of a week, participants were randomly prompted to
attend to and assess their current emotions. Findings show that attention to
and awareness of emotion were associated with higher levels of both positive
and negative emotions in the moment, meaning that increased awareness of
emotion elicited a higher intensity experience. Interestingly, they find that
attending to negative emotions over a period ranging from a few minutes to a
few hours dictated a decrease in intensity, which supports the premise that
emotional awareness is necessary for regulating and modulating emotion. This
aligns with Bugental's (1987) belief that increasing awareness of one's existence is accompanied by strong and painful emotions that must be moved
through for healing and transformation.

Alexithymia, which is conceptualized as a deficit in skill, involves difficulty
identifying, labeling, differentiating, and describing the emotions of oneself and
others and is associated with a variety of mental health conditions such as
trauma, substance use, mood disorders, eating disorders, panic disorders, psychosomatic disorders, anxiety, and personality disorders (Lane et al., 2022;
Peluso & Freund, 2018, 2019; Whelton, 2004). Additionally, it is related to poor
treatment outcomes in interpretive (i.e., psychodynamic) and supportive (i.e.,
skills based) forms of individual and group therapy (McCallum et al., 2003;
Ogrodniczuk et al., 2011). Higher levels of client alexithymia and less expression of positive emotion have also been associated with negative therapist reactions and poor therapeutic outcome, which highlights the importance of the
therapist's awareness of their own reactions, transference, and emotional
expression toward clients (Ogrodniczuk et al., 2008, 2011).

In terms of engagement, depth of experiencing is positively related to outcome across therapeutic orientations and is believed to be a common factor and
core change process (Pascual-Leone et al., 2016; Pascual-Leone & Yeryomenko,
2017; Whelton, 2004). Wiser and Goldfried (1998) explore the relationship
between transtheoretical interventions and depth of experiencing for clients
with depression and anxiety in cognitive behavior therapy (CBT) and
psychodynamic–interpersonal therapy (PI). They assess depth of experiencing
using the Experiencing Scale (Klein et al., 1986), which measures engagement,
productivity, and depth of experiencing and emotional processing. Interventions
associated with maintaining high levels of experiencing included affiliative (i.e.,

friendly) and noncontrolling stances, reflections and acknowledgements, and minimal, nonspecific comments (e.g., "Hmm, I see"). Interventions that elicited shifts to lower levels of experiencing included verbally lengthy interventions, moderately and highly controlling stances, close-ended questions, and interventions that avoided emotional content with some of these trends occurring more notably in the CBT interventions. This aligns with EH practices of helping clients to move in and out of the depths of experiencing using statements or summaries, reflection of emotions (i.e., a "felt" experience and depth of experiencing), and questions (i.e., a cognitive shift to less depth; Bugental, 1987).

Jeanne C. Watson and Bedard (2006) further explore depth of experiencing in CBT and process–experiential therapy (PET) for depression and find that higher levels of emotional processing and depth of experiencing predicted better outcomes. Clients with good outcomes were observed to engage in deeper exploration, refer to emotions more frequently, internally focus on their bodily experiences, examine and reflect on the experience, and create new meaning. In both CBT and PET good outcome groups, greater levels of emotional processing and depth of experiencing occurred as compared to the poor outcome groups. Although there was no difference observed in symptom reduction between CBT and PET therapies, clients who engaged in experiential therapy showed higher overall levels of depth of experiencing than those in the CBT group. These findings further highlight how experiential work and focusing on emotions is a fundamental cornerstone to depth therapies such as EH therapy.

Pos and colleagues (2003) compare depth of experiencing in early and late stages of experiential therapy in relation to outcomes for depression. They find that depth of experiencing increased over the course of therapy and note that clients arrived in therapy with different capacities to experience, express, and reflect on emotional experiences. Though this initial capacity was important, it was the depth of experiencing in later therapy that was deemed to be the sole independent predictor of outcome. Pos and colleagues (2009) build upon these findings by exploring the relationship between depth of experiencing and the working alliance across phases of therapy. They find that both depth of experiencing and the working alliance deepened over the course of therapy and, most notably, that depth of experiencing in the working phase of therapy was the best predictor of outcome above and beyond early levels of processing or the alliance. Pos and colleagues' contributions highlight the additive power and interactions of the working alliance, emotional processing, and depth work. More importantly, their message is rooted in hope that clients with limited capacity for depth of experiencing at the onset of therapy are not doomed to poor outcomes, but rather that their ability to grow and develop the capacity is the marker for successful outcome and transformation.

Arousal, Expression, and Enactment

There is no rulebook or general guidelines for the effective arousal and expression of emotion, as "it depends on what the emotion is, how it is expressed, by

whom, to whom, when, under what conditions, what the underlying therapeutic condition is" (Whelton, 2004, p. 60) in addition to the strength of the
therapeutic relationship. The expression and arousal of emotion is not always
therapeutically beneficial and depends on whether the emotion is over- or
underregulated and whether the emotion is a signal of overwhelming distress
or a marker of working through distress (Greenberg, 2002, as cited in Pascual-
Leone et al., 2016). The concept of catharsis, or experiencing high arousal for
high arousal's sake, is considered to be an incomplete and potentially antitherapeutic practice (Whelton, 2004), and Yalom (1980) would agree that arousing
affect for arousal's sake serves no therapeutic benefit. Furthermore, it is important to differentiate what type of emotion is being expressed, such as undifferentiated global distress, an emotion about an emotion (i.e., secondary emotion),
or whether the emotion moves a client toward or away from adaptive action.
EFT literature refers to adaptive and maladaptive emotions; however, EH therapists would conceptualize this as life-enhancing and life-constricting emotional experiences, or productive and unproductive emotional experiences.

Carryer and Greenberg (2010) explore the relationship between the amount
of time spent in high arousal and outcome for clients receiving EFT for depression using the Client Expressed Emotional Arousal Scale III—Revised (Warwar
& Greenberg, 1999) alongside session outcome and symptom outcome measures. Their landmark findings show that 25% of a session spent in highly
aroused emotional states was the optimal frequency that predicted good outcomes. Duration of high arousal greater than or less than 25% of a session
predicted poorer outcomes and highlighted the EH practice benefit of facilitating clients' movement in and out of heightened emotional states. Like someone
learning how to swim, allowing a client to come up for air from the depths of
emotional experiences is necessary and therapeutic, just as holding someone
underwater for extended periods of time is both antitherapeutic and harmful.

In a similar vein, Mackay and colleagues (2002) explore optimal times during session for arousal and find that productive arousal of unpleasant emotion
in sessions of psychodynamic–interpersonal therapy followed an inverted
U-shaped pattern, meaning the highest arousal of painful emotion occurred
during the middle of a session and tapered off or returned to baseline by the
session's end, thus allowing clients space and time to regulate and contain powerful affect before the end of the session. Similarly, McCarthy and colleagues
(2014) investigate differences in early-session dialogues between most improved
and least improved client–therapist dyads using the Therapeutic Cycles Model
(Mergenthaler, 1996) to analyze session transcripts. The most improved dyads
spent more time connecting highly aroused emotions with reflection and
meaning making during the first 40 minutes of the session. In contrast, the
least improved dyads spent time connecting arousal and meaning during the
last 20 minutes of the session, whereas the most improved dyads moved to a
lower aroused relaxing phase during this time. This emphasizes the importance
of awareness and time management to facilitate depths of experiencing and
heightened arousal in the constraints of a session.

In terms of productive and unproductive emotional arousal, Missirlian and colleagues (2005) find that high arousal in addition to high levels of reflection (i.e., meaning making) distinguished good and poor outcomes for clients receiving experiential therapy for depression. This combination was a stronger predictor of improvement than either process alone. They noted that high levels of arousal during early and working phases of therapy allowed clients' emotions to be readily accessible for reflection, and toward the end of therapy, levels of arousal were reduced and reflective processing increased. This supports the overarching premise of emotion-focused work and EH therapy: to assist clients with moving from a state of high arousal and low meaning to a place of high meaning and low arousal (Pascual-Leone & Greenberg, 2007).

Auszra and colleagues (2013) further explore the nuances of client emotional processing using the Client Emotional Productivity Scale—Revised (Auszra et al., 2010), which considers multiple factors, such as the level of arousal, type of emotion, and manner of processing (i.e., attending to emotion, symbolizing emotion in words, congruence of verbalization and experienced emotion, acceptance, regulation, agency, and differentiation). They find high productivity during the working phase of therapy to be the sole predictor of outcome beyond working alliance, high arousal, or baseline capacity for productivity. They note that clients whose productivity increased throughout treatment improved the most, which highlights that the ability to develop and grow capacity is a more important predictor of therapeutic progress than initial capacity.

In terms of the therapeutic relationship and therapist processes, two meta-analyses show that client expression and experiencing of emotion predicted a stronger therapeutic relationship and in-session progress (Peluso & Freund, 2018; 2019) and therapist facilitation of client emotional expression and experiencing increased client success rates from 35% to 65% in psychodynamic therapy (Diener et al., 2007). The more a therapist focuses on, attends to, and facilitates emotional expression, the more clients will experience growth, enduring change, and positive outcomes (Diener et al., 2007). Town and colleagues (2017) explore the relationship between affect experiencing (AE), distress, and therapeutic alliance in intensive short-term dynamic psychotherapy for depression. They discover that correlations between AE and distress could discriminate between good and poor outcome groups. Specifically, clients with good outcomes demonstrated higher in-session peak affect, which led to a reduction in distress seven days later. Furthermore, AE was associated with strengthening the therapeutic alliance, as was evidenced by client and therapist assessments of the bond. Iwakabe and colleagues (2000) caution that the arousal and expression of emotion alone does not facilitate change if the emotion is not fully and accurately received, attended to, and addressed by the therapist.

Regulation and Self-Soothing

Emotion regulation is considered to be foundational to working with emotions and is a measure of how individuals respond to and modify their emotional experiences through awareness, flexibility, modulation of arousal and expression, acceptance, and reflection (Sloan et al., 2017). The development of emotion regulation capacity is vital for depth of emotional processing (Greenberg & Pascual-Leone, 2006), and the therapeutic relationship is considered to be an affect-regulating bond that, over the course of therapy, becomes internalized by the client (Greenberg, 2014). There is a dynamic balance between facilitating intense but bearable emotional arousal, enhancing depth of experiencing and arousal for clients with emotional constriction (i.e., overregulated emotional experiencing), and helping clients regulate overwhelming emotions (i.e., underregulated emotional experiencing; Pascual-Leone et al., 2016). The short-term goal is to assist clients in gaining distance from or access to painful emotions, with the long-term goal of developing an internalized repertoire for coping (Greenberg & Pascual-Leone, 2006; Pascual-Leone et al., 2016). EH psychology would agree that until painful emotions can be tolerated, they will remain unexperienced, unarticulated, and without meaning, and thus they cannot be learned from to guide adaptive action (Kierkegaard, 1844/1944, 1844/1976; May, 1950/1977; Pascual-Leone et al., 2016).

Without sufficient regulation capacity, experiencing and expressing emotions may be too painful and overwhelming for clients (Hoffman, 2020). Emotional avoidance and suppression have been routinely linked to poor therapeutic outcomes and the maintenance of psychological distress and symptoms. Scherer and colleagues (2017) explore emotion regulation strategies (e.g., reappraisal, suppression, externalization) and outcomes in CBT in both inpatient and outpatient settings. They discover emotional suppression to be the predictor of therapeutic outcome beyond externalization and reappraisal, with high levels of suppression associated with poor outcome. They suggest that clients with higher levels of suppression may have difficulty forming a strong therapeutic alliance and tolerating emotional arousal. In their work with clients with Cluster C personality disorders, a population considered to struggle with emotional avoidance and suppression (i.e., affect phobia), Schanche and colleagues (2011) find that increases in activating affects (i.e., adaptive emotions, such as assertive anger, self-compassion, grief or hurt, acceptance, agency) and decreases in inhibiting affects (e.g., terror, shame, guilt) were significantly associated with increases in self-compassion and good outcomes in both cognitive therapy and short-term psychodynamic therapy. Importantly, it was not the experience and activation of emotion in general, but rather the activation of previously avoided affect and core pain that predicted increases in self-compassion. Ulvenes and colleagues (2014) further find that affect-focused therapy for clients living with Cluster C personality disorders may not lead to productive emotional experiences if clients are experiencing high levels of negativity and self-criticism. It is the combination of therapists orienting clients toward affect alongside the client's sense of self and self-compassion that predicts the activation of emotion.

Symbolizing the lived, visceral experience and making the implicit explicit has been regarded as a foundational component of EH therapy (Bugental,

1987). In terms of emotion regulation skills, fMRI studies have shown labeling emotions to be a form of emotion regulation, as it reduces the activity in the amygdala and limbic regions in the presence of negative emotional images and autobiographical memories (Lieberman et al., 2007). Extensions of this research have shown that putting feelings into words, though considered to be implicit emotion regulation, yields similar results as other forms of explicit regulation strategies such as reappraisal, problem solving, and acceptance (Torre & Lieberman, 2018).

In a systematic review of 67 studies, Sloan and colleagues (2017) investigate the role of emotion regulation and outcomes for anxiety, depression, substance use, eating disorders, and borderline personality disorder using both Gross's (1998) process model and Gratz and Roemer's (2004) deficit model to conceptualize emotion dysregulation. Sloan and colleagues find that regardless of intervention used, treatment modality, or disorder, maladaptive emotion regulation strategies (e.g., rumination, suppression, avoidance) and overall emotion dysregulation were seen to significantly decrease in all but two studies. They also note a parallel reduction in symptoms across all disorders. Similarly, in a meta-analysis of 38 studies, Iwakabe and colleagues (2023) find large gains in the ability to regulate emotions regardless of intervention and conclude that both exploratory (i.e., affect focused) and structured (i.e., skill building) interventions lead to improvements in regulation.

Reflection and Meaning Making

It is the reciprocal interaction and integration of emotion and narrative that leads to change in which "personal stories are given significance and salience when fused with emotions, and emotions are supplied with meaning when placed within a narrative context" (Angus & Greenberg, 2011, as cited in Carpenter et al., 2016, p. 70). It is this integration of felt experience with meaning making, a core concept of EH psychology, that defines successful emotional processing and transformation. The Narrative–Emotion Process Coding System (NEPCS; Angus et al., 2017; Boritz et al., 2014) identifies autobiographical memory and narrative organization, expression of emotion, and self-reflective processes. The system is built on research supporting the idea that processing emerging emotions in the context of personal autobiographical memories facilitates emotion regulation, meaning making, and the reformulation of self-identity and narratives. The NEPCS is composed of three types of narrative–emotion process markers and storytelling styles: problem markers associated with underregulated, overregulated, and unintegrated emotions and the maintenance of distress (e.g., same old, empty, unstoried, superficial storytelling); transition markers associated with movement toward narrative and emotion integration (e.g., competing plotlines, inchoate, experiential, reflective storytelling); and change markers denoted by narrative coherence, differentiated emotions, new meaning, and narrative reconstruction (i.e., unexpected outcome, discovery storytelling).

Carpenter and colleagues (2016) investigate narrative and emotion integration processes in experiential emotion-focused trauma therapy for complex trauma. NEPCS analysis revealed clients in the good outcome group were able to approach and regulate painful emotions (unstoried emotion) by verbally symbolizing, differentiating, and exploring painful emotions in the context of traumatic narratives (inchoate story). This enabled self-coherence and a deeper level of self-understanding (discovery story), which led to new adaptive ways of being and a restructuring of identity and self-narrative (unexpected outcome story) that challenged the problematic same old story (competing plotline story). Similar to the NEPCS analysis of depression (Boritz et al., 2014) and generalized anxiety disorder (GAD; Angus & Macaulay, 2023) across therapeutic modalities and theoretical orientations, clients in the poor outcome group articulated significantly more problem markers than recovered clients, and recovered clients evidenced significantly more change markers than their unchanged counterparts.

In a process–outcome study of complex trauma and emotion-focused trauma therapy, Khayyat-Abuaita and colleagues (2019) expand on previous NEPCS research to explore discrete moment-by-moment emotional experiences that occur in productive narratives. Utilizing Pascual-Leone and Greenberg's (2007) Sequential Model of Emotional Processing, which will be explored in the qualitative summary, the authors find significantly higher frequencies of adaptive emotional experiences (i.e., articulating existential needs, assertive anger, self-compassion, grief and hurt, acceptance, and agency) in late-session narratives of good outcome cases. Though both good outcome and poor outcome cases exhibited high levels of global, undifferentiated distress in early-session narratives, it was the ability of clients in good outcome cases to move from undifferentiated distress to highly aroused core pain to adaptive emotions that promote recovery, as proposed by May (1950/1977) and Kierkegaard's (1844/1944, 1844/1976) conceptualizations of healthy and unhealthy anxiety. The analysis emphasizes that as little as one minute of adaptive emotions during a session can double a client's potential for having a good treatment outcome (Khayyat-Abuaita et al., 2019).

Boritz and colleagues (2011) explore the relationship between autobiographical memory specificity and emotional intensity during sessions of EFT and cognitive therapy for depression. Clients with depression tend to demonstrate overgeneralized, nonspecific autobiographical memory narratives (i.e., summary memory), which align with Bortolan's (2017) phenomenological conceptualization of depression as a disturbance of the narrative self. Clients with good outcomes demonstrated higher proportions of specific autobiographical memories and peak emotional arousal across all stages of therapy, which was attributed to the evocation of experiential imagery that led to deeper levels of emotional intensity. Conversely, clients who continued to experience depression at termination showed lower levels of arousal during autobiographical narratives, which may indicate difficulty in tolerating the symbolization and expression of emotions. Most importantly, the study showed that neither narrative processes nor emotional processes alone were related to outcome but rather their integration facilitated therapeutic gains.

QUALITATIVE RESEARCH

Qualitative studies on emotions provide a nuanced, vivid, and in-depth exploration of therapeutic processes and give voice to the lived experiences of clients and therapists. In our review of qualitative research, we focus on narrative accounts, case studies, and phenomenological conceptualizations of emotional processes, emotional experiences, therapist characteristics, and experiential therapy.

Experiential Therapy

Marren and colleagues (2022) conducted a qualitative meta-analysis to explore clients' experiences with EFT to learn what they found helpful, difficult but helpful, and unhelpful. The analysis shows all clients found the experiential and emotionally evocative work to be powerful, with most describing it as helpful. For the few who found it unhelpful, reasons cited were inability to tolerate, engage with, or regulate during experiential interventions. A range of helpful experiences were identified, including awareness and differentiation of emotions, experiencing and processing emotions, and the relief and progress born from the difficult confrontation of previously ignored affects. In terms of the therapeutic relationship, emotional connection, support, validation, and understanding were commonly experienced as helpful. Their study highlights the dynamic integration of interwoven processes of emotional awareness, arousal, and regulation in the context of a strong therapeutic relationship.

In addition to difficulties with emotional awareness, regulation, and tolerating strong emotions, self-criticism has been shown to play a significant role in the etiology and maintenance of psychological distress. Bell and colleagues (2020) explore clients' lived experience of compassion-focused therapy's experiential chairwork for self-criticism and depression. Compassion-focused therapy's form of role-playing chairwork incorporates an additional chair for the compassionate self to interact with the critical and criticized selves when compared with traditional chairwork in EFT. In their interpretive phenomenological analysis, three superordinate themes emerged: embodiment and enactment, externalizing the self in physical form, and emotional intensity. In shifting between different forms of self, the participants expressed changes in mentality, affect, and somatic experiences that provided awareness of the presence, urges, purpose, and motivations of each self. Additionally, they highlighted accessing previously unavailable, vulnerable emotions. Externalization of the parts of self thus allowed participants to gain insight and draw connections between their intrapersonal and interpersonal ways of relating. All participants highlighted the intense, conflicting, and varied emotions they encountered and were observed to regulate their arousal by shifting in and out of heightened affect by moving chairs and engaging with another self. This led to a sense of agency and openness to experiencing emotions more fully, which aligns with previous research that experiential chairwork facilitates emotional regulation, self-efficacy, and resilience. Participants who previously engaged in CBT described that chairwork helped them link their head with their heart, which further supports existing research on the necessary presence of both cognition and the visceral felt experience for effective emotional processing (Teasdale, 1999). Henretty and colleagues (2008) also capture clients' paradoxical struggles with the benefit of exploring and experiencing sadness in therapy and the fear of vulnerability, discomfort, pathologization, and overwhelm. They also note a similar pattern of regulating arousal and overwhelm where clients would shift between varying levels of emotional intensity. Both studies highlight and emphasize Bugental's (1987) practice of helping clients move in and out of emotional arousal to facilitate regulation, curiosity, and meaning making. The ability to distance oneself temporarily from emotional arousal and respond flexibly to the ebb and flow of emotion during a session is believed to be productive to the therapy process and beneficial to the therapeutic relationship (Bugental, 1987). Henretty and colleagues (2008) also highlight how the stigmatization and pathologization of the ontological human experience of emotions (e.g., sadness) can perpetuate distress and emotional avoidance.

Timulak and colleagues (2017) conducted an exploratory study of EFT for GAD to assess the pre–post outcomes of 13 clients as well as their experience of the interventions and personal change. Quantitatively, the pre–post and 6 month follow-up data show large effect sizes, and these significant outcomes tentatively meet or exceed the findings from studies of other theoretical approaches. Qualitatively, all clients reported increased self-awareness and most noted less anxiety and improved emotional functioning. In terms of the therapeutic experience, clients indicate the soothing and validating nature of the therapeutic relationship as well as the experiential and in-depth work to be aspects they valued most, in light of describing the latter as difficult but helpful. The benefits of this shorter term therapy (16–20 sessions) extend far beyond mere symptom improvement to include a heightened sense of confidence, resilience, and self-compassion. This study also highlights the importance of identifying client capacity to tolerate and regulate emotions in service of facilitating exposure to painful but bearable affective experiences.

Therapist Characteristics

Few studies have explored clients' perceptions of and responses to therapists' emotional expression. Using a narrative thematic analysis of 10 semistructured interviews, Viou and colleagues (2018) identify two distinct functions of therapists' emotions and facial expressions: (a) facilitating connection and strengthening the therapeutic relationship and (b) providing alternative ways to experience emotions and motivating clients toward change. Analysis highlights six themes that emerged related to clients' assessment of therapist emotions and facial expressions: excitement (associated with joy and reassurance), calmness (associated with security and emotional regulation), affection (associated with trust and security), empathy and sadness (associated with genuine compassion and feeling understood), and anger. When therapists exhibited anger, an emotion that clients described as difficult to identify and express in their personal lives, clients stated it helped them better connect with and relate to their own feelings of anger. Viou and colleagues encourage therapists to consider emotional expression as part of the self-disclosure process that should be utilized in a way that is therapeutic, regulated, and professional. EH psychology emphasizes the importance of therapeutic presence, attunement, and the therapeutic relationship, which have been shown to have great impacts on emotional processes and emotional transformation in addition to the power of therapeutic disclosure in the here-and-now.

Additionally, therapist prosody (i.e., pitch, intonation, pitch accent, rhythm, and loudness of speech) directly impacts emotional processing during sessions. Through conversation analysis of 70 sessions of cognitive and psychoanalytic therapy, Weiste and Peräkylä (2014) identify two trajectories following therapist verbalizations of client's emotions: (a) validating trajectories marked by therapist's validation, understanding, and acceptance of the client's affect in addition to the therapist speaking with a quiet, low, level voice which matches the rhythm of the client's speech (i.e., prosodic continuity) and (b) challenging trajectories in which the therapist challenges the client's emotions, misattunes, or provides interpretation or evaluation in addition to the therapist speaking in a higher pitch, louder volume, and asynchronous rhythm when compared with the client's speech (i.e. prosodic disjuncture). Clients responded to the validating trajectory by staying with the emotion, feeling understood, and continuing to reflect on the experience and the challenging trajectory with silence, disagreement, and a sense of feeling misunderstood. Even when the expression of cognitive understanding of an emotional experience was present, it was not perceived as empathic communication without prosodic continuity. Absence of empathic responding and chronic misinterpreting, ignoring, and overlooking clients' emotions has been associated with the suppression of future emotional expressions, as posited by Anderson et al. (2008) as a possible explanation for low frequencies of verbalized emotional distress in patients with advanced cancer diagnoses. EH psychology places value on therapeutic presence and the "being" of a therapist rather than the "doing." The way therapists nonverbally respond to clients in how they convey empathy carries as much weight as what they express verbally. The lived and felt experience in the here-and-now is not confined solely to clients but rather includes the visceral experiences of empathy by EH therapists.

Therapeutic Relationship

Banerjee and Basu (2016) explore client and therapist perspectives on the transformational role of the therapeutic relationship. Through the interpretive phenomenological analysis of therapist–client dyads in India (CBT and psycho-analytic), five major themes emerge, as well as the processes resulting from them: listening, containment, reflection of past relationships (i.e., transference), surrender–obedience, and curative relational experience. Both therapists and clients associated listening with creating a space for emotional unburdening. In terms of containment, the dyads considered the therapist's understanding and tolerance of clients' emotions to facilitate the ability to accept, tolerate, and regulate difficult and previously unarticulated emotions. Whereas therapists believed that reflecting on past relationships (i.e., transference) bolstered insight, clients experienced this reflection to generate emotional strength and agency. Surrender–obedience captured the clients' trust in the therapist and motivation to engage in therapeutic processes (i.e., depth of experiencing). Whereas clients were comfortable with this culturally grounded model, thera-pists who studied under a Western and European model of psychotherapy expressed discomfort with this format in light of it yielding therapeutic gains. Lastly, both clients and therapists agreed that curative relational experiences in the therapy space led to the reformulation of self-identity and relationships as well as that the therapeutic relationship, as a whole, was both significant and necessary for emotional processing and enduring therapeutic change.

Emotional Avoidance, Suppression, and Alexithymia

Coggins and Fox (2009) seek to understand the development, maintenance, and consequences of emotional inhibition (EI) through the subjective experi-ence of 10 university students and conclude that EI is likely a function of nega-tive meaning and beliefs surrounding emotions. Using grounded theory, the researchers identify five experiential categories: experience of emotions in childhood, experience of basic emotions, coping with emotions, and the main-tenance and consequences of EI. All participants experienced a significant neg-ative event in childhood that impacted emotional development and contributed to patterned EI. In terms of relating to basic emotions, a consistent theme emerged regarding avoidance of anger, as it was believed to be toxic and sepa-rated from one's sense of self, and the avoidance of sadness, as it signified "weakness" and vulnerability to rejection. To cope with their emotional experi-ences, the participants engaged in a variety of behaviors, including rumination, detachment, food restriction, potentially addictive behaviors, social withdrawal, and emotional coupling (i.e., using a more palatable emotion to mask or inhibit a distressing emotion). Interpersonal factors such as judgment, misunderstand-ing, and rejection influenced emotional expression and were believed to con-tribute to the maintenance of EI. All participants experienced negative impacts of EI on their physiological, cognitive, and social functioning as well as the paradoxical amplification of the emotion, which served to reinforce negative beliefs about emotions and emotional experiences.

Difficulties with emotion regulation have long been associated with anorexia nervosa and are believed to be a mechanism that maintains illness. In a pilot study of Cognitive Remediation and Emotion Skills Training, a brief and low-intensity intervention designed for use in acute inpatient settings, Money and colleagues (2011) explore 28 patients' experiences of emotion-focused interventions (i.e., skills based and psychoeducation). Content analysis shows that half the patients recognized their avoidance and suppression of affect and reported future-oriented intentions of expressing their emotions in relationships. In terms of what patients found helpful, learning to label emotions and learning the function of emotions (i.e., expression of needs) were cited as the most beneficial. The researchers also note that patients experienced secondary benefits of improved assertiveness and self-confidence over the course of the program. This study highlights the effectiveness of emotion-focused interventions in acute settings and speaks to the importance of identifying patients' capacity for emotions, meeting them where they are, and bolstering regulation skills to facilitate future depth work. Once again, these studies highlight the importance of tailoring therapy to clients' needs and adapting skills-focused and education-focused interventions as needed in the facilitation of depth work and emotional transformation.

Alexithymia, which is associated with trauma, substance use, mood disorders, eating disorders, panic disorders, psychosomatic disorders, anxiety, and personality disorders, has historically been considered to be a trait-like quality (see Taylor & Bagby, 2013). A literature review of 23 studies finds that interventions that specifically targeted alexithymic symptoms versus nontargeted interventions yield improvement in alexithymia across therapeutic modality and clinical diagnosis (Cameron et al., 2014). The authors also identify the interventions of psychoeducation, skill building, and group therapy as those most commonly used for symptom reduction. Schneider's (2008) integrative model embraces these findings and encourages therapists to flexibly adapt interventions, such as skill building, upon the foundation of EH theory.

Emotional Transformation

Building upon Pascual-Leone and Greenberg's (2007) Sequential Model of Emotional Processing, a transtheoretical and empirically validated model that was originally developed to identify in-session processes of emotional transformation, Timulak and Pascual-Leone (2015) created an expanded framework for transformation both within and across sessions.

Phase 1: Approaching Emotion and Exploring Distress
A state of high arousal and global distress is experienced in response to a past or present situation. Global distress is identified as an overarching sense of hopelessness or helplessness, secondary emotions, undifferentiated affect, or rejecting anger (i.e., general irritation and rage). Negative self-treatment is believed to both fuel core emotional pain and contribute to anticipatory fear of painful situations which can catalyze behavioral and emotional avoidance.

Phase 2: Working Through Primary Maladaptive Emotions (i.e., Core Pain)

Through approaching and exploring the surface layer of distress, clients grow in their ability to access primary, core painful emotions rooted in loneliness, shame, and fear or terror. This core pain is often considered to be overwhelming, and it is not atypical to observe clients collapsing into global distress and earlier phases of processing, though these collapses become less frequent over the course of therapy as emotional range and flexibility are strengthened (Pascual-Leone, 2009). Alongside the capacity to access core pain is the growing ability to articulate unmet existential needs.

Phase 3: Facilitating Adaptive Emotions

Once able to access core pain and articulate unmet existential needs, clients are able to enact self-soothing (i.e., self-compassion) or protective anger en route to grieving the unmet needs and the situations that led to the core painful emotions. This process ultimately leads to relief, agency, empowerment, emotional resiliency, and enduring change.

Dillon and colleagues (2018) seek to further understand the process of emotional transformation of a woman who had recovered from depression over the course of 15 sessions of EFT. Alongside Timulak and Pascual-Leone's (2015) findings, Dillon and colleagues also note behavioral and emotional avoidance and identify loneliness as central to core pain.

O'Brien and colleagues (2019) conducted a descriptive–interpretive study of 14 clients' presentations and difficulties in the context of GAD and EFT. Their findings further support Timulak and Pascual-Leone's (2015) framework. Unique to their analysis is the finding that anticipatory fear or worry protected from core pain as a form of emotional avoidance; however, the attempt to chronically brace for unexpected emotional pain heightened rather than diminished anxiety. O'Brien and colleagues (2019) argue that anxiety is not a form of intolerance to emotional experiences but rather the inability to tolerate specific emotions related to core pain that are embedded in personal histories and earlier adverse experiences. Additionally, O'Brien and colleagues (2019) provide qualitative descriptions of emotional regulation styles for each client (i.e., overregulated, underregulated, and mixed) and tentatively propose that overregulated styles may be predominated by emotional and behavioral avoidance processes whereas underregulated styles are hallmarked by undifferentiated global distress.

The model of emotional transformation, alongside EH theory (Kierkegaard, 1844/1944, 1844/1976; May, 1950/1977), would argue the importance of differentiating healthy from unhealthy emotional experiences (i.e., life enhancing vs. life constricting) and that different presentations of the same emotion have different meanings, such as rejecting anger and assertive anger. This aligns with Diamond's (1996) concept of the daimonic and the potential for emotions to have both a constructive and destructive nature. Emotional distress, as discussed throughout this literature review and this conceptualization, is born from unproductive, stagnant emotional experiences that remain unproductive until core pain is accessed and learned from to inform the presence of underlying unmet existential needs and motivate adaptive action to fulfill those needs.

MULTICULTURAL CONSIDERATIONS

Although emotion, as an ontological given, is experienced by people regardless of culture, how emotion is experienced, expressed, and understood varies. It is important to not assume that the same emotion, such as anger, is experienced in the same manner across people from different cultures. A skilled therapist is able to work with emotions in various forms of embodiment and expression while avoiding imposing a particular language or form of expression (Vallejos & Johnson, 2019). From an EH perspective, what is vital is that clients and therapists are able to listen to the wisdom of emotions and allow space for one to experience the breadth and depth of emotion.

Granger (2011), for example, discusses that many individuals in the Black community work to suppress their emotions because of fear of how others will respond to their emotional expression. This is connected to an implicit, racially biased message that people of color are too emotional. When therapists explicitly or implicitly encourage clients to calm down or express their emotions in a less intense manner, they may be participating in *tone policing* (Hoffman, 2023), a practice in which a person in a position of privilege dictates what healthy emotional expression is to an individual from a different cultural group. This practice can be damaging to clients. Instead, it is the responsibility of the therapist to work to increase their own level of comfort, tolerance, and awareness of different forms of emotional expression.

A therapist's cultural insensitivity can directly and negatively affect the help-seeking behaviors and coping responses of marginalized communities experiencing emotional distress. Sisley and colleagues (2011) find that African Caribbean women, an underrepresented group in the United Kingdom mental health care system, experienced distress at the same levels as their White counterparts of European origin; however, cultural influences impacted their coping and help-seeking, such as the need to be strong, the pressure to mask their emotions, and varying generational perspectives and tolerance of difficult emotions. Whether or not the women sought help depended upon access, perceptions, and experiences of external support and resources, and many expressed feeling judged, misunderstood, and stigmatized by practitioners in both the medical and mental health care systems.

Brown and colleagues (2012) explore the interwoven physical, mental, spiritual, and cultural components of emotional distress in Aboriginal men in Australia. Although depressive symptoms were identifiable and congruent with symptom profiles of non-Aboriginal groups (i.e., a Western and European model of depression), "depression" both as a word and as a diagnostic construct was not used or recognized. Rather, depression was understood as being both a contributor to and a consequence of a weak or injured spirit (*kurunpa*) arising from the cumulative stressors of oppression, colonization, sociocultural change, and disadvantage as well as the subsequent feelings of disconnection, grief, and loss. The men identified sadness and worry (i.e., depressive rumination rather than anxiety) to be the most prominent emotions alongside self-destructive anger, emotional masking, and undifferentiated physical symptoms. Though there was no mention of hopelessness, a hallmark sign of depression from the Western medical model, its absence is best understood through the cultural linguistic lens that no Aboriginal word exists for "future" and that movement forward occurs by looking to the past.

Kang and colleagues (2003) note that Chinese individuals focus on more subtle and nuanced emotional expression. Furthermore, they indicate that different types of emotional expression may be healthier with individuals from different cultures. The focus on the nuanced approach to emotional expression in Asian and Asian American cultures can be a way of maintaining harmony.

These examples reveal divergent approaches to emotion, which are different from approaches to emotions common among White European and European-based American culture. It should be noted that most of these studies of marginalized populations were conducted by White researchers and therefore come with inherent biases. However, this bias can be mitigated, as therapists who are rooted in cultural humility can avoid assumptions that particular cultural approaches to emotion are appropriate or superior to other cultural approaches. Furthermore, they work to examine their assumptions about and reactions to different forms of emotional embodiment and expression while striving to not impose their preferences upon clients.

FUTURE RESEARCH NEEDS

The most obvious need involves the paucity of research of EH therapy and emotion across quantitative and qualitative studies. As discussed, the breadth of research for this chapter was drawn from EFT, humanistic, and experiential therapies, and future research specifically focusing on EH theory and therapy would serve to bolster its presence and legitimacy as an empirically grounded and evidence-based practice. Future directions for specific areas of study in the realm of emotion are so vast they would require a chapter (and potentially an entire book) solely dedicated to them. In their meta-analysis, Peluso and Freund (2018, 2019) provide a robust summary of gaps in existing research, citing inadequate reporting of demographic information (especially racial and ethnic identities as well as age) and an overrepresentation of White and European American participants, therapists, and researchers in studies where demographics were sufficiently reported. Additionally, they identified an overwhelming number of studies focused on clients with depression and the process of emotional expression. In our own literature review for this chapter, we observed a critical absence of cultural and contextual considerations in the majority of studies as well as a complete absence of representation of transgender, nonbinary, and genderfluid participants. These issues are reflections of the historical and systemic inequities in research across the field of psychology, which loudly demand attention and corrective action.

CONCLUSION

Emotions are an undeniable and ontological part of the human experience, and emotion-focused work is foundational to and embedded in EH practice. Emotional transformation occurs in the context of dynamic, multidimensional, and interacting processes, which are impacted and facilitated by therapist presence, the therapeutic relationship, and client characteristics. The nuances of emotion-focused work are unique to each client and must be understood and explored through a lens of contextual, multicultural awareness and humility. Despite a lack of direct research on EH therapy and emotions, there is a strong body of empirical evidence to support the way EH therapy approaches and works with emotions, as shown in the quantitative and qualitative studies of transtheoretical processes and clinical populations as well as experiential, emotion-focused, humanistic, psychodynamic, and cognitive behavior therapies.

REFERENCES

American Psychiatric Association. (2013). *Diagnostic and statistical manual of mental disorders* (5th ed.). https://doi.org/10.1176/appi.books.9780890425596

Anderson, W. G., Alexander, S. C., Rodriguez, K. L., Jeffreys, A. S., Olsen, M. K., Pollak, K. I., Tulsky, J. A., & Arnold, R. M. (2008). "What concerns me is...": Expression of emotion by advanced cancer patients during outpatient visits. *Supportive Care in Cancer, 16*(7), 803–811. https://doi.org/10.1007/s00520-007-0350-8

Angus, L. E., Boritz, T., Bryntwick, E., Carpenter, N., Macaulay, C., & Khattra, J. (2017). The Narrative–Emotion Process Coding System 2.0: A multi-methodological approach to identifying and assessing narrative–emotion process markers in psychotherapy. *Psychotherapy Research, 27*(3), 253–269. https://doi.org/10.1080/10503307.2016.1238525

Angus, L. E., & Macaulay, C. (2023). Tracking the interplay of narrative and emotion change processes in therapy sessions: The Narrative–Emotion Process Video Coding System 2.0. *Journal of Psychotherapy Integration, 33*(2), 185–200. https://doi.org/10.1037/int0000300

Auszra, L., Greenberg, L. S., & Herrmann, I. R. (2010). Client Emotional Productivity Scale—Revised [Unpublished manuscript]. York University.

Auszra, L., Greenberg, L. S., & Herrmann, I. (2013). Client emotional productivity—Optimal client in-session emotional processing in experiential therapy. *Psychotherapy Research, 23*(6), 732–746. https://doi.org/10.1080/10503307.2013.816882

Banerjee, P., & Basu, J. (2016). Therapeutic relationship as a change agent in psychotherapy: An interpretive phenomenological analysis. *Journal of Humanistic Psychology, 56*(2), 171–193. https://doi.org/10.1177/0022167814561547

Bell, T., Montague, J., Elander, J., & Gilbert, P. (2020). "A definite feel-it moment": Embodiment, externalisation and emotion during chair-work in compassion-focused therapy. *Counselling & Psychotherapy Research, 20*(1), 143–153. https://doi.org/10.1002/capr.12248

Boritz, T. Z., Angus, L., Monette, G., Hollis-Walker, L., & Warwar, S. (2011). Narrative and emotion integration in psychotherapy: Investigating the relationship between autobiographical memory specificity and expressed emotional arousal in brief emotion-focused and client-centred treatments of depression. *Psychotherapy Research, 21*(1), 16–26. https://doi.org/10.1080/10503307.2010.504240

Boritz, T. Z., Bryntwick, E., Angus, L., Greenberg, L. S., & Constantino, M. J. (2014). Narrative and emotion process in psychotherapy: An empirical test of the Narrative–Emotion Process Coding System (NEPCS). *Psychotherapy Research, 24*(5), 594–607. https://doi.org/10.1080/10503307.2013.851426

Bortolan, A. (2017). Affectivity and narrativity in depression: A phenomenological study. *Medicine, Health Care and Philosophy, 20*(1), 77–88. https://doi.org/10.1007/s11019-016-9735-0

Brown, A., Scales, U., Beever, W., Rickards, B., Rowley, K., & O'Dea, K. (2012). Exploring the expression of depression and distress in aboriginal men in central Australia: A qualitative study. *BMC Psychiatry, 12*(1), 97–97. https://doi.org/10.1186/1471-244X-12-97

Bugental, J. F. T. (1987). *The art of the psychotherapist.* W. W. Norton & Company.

Cameron, K., Ogrodniczuk, J., & Hadjipavlou, G. (2014). Changes in alexithymia following psychological intervention: A review. *Harvard Review of Psychiatry, 22*(3), 162–178. https://doi.org/10.1097/HRP.0000000000000036

Carpenter, N., Angus, L., Paivio, S., & Bryntwick, E. (2016). Narrative and emotion integration processes in emotion-focused therapy for complex trauma: An exploratory process–outcome analysis. *Person-Centered and Experiential Psychotherapies, 15*(2), 67–94. https://doi.org/10.1080/14779757.2015.1132756

Carryer, J. R., & Greenberg, L. S. (2010). Optimal levels of emotional arousal in experiential therapy of depression. *Journal of Consulting and Clinical Psychology, 78*(2), 190–199. https://doi.org/10.1037/a0018401

Coggins, J., & Fox, J. R. E. (2009). A qualitative exploration of emotional inhibition: A basic emotions and developmental perspective. *Clinical Psychology & Psychotherapy, 16*(1), 55–76. https://doi.org/10.1002/cpp.604

Diamond, S. A. (1996). *Anger, madness, and the daimonic: The psychological genesis of violence, evil, and creativity.* State University of New York Press.

Diener, M. J., Hilsenroth, M. J., & Weinberger, J. (2007). Therapist affect focus and patient outcomes in psychodynamic psychotherapy: A meta-analysis. *The American Journal of Psychiatry, 164*(6), 936–941. https://doi.org/10.1176/ajp.2007.164.6.936

Dillon, A., Timulak, L., & Greenberg, L. S. (2018). Transforming core emotional pain in a course of emotion-focused therapy for depression: A case study. *Psychotherapy Research, 28*(3), 406–422. https://doi.org/10.1080/10503307.2016.1233364

Ekman, P., Friesen, W. V., & Ellsworth, P. (1972). *Emotion in the human face: Guidelines for research and an integration of findings.* Pergamon Press.

Ghaemi, S. N. (2006). Feeling and time: The phenomenology of mood disorders, depressive realism, and existential psychotherapy. *Schizophrenia Bulletin, 33*(1), 122–130. https://doi.org/10.1093/schbul/sbl061

Granger, N., Jr. (2011). *Perceptions of racial microaggressions among African American males in higher education: A heuristic inquiry* (UMI No. 3453836) [Doctoral dissertation, University of the Rockies]. ProQuest Dissertations & Theses. https://www.proquest.com/openview/875f86c038c19554d7392b56e74c4a16/1?pq-origsite=gscholar&cbl=18750

Gratz, K. L., & Roemer, L. (2004). Multidimensional assessment of emotion regulation and dysregulation: Development, factor structure, and initial validation of the difficulties in emotion regulation scale. *Journal of Psychopathology and Behavioral Assessment, 26*(1), 41–54. https://doi.org/10.1023/B:JOBA.0000007455.08539.94

Greenberg, L. (2014). The therapeutic relationship in emotion-focused therapy. *Psychotherapy*, *51*(3), 350–357. https://doi.org/10.1037/a0037336

Greenberg, L. S. (2017). *Emotion-focused therapy* (Rev. ed.). American Psychological Association. https://doi.org/10.1037/15971-000

Greenberg, L. S., Malberg, N. T., & Tompkins, M. A. (2019). *Working with emotion in psychodynamic, cognitive behavior, and emotion-focused therapy*. American Psychological Association. https://doi.org/10.1037/0000130-000

Greenberg, L. S., & Pascual-Leone, A. (2006). Emotion in psychotherapy: A practice-friendly research review. *Journal of Clinical Psychology*, *62*(5), 611–630. https://doi.org/10.1002/jclp.20252

Gross, J. J. (1998). The emerging field of emotion regulation: An integrative review. *Review of General Psychology*, *2*(3), 271–299. https://doi.org/10.1037/1089-2680.2.3.271

Heavey, C. L., Hurlburt, R. T., & Lefforge, N. L. (2012). Toward a phenomenology of feelings. *Emotion*, *12*(4), 763–777. https://doi.org/10.1037/a0026905

Henretty, J. R., Levitt, H. M., & Mathews, S. S. (2008). Clients' experiences of moments of sadness in psychotherapy: A grounded theory analysis. *Psychotherapy Research*, *18*(3), 243–255. https://doi.org/10.1080/10503300701765831

Hoffman, L. (2019). Introduction to existential–humanistic psychology in a cross-cultural context. In L. Hoffman, M. Yang, F. J. Kaklauskas, A. Chan, & M. Mansilla (Eds.), *Existential psychology East–West* (Vol. 1, Rev. ed., pp. 1–72). University Professors Press.

Hoffman, L. (2020). Existential–humanistic therapy and disaster response: Lessons from the COVID-19 pandemic. *Journal of Humanistic Psychology*, *61*(1), 33–54. https://doi.org/10.1177/0022167820931987

Hoffman, L. (2023). White privilege, social justice, and existential psychology. *Journal of Constructivist Psychology*, *36*(2), 154–167. https://doi.org/10.1080/10720537.2022.2068705

Hoffman, L., Vallejos, L., Cleare-Hoffman, H. P., & Rubin, S. (2015). Emotion, relationship, and meaning as core existential practice: Evidence-based foundations. *Journal of Contemporary Psychotherapy*, *45*(1), 11–20. https://doi.org/10.1007/s10879-014-9277-9

Iwakabe, S., Nakamura, K., & Thoma, N. C. (2023). Enhancing emotion regulation. *Psychotherapy Research*, *33*(7), 918–945. https://doi.org/10.1080/10503307.2023.2183155

Iwakabe, S., Rogan, K., & Stalikas, A. (2000). The relationship between client emotional expressions, therapist interventions, and the working alliance: An exploration of eight emotional expression events. *Journal of Psychotherapy Integration*, *10*(4), 375–401. https://doi.org/10.1023/A:1009479100305

Kang, S.-M., Shaver, P. R., Sue, S., Min, K.-H., & Jing, H. (2003). Culture-specific patterns in the prediction of life satisfaction: Roles of emotion, relationship quality, and self-esteem. *Personality and Social Psychology Bulletin*, *29*(12), 1596–1608. https://doi.org/10.1177/0146167203255986

Khayyat-Abuaita, U., Paivio, S., Pascual-Leone, A., & Harrington, S. (2019). Emotional processing of trauma narratives is a predictor of outcome in emotion-focused therapy for complex trauma. *Psychotherapy*, *56*(4), 526–536. https://doi.org/10.1037/pst0000238

Kierkegaard, S. (1944). *The concept of dread* (W. Lowrie, Trans.). Princeton University Press. (Original work published 1844)

Kierkegaard, S. (1976). *The concept of anxiety* (A. Hannay, Ed. & Trans.). Liveright Publishing Company. (Original work published 1844)

Klein, M. H., Mathieu-Coughlan, P., & Kiesler, D. J. (1986). The experiencing scales. In L. S. Greenberg & W. M. Pinsof (Eds.), *The psychotherapeutic process: A research handbook* (pp. 21–71). Guildford Press.

Lane, R. D., Quinlan, D. M., Schwartz, G. E., Walker, P. A., & Zeitlin, S. B. (1990). The Levels of Emotional Awareness Scale: A cognitive–developmental measure of emotion. *Journal of Personality Assessment, 55*(1–2), 124–134. https://doi.org/10.1080/00223891.1990.9674052

Lane, R. D., Subic-Wrana, C., Greenberg, L., & Yovel, I. (2022). The role of enhanced emotional awareness in promoting change across psychotherapy modalities. *Journal of Psychotherapy Integration, 32*(2), 131–150. https://doi.org/10.1037/int0000244

Lieberman, M. D., Eisenberger, N. I., Crockett, M. J., Tom, S. M., Pfeifer, J. H., & Way, B. M. (2007). Putting feelings into words. *Psychological Science, 18*(5), 421–428. https://doi.org/10.1111/j.1467-9280.2007.01916.x

Mackay, H. C., Barkham, M., Stiles, W. B., & Goldfried, M. R. (2002). Patterns of client emotion in helpful sessions of cognitive-behavioral and psychodynamic-interpersonal therapy. *Journal of Counseling Psychology, 49*(3), 376–380. https://doi.org/10.1037/0022-0167.49.3.376

Marren, C., Mikoška, P., O'Brien, S., & Timulak, L. (2022). A qualitative meta-analysis of the clients' experiences of emotion-focused therapy. *Clinical Psychology & Psychotherapy, 29*(5), 1611–1625. https://doi.org/10.1002/cpp.2745

May, R. (1977). *The meaning of anxiety.* W. W. Norton & Company. (Original work published 1950)

McCallum, M., Piper, W. E., Ogrodniczuk, J. S., & Joyce, A. S. (2003). Relationships among psychological mindedness, alexithymia and outcome in four forms of short-term psychotherapy. *Psychology and Psychotherapy, 76*(2), 133–144. https://doi.org/10.1348/147608303765951177

McCarthy, K. L., Mergenthaler, E., & Grenyer, B. F. S. (2014). Early in-session cognitive-emotional problem-solving predicts 12-month outcomes in depression with personality disorder. *Psychotherapy Research, 24*(1), 103–115. https://doi.org/10.1080/10503307.2013.826834

Mergenthaler, E. (1996). Emotion–abstraction patterns in verbatim protocols: A new way of describing psychotherapeutic processes. *Journal of Consulting and Clinical Psychology, 64*(6), 1306–1315. https://doi.org/10.1037/0022-006X.64.6.1306

Missirlian, T. M., Toukmanian, S. G., Warwar, S. H., & Greenberg, L. S. (2005). Emotional arousal, client perceptual processing, and the working alliance in experiential psychotherapy for depression. *Journal of Consulting and Clinical Psychology, 73*(5), 861–871. https://doi.org/10.1037/0022-006X.73.5.861

Money, C., Genders, R., Treasure, J., Schmidt, U., & Tchanturia, K. (2011). A brief emotion focused intervention for inpatients with anorexia nervosa: A qualitative study. *Journal of Health Psychology, 16*(6), 947–958. https://doi.org/10.1177/1359105310396395

O'Brien, K., O'Keeffe, N., Cullen, H., Durcan, A., Timulak, L., & McElvaney, J. (2019). Emotion-focused perspective on generalized anxiety disorder: A qualitative analysis of clients' in-session presentations. *Psychotherapy Research, 29*(4), 524–540. https://doi.org/10.1080/10503307.2017.1373206

Ogrodniczuk, J. S., Piper, W. E., & Joyce, A. S. (2008). Alexithymia and therapist reactions to the patient: Expression of positive emotion as a mediator. *Psychiatry, 71*(3), 257–265. https://doi.org/10.1521/psyc.2008.71.3.257

Ogrodniczuk, J. S., Piper, W. E., & Joyce, A. S. (2011). Effect of alexithymia on the process and outcome of psychotherapy: A programmatic review. *Psychiatry Research, 190*(1), 43–48. https://doi.org/10.1016/j.psychres.2010.04.026

Pascual-Leone, A. (2009). Dynamic emotional processing in experiential therapy: Two steps forward, one step back. *Journal of Consulting and Clinical Psychology, 77*(1), 113–126. https://doi.org/10.1037/a0014488

Pascual-Leone, A., & Greenberg, L. S. (2007). Emotional processing in experiential therapy: Why "the only way out is through." *Journal of Consulting and Clinical Psychology, 75*(6), 875–887. https://doi.org/10.1037/0022-006X.75.6.875

Pascual-Leone, A., Paivio, S., & Harrington, S. (2016). Emotion in psychotherapy: An experiential–humanistic perspective. In D. J. Cain, K. Keenan, & S. Rubin (Eds.),

Humanistic psychotherapies: Handbook of research and practice (2nd ed., pp. 147–181). American Psychological Association. https://doi.org/10.1037/14775-006

Pascual-Leone, A., & Yeryomenko, N. (2017). The client "experiencing" scale as a predictor of treatment outcomes: A meta-analysis on psychotherapy process. *Psychotherapy Research, 27*(6), 653–665. https://doi.org/10.1080/10503307.2016.1152409

Peluso, P. R., & Freund, R. R. (2018). Therapist and client emotional expression and psychotherapy outcomes: A meta-analysis. *Psychotherapy, 55*(4), 461–472. https://doi.org/10.1037/pst0000165

Peluso, P. R., & Freund, R. R. (2019). Emotional expression. In J. C. Norcross & M. J. Lambert (Eds.), *Psychotherapy relationships that work: Vol. 1. Evidence-based therapist contributions* (3rd ed., pp. 421–460). Oxford University Press. https://doi.org/10.1093/med-psych/9780190843953.003.0012

Porges, S. (2011). *The polyvagal theory: Neurophysiological foundations of emotions, attachment, communication, self-regulation.* W. W. Norton & Company.

Pos, A. E., & Greenberg, L. S. (2007). Emotion-focused therapy: The transforming power of affect. *Journal of Contemporary Psychotherapy, 37*(1), 25–31. https://doi.org/10.1007/s10879-006-9031-z

Pos, A. E., Greenberg, L. S., Goldman, R. N., & Korman, L. M. (2003). Emotional processing during experiential treatment of depression. *Journal of Consulting and Clinical Psychology, 71*(6), 1007–1016. https://doi.org/10.1037/0022-006X.71.6.1007

Pos, A. E., Greenberg, L. S., & Warwar, S. H. (2009). Testing a model of change in the experiential treatment of depression. *Journal of Consulting and Clinical Psychology, 77*(6), 1055–1066. https://doi.org/10.1037/a0017059

Salovey, P., Mayer, J. D., Goldman, S. L., Turvey, C., & Palfai, T. P. (1995). Emotional attention, clarity and repair: Exploring emotional intelligence using the Trait Meta-Mood Scale. In J. W. Pennebaker (Ed.), *Emotion, disclosure, and health* (pp. 125–154). American Psychological Association. https://doi.org/10.1037/10182-006

Schanche, E., Stiles, T. C., McCullough, L., Svartberg, M., & Nielsen, G. H. (2011). The relationship between activating affects, inhibitory affects, and self-compassion in patients with cluster C personality disorders. *Psychotherapy, 48(3), 293–303.* https://doi.org/10.1037/a0022012

Scherer, A., Boecker, M., Pawelzik, M., Gauggel, S., & Forkmann, T. (2017). Emotion suppression, not reappraisal, predicts psychotherapy outcome. *Psychotherapy Research, 27*(2), 143–153. https://doi.org/10.1080/10503307.2015.1080875

Schneider, K. J. (2008). *Existential–integrative psychotherapy: Guidepost to the core of practice.* Routledge.

Schneider, K. J., & Krug, O. T. (2017). *Existential–humanistic therapy* (2nd ed.). American Psychological Association. https://doi.org/10.1037/0000042-000

Schore, A. (1994). *Affect regulation and the origin of the self: The neurobiology of emotional development.* Lawrence Erlbaum Associates.

Sisley, E. J., Hutton, J. M., Louise Goodbody, C., & Brown, J. S. L. (2011). An interpretative phenomenological analysis of African Caribbean women's experiences and management of emotional distress. *Health & Social Care in the Community, 19*(4), 392–402. https://doi.org/10.1111/j.1365-2524.2010.00986.x

Sloan, E., Hall, K., Moulding, R., Bryce, S., Mildred, H., & Staiger, P. K. (2017). Emotion regulation as a transdiagnostic treatment construct across anxiety, depression, substance, eating and borderline personality disorders: A systematic review. *Clinical Psychology Review, 57,* 141–163. https://doi.org/10.1016/j.cpr.2017.09.002

Taylor, G. J., & Bagby, R. M. (2013). Psychoanalysis and empirical research: The example of alexithymia. *Journal of the American Psychoanalytic Association, 61*(1), 99–133. https://doi.org/10.1177/0003065112474066

Teasdale, J. D. (1999). Emotional processing, three modes of mind and the prevention of relapse in depression. *Behaviour Research and Therapy, 37*(7, Suppl. 1), S53–S77. https://doi.org/10.1016/S0005-7967(99)00050-9

Thompson, R. J., Mata, J., Jaeggi, S. M., Buschkuehl, M., Jonides, J., & Gotlib, I. H. (2011). Concurrent and prospective relations between attention to emotion and affect intensity: An experience sampling study. *Emotion, 11*(6), 1489–1494. https://doi.org/10.1037/a0022822

Timulak, L., McElvaney, J., Keogh, D., Martin, E., Clare, P., Chepukova, E., & Greenberg, L. S. (2017). Emotion-focused therapy for generalized anxiety disorder: An exploratory study. *Psychotherapy, 54*(4), 361–366. https://doi.org/10.1037/pst0000128

Timulak, L., & Pascual-Leone, A. (2015). New developments for case conceptualization in emotion-focused therapy. *Clinical Psychology & Psychotherapy, 22*(6), 619–636. https://doi.org/10.1002/cpp.1922

Torre, J. B., & Lieberman, M. D. (2018). Putting feelings into words: Affect labeling as implicit emotion regulation. *Emotion Review, 10*(2), 116–124. https://doi.org/10.1177/1754073917742706

Town, J. M., Salvadori, A., Falkenström, F., Bradley, S., & Hardy, G. (2017). Is affect experiencing therapeutic in major depressive disorder? Examining associations between affect experiencing and changes to the alliance and outcome in intensive short-term dynamic psychotherapy. *Psychotherapy, 54*(2), 148–158. https://doi.org/10.1037/pst0000108.

Ulvenes, P. G., Berggraf, L., Wampold, B. E., Hoffart, A., Stiles, T., & McCullough, L. (2014). Orienting patient to affect, sense of self, and the activation of affect over the course of psychotherapy with cluster C patients. *Journal of Counseling Psychology, 61*(3), 315–324. https://doi.org/10.1037/cou0000028

Vallejos, L., & Johnson, Z. (2019). Multicultural competencies in humanistic psychology. In. L. Hoffman, H. Cleare-Hoffman, N. Granger, Jr., & D. St. John (Eds.), *Humanistic approaches to multiculturalism and diversity: Perspectives on existence and difference* (pp. 63–75). Routledge. https://doi.org/10.4324/9781351133357-6

Viou, M., Moschakis, C., & Nikolaou, A. (2018). Love in therapy: A qualitative study of how clients perceive their therapists' emotions. *European Journal of Psychotherapy & Counselling, 20*(4), 450–467. https://doi.org/10.1080/13642537.2018.1529692

Vodušek, V. V., Parnas, J., Tomori, M., & Škodlar, B. (2014). The phenomenology of emotion experience in first-episode psychosis. *Psychopathology, 47*(4), 252–260. https://doi.org/10.1159/000357759

Warwar, S. H., & Greenberg, L. S. (1999). Client Emotional Arousal Scale—III [Unpublished manuscript]. York University.

Watson, D., Clark, L. A., & Tellegen, A. (1988). Development and validation of brief measures of positive and negative affect: The PANAS scales. *Journal of Personality and Social Psychology, 54*(6), 1063–1070. https://doi.org/10.1037/0022-3514.54.6.1063

Watson, J. C., & Bedard, D. L. (2006). Clients' emotional processing in psychotherapy: A comparison between cognitive-behavioral and process-experiential therapies. *Journal of Consulting and Clinical Psychology, 74*(1), 152–159. https://doi.org/10.1037/0022-006X.74.1.152

Weiste, E., & Peräkylä, A. (2014). Prosody and empathic communication in psychotherapy interaction. *Psychotherapy Research, 24*(6), 687–701. https://doi.org/10.1080/10503307.2013.879619

Whelton, W. (2004). Emotional processes in psychotherapy: Evidence across therapeutic modalities. *Clinical Psychology & Psychotherapy, 11*(1), 58–71. https://doi.org/10.1002/cpp.392

Wiser, S., & Goldfried, M. R. (1998). Therapist interventions and client emotional experiencing in expert psychodynamic-interpersonal and cognitive-behavioral therapies. *Journal of Consulting and Clinical Psychology, 66*(4), 634–640. https://doi.org/10.1037/0022-006X.66.4.634

World Health Organization. (2019). *International statistical classification of diseases and related health problems* (11th ed.). https://icd.who.int

Yalom, I. D. (1980). *Existential psychotherapy*. Basic Books.

Yalom, I. D. (1989). *Love's executioner*. Basic Books.

7

Authenticity, Self-Awareness, and Facing Life Directly in Existential–Humanistic Psychotherapy

Drake Spaeth, Joseph Alexander Vanderhoff, Marguerite Pintauro, and Louis Hoffman

Authenticity, self-awareness, and facing life directly (i.e., being honest about the human condition) are closely related in existential–humanistic (EH) psychology. In this chapter, we begin with some general considerations of these concepts in psychotherapy before considering how they are worked with specific to an EH context. Next, we consider quantitative and qualitative research related to these topics. As there is the potential for an individualist bias with authenticity definitions and applications, it is particularly important to consider how EH therapy may need to be cautious (and potentially be adapted) when working with people from collectivist backgrounds. We examine this and other issues after the research is considered. Last, we give a brief discussion of future research directions.

DEFINITIONS

In the *APA Dictionary of Psychology*, self-awareness is simply defined as "self-focused attention or knowledge" (American Psychological Association [APA], n.d.-c). The importance of self-awareness varies across therapy modalities. Solution focused therapies, for example, place less emphasis on the value of self-awareness. The various depth psychologies, including psychoanalytic/psychodynamic, Jungian, existential, humanistic, and other psychologies, place a

We would like to acknowledge Emanuel Hermosillo and Arielle Kahana, who assisted with locating articles and other scholarly resources cited in the chapter.

https://doi.org/10.1037/0000446-008
The Evidence-Based Foundations of Existential–Humanistic Therapy, L. Hoffman and V. Lac (Editors)

great value on self-awareness; however, there are still discrepancies in what it means. For example, although many of these approaches purport the existence of an unconscious, some existential approaches do not (see Wyschogrod, 1961). Among existentialists, there is often a preference for the idea of the subconscious, as this does not suggest a separate consciousness. Regardless of the view of the unconscious and subconscious, depth psychologies generally believe that making the unconscious or subconscious conscious is beneficial for psychological well-being and, at times, ethical well-being (see Riker, 1997).

Though facing life directly or honestly is a concept developed primarily within existential literature, there are parallels in other psychological theories. For example, concepts such as repression, suppression, and cognitive distortion all imply that not being honest about aspects of one's life or experience is problematic. These, however, do not necessarily imply the broader conception of facing one's life directly or honestly in the context of one's broader existence.

The *APA Dictionary of Psychology* offers two definitions of authenticity, one that is existential and another that is general. The general definition of authenticity is,

> in psychotherapy and counseling, genuineness and caring demonstrated by the therapist or counselor through a down-to-earth attitude that the client senses to be a reflection of the true person and not simply of a professional acting in their professional role. (APA, n.d.-a)

In this general definition, authenticity is essentially synonymous with genuineness and understood primarily in an interpersonal context. Implicit in this definition is that there is a real self, which in psychology often suggests a stable self that can be discovered. This contrasts with an existential view of self that views the self as more fluid or changing and as a product of self-creation (see Chapter 13 of this volume). This general definition of authenticity also is commonly used in humanistic psychology. Thus, the humanistic and existential definitions of authenticity often are not in alignment, which is consistent with how mainstream psychology's view of the self is in conflict with the existential understanding.

CONTEXTUALIZING FACING LIFE DIRECTLY, SELF-AWARENESS, AND AUTHENTICITY IN AN EH CONTEXT

The idea of facing life directly or honestly is deeply embedded in existential thought and can be traced back to existential philosophy. For Nietzsche (1892/1966), facing life directly is something that people ought to strive to achieve. Yet Nietzsche also recognizes that this is not something that is readily achieved. He states, "I call a lie: wanting *not* to see something one does see, wanting not to see something *as* one sees it. . . . The most common lie is the lie one tells to oneself; lying to others is relatively the exception" (Nietzsche, 1894/1990, p. 185). For Nietzsche, facing life directly is not about living a happy life; rather, it is an essential component of an ethical life.

Yalom (1980), who has influenced existential psychology, is known by his advocacy for the concept that facing four existential givens—death, freedom, isolation, and meaninglessness—is psychologically beneficial. He is not the first to introduce the ideas of the givens. The idea of there being innate aspects of human existence that provide challenges has been variously labeled, discussed, and categorized (e.g., ontological or existential challenges) in the history of existential thought. Although these represent universal challenges, Hoffman (2019a) advocates that these universal challenges require a personally and culturally informed response.

Zhi mian therapy, which was developed by Xuefu Wang and has been identified as an Indigenous Chinese existential therapy, similarly purports the idea of facing life directly (Dueck & Wei, 2019; Wang, 2019). *Zhi mian* is not easily translated into English, but it roughly means "face to face" or "to face directly." According to Wang, this can mean to face oneself directly, to face others directly, or to face the world directly. Developing self-awareness in the context of facing life directly is a foundation of this approach to therapy.

Although facing life directly can be valuable, cautions also need to be considered. Often, existential givens or realities elicit negative or overwhelming aemotions. As noted by Vos (see Chapter 2 of this volume), encouraging clients to face existential givens directly can have harmful implications. Similarly, Ernest Becker (1973), in the context of discussing the harms of the denial of death, emphasizes caution and consideration of the context. For example, Becker notes that "man [*sic*] cannot endure his own littleness unless he can translate it into meaningfulness on the largest possible level" (p. 196). It is not that the initial awareness brings about the benefits, but rather that what is done with this awareness holds the potential for benefit. As noted by Yalom (1980), "though the physicality of death destroys us, the idea of death saves us" (p. 7). Therapists must be aware of the client's resources, such as meaning, when delving into the challenges of givens. Similarly, Hoffman (2019b, 2021) advocates for maintaining awareness of the relational context and client's resources (including emotional regulation). When the resources are in place and an appropriate context is provided, then facing life directly can bring about a host of benefits, including deeper engagement with life, relationships, and meaning. It is these secondary benefits that are sought. Therapists must hold appropriate awareness and reverence for the risks of facing life directly and should never seek it simply for the sake of doing so. Rather, this technique is engaged at the proper time in therapy to help clients develop a greater resilience to the inevitability of facing these givens while also seeking the potential benefits from how clients learn to live in the face of such realities.

Self-awareness is closely related to facing life honestly. It could even be considered an aspect of self-awareness. One complexity in researching the effects of insight and awareness is the way that insight may affect therapeutic change. At times, insight and self-awareness can bring about "Aha!" moments that are pivotal in change. These moments are described as instances of sudden, profound insight that bring about an emotional reaction or relief. At times, "Aha!" moments lead directly to change. Other times, they are the start of the change process. It is more common for insight to occur slowly over time in therapy—at times, clients and therapists may not even be able to pinpoint when the insight occurred because of its gradual emergence. Both sudden and gradual insight can lead to direct change; however, their impact often may be through empowering other agents of change, rendering the role of insight to a necessary but indirect role. Given that insight can be sudden or gradual and contribute to direct and indirect change, the role of insight and self-awareness is difficult to assess through typical randomized clinical trials. Instead, structural equations or qualitative research may be more effective in researching insight and awareness.

EH therapy brings an added dimension to understanding self-awareness that can be illustrated in the dialogue between Carl Rogers and Rollo May on the topic of evil.[1] The exchange begins with Rogers (1982) publishing a short article on May in which he identifies the key difference between May and himself as being related to May seeing "the demonic as a basic element in the human makeup" (p. 8). Although May (1982) clarifies that his term was the daimonic, not demonic, he agrees that the perspective on human nature in regard to evil or the potential for evil is a key difference. For May, awareness of one's potential for evil is key to preventing evil—if we are unaware of our potential for evil, we are more likely to participate in it. Therefore, whereas both humanistic and existential perspectives believe in the value of self-awareness, EH approaches place greater emphasis on the importance of looking at our destructive potential.

When working with self-awareness in EH therapy, it is not the therapist's job to force self-awareness. Rather, the EH therapist works to gently guide or invite the client into self-exploration in order to increase self-awareness. This should be a gradual process that occurs in a supportive, compassionate, and relational context. At times, it may even be valuable to slow the client down on their journey into self-awareness to avoid it overwhelming them or becoming harmful. Moreover, this ensures that the journey is an authentic one for the client, illuminating the connection of facing life directly and deepening self-awareness to authenticity.

Authenticity requires an introduction before discussing in greater depth its relationship to facing life directly and self-awareness. First, it is important to recognize that there are various definitions and understandings of authenticity in humanistic and existential psychology (see Cleary, 2022; DuBose, 2026; Gordon, 1999/2013; Hayes & Adams, 2019; Holzhey-Kunz, 2019). One existential definition of authenticity is included in the *APA Dictionary of Psychology* (APA, n.d.-a): "a mode of being that humans can achieve by accepting the burden of freedom, choice, and responsibility and the need to construct their own values and meanings in a meaningless universe." For this chapter, we will draw on perspectives that have been particularly influential on EH psychology. Ellenberger (1958) provides a succinct description of authenticity: "Inauthentic existence is the modality of the man [*sic*] who lives under the tyranny of the

---

[1]Evil, here, is not seen as an external entity for force, or a categorization of people, but rather a label applied to harmful or destructive behaviors or occurrences.

plebs (the crowd, i.e., the anonymous collectivity). Authentic existence is the modality in which a man assumes the responsivity of his own existence" (p. 118). Though there is a potential individualist bias in both statements, it is important to clarify that aligning with the collective as a value is not the same as living under the tyranny of the plebs. The distinguishing factors are self-reflection and choice. For Bugental (1965), authenticity also entails one living "in accord with the givenness of his [*sic*] own nature and the world" (p. 32). Although at first glance this can sound as if it conflicts with assuming responsibility for one's life, Bugental goes on to identify four givens of awareness: (a) finiteness, (b) potential to act, (c) choice, and (d) separateness. Building from this, he states that authentic awareness "fully confronts the existential anxieties of being and affirms its own being by incorporating those anxieties while yet avoiding their distortion" (p. 40). Here it is demonstrated how authenticity is connected with self-awareness and facing life directly.

Although some existentialists, such as Martin Heidegger, view authenticity as morally neutral, others, including Bugental, Jean-Paul Sartre, and Simone de Beauvoir, understand authenticity as having an ethical component (Gordon, 1999/2013). We have freedom and choice, but with this comes responsibility—responsibility for our choices as well as responsibility for the values we choose to live by (and how well we live in accordance with those values). In considering values, it is important to consider Beauvoir's contributions. Cleary (2022), in discussing Beauvoir, states,

> To become authentic means to create our own essence. It's the creation that is vital here. We don't discover ourselves, we make ourselves. Authenticity is a way of expressing our freedom: to realize and accept that we are free; to be lucid about what we can and can't choose about ourselves, our situation, and others; and to use our freedom as a tool to shape ourselves. (p. x)

For Beauvoir (1948/1976), one cannot be authentic in isolation. Authenticity embraces freedom and responsibility, and responsibility entails a recognition that we are interconnected, which adds an important dimension to the previously noted definitions. Beauvoir captures this with her understanding of intersubjectivity, which entails "the mutual recognition and respect for one another's freedom" (Cleary, 2022, p. xii). This, too, involves the recognition of other people in their fullness or their full humanity. Through this, our freedom, dignity, and humanity are connected to the freedom, dignity, and humanity of others. If we treat others as less than human, we devalue our own dignity and are not being authentic.

Authenticity, then, is not a state we achieve, but something we strive toward. It is not possible to be authentic all the time (Bugental, 1965; Cleary, 2022; Gordon, 1999/2013). It is strived toward by taking responsibility for our self-creation and choice, being aware of our intersubjective and interconnected nature, and pursuing living in harmony with our nature, including our contingencies. When we live passively and without reflection, and when we are not taking responsibility for our lives, we are living in bad faith or inauthentically (see Cleary, 2022; Gordon, 1999/2013).

According to May (1981), "the purpose of [EH] psychotherapy is to set people free" (p. 19). Similarly, Bugental (1965) notes,

> The main undertaking of psychotherapy is that of aiding the patient in his [*sic*] efforts, (a) to discard the distortions of awareness which arose to forestall existential anxiety, and (b) to accept the responsibilities and opportunities of authentic being in the world. (p. 31)

Within both of these quotes, there is a connection among freedom, awareness, and choice. To help clients seek authenticity, therapists must also pursue authenticity in their own lives and their work with clients. In EH therapy, therapists seek to create a space where clients are able to engage in self-reflection in the context of their broader existence. This is done in order to pursue a more authentic, and therefore free, existence in the context of responsibility, which exists within the context of intersubjectivity and interconnectedness. As previously discussed, it is essential to remain aware that this can be a difficult process. It is not the job of the therapist to thrust the client into authenticity. It is important that this is a gentle process embedded in a supportive relationship. Furthermore, therapists must continually be aware if the client lacks the resources for this work, is becoming overwhelmed, or is not ready or interested in the deeper explorations. Readiness can be difficult to assess as it can vary from client to client, but aspects to consider are the strength of the therapy relationship; the client's ability to stay with the here-and-now, especially with difficult topics; client personal resources (e.g., coping mechanisms, insight); client resilience; client social support; and client willingness to engage in these explorations.

RESEARCH SUPPORT

Research on authenticity, self-awareness, and facing life directly and honestly is complex. It ought not to be expected that these will always readily and directly correlate with psychological well-being, especially in regard to self-awareness and facing life directly. Rather, there is a complex relationship in which these serve vital roles in working toward a heartier, more resilient well-being.

Quantitative Research

There is a wealth of quantitative research relevant to authenticity, self-awareness, and facing life directly, even if often not using this terminology. A challenge is that many of the research measures may approach these topics somewhat differently than an approach dictated by the philosophical understanding of EH therapy, which creates some limitations in the research. Despite this, there is significant research support for the relevance of these concepts in EH therapy that is considered in this section.

Authenticity

In evaluating quantitative research studies on authenticity, we are faced with a dilemma: The very nature of EH approaches, including authenticity, endeavor to embody something that transcends typical categorization. However, it remains important to evaluate efficacy. In this first section, we will investigate the salient quantitative research studies regarding authenticity.

Two seminal figures in this literature on authenticity are Michael Kernis and Brian Goldman (2006), who developed "a multicomponent conceptualization of authenticity" (p. 283). They define authenticity as "the unobstructed operation of one's true- or core-self in one's daily enterprise" (p. 294) and break it down into four subcategories: awareness, unbiased processing, behavior, and relational orientation. Authenticity scores were calculated using a 45 item scale with questions addressing each of the aforementioned categories: "Awareness: 12 items, Unbiased Processing: 10 items, Behavior: 11 items, and Relational Orientation: 12 items" (p. 303). They find authenticity to be positively related to level of self-esteem and life satisfaction, as well as negatively related to self-esteem contingency and net negative affect. Not only are the total authenticity scores related to these factors, but each of the four subcategories shows relationships of magnitude with all four well-being measures. Awareness is shown to be positively related to higher life satisfaction and self-esteem while being negatively related to lower net negative affect. Unbiased processing is positively related to greater life satisfaction. *Behavior*, defined as "acting in ways congruent with one's values, preferences, and needs" (p. 302), is demonstrated as being positively related to self-esteem and negatively related to less contingent self-esteem. Finally, relational orientation is positively correlated with higher life satisfaction and negatively correlated with less net negative affect.

Kernis and Goldman's (2006) research shows that the higher the self-reported level of authenticity, the less frequently one experiences negative emotions (less net negative affect) and the more a person perceives satisfaction in their life. Additionally, the feelings of self-worth related to authenticity are not only more positive but also more secure—meaning that they are less dependent on specific outcomes (Goldman & Kernis, 2002). The findings of Kernis and Goldman's research (2002, 2006) provide empirical data to substantiate authenticity's relationship to healthy psychological functioning and positive subjective well-being. Unfortunately, minimal consideration was given to race, ethnicity, and gender, and a significant portion of their research summaries were drawn from unpublished data.

Sohal and Murphy (2023) conduct a quantitative, longitudinal study that examines the relationship between clients expressing suicidal thoughts who were receiving person-centered therapy and their levels of authenticity, well-being, and psychological distress. They measured authenticity using the Authenticity Scale (Wood et al., 2008), which is divided equally into three subcategories: self-alienation, accepting external influence, and authentic living. The data show statistically significant improvements in levels of authenticity, well-being, and psychological distress over the 20 therapy sessions with a minimum of 15 sessions required to detect significant change. The results from their study reveal that there are significant positive associations between authenticity and well-being and that these levels predict, and are negatively associated with, levels of psychological distress. In this study, over 50% of the participants were White and British, and 26.8% were identified as other or unspecified. Gender was not reported.

A meta-analysis was conducted, examining authenticity's relationship to well-being and engagement while evaluating the effect of variables such as age, gender, sample type, conceptual measure, and individual versus collectivist cultures (Sutton, 2020). This meta-analysis is particularly comprehensive in that it explicates both different definitions of authenticity (i.e., trait versus existential, congruence, and coherence) and disparate categories of measurement (e.g., authenticity scale, authenticity inventory, authenticity in relationships scale). The meta-analysis includes 75 independent samples resulting in a total international sample size of 36,533 participants. The data show all five categories of authenticity measurements to possess medium to large positive relationships with well-being and engagement, with Kernis and Goldman's (2006) Authenticity Inventory being the strongest. Sutton (2020) concludes that these relationships are "remarkably robust, showing no moderation by gender, age, or type of sample" (p. 10). The study does, however, find individualist cultures to be a positive moderator between authenticity and well-being, believing that collectivist cultures may influence people to value the group interest above their own interest. This may suggest a different understanding of authenticity than the EH approach, particularly Beauvoir's understanding of empathy.

Myriad studies have found authenticity to be positively related to self-esteem and life satisfaction while being negatively related to negative affect (Kernis & Goldman, 2006) and psychological distress (Sohal & Murphy 2023). Additionally, other research has found authenticity to be positively related to higher performance and job satisfaction (van den Bosch & Taris, 2014), increased commitment to work, lower turnover (Cable, Gino, & Staats, 2013), and employee engagement (Glavas, 2016). Although authenticity shares a diversity of experience, quantitative research has supported authenticity's significance to well-being and psychological health.

Self-Awareness

In this section, we will explore the constituents of self, self-consciousness, and self-awareness and the conclusions of their relevant quantitative research studies. Seghezzi and colleagues (2019) conducted a meta-analysis exploring the relationship between body ownership and agency. Postulating that the minimal self, defined as "the consciousness of oneself as an immediate subject of an experience" (p. 170), contains both body ownership and a sense of agency—two essential levels for self-awareness—they utilize neuroimaging to locate the brain regions associated with these parts, finding support for a relationship between the two, which are "operating in partially distinct brain networks" in the insular cortex (p. 176). Martial and colleagues (2018) found evidence that the self-concept, conceived of as a general context-independent self-representation as well as a set of context-dependent selves that represent personal attributes, was evident in the medial prefrontal cortex, with the bulk of activity occurring during general self-judgements rooted in preexisting knowledge affiliated with representations of self and other. The results of this study show that both "context-independent and context-dependent self-referential judgements" (p. 23) have shared and separate patterns of brain activation, bolstering evidence that the self-concept is a multidimensional construct that includes both general and context specific selves. Fingelkurts and colleagues (2012) utilized an electroencephalogram to investigate neurological aspects of self-consciousness. They measured the strength of operational synchrony within the default mode network (DMN) in individuals with varying levels of conscious states, finding that it was "smallest or even absent in patients in vegetative state, intermediate in patients in minimally conscious state and highest in healthy fully self-conscious subjects" (p. 55). They found that the strength of the DMN was correlated with the strength of self-consciousness expression, concluding that coordinated activity within the DMN is essential for integrating self-representational processes within a coherent model of the subjectively experienced self and protecting said self-model from disintegration. Additionally, Fingelkurts and colleagues speculated that "DMN persistent operational integrity" (p. 64) may permit experiences of our minimal self in the present to be connected and integrated with our self-experiences of the past and future. These studies are significant in their potential contribution to a biological foundation of a holistic, biopsychosocial framework of the nature of conscious self-awareness, providing fertile ground for future research endeavors.

Anna Sutton (2016) sought to measure the effects of self-awareness and parse out the unique outcomes of its constituents. She identified four main themes of self-awareness—insight, reflection, rumination, and mindfulness—and identified four factors that emerged from her statistical analysis: reflective self-development, acceptance of self and others, proactivity at work, and emotional costs. The first study was used to develop the Self-Awareness Outcomes Questionnaire originally consisting of 61 items but truncated to 38 items for its final form. The second study "aimed to refine the items from the first study into a psychometrically sound self-report questionnaire that could be used to measure the outcomes self-awareness" (p. 649). Sutton concludes that the Self-Awareness Outcomes Questionnaire "captures both statistically sound and qualitatively meaningful outcomes of self-awareness" (p. 654). Evaluating the outcomes showed that "self-reflection and insight predicted beneficial outcomes, rumination predicted reduced benefits and increased costs, and mindfulness predicted both increased proactivity and costs" (p. 645). In Sutton's study, 76% of participants were female; no gender differences were reported. Race and ethnicity were not reported.

In evaluating the salience of self-awareness, it is equally important to examine the impact of its absence. A meta-analysis by Mund and Mitte (2012) examines the relationship between repressive coping—trying to "avoid the conscious perception of negative feelings" (p. 640)—and somatic diseases. The meta-analysis includes 22 studies and a total of 6,775 participants (57% female; race and ethnicity are not reported). People labeled "repressive copers" are found to have elevated heart rate and skin conductance levels compared with nonrepressors when presented with a stressful task (Mund & Mitte, 2012, p. 641; see also Asendorpf & Scherer, 1983). This self-deception rather than self-awareness proves to have additional pernicious effects: Data gleaned from the meta-analysis found participants utilizing repression to be at an especially higher risk for cancer and hypertension while also being significantly associated with cardiovascular diseases.

Despite disparate views of the self, evidence from the aforementioned studies support the notion of the self as a multidimensional construct with the insular cortex and DMN being integral to the self-experience. Additionally, people lacking self-awareness (repressive copers) are at a significantly higher risk for cancer, hypertension, and cardiovascular diseases. These studies highlight and support the importance of self-awareness in living a psychologically and physiologically healthy and full life.

Facing Life Directly and Honestly

Integral to EH psychology is the notion that congruence between one's internal experience and the external world bolsters psychological health. The deleterious effects of avoiding emotions are accepted and espoused by multifarious modalities. For EH therapists, the ability to be with phenomenological emotional experience is essential. The quality of acceptance and its salubrious effects has been the subject of more recent investigation. Ford and colleagues (2018) find that participants who persistently accepted their emotions and thoughts without judgement experienced less negative emotion during stressful events and on a daily basis while also being negatively correlated with rumination. Additionally, the relationship between acceptance and psychological health proved to remain robust across disparate demographics of gender, ethnicity, and socioeconomic status. Facing life directly involves acceptance and honesty with ourselves about situations in our lives and our internal responses to them. Being with our emotions actually ameliorates negative affect. The Ford and colleagues study provides quantitative data to support ideas espoused by EH therapists and shines light on a salient paradox: Accepting negative emotions assuages negative affect while avoiding negative emotions bolsters them. The extent to which this paradox applies to deeper existential questions is an intriguing one.

Although human beings tend to avoid awareness of their own finitude and mortality in an effort to protect themselves (Dor-Ziderman and colleagues, 2019), EH theorists posit that awareness and reflection on the existential givens of life can lead to more propitious and fully lived life outcomes. Poppelaars and colleagues (2020) investigate the relationship between four existential threat conditions—mortality salience, freedom restriction, uncontrollability, and uncertainty—and their effect on emotions and physiological activation. They find that reflecting on these existential threats had a significant influence on negative affect, but not on positive affect, subjective arousal, or physiological activation. The results show that even when compared with a control condition, reflecting on existential threat conditions elicits an increase in self-reported negative affect without producing change in self-reported positive affect and physiological activation. Ford and colleagues' (2018) study shows how accepting negative emotions produces psychological health benefits. Therefore, it is a possibility that the elevation of negative affect elicited by honest reflection of existential givens can in some situations engender a healthier psychological life. However, as discussed by Vos (Chapter 2 of this volume), there are risks associated with this. More research is needed to determine whether positive versus negative outcomes in facing the existential givens are more prominent under different conditions, such as gradual exposure in an established, supportive environment.

In order to face life directly and honestly, we must first be honest with confronting ourselves. A contemporary quantitative research study investigated participants' likelihood of being honest about racial bias or inappropriate sexual arousal and whether a period of self-reflection would influence the outcome (Burum et al., 2016). The results indicate that participants who were informed by researchers that they had objective evidence about their thoughts and feelings (i.e., participants were falsely told that researchers secretly measured their galvanic skin response) were less likely to admit to bias and inappropriate responses. Allowing participants to engage in self-reflection only mediated results when they were informed of this "objective evidence" before a period of self-reflection. Of the participants, 54% were female; all participants were White. This study provides evidence for an extremely salient and topical point: When we directly confront others, we are likely to elicit defensive and protective responses; however, by providing people with the opportunity for self-reflection and a chance to be with themselves, we are more likely to inspire human beings to face life directly and honestly by fostering interpersonal and intrapersonal growth.

Since its publication in 1973, Ernest Becker's *The Denial of Death* has been largely influential and embraced by existential thinkers. Becker posits an existential dilemma: Human beings strive for self-preservation while possessing the cognitive fortitude to ascertain their own mortality that elicits a paralyzing terror (Klackl et al., 2014). Contemporary researchers have investigated the brain regions involved in processing death, self-esteem, and existential anxiety. They find that when participants were processing death-related sentences, the bilateral insula regions were less active (Klackl et al., 2014). This is especially significant because prior research shows that the insula may be responsible for our "representation of a sentient self" (Klackl et al., 2014, p. 1759) and helps placate existential anxiety (Craig, 2002, 2009; Klackl et al., 2014).

Previous research has shown self-reported death anxiety to be negatively correlated to self-esteem (Davis et al., 1983). In their research, Klackl and colleagues (2014) look at the specific brain regions activated in participants with high self-esteem and low self-esteem. Individuals with high self-esteem showed deactivation in their right anterior insula when confronted with death-related sentences, which may be a kind of coping mechanism to existential anxiety by reducing a person's self-related awareness and helping them to feel less exposed. Individuals with low self-esteem had activation in copious brain regions not seen in the former: bilateral ventrolateral prefrontal cortex and lateral orbitofrontal cortex, left ventromedial prefrontal cortex, and left anterior insula. These data lead to an important potential conclusion: Those with low self-esteem may have to put more effort into suppressing negative emotions in the face of existential anxiety as seen by the activation of multiple prefrontal regions when processing death-related sentences, demonstrating that they depend more on emotional regulation when threatened (Klackl et al., 2014). Ergo, when one does not face life honestly and directly, they are required to exert more effort for a less satisfactory and incongruent lived experience.

The existential theory that likely has the most empirical research supporting it is terror management theory (TMT; Burke et al., 2010). A foundational component of TMT is mortality salience, which is understood anxiety resultant from the inevitable awareness of death. Building from this, the mortality salience hypothesis suggests that

> to the extent a psychological structure (self-esteem, cultural worldview, interpersonal attachments) provides protection against death anxiety, reminders of death should intensify one's need for this structure, and therefore lead to more positive reactions to people and ideas that support that structure and more negative reactions to those that threaten it. (Pyszczynski & Diarra, 2026, Chap. 17)

Death and death anxiety are inevitable. This awareness can lead to positive or negative consequences (Vail et al., 2012). For example, mortality salience can lead to antagonistic attitudes toward people or occurrences that pose a threat to one's worldview or self-esteem, resulting in support for violence toward what is deemed as an outgroup or threat to one's worldview (Hirschberger et al., 2015, Pyszczynski et al., 2006) or increased implicit bias (Bradley et al., 2012).

Drawing from TMT, it is not that facing life directly itself leads to psychological benefits. Rather, death as an existential given is something that people will inevitably face at conscious or unconscious levels. This awareness and the anxiety it produces has the potential to impact people negatively. From a therapeutic perspective, then, what is important is helping people face these givens in a constructive manner. This reduces the likelihood of negative consequences. TMT focuses on three strategies: self-esteem, cultural worldview, and interpersonal attachments (Pyszczynski & Diarra, 2026). From an EH perspective, each of these can be seen as sources of meaning. Other research has suggested additional ways to constructively cope with death anxiety, including creativity (Perach & Wisman, 2019) and intrinsic religion (Vail et al., 2010). The results of TMT research have been fairly consistent across racial and ethnic identities and gender.

Schneider (2023) proposes that the surge of anxiety in our time is not a problem of excessive anxiety, but rather a problem of not facing anxiety directly and honestly. One inspiration for his work on life-enhancing anxiety is *psychological hardiness*, which is conceptualized as having three components: commitment, control, and challenge (Maddi, 2006). Maddi defines psychological hardiness as "a combination of attitudes that provides the courage and motivation to do the hard, strategic work of turning stressful circumstances from potential disasters into growth opportunities" (p. 160). Research has demonstrated that participants high in psychological hardiness deal with stressful situations by facing them directly and accepting responsibility for themselves (Maddi, 2006).

Viktor Frankl (1946/1984) asserts that happiness is best attained as a side effect of a well-lived life, which implies a paradoxical nature to happiness. This postulation was put to the test by researchers who wanted to know if valuing happiness could sometimes be self-defeating (Mauss et al., 2011). First, researchers tested to see if there was an association between valuing happiness and being happy. Then, they analyzed the effect of participants' happiness values. The results from the first study find that "female participants who valued happiness more (vs. less) reported lower happiness when under conditions of low, but not high, life stress" (p. 807). Similarly, the data from the second study show that "female participants who were experimentally induced to value happiness reacted less positively to a happy, but not a sad, emotion induction" (p. 807), which was mediated by "participants' disappointment at their own feelings" (p. 807). The researchers concluded that valuing happiness could have deleterious effects under certain circumstances.

Ruan and colleagues (2020) use "real-time experience sampling data" (p. 427) to examine whether suppressing negative emotions had an impact on successive emotions. Preceding the studies, participants completed an intake session to measure their levels of trait anxiety, neuroticism, and baseline positive and negative affect. Participants were then paged 10 times a day for three days, at which points they were required to answer questions about emotional suppression in the time since the last page and current affect using the Positive and Negative Affect Scale. After reviewing the data, researchers conclude "that naturally occurring suppression adversely affects subsequent emotions" (p. 433) and "that suppressing negative emotions at one signal significantly predicted more negative emotions at the next signal, for both high-arousal and low-arousal negative emotion" (p. 433) even when controlling for prospective moderators. These findings show that not facing life directly and honestly by suppressing our emotions is not only inefficacious but also emotionally taxing.

It is clear that this is a nuanced and complex subject, yet data seems to corroborate EH theorists' emphasis on choosing to face life directly and honestly; however, there are exceptions. The data is clearer with regard to the negative effects with the suppression of negative emotions. With regard to other ways of facing life directly, more research is needed to parse out potential risks and benefits of facing life directly.

Qualitative Research

Given the complexities of these topics, qualitative research may be better suited to address the various nuances of authenticity, self-awareness, and facing life directly and honestly. Often, EH psychological concepts are explored through qualitative methods, which seek to interpret the lived reality of human experience. Qualitative research methods can offer an in-depth understanding of human experience and bring to light the existential aspects of human life. By exploring the intricacies and nuances of human behavior, these methods can shed light on "the choices that one can make in the face of one's circumstances" (Churchill, 2021, p. 24). Surprisingly, however, specific qualitative research in this field is limited and lacking when exploring the applications of EH notions of authenticity, self-awareness, and facing the world directly as well as their relationship to one another within therapy. Indeed, when comparing narrative themes to existing self-report measures of authenticity (discussed earlier, i.e., Kernis & Goldman, 2006), there is conceptual overlap but not redundancy, supporting that the qualitative narrative approach to exploring authenticity may provide unique information not fully accessible through mainstream self-report measures and likely could be expanded to support other qualitative designs (Wilt et al., 2019). In this section, we consider the qualitative research support for these themes related to EH psychotherapy.

Authenticity in Therapy
Research exploring authenticity within social roles has increased since the early 2010s, particularly in therapeutic settings. Within a psychotherapeutic context, phenomenological research on psychologists by Burks and Robbins (2011, 2012) demonstrated the fluidness of authenticity; authenticity is an evolving process expressed in varying degrees across different social roles. This is further supported by the central theme of congruence (described as a facet of authenticity) as a life-lasting process regarding person-centered therapists' perspectives as studied by Kaimaxi and Lakioti (2021). In addition, Burks and Robbins (2011, 2012) demonstrate self-awareness and self-reflection as essential, especially in balancing periods of inauthenticity. Participants noted that core components of authenticity within the therapeutic relationship included humility and allowing authenticity to emerge naturally rather than forced. In this study, non–humanistically oriented therapists valued authenticity as much as humanistic-minded therapists.

Beaton and Thielking's (2020) research includes similar themes. The establishment of trust between young women with a history of childhood maltreatment and their psychological service providers was essential to the therapeutic process. As supported by the themes from semistructured interviews conducted with 10 experienced psychologists, the practice of authenticity helped establish a trusting therapeutic relationship with the young women. Further, when ruptures in the therapeutic relationship occurred, re-demonstrating authenticity helped restore trust.

Schnellbacher and Leijssen (2009) study authenticity from the client's perspective. All participants were female clients from Belgium; no other race or ethnicity information was provided. They conclude that while therapist authenticity and genuineness may not be the most crucial therapeutic process, it was a significant therapeutic factor for five of six case studies. As research in therapeutic practice expands, EH values have an evident growing influence on other therapeutic practices and diverse orientations (Shahar & Schiller, 2016). In order to develop more meaningful practices in therapy, it is essential to ground authenticity within EH principles.

Additional qualitative research explores the role of authenticity in trainees (Swaby, 2020; Yang et al., 2022). Swaby (2020) conducts semistructured interviews with five integrative trainee psychotherapists in the United Kingdom. The only demographic information provided is that participants were third year or higher in a developmental–relational psychotherapy course in the United Kingdom. Through interpretative phenomenological analysis, two primary themes emerged. The first involved trainees' difficulty balancing their personal identity with the professional expectations to be an authentic therapist. In this regard, trainees shared feeling a sense of pressure to present themselves in a manner that matched the expectations of their program and role—where authenticity was highly regarded—leading to a false presentation of the self. This situation creates a complex and contradictory dynamic that can be challenging to navigate as trainees work toward becoming effective therapists. The second theme included developing an identity as a psychotherapist through self-awareness and acceptance. Notably, this study lacked diversity among participants.

In expanding on this work, Yang and colleagues (2022) explore counseling doctoral students' experiences of authenticity throughout all aspects of training in a collaborative autoethnography study. Emerging themes reveal that program messages about authenticity were overall mixed and the capacity to be authentic differed according to the role (i.e., researcher, therapist, teacher, and student). Several influences became known that either promoted or impeded the ability to be authentic, including interactions with family and peers, as well as the hierarchical structures and social identities of privilege or marginalization. Research in this regard highlights the importance of how concepts of authenticity are taught within therapy training programs.

Barriers to Collective Authenticity

Although Yang and colleagues (2022) touch upon potential barriers to authenticity, Quade and colleagues (2019) explore the experience of scapegoating and the impact of traumatic events on one's ability to remain authentic. This qualitative descriptive study focused on 12 female leaders and their descriptions of authenticity in the face of being a recipient of scapegoating behavior. All participants shared that, in the moment, it was difficult to maintain authenticity. However, in exploring the posttraumatic growth from this experience, many of the women reported the role of being blamed in the overall transformative process of becoming authentic.

This research touches upon a salient point when attempting to understand authenticity: the influence of trauma on interrupting and transforming one's authentic self. This is crucial when discussing issues of culture and race.

Individuals with marginalized or oppressed identities may have to overcome more complexities in being authentic than their privileged counterparts (Yang et al., 2022). Collective aspects of authenticity, expanding beyond the seemingly individualistic bias in authenticity, is an essential area of research within EH therapy. Assisting clients in developing cultural authenticity is an essential aspect of therapy, as it "honors ancestral wisdom, cultural knowledge, and self-definition instead of being defined by oppressors or what liberation psychology theorists describe and the recovery of historical memory" (Adames et al., 2023, p. 41). Adames and colleagues (2023) conduct a case study that explores a client's path to healing, which involved increasing her self-awareness toward the complexities of her identity as a Black woman. This process of self-discovery enabled her to acknowledge the harm and damage caused by oppression while also recognizing the strengths of her community and the authenticity of her cultural heritage. Additional research on collective authenticity through in-depth interviews with Potawatomi Indians and Mexican Americans by researchers Vasquez and Wetzel (2009) finds that through prioritizing authentic traditions as valuable and integral components of their cultural identity, historically marginalized racial groups are able to differentiate themselves from the dominant American culture. By framing discussions of mortality and race around concepts of authenticity, these minoritized groups can reassess their place in society and empower their communities with greater esteem, a form of resistance to institutional racism.

MULTICULTURAL CONSIDERATIONS

It is critical that all therapy strategies, stances, and techniques are considered in the context of multicultural considerations with cultural humility. It is unlikely that any therapy strategy does not require, at least in some situations, adaptation for individual or cultural differences. In this section, we provide some considerations on working with authenticity, self-awareness, and facing life directly with minoritized clients.

The pursuit of authenticity has the potential to embody an individualistic bias. With the focus on self-creation and concerns about conformity, EH therapy can be applied in a manner that is insensitive to individuals from collectivist backgrounds. Fortunately, collectivistic and prosocial elements are also inherent in EH theory and therapy, even as the paradigm has certainly celebrated individualism and self-expression for its own sake. For instance, Rogers (1961, 1964) emphasizes how increasing self-acceptance and investing in one's own process of growth and becoming a fully functioning person tends to organically engender a sense of compassion, concern for the well-being and flourishing of others, and an orientation toward what is commonly regarded as global social justice. Sartre (1943/2021), known and well-regarded for his ideas about the paradoxical nature of freedom and whose work is foundational to existential philosophy and later psychology, asserts that no one can be understood to be free until everyone is free. Sartre's words call to mind Martin Luther King Jr. (1963), who independently articulates this idea in "Letter From a Birmingham Jail," published in *The Atlantic Monthly*—a correspondence that helps illuminate collectivist concepts in existential philosophy that had an impact on existential psychology. If freedom is a core component of authentic self-expression and the ability and willingness to face life directly, this notion illuminates a collective aspect of authenticity and facing life directly. Returning to these potential collective foundational aspects thus also constitutes an honoring of the legacy of the founders of the EH paradigm. However, it could be noted that this type of collectivism may be different from some forms of collectivism common within some cultures.

Building from Sartre's conceptions of freedom as interconnected and Beauvoir's recognition of intersubjective aspects of freedom and dignity, Frantz Fanon (1952/2008) advocates for a new humanism in which full subjectivity, agency, and dignity is recognized, respected, and responded to in all people. To not recognize these, or to treat someone as an other, is inauthentic (Cleary, 2022). Thus, it can be recognized that any psychotherapy that takes authenticity seriously must be rooted in social justice perspectives. If a therapist is working with a client who engages in sexism, racism, homophobia, or transphobia, this has implications for the client's authenticity and may impact their psychological and interpersonal health. This may also negatively affect the therapist. Many therapists avoid addressing clients' implicit or explicit prejudices in therapy, even if directed at the therapist, often justifying this by stating that addressing prejudice, discrimination, and microaggressions are not the client's presenting issues. However, a therapy rooted in authenticity requires engagement with these. At times, this may be addressing the prejudice directly, potentially even through a confrontation. Often, this may entail helping clients explore their prejudicial beliefs and their personal and interpersonal consequences.

It is important to consider cultural adaptations necessary for working with authenticity, self-awareness, and facing life directly in a culturally sensitive manner rooted in cultural humility. For example, even with the recognition of how our freedoms are connected, there can remain an individualist bias. It is common for therapists, including EH therapists, to encourage clients to do what is best for themselves, potentially even pathologizing making decisions from a more collectivist mindset. Concepts such as individuation, codependency, and enmeshment often contain an individualist bias. Although authenticity is connected with freedom and choice, this does not necessitate that freedom and choice must be toward the individual. In exploring choices, reflections made and questions asked can give the impression to clients that they should focus decisions more on their own desires and needs. This may be one example of why, as the qualitative research suggests, that minoritized clients face more challenges in pursuing authenticity. For example, frequent reflections or questions around what the client wants can lead to such an impression without explicitly or directly encouraging clients to make choices based upon what is best for them.

W. E. B. Du Bois (1903/2003) discusses the concepts of *code switching* and *dual consciousness*. Code switching refers to shifting between two or more dialects or ways of communicating as influenced by context. Dual consciousness (also called *double consciousness*) refers to the experience of Black Americans viewing themselves "through their own consciousness as well as through their awareness of how they are perceived by White Americans" (APA, n.d.-b). Similar experiences can also occur with other minoritized groups. Smith (2021) uses qualitative methods to explore the impact of code switching, which includes "preoccupation with presentation and perception," the "loss of Black identity," and "a negative emotional impact of code switching," among other consequences (p. iv). Though many of the themes from Smith's research are important, the loss of identity and its connection with a negative psychological impact is particularly relevant for authenticity—for both therapist and client. Black therapists, indigenous therapists, and therapists of color may also need to code switch with some of their clients. For White therapists, it is important to be aware that clients may be code switching. It may be valuable to gently explore this. Although it may be beneficial to invite clients to be themselves, it is important not to push for this if the client is not ready as this may not feel safe. For White, Black, and Indigenous therapists and therapists of color, it can be valuable to help clients explore their use of code switching and dual consciousness, including the impact of this on their identity and psychological health.

An important aspect of self-awareness includes cultural identity development. This includes helping individuals explore their own racial and cultural background and their relationships with their own cultural group. As part of this, it is important for therapists to be aware of different cultural identity development models. Although awareness of these models is important, this is not to suggest that these models apply to all clients or apply the same way across clients. Each person has a unique journey with their cultural identity development. Additionally, working with self-awareness may entail helping clients to recognize the presence and impact of prejudices, discrimination, and microaggressions. For minoritized clients, this may be, at times, helping clients recognize the impact these have upon them and considering how or if they want to respond in the presence of these. For others, particularly individuals with more types of privilege, it may entail helping them recognize their prejudices and microaggressions, including how it impacts others, themselves, and their relationships. Similarly, it may involve helping them recognize the impact of their privileges, such as White privilege.

FUTURE RESEARCH NEEDS

A primary need for future research is an exploration of authenticity, self-awareness, and facing life directly and honestly in the context of EH therapy. There are no studies to date that consider these qualities specifically within the context of EH therapy. This may require improved measures. For example, though the authenticity measures reflect an understanding of authenticity that overlaps with EH perspectives, they may lack some of the nuance of EH conceptual frameworks, particularly Beauvoir's articulation of the intersubjective and interconnected aspects of authenticity.

With the exception of TMT research reviewed, it is striking that most of the studies do not consider race or ethnicity, and many do not consider gender. It is critical that this is addressed in future research. With TMT research, in general, there are some consistencies across cultures; however, there are also some interesting findings regarding how this may play out differently due to context. For example, in research comparing samples between the United States and Iran, the impact of mortality salience is consistent regarding violence and justice themes; however, it suggests that the type of violence may be different based upon the culture (Hirschberger et al., 2015; Pyszczynski et al., 2006). This makes sense given the perceived power differences between countries. Overall, it suggests general consistency in the implications of mortality salience on violence.

Authenticity research should explore the unique challenges for minoritized groups, such as code switching and dual consciousness. There are many aspects of this that need further consideration, including the impact on cultural identity development, authenticity, and psychological health. It is important to further develop research on how White therapists can work with this more effectively. Additionally, research on the impact of code switching and dual consciousness on Black therapists, indigenous therapists, and therapists of color, including the psychological impact and their professional identity development, is also needed.

With facing life directly, there is some research that strongly attests to the risks of emotional repression. Research on the benefits of facing life directly and honestly is more mixed, including some potential risks and benefits. From an EH perspective, this is not surprising. It is important that these are faced in a supportive, compassionate relationship with consideration to timing. To push for facing the givens before a client is ready is harmful. Thus, timing and context are essential to facing life directly and honestly. Yet this is difficult to research. A research agenda moving back and forth between qualitative and quantitative studies over time may be the best strategy for clarifying when and how facing the givens is most beneficial. For quantitative research, it is necessary to utilize more complex models, such as path analysis and structural equationing that are better able to parse out complex relationships.

Research that is making progress in identifying areas, pathways, and networks in the brain that are pertinent to self-awareness and self-consciousness is intriguing and critical to a sophisticated and thorough biopsychosocial understanding of these phenomena. More investigation of these biological aspects is certainly warranted as conceptual understanding of relationship among self-awareness, facing life directly, and authenticity also evolves.

CONCLUSION

Authenticity, self-awareness, and facing life directly and honestly are foundations of existential therapy. However, these are also complex concepts. Authenticity is understood variously, even within existential approaches. This provides
inherent limitations in much of the research on authenticity as studies often
measure a less nuanced understanding of the construct. Yet there is some
research support that helping clients become more authentic is valuable, despite
some limitations in this research. To help clients in this pursuit, it is important
that therapists are also pursuing authenticity in their own lives. Research on
self-awareness supports that the avoidance of awareness, particularly through
repression and suppression, has negative consequences; however, the research
on it constructively contributing to well-being is mixed. This may be in part
because self-awareness and facing life directly often cause some initial discomfort and even distress, especially at first. From an EH perspective, self-awareness
and facing life directly are not an end in themselves; rather, they are an important part of the journey. Furthermore, an essential aspect of facing life directly
relates to the existential givens, which are inherent in the human condition,
and therefore something that clients will inevitably face—consciously, unconsciously, or subconsciously. It is critical that therapists consider the strength of
the alliance, client resources, and timing in working with self-awareness and,
in particular, facing life directly. This awareness should be encouraged in a sensitive, gentle, and gradual manner. This caution is important given there is
some evidence that when this is not done, it can cause harm. However, an
extensive body of research in TMT supports that attempts to avoid one of these
givens—death—is not possible. Even if not consciously facing death, death
awareness and reminders still affect beliefs, emotions, and behaviors. Working
with self-awareness and facing life directly requires therapeutic skills that may
take longer to develop than many other therapeutic skills.

REFERENCES

Adames, H. Y., Chavez-Dueñas, N. Y., Lewis, J. A., Neville, H. A., French, B. H., Chen,
G. A., & Mosley, D. V. (2023). Radical healing in psychotherapy: Addressing the
wounds of racism-related stress and trauma. *Psychotherapy, 60*(1), 39–50. https://doi.
org/10.1037/pst0000435

American Psychological Association. (n.d.-a). Authenticity. In *APA dictionary of psychology*.
Retrieved June 21, 2024, from https://dictionary.apa.org/authenticity

American Psychological Association. (n.d.-b). Double consciousness. In *APA dictionary of
psychology*. Retrieved June 21, 2024, from https://dictionary.apa.org/double-
consciousness

American Psychological Association. (n.d.-c). Self-awareness. In *APA dictionary of psychology*. Retrieved June 21, 2024, from https://dictionary.apa.org/self-awareness

Asendorpf, J. B., & Scherer, K. R. (1983). The discrepant repressor: Differentiation
between low anxiety, high anxiety, and repression of anxiety by autonomic-facial-
verbal patterns of behavior. *Journal of Personality and Social Psychology, 45*(6), 1334–
1346. https://doi.org/10.1037/0022-3514.45.6.1334

Beaton, J., & Thielking, M. (2020). Chronic mistrust and complex trauma: Australian psychologists' perspectives on the treatment of young women with a history of childhood maltreatment. *Australian Psychologist, 55*(3), 230–243. https://doi.org/10.1111/ap.12430

Beauvoir, S. (1976). *The ethics of ambiguity*. Kensington Publishing. (Original work published 1948)

Becker, E. (1973). *The denial of death*. Free Press.

Bradley, K. I., Kennison, S. M., Burke, A. L., & Chaney, J. M. (2012). The effect of mortality salience on implicit bias. *Death Studies, 36*(9), 819–831. https://doi.org/10.1080/07481187.2011.605987

Bugental, J. F. T. (1965). *The search for authenticity*. Holt, Rinehart & Winston.

Burke, B. L., Martens, A., & Faucher, E. H. (2010). Two decades of terror management theory: A meta-analysis of mortality salience research. *Personality and Social Psychology Review, 14*(2), 155–195. https://doi.org/10.1177/1088868309352321

Burks, D. J., & Robbins, R. (2011). Are you analyzing me? A qualitative exploration of psychologists' individual and interpersonal experiences with authenticity. *The Humanistic Psychologist, 39*(4), 348–365. https://doi.org/10.1080/08873267.2011.620201

Burks, D. J., & Robbins, R. (2012). Psychologists' authenticity: Implications for work in professional and therapeutic settings. *Journal of Humanistic Psychology, 52*(1), 75–104. https://doi.org/10.1177/0022167810381472

Burum, B. A., Gilbert, D. T., & Wilson, T. D. (2016). Caught red-minded: Evidence-induced denial of mental transgressions. *Journal of Experimental Psychology: General, 145*(7), 844–852. https://doi.org/10.1037/xge0000174

Cable, D. M., Gino, F., & Staats, B. R. (2013). Breaking them in or eliciting their best? Reframing socialization around newcomers' authentic self-expression. *Administrative Science Quarterly, 58*(1), 1–36. https://doi.org/10.1177/0001839213477098

Churchill, S. D. (2021). *Essentials of existential phenomenological research*. American Psychological Association.

Cleary, S. (2022). *How to be authentic: Simone de Beauvoir and the quest for fulfillment*. St. Martin's Essentials.

Craig, A. D. (2002). How do you feel? Interoception: The sense of the physiological condition of the body. *Nature Reviews Neuroscience, 3*(8), 655–666. https://doi.org/10.1038/nrn894

Craig, A. D. (2009). How do you feel—Now? The anterior insula and human awareness. *Nature Reviews Neuroscience, 10*(1), 59–70. https://doi.org/10.1038/nrn2555

Davis, S. F., Bremer, S. A., Anderson, B. J., & Tramill, J. L. (1983). The interrelationships of ego strength, self-esteem, death anxiety, and gender in undergraduate college students. *The Journal of General Psychology, 108*(1), 55–59. https://doi.org/10.1080/00221309.1983.9711478

Dor-Ziderman, Y., Lutz, A., & Goldstein, A. (2019). Prediction-based neural mechanisms for shielding the self from existential threat. *NeuroImage, 202*, 116080. https://doi.org/10.1016/j.neuroimage.2019.116080

Du Bois, W. E. B. (2003). *The souls of black folks*. Barnes & Noble. (Original work published 1903)

DuBose, T. (2026). Authenticity and genuineness. In L. Hoffman (Ed.), *APA handbook of humanistic and existential therapy: Vol. 1. History, research, philosophy, and theory* (pp. 545–564). American Psychological Association. https://doi.org/10.1037/0000431-023

Dueck, A., & Wei, G. Q. (2019). The indigenous psychology of Lu Xun and Xuefu Wang. In L. Hoffman, M. Yang, M. Mansilla, J. Dias, M. Moats, & T. Claypool (Eds.), *Existential psychology East–West* (Vol. 2, pp. 17–46). University Professors Press.

Ellenberger, H. F. (1958). A clinical introduction to psychiatric phenomenology and existential analysis. In R. May, E. Angel, & H. F. Ellenberger (Eds.), *Existence: A new dimension in psychiatry and psychology* (pp. 92–124). Jason Aronson.

Fanon, F. (2008). *Black skin, white masks* (R. Philcox, Trans.). Grove Press. (Original work published 1952)

Fingelkurts, A. A., Fingelkurts, A. A., Bagnato, S., Boccagni, C., & Galardi, G. (2012). DMN operational synchrony relates to self-consciousness: Evidence from patients in vegetative and minimally conscious states. *The Open Neuroimaging Journal, 6,* 55–68. https://doi.org/10.2174/1874440001206010055

Ford, B. Q., Lam, P., John, O. P., & Mauss, I. B. (2018). The psychological health benefits of accepting negative emotions and thoughts: Laboratory, diary, and longitudinal evidence. *Journal of Personality and Social Psychology, 115*(6), 1075–1092. https://doi.org/10.1037/pspp0000157

Frankl, V. E. (1984). *Man's search for meaning: An introduction to logotherapy.* Simon & Schuster. (Original work published 1946)

Glavas, A. (2016). Corporate social responsibility and employee engagement: Enabling employees to employ more of their whole selves at work. *Frontiers in Psychology, 7,* 796. https://doi.org/10.3389/fpsyg.2016.00796

Goldman, B. M., & Kernis, M. H. (2002). The role of authenticity in healthy psychological functioning and subjective well-being. *Annals of American Psychotherapy, 5*(6), 18–20.

Gordon, H. (2013). Authenticity. In H. Gordon (Ed.), *Dictionary of existentialism.* Routledge. https://doi.org/10.4324/9781315062716 (Original work published 1999)

Hayes, H., & Adams, M. (2019). Existential phenomenological therapy: Philosophy and theory. In E. van Deurzen, E. Craig, A. Längle, K. J. Schneider, D. Tantam, & S. du Plock (Eds.), *The Wiley world handbook of existential therapy* (pp. 154–166). John Wiley & Sons. https://doi.org/10.1002/9781119167198.ch8

Hirschberger, G., Pyszczynski, T., & Ein-Dor, T. (2015). Why does existential threat promote intergroup violence? Examining the role of retributive justice and cost–benefit utility motivations. *Frontiers in Psychology, 6,* 1761. https://doi.org/10.3389/fpsyg.2015.01761

Hoffman, L. (2019a). Gordo's ghost: An introduction to existential–humanistic perspectives on myth. In L. Hoffman, M. Yang, F. J. Kaklauskas, A. Chan, & M. Mansilla (Eds.), *Existential psychology East–West* (Vol. 1, Rev. ed., pp. 273–288). University Professors Press.

Hoffman, L. (2019b). Introduction to existential-humanistic psychology in a cross-cultural context. In L. Hoffman, M. Yang, F. J. Kaklauskas, A. Chan, & M. Mansilla (Eds.), *Existential psychology East–West* (Vol. 1, Rev. ed., pp. 1–72). University Professors Press.

Hoffman, L. (2021). Existential–humanistic therapy and disaster response: Lessons from the COVID-19 pandemic. *Journal of Humanistic Psychology, 61*(1), 33–54. https://doi.org/10.1177/0022167820931987

Holzhey-Kunz, A. (2019). Philosophy and theory: Daseinsanalysis—An ontological approach to psychic suffering based on the philosophy of Martin Heidegger. In E. van Deurzen, E. Craig, A. Längle, K. J. Schneider, D. Tantam, & S. du Plock (Eds.), *The Wiley world handbook of existential therapy* (pp. 55–67). John Wiley & Sons. https://doi.org/10.1002/9781119167198.ch2

Kaimaxi, D., & Lakioti, A. (2021). The development of congruence: A thematic analysis of person-centered counselors' perspectives. *Person-Centered and Experiential Psychotherapies, 20*(3), 232–249. https://doi.org/10.1080/14779757.2021.1938179

Kernis, M. H., & Goldman, B. M. (2006). A multicomponent conceptualization of authenticity: Theory and research. *Advances in Experimental Social Psychology, 38,* 283–357. https://doi.org/10.1016/S0065-2601(06)38006-9

King, M. L., Jr. (1963). Letter from a Birmingham Jail. *Atlantic Monthly, 212*(2), 78–88.

Klackl, J., Jonas, E., & Kronbichler, M. (2014). Existential neuroscience: Self-esteem moderates neuronal responses to mortality-related stimuli. *Social Cognitive and Affective Neuroscience, 9*(11), 1754–1761. https://doi.org/10.1093/scan/nst167

Maddi, S. R. (2006). Hardiness: The courage to grow from stresses. *The Journal of Positive Psychology, 1*(3), 160–168. https://doi.org/10.1080/17439760600619609

Martial, C., Stawarczyk, D., & D'Argembeau, A. (2018). Neural correlates of context-independent and context-dependent self-knowledge. *Brain and Cognition, 125*, 23–31. https://doi.org/10.1016/j.bandc.2018.05.004

Mauss, I. B., Tamir, M., Anderson, C. L., & Savino, N. S. (2011). Can seeking happiness make people unhappy? Paradoxical effects of valuing happiness. *Emotion, 11*(4), 807–815. https://doi.org/10.1037/a0022010

May, R. (1981). *Freedom and destiny*. W. W. Norton & Company.

May, R. (1982). The problem of evil: An open letter to Carl Rogers. *Journal of Humanistic Psychology, 22*(3), 10–21. https://doi.org/10.1177/0022167882223003

Mund, M., & Mitte, K. (2012). The costs of repression: A meta-analysis on the relation between repressive coping and somatic diseases. *Health Psychology, 31*(5), 640–649. https://doi.org/10.1037/a0026257

Nietzsche, F. (1966). *Thus spoke Zarathustra: A book for all and none* (W. Kauffman, Trans.). Penguin Books. (Original work published 1892)

Nietzsche, F. (1990). *Twilight of the idols and the anti-Christ* (R. J. Hollingdale, Trans.). Penguin Books. (Original works published 1889 & 1894).

Perach, R., & Wisman, A. (2019). Can creativity beat death? A review and evidence on the existential anxiety buffering functions of creative achievement. *The Journal of Creative Behavior, 53*(2), 193–210. https://doi.org/10.1002/jocb.171

Poppelaars, E. S., Klackl, J., Scheepers, D. T., Mühlberger, C., & Jonas, E. (2020). Reflecting on existential threats elicits self-reported negative affect but no physiological arousal. *Frontiers in Psychology, 11*, 962. https://doi.org/10.3389/fpsyg.2020.00962

Pyszczynski, T., Abdollahi, A., Solomon, S., Greenberg, J., Cohen, F., & Weise, D. (2006). Mortality salience, martyrdom, and military might: The great Satan versus the axis of evil. *Personality and Social Psychology Bulletin, 32*(4), 525–537. https://doi.org/10.1177/0146167205282157

Pyszczynski, T., & Diarra, M. (2026). Terror management theory: Toward a merger of existential and experimental approaches to understanding human behavior and experience. In L. Hoffman (Ed.), *APA handbook of humanistic and existential psychology: Vol. 1. History, research, philosophy, and theory* (pp. 405–429). American Psychological Association. https://doi.org/10.1037/0000431-017

Quade, K., Beaver, A. K., Fry, L., Bulmini, D., & Miller, E. (2019). Being thrown under the bus and rising above the fray: Maintaining authenticity. *Journal of Institutional Research, 8*(1), 92–98. https://doi.org/10.9743/JIR.2019.1.9

Riker, J. H. (1997). *Ethics and the discovery of the unconscious*. State University of New York Press.

Rogers, C. (1961). *On becoming a person: A therapist's view of psychotherapy*. Constable.

Rogers, C. (1982). Notes on Rollo May. *Journal of Humanistic Psychology, 22*(3), 8–9. https://doi.org/10.1177/0022167882223002

Rogers, C. R. (1964). Toward a modern approach to values: The valuing process in a mature person. *Journal of Abnormal Psychology, 68*(2), 160–167. https://doi.org/10.1037/h0046419

Ruan, Y., Reis, H., Zareba, W., & Lane, R. (2020). Does suppressing negative emotion impair subsequent emotions? Two experience sampling studies. *Motivation and Emotion, 44*(3), 427–435. https://doi.org/10.1007/s11031-019-09774-w

Sartre, J. P. (2021). *Being and nothingness*. Washington Square Press. (Original work published 1943)

Schneider, K. J. (2023). *Life-enhancing anxiety: Key to a sane world*. University Professors Press.

Schnellbacher, J., & Leijssen, M. (2009). The significance of therapist genuineness from the client's perspective. *Journal of Humanistic Psychology, 49*(2), 207–228. https://doi.org/10.1177/0022167808323601

Seghezzi, S., Giannini, G., & Zapparoli, L. (2019). Neurofunctional correlates of body-ownership and sense of agency: A meta-analytical account of self-consciousness. *Cortex, 121*, 169–178. https://doi.org/10.1016/j.cortex.2019.08.018

Shahar, G., & Schiller, M. (2016). A conqueror by stealth: Introduction to the special issue on humanism, existentialism, and psychotherapy integration. *Journal of Psychotherapy Integration, 26*(1), 1–4. https://doi.org/10.1037/int0000024

Smith, K. S. (2021). The psychological impact of code-switching behavior in African Americans: A qualitative study [Doctoral dissertation, National University]. ProQuest Dissertations and Theses. https://www.proquest.com/docview/2755892393

Sohal, A., & Murphy, D. (2023). A longitudinal analysis of person-centred therapy with suicidal clients. *Counselling & Psychotherapy Research, 23*(1), 20–30. https://doi.org/10.1002/capr.12588

Sutton, A. (2016). Measuring the effects of self-awareness: Construction of the Self-Awareness Outcomes Questionnaire. *Europe's Journal of Psychology, 12*(4), 645–658. https://doi.org/10.5964/ejop.v12i4.1178

Sutton, A. (2020). Living the good life: A meta-analysis of authenticity, well-being and engagement. *Personality and Individual Differences, 153*, 109645. https://doi.org/10.1016/j.paid.2019.109645

Swaby, H. (2020). Learning to "live upside down": Experiencing the true and false self in psychotherapy training. *Psychotherapy and Politics International, 18*(2), Article e1531. https://doi.org/10.1002/ppi.1531

Vail, K. E., III, Juhl, J., Arndt, J., Vess, M., Routledge, C., & Rutjens, B. T. (2012). When death is good for life: Considering the positive trajectories of terror management. *Personality and Social Psychology Review, 16*(4), 303–329. https://doi.org/10.1177/1088868312440046

Vail, K. E., III, Rothschild, Z. K., Weise, D. R., Solomon, S., Pyszczynski, T., & Greenberg, J. (2010). A terror management analysis of the psychological functions of religion. *Personality and Social Psychology Review, 14*(1), 84–94. https://doi.org/10.1177/1088868309351165

van den Bosch, R., & Taris, T. W. (2014). Authenticity at work: Development and validation of an individual authenticity measure at work. *Journal of Happiness Studies, 15*(1), 1–18. https://doi.org/10.1007/s10902-013-9413-3

Vasquez, J. M., & Wetzel, C. (2009). Tradition and the invention of racial selves: Symbolic boundaries, collective authenticity, and contemporary struggles for racial equality. *Ethnic and Racial Studies, 32*(9), 1557–1575. https://doi.org/10.1080/01419870802684232

Wang, X. (2019). The symbol of the iron house: From survivalism to existentialism. In L. Hoffman, M. Yang, M. Mansilla, J. Dias, M. Moats, & T. Claypool (Eds.), *Existential psychology East–West* (Vol. 2, pp. 3–16). University Professors Press.

Wilt, J. A., Thomas, S., & McAdams, D. P. (2019). Authenticity and inauthenticity in narrative identity. *Heliyon, 5*(7), e02178. https://doi.org/10.1016/j.heliyon.2019.e02178

Wood, A. M., Linley, P., Maltby, J., Baliousis, M., & Joseph, S. (2008). The authentic personality: A theoretical and empirical conceptualization and the development of the Authenticity Scale. *Journal of Counseling Psychology, 55*(3), 385–399. https://doi.org/10.1037/0022-0167.55.3.385

Wyschogrod, M. (1961). Sartre, freedom and the unconscious. *Review of Existential Psychology and Psychiatry, 1*(3), 179–188.

Yalom, I. D. (1980). *Existential psychotherapy.* Basic Books.

Yang, N., Jankauskaite, G., Gerstenblith, J. A., Hillman, J. W., Wang, R. J., Le, T. P., & Hill, C. E. (2022). Counseling psychology doctoral students' experiences of authenticity: A collaborative autoethnography. *Counselling Psychology Quarterly, 36*(1), 89–111. https://doi.org/10.1080/09515070.2022.2063260

8

Here-and-Now Work in Existential–Humanistic Psychotherapy

Justin J. Underwood

The here-and-now, in the context of psychotherapy, is what happens during the therapeutic hour between the client and the therapist. Some therapeutic skills encourage mindful awareness in the present moment, but the here-and-now is about attending to the interaction between two people. Other terms are commonly used to capture this phenomenon, such as immediacy, therapeutic immediacy, or therapist self-involved disclosures. It occurs when therapists engage in discussions with clients about their responses to the client or the therapeutic relationship (Hill & O'Brien, 1999; Kuutmann & Hilsenroth, 2012; Mayotte-Blum et al., 2012; McCarthy & Betz, 1978; Yalom, 2002). Therapy most often includes two people sharing space and time (Elkins, 2016). Thoughts, emotional responses, and beliefs conceptually take clients into their past and project into their future, yet this all takes place in the present moment. Memories and fantasies of countless others often permeate hour-long sessions, but the discussions occur between two people, a therapist and a client, in real time: the here-and-now.

DEFINING THE HERE-AND-NOW

The relationship between the client and therapist is part of the unavoidable reality of therapy. In the earliest days of psychoanalytic psychotherapy, this relationship was something to be overcome as the therapist would attempt to take the position of a blank screen and be as objective as possible (Cooper,

https://doi.org/10.1037/0000446-009
The Evidence-Based Foundations of Existential–Humanistic Therapy, L. Hoffman and V. Lac (Editors)

1987; Henretty & Levitt, 2010). Later, the therapeutic relationship was recognized as not only something to be addressed but a fundamental aspect of change (Stolorow, 2004; Strupp & Binder, 1984). Interactions between therapists and clients have been central to theories of therapeutic change since Freud first conceptualized transference and then countertransference. Transference describes clients relating to the therapist, yet through their experiences of others, they project this relationship onto the therapist. An example may be a client relating to the therapist as they would to an authoritative parent (Cooper, 1987). Countertransference is similar but typically means that it is based on the reactions of the therapist toward clients. These reactions are based on figures from the therapist's past instead of the client in front of them (Hayes et al., 2011). In these instances, the focus is not quite on the relationship but instead is concerned with unpacking how the relationship is impacted by experiences with others.

In contrast, the here-and-now of psychotherapy focuses on the reactions of both the therapist and the client in the immediate moment and them genuinely relating to one another rather than vicariously reenacting past reactions and relationships (Cooper, 1987; Safran & Muran, 2000; Wachtel, 1993, 2008). Therapists sharing their immediate reactions, particularly negative reactions, with clients appears to be common. According to Henretty and colleagues (2014), more than 50% of therapists surveyed shared feelings of disappointment with their clients while 90% shared feelings of anger with them. In these cases, here-and-now work is used to encourage a corrective emotional experience by bringing awareness to feelings between the client and therapist instead of attributing the genesis of thoughts and feelings to outside forces.

Here-and-now work also differs from giving feedback to clients. Where feedback is unidirectional from the therapist to the client who receives the feedback, the here-and-now is dyadic and bidirectional. It includes bringing attention to emotional reactions in the session, asking the client directly about their experience of therapy, sharing experiences of each other, validating the client's feelings during the session, and even expressing gratitude toward one another (Mayotte-Blum et al., 2012). The here-and-now may be considered a type of self-disclosure; however, it is distinguished from other types of self-disclosures that consist of sharing historical data or information about the therapist outside of the therapeutic situation (H. Berg et al., 2016; Henretty et al., 2014, Henretty & Levitt, 2010; Hill & O'Brien, 1999; Jowers et al., 2019).

Here-and-now work promotes insight by informing clients how other people may perceive them, identifying and intensifying feelings that can be addressed in the session, making covert communication more direct, identifying adaptive and maladaptive relationship skills, and addressing issues that may be hindering the process, such as ruptures in the therapeutic relationship (Hill & O'Brien, 1999; Jowers et al., 2019). When therapists disclose how they are impacted by the client and their responses to their actions, they are likely encouraging reflection and insight that they rarely get in other types of relationships (Kiesler & Van Denburg, 1993). This helps clients develop a deeper understanding of what they are doing and how they are perceived in their interactions with other people in the client's outside world (Hill & O'Brien, 1999). The benefits of here-and-now work are recognized across theories from diverse contemporary psychoanalytic schools, feminist theory, cognitive behavior theory, and humanistic–existential theory (Ziv-Beiman, 2013).

CONTEXTUALIZING THE HERE-AND-NOW IN AN EXISTENTIAL–HUMANISTIC CONTEXT

Using the here-and-now in psychotherapy fits firmly within the existential–humanistic (EH) framework. In fact, EH theory is often credited with the field's first use and advocacy of this focus that is now used broadly (H. Berg et al., 2016; Henretty & Levitt, 2010; Hill et al., 2020). Here-and-now work animates the basic EH assumptions that the authentic encounter is vital for healing and cultivating presence in the client will help set clients free, which is the goal of EH therapy (Jourard, 1971; May, 1939/1967; Rogers, 1967; Schneider & Krug, 2010; Yalom, 2002).

The authentic encounter is central to EH psychotherapy (see also Chapter 12 of this volume). Human beings are relational beings, and it is through relationships that people are healed (Elkins, 2016). Given this, EH therapists are real, genuine, and open with their clients. Carl Rogers calls this *congruence* and finds that it is one of the three necessary and sufficient conditions for psychological growth. According to Rogers (1967), "it is the quality of the interpersonal encounter with the client which is the most significant element in determining effectiveness" (p. 89). The therapist is emotionally involved, and this involvement creates a bond that includes responsiveness in both the client and the therapist (Rogers, 1942). Engagement with clients in the present moment as a genuine encounter eschews any attempt to manipulate the client's behavior or coyly play a role to discover the client's hidden motives. This honest, respectful relationship between equals is reflected in Martin Buber's I-and-thou conceptualization of relationships that influenced many theorists under the EH umbrella and beyond. I-and-thou relating demands that dialogue respects the personhood of both the therapist and the client. This is a bidirectional relationship that impacts both parties. The therapist is impacted by the client and the client is impacted by the therapist (Adame, 2020; Elkins, 2016; Jourard, 1971; Yalom, 2002). Respectful relationships between equals include affirmations and building up one another, and it also includes things that may be difficult to hear. The therapist must be a person first, instead of faking cordiality or playing the role of what one would expect a therapist to be (May, 1939/1967).

People often hide parts of themselves from their friends, coworkers, families, and even themselves because being seen as they truly are leaves them vulnerable and exposed. However, this hiding causes incongruence and dysfunction within us and in our relationships. Here-and-now work invites clients to reveal themselves within the authentic relationship. Jourard (1971) states,

> When a man [sic] does not acknowledge to himself who, what, and how he is, he is out of touch with reality, and he will sicken . . . no man can come to know himself except as an outcome of disclosing himself to another person. (p. 6)

In psychotherapy, that other person is the therapist. Yalom (2002) further emphasizes this point, stating, "Our self-image is formulated to a large degree upon the reflected appraisals we perceive in the eyes of the important figures in our lives" (p. 47). Being seen is risky. It is frightening to be unarmed and without pretense as a defense, but disclosing what we think about clients in the moment increases trust and ushers them into that process. The therapist is real and has real reactions moment to moment. Shielding thoughts, feelings, and responses hides therapists from clients and is more akin to an inhuman machine with the goal of having clients accept thoughts, behaviors, and actions that the therapist prefers. A more authentic relationship avoids even well-intentioned manipulation (Jourard, 1971).

Focusing on the here-and-now also models for the client what healthy relationships look like. Close, healing relationships require this vulnerability. Being intimate means being willing to be hurt because responses can be unpredictable in authentic relationships. Therapy provides a place where this can be practiced with a caring person. Yalom (2002) describes the therapeutic situation as a "social microcosm" that parallels the client's behavior outside the treatment room (p. 47). If the client is regularly arrogant, self-critical, or hostile, then this will show up in a genuine therapeutic relationship. Bringing the client to the here-and-now adds the advantage of in vivo reactions. Instead of postulating how the client may impact others, the client and therapist share in how they are both impacted in that very moment. This moves psychotherapy from being an academic exercise of recounting the past or events outside of therapy to a lively experience in the present moment; in other words, it allows for the change to begin in the therapy room. The therapist uses their own feelings as data and shares that data in the immediate moment, bringing the client to address that very moment instead of describing past thoughts or feelings. Surfers know that seeing photos or hearing descriptions of the perfect wave cannot compare to the experience of riding it themselves. In the same way, the experience in the therapy room is more potent than recounting the past or projecting into the future. The here-and-now animates and energizes the therapeutic situation (Yalom, 2002).

Another central concern of existential therapy is the present moment. As the present moment includes mindful awareness of the present, a focus on the here-and-now engages clients in the present moment person to person. Existential therapy generally takes an ahistorical approach (Schneider & Krug, 2010). This means that while the experience of the past and goals for the future are important, what is more important is understanding how the client is in the present moment, here-and-now. How is the client coping with their past or impacted by their thoughts of the future right now? This implicit process and what the client is experiencing right now is more of a concern than the explicit content, uncovering drives, or examining patterns of behavior (Schneider & Krug, 2010).

Here-and-now work with clients encourages them to cultivate presence in their own lives (see Chapter 4 of this volume). When in the present moment and not stuck in the past or frozen by fear of the future, people have more agency and are better able to make decisions while taking responsibility for them (May, 1983). Focus on the here-and-now does not devalue past relationships or developmental processes. Instead, it encourages exploration of how those relationships and processes are impacting the client in the moment. This may uncover a deeper understanding of how or why the past or future impacts clients in the moment. One possible explanation for pining for the past or escaping into the future is that doing so protects people from experiencing the full breadth of what it means to be alive right now. This escape prevents people from experiencing the awes and terrors that come with realizing that we exist for only a finite amount of time. The past or an imagined future may seem safer than the reality of temporality (Schneider, 2004). Engagement of the here-and-now interrupts the escape into the past or into the future and helps clients accept what they are feeling, gives insight into how they have blocked what they are feeling, and encourages taking responsibility for their experience to make an informed choice of how they will live life from here on out (Schneider & Krug, 2010). EH therapists use here-and-now work to activate this presence in their clients instead of attempting to interpret or explain their actions and beliefs. This puts clients in the driver's seat of their own lives (Bugental, 1987).

RESEARCH SUPPORT FOR HERE-AND-NOW WORK

The available research supports the use of here-and-now work. Quantitative research, through standardized methods and statistical analysis, shows measurable reductions in symptoms and statistically significant improvements in the therapeutic relationship. Qualitative research documents the clients' perceptions of symptom relief, poignancy of the intervention, and perceived alliance with the therapist.

Quantitative Research

The evidence for the efficacy of using here-and-now work in psychotherapy from experimental or quasi-experimental research is lacking due to scarcity of these types of studies on the topic. A meta-analysis of 184 quantitative studies ranging from 1968 to 2013 found only eight studies assessing the impact of working in the here-and-now (Henretty et al., 2014). However, the evidence to date supports the value of here-and-now focused interventions. These interventions may reduce common symptomatic presentations of depression and anxiety such as sleep difficulty, depressed mood, fatigue, restlessness, muscle tension, and irritability (Barrett & Berman, 2001). Furthermore, through improving the therapeutic relationship, these interventions empower therapy and contribute to better therapeutic outcomes including reducing overall distress and improving the alliance between therapist and client (Barrett & Berman, 2001; Kuutmann & Hilsenroth, 2012).

Research suggests that focusing on the here-and-now with clients reduces symptoms. Early research on therapeutic effectiveness shows that when therapists disclosed their feelings and reactions to clients in the moment, clients' symptoms and their tendency to procrastinate reduced (Hoffman & Spencer, 1977). Barrett and Berman (2001) show that clients' distress greatly reduced on a range of mental health symptoms as measured by the Hopkins Symptom Checklist when the therapist focused clients to the here-and-now. Barrett and Berman (2001) compared therapists using here-and-now engagement with clients with therapists who did not. While both groups' symptoms reduced, the clients' symptoms in the group receiving here-and-now feedback were significantly lower at the completion of the study. Kuutmann and Hilsenroth (2012) found that an increased focus on here-and-now work had a large, significant impact on self-esteem while also improving a cold and distant style of relating to others that has been shown to be a therapy-interfering quality in clients (Beretta et al., 2005). Avoidance, another therapy-interfering behavior, reduced in group therapy and thus improved the therapeutic outcomes (Speckhart, 1999). Research consistently shows that utilizing the here-and-now intensifies emotions and that when emotions are expressed in psychotherapy, whether positive or negative, it leads to improved emotional well-being (Bareket-Bojmel & Shahar, 2011; MacCluskie, 2010; Zech & Rime, 2005).

Research suggests that here-and-now work improves the therapeutic relationship. Therapists are viewed as warmer and more caring when engaging the here-and-now, resulting in clients rating the quality of the relationship with their therapists higher (VandeCreek & Angstadt, 1985). Based on standardized measures (McCarthy, 1979, 1982), when therapists share here-and-now feelings and responses to their clients, clients in turn rate them as more trustworthy and view them more as experts in their field compared with those who do not share feelings and responses or only share their backgrounds. Meta-analysis shows that immediacy increases the likelihood a client will refer a friend to the therapist and decreases premature dropouts of therapy (Henretty & Levitt, 2010). Here-and-now disclosures about the therapeutic relationship show that clients perceive their therapists as more professional and skilled compared to those who do not discuss their personal reactions to the client (Diener et al., 2009; Hill et al., 2020). Findings that the impact of using the here-and-now improve the therapeutic relationship are particularly salient because it is well-established that the therapeutic relationship is the most potent factor in therapeutic effectiveness involving the therapist (Anker et al., 2009; Del Re et al., 2021; Lambert & Barley, 2001; Norcross & Lambert, 2011; Wampold, 2001).

Qualitative Research

In-depth qualitative research supports the available quantitative data on the use of here-and-now work. Information gathered qualitatively also finds that this emphasis decreases symptoms and improves the therapeutic relationship (Hill et al., 2003; Hill et al., 2018; Mayotte-Blum et al. 2012; McCarthy & Betz, 1978). Furthermore, this research suggests that emphasis on the here-and-now improves outcomes by reducing premature terminations (Audet, 2011; H. Berg et al., 2016; Hill et al., 2008).

Audet (2011) interviewed nine clients presenting with depression, anxiety, bipolar disorder, low self-esteem, relationship and family issues, and substance use. Therapists used here-and-now statements such as, "As you continue to show up late for our sessions, I am feeling increasingly frustrated" (p. 86). All nine clients reported a reduction in their presenting issues. Hill and colleagues (2003) found that similar statements reduced clients' self-reported anger. Here-and-now disclosures may reduce symptoms by honing the focus of treatment. Another interesting study compares types of therapeutic disclosures (McCarthy & Betz, 1978). The researchers found that when therapists only disclosed historical data about themselves, clients continued asking the therapist to divulge more, therefore shifting the focus of psychotherapy to the therapist. Conversely, when therapists focused on the here-and-now of psychotherapy, clients increased their own introspective curiosity instead of the curiosity about their therapist.

Three notable case studies use a mixed methods approach to assess the impact of integrating here-and-now work into their treatment by assessing quantitative information regarding symptom reduction and investigating the characteristics of the treatment that both the therapist and client found important (Hill et al., 2008; Kasper et al., 2008, Mayotte-Blum et al., 2012). Both Mayotte-Blum and colleagues (2012) and Hill and colleagues (2008) found a significant decrease in symptomatology after 16 sessions and 17 sessions, respectively. Mayotte-Blum and colleagues (2012) found a powerful change in overall symptomatology. The client initially presented with severe symptoms, then exhibited an overall change on these measures close to three standard deviations posttreatment. Hill and colleagues (2008) found a significant change in symptoms, interpersonal functioning, and social functioning as measured by the Outcome Questionnaire and the Index of Industrial Production. While Kasper and colleagues (2008) failed to replicate the quantitative findings regarding symptomatology after 12 sessions, they did find that therapy focusing on the here-and-now profoundly increased the client's reported depth and importance of each session, the client's assessment of the working alliance, and the client's self-reported increase in self-understanding. Using these same process measures, Hill and colleagues (2008) found that the client in their study also reported the increased depth of each session, profoundly impacted the working alliance and increased her self-understanding. A client in Mayotte-Blum and colleagues' (2012) study "rated her sessions as possessing a high level of 'depth' . . . [and] considered the session process to be 'powerful,' 'valuable,' 'deep,' 'full,' and 'special'" (p. 31).

Several other case studies analyzing the alliance and bond between client and therapist found that immediacy strengthens the working alliance among clients presenting with diverse symptoms including anxiety and depression (Agnew et al., 1994; Friedlander et al., 2018), anorexia (Berman et al., 2012), and interpersonal difficulties (Li et al., 2016). Bennett and colleagues (2006) found that here-and-now work was extremely important in creating a strong therapeutic bond with clients diagnosed with borderline personality disorder. In a mixed method study, the qualitative findings focusing on working alliance showed a significant increase on both therapist- and client-rated working alliance following therapists' training on implementing here-and-now skills into their treatment (Hill et al. 2020).

Henrik Berg and colleagues (2016) interviewed 10 therapists with a median of 28 years of experience working with clients. A consistent theme of "At this point it is right to tell you how I really feel" (p. 254) was rated one of the most potent interventions used in their treatment. These interventions prevented early termination of treatment, clarified misunderstandings between the client and therapist, and reinvigorated stagnant therapeutic situations. Repairing ruptures that are common in therapeutic situations is one of the most often cited benefits of using here-and-now work (Hill et al., 2014; Rhodes et al., 1994; Safran & Muran, 1996). Repairing ruptures in the therapeutic situation not only allows for continuation of therapy by preventing premature dropout but it also has significant benefits to the client after the repair (Duncan et al., 2021; Zlotnick et al., 2020). Clients confirm that using the here-and-now fosters a corrective experience, increases depth of experiencing, and allows them to see therapists as engaged and caring (Friedlander et al., 2018; Hanson, 2005; Hill, Mahalik, & Thompson, 1989; Hill et al., 2003).

MULTICULTURAL CONSIDERATIONS

Using here-and-now work multiculturally requires more attention as the benefits are not as universal as described earlier when using it across cultures. This is particularly important when a therapist who holds historical power and privilege, such as White ethnicity or heterosexual identity, is engaged in psychotherapy with clients who do not share that power and privilege. As we are all cultural and multicultural beings, we are always working multiculturally. Cultural humility, a stance of recognizing what you do not know about the culture of another person and learning directly from others, helps avoid stereotyping and being a wiseacre of cultural expertise. Therapists in positions of privilege are often rated low on measures of cultural humility and frequently rely on broad assumptions about differences that negatively impact the treatment and well-being of groups without historical privilege (Hook et al., 2016; Patallo, 2019). Yet this stance of cultural humility does not excuse cultural ignorance about common experiences and impacts of diverse cultural representations, and there is value in understanding these common experiences to help guide clinical work (Sue, 2001).

This section considers theory and research over the past few decades that examines focusing clients on the here-and-now while working across our cultural representations. Two intersections of culture explored here are sexual diversity and racial or ethnic diversity. Lesbian, gay, bisexual, transgender, and queer (LGBTQ+) clients have long sought out LGBTQ+ therapists to work with to avoid culturally ingrained heterosexism that often shows itself in the therapy room in the form of pathologizing behaviors, negative assumptions, or heteronormalizing worldviews that have long been the standard in the field (Cole & Drescher, 2006; Guthrie, 2006). The common assumption is that with LGBTQ+ therapists it will be easier to develop a safe, trusting relationship that is free from common homophobia. There is also a long history of Black clients seeking other Black professionals for similar reasons; cultural expressions in the Black community have long been pathologized while psychological health has been normed to Eurocentric values. Clients of color have expressed wanting to find a harbor, safe from White supremacy that finds its way into the therapeutic situation (Atkinson et al., 1981; Carkhuff & Pierce, 1967; Carroll et al., 2011; Liddle, 1996; Sladen, 1982).

Around the same time that existential psychologists began to challenge the need for therapists to remain distant and nonresponsive, gay therapists also began to question the superiority of nondisclosure (Cole & Drescher, 2006). This was primarily done by sharing their own sexual identities with clients. Many therapists found maintaining the blank screen approach detrimental to therapy with their gay clients (Cole, 2006, Cole & Drescher, 2006; Frommer, 2000). However, working with the here-and-now may present challenges. According to Cabaj (1996), gay clients may seek gay therapists to avoid exploring powerful material, expecting the therapist to collude with ignoring impactful content and express total acceptance of even problematic beliefs and behaviors. When this does not occur and therapists share critical responses, some clients feel a sense of betrayal. This may in turn create feelings of being unsafe for both the therapist and client (Cabaj, 1996; Guthrie, 2006; Herlands, 2006; Mathy, 2006).

It has also been found that when lesbian, gay, and bisexual therapists disclose their immediate reactions with their among-group clients, this enables "normalizing the clients' experiences, demonstrating the range of feelings for modeling purposes" (Kronner & Northcut, 2015, p. 177). This can be vital, as many in the LGBTQ+ community share a history of needing to hide their sexual identity from family and peers at some point or throughout their lives, particularly during developmentally sensitive times throughout childhood and adolescence when these skills are typically developed (Guthrie, 2006). When therapists share responses, both positive and critical, it allows the expression of a real relationship and fosters both relational skills and depth of relating to encourage healing (Frost, 1998; Kronner & Northcut, 2015). Here-and-now emphasis is not only helpful for LGBTQ+ therapists, but it also has also been shown to be beneficial for straight therapists working with LGBTQ+ clients in psychotherapy. A genuine relationship that is accepting and challenging fosters trust and even displays competence that may serve as a corrective emotional experience to clients who have experienced damaging impacts of a culture saturated in homophobia and heteronormativity (Atkinson et al., 1981; Liddle, 1996).

A complex history is reflected in the research on therapy across racial and ethnic differences. Of the research available, the focus is on disclosures. While research in this area is narrow overall, discussion of this topic by therapists of color is even more limited. In looking at overall disclosures, research suggests that Black clients are more open when Black therapists share about themselves but are more inhibited when White therapists engage in more personal discussions (Wetzel & Wright-Buckley, 1988). Studies also show that many Latinos see therapist sharing as unprofessional and arouses questions regarding the motives of therapists' immediacy (Borrego, et al., 1982; Cherbosque, 1987). While this research is older, it points to cultural expectations to be explored. Likewise, research indicates that Black clients may be suspicious of the motives of White therapists when they disclose feelings and responses (Ridley, 1984). Wetzel and Wright-Buckley (1988) find some sharing to be "condescending, paternalistic, and ingratiating" (p. 284). Given the condescending, paternalistic, and ungenuine history of racism and bias throughout psychology's history, this may well be a fair evaluation of their therapists' values and assumptions. This is not necessarily a case against here-and-now reflections with clients but is rather a case against responses that betray condescending, paternalistic, and ungenuine attitudes many therapists hold. This may explain the contradicting findings in cross-racial therapy showing Black clients' preference for White therapists sharing their thoughts and feelings in the present moment. These findings also show that therapists convey warmth and acceptance when utilizing here-and-now work (J. H. Berg & Wright-Buckley, 1988; Cashwell et al., 2003; Sue & Sue, 1999).

Based on their experimental research, along with their review of literature, Cashwell and colleagues (2003) go as far as to suggest that White therapists use a "trial disclosure" (p. 199) early in therapy focused on immediacy while assessing verbal and nonverbal responses of Black clients. This suggestion is based on the beneficial outcomes in the therapeutic relationship, while acknowledging the potential for here-and-now work to be objectionable based on well-deserved skepticism due to historic racism experienced in their lives. Sladen (1982) phrases this as "clients' biased estimate of differences" (p. 564), yet it might be telling that research indicating that here-and-now discussions are problematic and do not tend to show these results when Black therapists bring immediacy into the therapeutic situation (Carkuff & Pierce, 1967; Sladen, 1982; Wetzel & Wright-Buckley, 1988). This suggests that it is not the use of the here-and-now but violations in the protocol that here-and-now work must always be used for the benefit of the client and not the therapist (Jourard, 1971; Yalom, 2002).

This research suggests that here-and-now work in psychotherapy is complex in the context of cultural differences. There is evidence that it benefits the therapeutic relationship and may lead to better therapeutic outcomes such as clients feeling more connected to their therapists and increasing their own intimate disclosures in session (Berg & Wright-Buckley, 1988; Kronner & Northcut, 2015; Sue & Sue, 1999). Other evidence suggests that it may hinder the alliance between client and therapist, leading some clients to question their professionalism and, in some cases, negatively impacting the trust clients have in their therapists (Cabaj, 1996; Cherbosque, 1987; Wetzel & Wright-Buckley, 1988). Even though this research seems to conflict, it emphasizes the need for therapists to be flexible and adapt their use of the here-and-now. Therapists must be able to recognize when it may not be effective or may be potentially harmful to the therapeutic relationship.

FUTURE RESEARCH NEEDS

The benefits of using here-and-now work appear overwhelming, with the exception of expressed attention given to working across cultures, particularly when therapists of historical privilege work with clients without historical privilege. Given this conflicting data, further research should focus on the impact of using here-and-now work cross-culturally. The power differential that already exists between therapists and clients is exacerbated by privilege, and it should be well understood how this impacts clients. Does it help set them free and increase agency, or does it serve to oppress in other ways? The historical power differentials need to be explored in multiple ways given our intersectional privileges and lack of privileges. It may also be helpful to differentiate and clarify what types of here-and-now work and disclosures are beneficial or even potentially harmful when privileged therapists are working with historically marginalized groups. While there is some support in the literature to encourage certain types of disclosures by therapists of color, more attention should be given to this area centering therapists of color and distinct here-and-now work that includes attending to somatic experiences moment to moment.

Further experimental research in naturalistic settings would also benefit the field to either confirm or disconfirm the considerable qualitative data on the use of here-and-now work. Mixed methods studies are powerful approaches to gathering these data. This would allow comparing specific questions such as reducing symptoms while also gaining a deeper understanding on the impact of using here-and-now from clients' perspectives and therapists' perspectives and analyzing that match as well.

Using the here-and-now appears to be beneficial in psychotherapy. However, it is not clear whether its use aids clients and therapists in achieving the aims of EH psychotherapy, such as increasing autonomy and engaging authentically in the world. Further research on the effectiveness of the here-and-now specifically in EH therapy would be helpful in understanding potential benefits or risks in achieving these goals in an EH context.

The findings should also be applied to training therapists in their use of the here-and-now focus in psychotherapy. The field would benefit from understanding how teachable these skills are and how much time and effort should be dedicated to improving them.

CONCLUSION

Therapists and clients engaging in discussions about what is happening in the present moment is powerful and recognized by multiple established theoretical orientations in psychology. It moves clients from a theoretical stance about what their beliefs and actions mean to feeling and acting in the presence of their therapist. While this may be frightening, when done in the right way, the feeling and acting can be done in a protected place. Clients can use this opportunity to understand how they are perceived by their world, and it allows them to interact authentically with a person of goodwill. Interacting in a real relationship focused on their own well-being can correct negative experiences of relationships that hurt or harmed them. Interacting with therapists in this way improves clients' ability to relate and creates deep, meaningful relationships that in turn reduce their constellations of negative symptoms that distress them and those around them. This comes as no surprise to EH practitioners who have long advocated for using here-and-now work to develop relationships that heal and allow clients to use the present moment to expose the choice and freedom they already possess.

REFERENCES

Adame, A. L. (2020). Self-in-relation: Martin Buber and D. W. Winnicott in dialogue. *The Humanistic Psychologist*. Advance online publication. https://doi.org/10.1037/hum0000203

Agnew, R. M., Harper, H., Shapiro, D. A., & Barkham, M. (1994). Resolving a challenge to the therapeutic relationship: A single-case study. *The British Journal of Medical Psychology*, 67(2), 155–170. https://doi.org/10.1111/j.2044-8341.1994.tb01783.x

Anker, M. G., Duncan, B. L., & Sparks, J. A. (2009). Using client feedback to improve couple therapy outcomes: A randomized clinical trial in a naturalistic setting. *Journal of Consulting and Clinical Psychology*, 77(4), 693–704. https://doi.org/10.1037/a0016062

Atkinson, D. R., Brady, S., & Casas, T. G. (1981). Sexual preference similarity, attitude similarity, and perceived counselor credibility and attractiveness. *Journal of Counseling Psychology*, 28(6), 504–509. https://doi.org/10.1037/0022-0167.28.6.504

Audet, C. T. (2011). Client perspectives of therapist self-disclosure: Violating boundaries or removing barriers? *Counselling Psychology Quarterly*, 24(2), 85–100. https://doi.org/10.1080/09515070.2011.589602

Bareket-Bojmel, L., & Shahar G. (2011). Emotional and interpersonal consequences of self-disclosure in a lived, online interaction. *Journal of Social and Clinical Psychology*, 30(7), 732–759. https://www.researchgate.net/publication/270540732_Emotional_and_Interpersonal_Consequences_of_Self-Disclosure_in_a_Lived_Online_Interaction

Barrett, M. S., & Berman, J. S. (2001). Is psychotherapy more effective when therapists disclose information about themselves? *Journal of Consulting and Clinical Psychology*, 69(4), 597–603. https://doi.org/10.1037/0022-006X.69.4.597

Bennett, D., Parry, G., & Ryle, A. (2006). Resolving threats to the therapeutic alliance in cognitive analytic therapy of borderline personality disorder: A task analysis. *Psychology and Psychotherapy: Theory, Research and Practice, 79*(3), 395–418. https://doi.org/10.1348/147608305X58355

Beretta, V., de Roten, Y., Stigler, M., Drapeau, M., Fischer, M., & Desplan, J.-N. (2005). The influence of patient's interpersonal schemas on early alliance building. *Swiss Journal of Psychology, 64*(1), 13–20. https://doi.org/10.1024/1421-0185.64.1.13

Berg, H., Antonsen, P., & Binder, P.-E. (2016). Sediments and vistas in the relational matrix of the unfolding "I": A qualitative study of therapists' experiences with self-disclosure in psychotherapy. *Journal of Psychotherapy Integration, 26*(3), 248–258. https://doi.org/10.1037/a0040051

Berg, J. H., & Wright-Buckley, C. (1988). Effects of racial similarity and interviewer intimacy in a peer counseling analogue. *Journal of Counseling Psychology, 35*(4), 377–384. https://doi.org/10.1037/0022-0167.35.4.377

Berman, M. I., Hill, C. E., Liu, J., Jackson, J., Sim, W., & Spangler, P. (2012). Relational events in acceptance and commitment therapy for three clients with anorexia nervosa: What is corrective? In L. G. Castonguay & C. E. Hill (Eds.), *Transformation in psychotherapy: Corrective experiences across cognitive behavioral, humanistic, and psychodynamic approaches* (pp. 215–244). American Psychological Association.

Borrego, R. L., Chavez, E. L., & Titley, R. W. (1982). Effect of counselor technique on Mexican-American and Anglo-American self-disclosure and counselor perception. *Journal of Counseling Psychology, 29*(5), 538–541. https://doi.org/10.1037/0022-0167.29.5.538

Bugental, J. F. T. (1987). *The art of the psychotherapist.* W. W. Norton & Company.

Cabaj, R. P. (1996). Sexual orientation of the therapist. In R. P. Cabaj & T. S. Stein (Eds.), *Textbook of homosexuality and mental health* (pp. 513–517). American Psychiatric Association.

Carkhuff, R. R., & Pierce, R. (1967). Differential effects of therapist race and social class upon patient depth of self-exploration in the initial clinical interview. *Journal of Consulting Psychology, 31*(6), 632–634. https://doi.org/10.1037/h0025163

Carroll, L., Gauler, A. A., Relph, J., & Hutchinson, K. S. (2011). Counselor self-disclosure: Does sexual orientation matter to straight clients? *International Journal for the Advancement of Counseling, 33*(2), 139–148. https://doi.org/10.1007/s10447-011-9118-4

Cashwell, C. S., Shcherbakova, J., & Cashwell, T. H. (2003). Effect of client and counselor ethnicity on preference for counselor disclosure. *Journal of Counseling and Development, 81*(2), 196–201. https://doi.org/10.1002/j.1556-6678.2003.tb00242.x

Cherbosque, J. (1987). Differential effects of counselor self-disclosure statements on perception of the counselor and willingness to disclose: A cross-cultural study. *Psychotherapy, 24*(3), 434–437. https://doi.org/10.1037/h0085736

Cole, G. W. (2006). Disclosure, HIV, and the dialectic of sameness and difference. *Journal of Gay & Lesbian Psychotherapy, 10*(1), 7–25. https://doi.org/10.1300/J236v10n01_02

Cole, G. W., & Drescher, J. (2006). Do tell: Queer perspectives on therapist self-disclosure: Introduction. *Journal of Gay & Lesbian Psychotherapy, 10*(1), 1–6. https://doi.org/10.1300/J236v10n01_01

Cooper, A. M. (1987). Changes in psychoanalytic ideas: Transference interpretation. *Journal of the American Psychoanalytic Association, 35,* 77–98.

Del Re, A. C., Flückiger, C., Horvath, A. O., & Wampold, B. E. (2021). Examining therapist effects in the alliance–outcome relationship: A multilevel meta-analysis. *Journal of Consulting and Clinical Psychology, 89*(5), 371–378. https://doi.org/10.1037/ccp0000637

Diener, M. J., Hilsenroth, M. J., & Weinberger, J. (2009). A primer on meta-analysis of correlation coefficients: The relationship between patient-reported therapeutic alliance and adult attachment style as an illustration. *Psychotherapy Research, 19*(4–5), 519–526. https://doi.org/10.1080/10503300802491410

Duncan, B. L., Reese, R. J., Lengerich, A. J., DeSantis, B., Comeau, C. V., & Johnson-Esparza, Y. (2021). Measurement-based care in integrated health care: A randomized clinical trial. *Families, Systems & Health, 39*(2), 259–268. https://doi.org/10.1037/fsh0000608

Elkins, D. N. (2016). *The human elements of psychotherapy: A nonmedical model of emotional healing.* American Psychological Association. https://doi.org/10.1037/14751-000

Friedlander, M. L., Angus, L., Wright, S. T., Günther, C., Austin, C. L., Kangos, K., Barbaro, L., Macaulay, C., Carpenter, N., & Khattra, J. (2018). "If those tears could talk, what would they say?": Multi-method analysis of a corrective experience in brief dynamic therapy. *Psychotherapy Research, 28*(2), 217–234. https://doi.org/10.1080/10503307.2016.1184350

Frommer, M. S. (2000). Reflections on self-disclosure, desire, shame and emotional engagement in the gay male psychoanalytic dyad. *Journal of Gay & Lesbian Psychotherapy, 3*(1), 53–65. https://doi.org/10.1300/J236v03n01_07

Frost, J. C. (1998). Countertransference considerations for the gay male when leading psychotherapy groups for gay men. *International Journal of Group Psychotherapy, 48*(1), 3–24. https://doi.org/10.1080/00207284.1998.11491517

Guthrie, C. (2006). Disclosing the therapist's sexual orientation: The meaning of disclosure in working with gay, lesbian, and bisexual patients. *Journal of Gay & Lesbian Psychotherapy, 10*(1), 63–77. https://doi.org/10.1300/J236v10n01_07

Hanson, J. (2005). Should your lips be zipped? How therapist self-disclosure and non-disclosure affects clients. *Counselling & Psychotherapy Research, 5*(2), 96–104. https://doi.org/10.1080/17441690500226658

Hayes, J. A., Gelso, C. J., & Hummel, A. M. (2011). Managing countertransference. *Psychotherapy, 48*(1), 88–97. https://doi.org/10.1037/a0022182

Henretty, J. R., Currier, J. M., Berman, J. S., & Levitt, H. M. (2014). The impact of counselor self-disclosure on clients: A meta-analytic review of experimental and quasi-experimental research. *Journal of Counseling Psychology, 61*(2), 191–207. https://doi.org/10.1037/a0036189

Henretty, J. R., & Levitt, H. M. (2010). The role of therapist self-disclosure in psychotherapy: A qualitative review. *Clinical Psychology Review, 30*(1), 63–77. https://doi.org/10.1016/j.cpr.2009.09.004

Herlands, N. (2006). Gay patient, gay analyst: Is it all about sex? Clinical case notes from a contemporary Freudian view. *Journal of Gay & Lesbian Psychotherapy, 10*(1), 95–108. https://doi.org/10.1300/J236v10n01_09

Hill, C. E., Gelso, C. J., Chui, H., Spangler, P. T., Hummel, A., Huang, T., Jackson, J., Jones, R. A., Palma, B., Bhatia, A., Gupta, S., Ain, S. C., Klingaman, B., Lim, R. H., Liu, J., Hui, K., Jezzi, M. M., & Miles, J. R. (2014). To be or not to be immediate with clients: The use and perceived effects of immediacy in psychodynamic/interpersonal psychotherapy. *Psychotherapy Research, 24*(3), 299–315. https://doi.org/10.1080/10503307.2013.812262 (Retraction published 2012, *Psychotherapy Research, 34*[3], 415, https://doi.org/10.1080/10503307.2024.2313421)

Hill, C. E., Kellems, I. S., Kolchakian, M. R., Wonnell, T. L., Davis, T. L., & Nakayama, E. Y. (2003). The therapist experience of being the target of hostile versus suspected–unasserted client anger: Factors associated with resolution. *Psychotherapy Research, 13*(4), 475–491. https://doi.org/10.1093/ptr/kpg040

Hill, C. E., Kivlighan, D. M., Rousmaniere, T., Kivlighan, D. M., Gerstenblith, J. A., & Hillman, J. W. (2020). Deliberate practice for the skill of immediacy: A multiple case study of doctoral student therapists and clients. *Psychotherapy, 57*(4), 587–597. https://doi.org/10.1037/pst0000247

Hill, C. E., Knox, S., & Pinto-Coelho, K. G. (2018). Therapist self-disclosure and immediacy: A qualitative meta-analysis. *Psychotherapy, 55*(4), 445–460. https://doi.org/10.1037/pst0000182

Hill, C. E., Mahalik, J. R., & Thompson, B. J. (1989). Therapist self-disclosure. *Psychotherapy, 26*(3), 290–295. https://doi.org/10.1037/h0085438

Hill, C. E., & O'Brien, K. M. (1999). *Helping skills: Facilitating exploration, insight, and action.* American Psychological Association.

Hill, C. E., Sim, W., Spangler, P., Stahl, J., Sullivan, C., & Teyber, E. (2008). Therapist immediacy in brief psychotherapy: Case study II. *Psychotherapy, 45*(3), 298–315. https://doi.org/10.1037/a0013306

Hoffman, M. A., & Spencer, G. P. (1977). Effect of interviewer self-disclosure and interviewer–subject sex pairing on perceived and actual subject behavior. *Journal of Counseling Psychology, 24*(5), 383–390. https://doi.org/10.1037/0022-0167.24.5.383

Hook, J. N., Farrell, J. E., Davis, D. E., DeBlaere, C. Van Tongeren, D. R., & Utsey, S. O. (2016). Cultural humility and racial microaggressions in counseling. *Journal of Counseling Psychology, 63*(), 269-277. https://doi.org/10.1037/cou0000114

Jourard, S. (1971). *The transparent self.* Van Norstrand Reinhold.

Jowers, C. E., Cain, L. A., Hoffman, Z. T., Perkey, H., Stein, M. B., Widner, S. C., & Slavin-Mulford, J. (2019). The relationship between trainee therapist traits with the use of self-disclosure and immediacy in psychotherapy. *Psychotherapy, 56*(2), 157–169. https://doi.org/10.1037/pst0000225

Kasper, L. B., Hill, C. E., & Kivlighan, D. M., Jr. (2008). Therapist immediacy in brief psychotherapy: Case study I. *Psychotherapy, 45*(3), 281–297. https://doi.org/10.1037/a0013305

Kiesler, D. J. & Van Denburg, T. F. (1993). Therapeutic impact disclosure: A last taboo in psychoanalytic theory and practice. *Clinical Psychology & Psychotherapy, 1*(1), 3–13. https://doi.org/10.1002/cpp.5640010103

Kronner, H. W., & Northcut, T. (2015). Listening to both sides of the therapeutic dyad: Self-disclosure of gay male therapists and reflections from their gay male clients. *Psychoanalytic Social Work, 22*(2), 162–182. https://doi.org/10.1080/15228878.2015.1050746

Kuutmann, K., & Hilsenroth, M. J. (2012). Exploring in-session focus on the patient–therapist relationship: Patient characteristics, process and outcome. *Clinical Psychology & Psychotherapy, 19*(3), 187–202. https://doi.org/10.1002/cpp.743

Lambert, M. J., & Barley, D. E. (2001). Research summary on the therapeutic relationship and psychotherapy outcome. *Psychotherapy, 38*(4), 357–361. https://doi.org/10.1037/0033-3204.38.4.357

Li, X., Jauquet, C. A., & Kivlighan, D. M. (2016). When is therapist metacommunication followed by more client collaboration? The moderation effects of timing and contexts. *Journal of Counseling Psychology, 63*(6), 693–703. https://doi.org/10.1037/cou0000162

Liddle, B. J. (1996). Therapist sexual orientation, gender, and counseling practices as they relate to ratings of helpfulness by gay and lesbian clients. *Journal of Counseling Psychology, 43*(4), 394–401. https://doi.org/10.1037/0022-0167.43.4.394

MacCluskie, K. (2010). *Acquiring counseling skills: Integrating theory, multiculturalism, and self-awareness.* Pearson.

Mathy, R. M. (2006). Self-disclosure: A dance of the heart and a ballet of the mind. *Journal of Gay & Lesbian Psychotherapy, 10*(1), 109–121. https://doi.org/10.1300/J236v10n01_10

May, R. (1967). *The art of counseling: A practical guide with case studies and demonstrations.* Abingdon Press. (Original work published 1939)

May, R. (1983). *The discovery of being: Writings in existential psychology.* W. W. Norton & Company.

Mayotte-Blum, J., Slavin-Mulford, J., Lehmann, M., Pesale, F., Becker-Matero, N., & Hilsenroth, M. (2012). Therapeutic immediacy across long-term psychodynamic psychotherapy: An evidence-based case study. *Journal of Counseling Psychology, 59*(1), 27–40. https://doi.org/10.1037/a0026087

McCarthy, P. R. (1979). Differential effects of self-disclosing versus self-involving counselor statements across counselor–client gender pairings. *Journal of Counseling Psychology, 26*(6), 538–541. https://doi.org/10.1037/0022-0167.26.6.538

McCarthy, P. R. (1982). Differential effects of counselor self-referent responses and counselor status. *Journal of Counseling Psychology, 29*(2), 125–131. https://doi.org/10.1037/0022-0167.29.2.125

McCarthy, P. R., & Betz, N. E. (1978). Differential effects of self-disclosing versus self-involving counselor statements. *Journal of Counseling Psychology, 25*(4), 251–256. https://doi.org/10.1037/0022-0167.25.4.251

Norcross, J. C., & Lambert, M. J. (2011). Psychotherapy relationships that work II. *Psychotherapy, 48*(1), 4–8. https://doi.org/10.1037/a0022180

Patallo, B. J. (2019). The multicultural guidelines in practice: Cultural humility in clinical training and supervision. *Training and Education in Professional Psychology, 13*(3), 227–232. https://doi.org/10.1037/tep0000253

Rhodes, R., Hill, C. E., Thompson, B. J., & Elliott, R. (1994). Client retrospective recall of resolved and unresolved misunderstanding events. *Journal of Counseling Psychology, 41*(4), 473–483. https://doi.org/10.1037/0022-0167.41.4.473

Ridley, C. R. (1984). Clinical treatment of the nondisclosing black client: A therapeutic paradox. *American Psychologist, 39*(11), 1234–1244. https://doi.org/10.1037/0003-066X.39.11.1234

Rogers, C. R. (1942). *Counseling and psychotherapy*. Houghton Mifflin.

Rogers, C. R. (1967). The interpersonal relationship. In C. R. Rogers & B. Stevens (Eds.), *Person to person: The problem with being human*. Pocket Books.

Safran, J. D., & Muran, J. C. (1996). The resolution of ruptures in the therapeutic alliance. *Journal of Consulting and Clinical Psychology, 64*(3), 447–458. https://doi.org/10.1037/0022-006X.64.3.447

Safran, J. D., & Muran, J. C. (2000). *Negotiating the therapeutic alliance: A relational treatment guide*. Guilford Press

Schneider, K. J. (2004). *Rediscovery of awe: Splendor, mystery, and the fluid center of life*. Paragon House.

Schneider, K. J., & Krug, O. T. (2010). *Existential–humanistic therapy*. American Psychological Association. https://doi.org/10.1037/12050-000

Sladen, B. J. (1982). Effects of race and socioeconomic status on the perception of process variables in counseling. *Journal of Counseling Psychology, 29*(6), 560–566. https://doi.org/10.1037/0022-0167.29.6.560

Speckhart, D. S. (1999). *An investigation of the experiential component in group leader trainees' acquisition of "here-and-now" intervention skills* (UMI No. 9942853) [Doctoral dissertation, University of Indiana]. ProQuest Dissertations & Theses. https://www.proquest.com/pqdtglobal/docview/304509009/B09EB2D365514508PQ/

Stolorow, R. D. (2004). The intersubjective context of intrapsychic experience. In R. D. Stolorow, G. E. Atwood, & B. Brandchaft (Eds.), *The intersubjective perspective* (pp. 3–14). Rowman & Littlefield.

Strupp, H. H., & Binder, J. L. (1984). *Psychotherapy in a new key*. Basic Books.

Sue, D. W. (2001). Multidimensional facets of cultural competence. *The Counseling Psychologist, 29*(6), 790–821. https://doi.org/10.1177/0011000001296002

Sue, D. W., & Sue, D. (1999). *Counseling the culturally different: Theory and practice* (3rd ed.). John Wiley & Sons.

VandeCreek, L., & Angstadt, L. (1985). Client preferences and anticipations about counselor self-disclosure. *Journal of Counseling Psychology, 32*(2), 206–214. https://doi.org/10.1037/0022-0167.32.2.206

Wachtel, P. L. (1993). *Therapeutic communication*. Guilford Press.

Wachtel, P. L. (2008). *Relational theory and the practice of psychotherapy*. Guilford Press.

Wampold, B. E. (2001). *The great psychotherapy debate: Models, methods, and findings*. Erlbaum.

Wetzel, C. G., & Wright-Buckley, C. (1988). Reciprocity of self-disclosure: Breakdowns of trust in cross-racial dyads. *Basic and Applied Social Psychology, 9*(4), 277–288. https://doi.org/10.1207/s15324834basp0904_3

Yalom, I. D. (2002). *The gift of therapy*. Harper.

Zech, E., & Rime, B. (2005). Is talking about an emotional experience helpful? Effects on emotional recovery and perceived benefits. *Clinical Psychology & Psychotherapy, 12*(4), 270–287. https://doi.org/10.1002/cpp.460

Ziv-Beiman, S. (2013). Therapist self-disclosure as an integrative intervention. *Journal of Psychotherapy Integration, 23*(1), 59–74. https://doi.org/10.1037/a0031783

Zlotnick, E., Strauss, A. Y., Ellis, P., Abargil, M., Tishby, O., & Huppert, J. D. (2020). Reevaluating ruptures and repairs in alliance: Between- and within-session processes in cognitive–behavioral therapy and short-term psychodynamic psychotherapy. *Journal of Consulting and Clinical Psychology, 88*(9), 859–869. https://doi.org/10.1037/ccp0000598

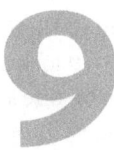

9

Working With Meaning in Life in Existential–Humanistic Psychotherapy

Joel Vos

There are few topics in history about which so many books have been written and about which so many wars have been fought as meaning in life. However individuals define their personal meanings, they seem to share that they regard certain activities and experiences in their life as more meaningful than others. This also applies to readers of this chapter: The fact that they are spending their time reading this chapter seems to indicate that, at least at this moment, they prefer reading over other activities such as going to the gym or pub; thus, readers may have an implicit hierarchy of meanings. Like the readers who have most likely not intentionally reflected on the decision whether to read this chapter, most individuals seem to make meaningful decisions and live a meaningful daily life without explicit deliberation. It seems, therefore, more appropriate to use "meaning" as an adjective (e.g., "living a meaningful life") rather than a noun (e.g., "the meaning of life"). This is because the nuanced adjectival form acknowledges meaning as a subjective, dynamic, and contextual process instead of a reified, static, predetermined, and theoretical concept. The adjective emphasizes personal agency and allows for multiple types and approaches to meaning, reflecting the diverse ways individuals experience meaning, just as Victor Frankl (1946/1985) wrote:

> The meaning of life differs from man to man [*sic*], from day to day and from hour to hour. What matters, therefore, is not the meaning of life in general but rather the specific meaning of a person's life at a given moment. (p. 56)

https://doi.org/10.1037/0000446-010
The Evidence-Based Foundations of Existential–Humanistic Therapy, L. Hoffman and V. Lac (Editors)

Individuals often only become aware of and reflect on what has been meaningful to them when they face boundaries in life, such as a disruption of their daily meaningful activities due to physical or mental disease or COVID-19 lockdowns (Vos, 2016a, 2016b, 2018b, 2020). This sudden disruption of one's habitual meanings and unexpected existential reflection may coincide with or cause psychological problems such as anxiety and depression (Vos, 2016a, 2016b). Therefore, it is understandable that clients often raise explicit questions about meaning when they see a psychological therapist for their mental health problems or, after some sessions, the therapist may become aware of their client's unresolved quests for meaning underlying their psychopathology and stress (Vos, 2016a, 2016b). Consequently, many mental health care clients describe living a meaningful life despite life's challenges as a critical outcome of their recovery (Andresen et al., 2011). Whereas learning to live a meaningful daily life may improve one's mental and physical well-being, an unaddressed quest for meaning may decrease one's well-being and lead to demoralization, despair, and a search for ineffective or harmful resources outside the therapy room (Vos, 2018b).

Given the importance of meaning in therapy, it is understandable that meaning has a central role in existential–humanistic (EH) therapies, highlighting the twin questions "How is one presently living?" and "How is one willing to live?" (Schneider, 2003; cf. Hoffman et al., 2015). Ultimately, EH therapists aim to set clients free (May, 1981) so that they can freely decide their own meanings and how they strive toward these meanings, experience them, and enjoy them. Clients need to take responsibility for their liberation, including facing resistance and protection mechanisms. Therapists may support clients in their in-depth inquiries via their presence, attunement, and supportive therapeutic relationship. EH therapists also highlight life's paradoxes and ambiguities, as the personal quest for meaning happens in the context of biological, emotional, socioeconomic, and existential limitations and uncertainties. Instead of denying these limits, individuals may find that slowing down, staying with their struggles, and fully experiencing the present may help them tolerate difficult feelings and find new ways to live meaningful lives despite life's challenges. By exploring, deepening, vivifying, and confronting their experiences of struggle, clients may become more fully aware of what really matters, from which a sense of meaning, intentionality, and awe may arise (cf. Schneider, 2003). This sense of direction in life may emerge in many forms, such as stories and myths (May, 1991).

This chapter offers an overview of how therapists can help clients live more meaningful and fulfilling lives despite life's challenges, focusing on EH therapies while integrating evidence-based findings and best practices from other therapeutic approaches (cf. existential–integrative therapies; Schneider, 2011a). This chapter starts with a definition of meaning in life and an overview of the types and approaches to meaning that clients benefit most from. Subsequently, we will explore the context of meaning in EH therapies, which will include a brief overview of components that may be integrated from other therapies (the word "therapeutic" refers to any form of helping clients via talking, such as psychotherapy, counseling, coaching, etc.). The remainder of the chapter will focus on qualitative and quantitative research on meaning in EH therapies.

DEFINITIONS

Meaning in life describes a set of psychological experiences that are empirically distinguished from phenomena such as happiness, meaninglessness, and daily life (Vos, 2016b, 2018b). Psychological research has shown that most individuals do not experience one absolute ultimate meaning of life, although some say they do. Rather, they experience multiple simultaneous meanings that can change over time and do not need to be religious or spiritual. The experience of meaning can involve smaller as well as larger events, such as listening to a bird in a park or marriage. Meaning seems to involve an experience of transcendence and significance that deviates from mundane daily life, just like the meaning of a sentence transcends its grammar and spelling. The experience of meaning also seems to require individuals to take up their personal responsibility to discover what is meaningful for them and translate this into daily life actions.

Although philosophers and psychologists differ in their theoretical definitions of meaning, a review of 37 empirical studies has identified seven common components to define meaning in life (Vos, 2016b, 2018b).

1. **Motivation (e.g., purpose, goals, directionality)**: An individual's motivation describes how individuals move toward directions, goals, or purposes in life (the word "motivation" is etymologically derived from *movere*, to move). For example, a client may initially strive toward professional success but may learn to shift toward social and ethical goals in therapy. Thus, there is a directionality in the experience of meaning. However, this directionality does not need to be in the form of specific future goals that individuals move toward in a linear path, as individuals may experience meaning in the process of moving through life and not merely in achieving the goals in the most efficient way possible (this is sometimes described as the difference between teleological versus nonteleological approaches, referring to Aristotle's term for goal or purpose, "telos"; Vos, 2018b, 2021c).

2. **Values**: Most individuals do not seem to move randomly through life but instead follow norms and values, which are their subjective and intersubjective principles about realizing their motivations. For example, individuals may be ethical in how they strive toward goals.

3. **Understanding (e.g., coherence)**: The experience of meaning often involves an understanding of self, life, world, and events, such as a sense of coherence of one's life history and situation. For example, a life-threatening illness can make patients reflect on the legacy they were given (i.e., where

they come from), the legacy they live (i.e., where they are now), and the legacy they still want to live and that they want to give to those remaining after their death (Vos, 2016a).

4. **Self-worth and significance**: Individuals need to feel worthy to follow their own meaning in life, and their own meaning needs to feel significant instead of them robotically following the expectations of family, friends, and society. For example, individuals may first need to go through separation–individuation, emotionally process early life traumas, and develop self-compassion before they can listen to their own critical intuition telling them what is meaningful in life.

5. **Goal-management and self-regulation skills**: Living a meaningful life also includes practical skills. Individuals need to translate their sense of meaning into specific steps, actions, and goals. Therefore, research has shown how goal management and affective self-regulation skills are strongly positively correlated with a sense of meaningfulness in life (Vos, 2016a).

6. **Existential skills**: Individuals will inevitably face challenges and human limitations, such as mortality, freedom, and responsibility. Individuals may need existential competencies to cope with life's challenges and limits, such as meaning-centered coping, coping flexibility, and psychological resilience and hardiness.

7. **Commitment**: The seventh component of the experience of meaning in life follows from the clinical observation that some clients seem to have all the previous six components, but they still sit on the shore looking at other people sailing meaningfully through life without taking their own sailing boat onto the water. Thus, the experience of meaningfulness in life requires a commitment to actually striving toward realizing their meaning in daily life.

In sum, the general experience of meaning in life may be defined as the subjective experience of being motivated and committed to moving in a self-regulated and existentially competent way toward self-determined directions, goals, or purposes in life, in line with one's values and understanding of the world and significance of oneself (Vos, 2023b). Consequently, when clients share that they struggle with meaning, the therapist may explore what they mean by meaning and which components they particularly struggle with.

Types and Approaches to Meaning

Sigmund Freud allegedly stated that clients should learn to love and to work, assuming that love and work are the two most important types of meaning. Frankl described three pathways to meaning (sometimes inaccurately translated as "sources of meaning"; Vos, 2023c): experience, creative productivity, and our inner attitude. These examples show how therapists may differ in what they think are beneficial meanings for their clients.

Therefore, a systematic literature review was conducted to examine which types and subtypes of meaning may be the most helpful to discuss in therapy (Vos, 2023a). This included 107 studies in which 45,710 participants were asked what they experienced as meaningful, important, or valuable in life. The participants' answers were categorized via reflexive thematic analysis into types and subtypes of meaning (Vos, 2023b):

> A type of meaning describes *what* group or pattern of frequent activities or experiences give an individual an overall sense of meaningfulness in life. For example, when individuals say that they orient themselves around "social types of meaning", they mean that their intentions and actions in many life situations focus on finding meaning in relationships with other people, such as altruism, belonging to a community, etc. (p. 205, italics in original)

This study indicates the existence of a universal typology of meaning in life, consisting of six types and 29 subtypes of meaning: (a) *materialistic types of meaning* (i.e., material conditions, professional–educational success), (b) *hedonistic types* (i.e., enjoying hedonistic or physical experiences and health and sports), (c) *self-oriented types* (i.e., resilience and coping, self-insight, self-efficacy, self-acceptance, autonomy, creative self-expression, and self-care), (d) *social types* (i.e., social connections, belonging, conformism, altruism, and giving birth and looking after young generations), (e) *larger types* (i.e., specific purposes, personal growth, a sense of one's temporality or past-present-future, justice and ethics, and spirituality or religion), and (f) *existential–philosophical types* (i.e., being alive and mortality awareness, uniqueness, freedom and responsibility, connections, gratitude, and responsibility). For example, therapists may ask clients to explore experientially after an introductory mindfulness exercise to let any examples intuitively arise for each type and subtype in their past, present, or possible future (Vos, 2018b).

These six types of meaning were also found in a thinking aloud and interview study and were subsequently operationalized in the new Meaning Sextet Questionnaire. The universality of this meaning sextet was confirmed in 1,281 participants in 49 countries with factor structure and correlations as expected with other questionnaires (this questionnaire can be downloaded for therapeutic use from https://joelvos.com/). Meta-analyses indicated that materialistic, hedonistic, and self-oriented meanings correlated with low psychological well-being, whereas social and larger meanings correlated with greater psychological well-being, similar to previous studies (e.g., Baumeister et al., 2013; Nielsen et al., as cited in Batthyany & Russo-Netzer, 2014). The meaning sextet was again validated in a longitudinal survey during the COVID-19 pandemic across 1,479 individuals in 40 countries, showing how individuals reported worse mental and physical health and were more likely to report COVID-19 symptoms if they said that they only focused on a small number of meanings in life; experienced that the pandemic restrictions prevented them from realizing their important meanings in life; lacked the flexibility to shift their focus to a different meaning; and dominantly focused on materialistic, hedonistic, and self-oriented meanings instead of social or larger types (Vos, 2021b).

Clients seem to benefit from systematically exploring as many types and subtypes of meaning in therapy: the more types and subtypes they explore, the more effective the therapy becomes (Vos & Vitali, 2018). This is understandable, as a client is more likely to find something meaningful when a broad range of meanings is discussed, like how a person fishing is more likely to catch fish with a wide net than a tiny fishing rod (Vos, 2018b). Furthermore, research indicates that individuals experienced better mental and physical well-being if they dominantly focused on social and larger types of meaning, whereas their mental and physical well-being was worse if they dominantly focused on materialistic, hedonistic, and self-oriented types of meaning (Vos, 2023a, in press). It has also been suggested that there is benefit for an individual to have between three and six important meanings in life, particularly different types, as this could make individuals more resilient if they cannot realize one example of meaning (Lukas, 2014). For instance, individuals who had dominantly focused on a single meaning in life, such as going to a football stadium for a game, struggled with their mental health when a COVID-19 lockdown prevented them from attending the game at the stadium (Vos, 2020).

What is the most beneficial way for individuals to discover what they experience as meaningful in life? Individuals differ in how they approach meaning in life. For example, they could use a traditional approach by following religions or societal expectations to discover what type of meaning they want to follow; they could use a functionalistic or mechanistic approach by controlling their life and striving in the most linear way possible to achieve ambitious self-set goals; or they may apply a phenomenological approach by critically intuiting what is meaningful to them (Vos, 2018b, 2020, 2021a, 2021b, in press). A study with 1,281 participants in 49 countries using the Meaning Approach Questionnaire indicates that there are three distinct approaches (Vos, 2023a; this questionnaire can be downloaded for therapeutic use from https://joelvos.com/). Traditional and functionalistic approaches to meaning in life have moderately strong correlations with poor mental well-being, whereas phenomenological approaches correlate strongly with good mental well-being (Vos, 2023a). Research indicates that clients benefit from therapists who use phenomenological and experiential methods to explore their sense of meaning in life (Vos & Vitali, 2018). For example, experiential approaches to meaning in life, such as focusing on our embodied felt sense and mindfulness, are associated with large satisfaction about decisions and life and good mental and physical health (Chu & Mak, 2020; L. S. Greenberg et al., 1994; Kim et al., 2022; Remmers et al., 2016; Vanhooren et al., 2022). Having a sense of meaning may also help with accepting and exploring difficult experiences (Kelso et al., 2020; Ostafin & Proulx, 2020). Vos (2016a, 2016b, 2023c) effectively used these systematic reviews to develop the 10-session Systematic Meaning in Life Therapy to invite clients to systematically investigate all types and subtypes of meaning with their experiences and intuitions (the 10-session treatment manual can be found in Vos, 2018b).

CONTEXTUALIZING MEANING IN AN EH CONTEXT

The topic of meaning may be relevant for psychological therapists for several reasons. First, many clients explicitly ask meaning-oriented questions. Over 70 qualitative studies have shown that living a meaningful life is one of the key outcomes that clients want to achieve in therapy: "Recovery is about building a meaningful and satisfying life, as defined by the person themselves, whether or not there are ongoing or recurring symptoms or problems" (Andresen et al., 2011, p. 2). Clients may not recover from their psychological problems, but they may still be helped to live a meaningful and fulfilling life. Research indicates that individuals particularly ask questions about meaning in life in boundary situations when confronted with life's limitations, such as suffering, grief, illness, and death (Vos, 2016a, 2016b).

Second, meaning in life and mental health seem to be intertwined. In general, questionnaire research suggests that most people search for or experience meaning, purpose, or coherence in life, although the precise percentages differ by instrument, population, and study (e.g., Eriksson, 2022; see also Brandstätter et al., 2012; Shin & Steger, 2014; Steger, 2012). When individuals lack a sense of meaning, they seem more prone to developing depression, anxiety, and other psychological problems (e.g., Reker & Chamberlain, 1999; Shin & Steger, 2014; Steger, 2012). When individuals feel frustrated in roles and activities they highly value, they seem to experience lower psychological and physical well-being (Krause, 2004); for example, during the COVID-19 pandemic, individuals who experienced that the pandemic limited their ability to live a meaningful life experienced poor mental health (Vos, 2021c). Several studies have described how individuals can feel frustrated in experiencing meaning in life and how an *existential vacuum* may lead to mental health problems (Marshall & Marshall, 2012; Reker et al., 1987). However, most of this evidence comes from studies with nonexperimental designs, and these studies have not clarified the causal direction (e.g., King et al., 2006). Some evidence for causality can be found in cross-sectional studies showing how meaning-based coping contributes to better psychological adjustment during or after stressful events (e.g., Henoch & Danielson, 2009; Park, 2010; Park & Folkman, 1997). Clinical trials have also shown that by improving an individual's sense of meaning in their life, their mental health improves (Vos & Vitali, 2018); furthermore, clients seem to view finding new ways to live a meaningful life as an important aspect of therapeutic recovery (Bennett et al., 2014).

Third, an emerging field of research shows the relationship between meaning and physical health. For example, the experience that life is meaningful correlates with a range of biomarkers, such as stress hormones, immune system functioning, physical energy, slower growth of tumor cells, and longer survival (Bower et al., 2003; Ryff et al., 2004, 2006; Vos, 2016a). A systematic review of 113 qualitative and quantitative studies showed how many cardiovascular disease patients report explicit questions about meaning in life and how a sense of meaningfulness is correlated with a lower risk for cardiovascular events (Vos,

2021a). A sense of meaningfulness also seems to function as a source of resilience in coping with chronic or life-threatening physical disease, which suggests its societal relevance: More than 30% of the population live with a chronic or life-threatening disease, of whom over 40% also experience mental health problems and stress that exacerbate their physical problems and health care costs (Vos, 2016a). It seems that the stress levels in physically ill patients are related to their sense of meaning, as a review of 47 studies in physically ill patients showed moderately strong correlations between meaning in life and the level of psychological stress and psychopathology (Steger, 2012; Winger et al., 2016). Surveys have also shown that a majority of patients with a chronic or life-threatening disease ask questions about meaning; for instance, because they cannot do previous meaningful activities, they start to reflect on priorities in life and may question assumptions that they formerly had about their life (e.g., Henoch & Danielson, 2009; Lee et al., 2004; Schulenberg et al., 2014). Meaning has been given an essential role in many influential models in health and medical psychology (Vos, 2016a):

> The disease can challenge everyday assumptions about the world, life, the self and meaning, which can lead to the question: "How can I live a meaningful and satisfying life despite the physical, psychological, social and existential limitations of my disease?" Patients subsequently appraise their situation and assimilate the disease experience within their existing assumptions, transcend the situation by flexibly experiencing meaning despite being ill, change specific meanings in their lives, or change their general perspective on life. These appraisal processes could lead to motivated lifestyle changes, psychological symptoms and a request for professional support. (p. 86)

Furthermore, a meta-analysis (Vos & Vitali, 2018) has indicated that psychological therapies that focus on meaning in life have large short-term effects and moderate long-term effects on self-reported physical well-being ($g = 0.81$, $SE = 0.29$, $k = 8$; $g = 0.53$, $SE = 0.11$, $k = 4$), possibly via large effects on blood pressure, stress hormones, and survival time both immediately and at follow-up ($g = 0.86$, $SE = 0.31$, $k = 3$; $g = 1.20$, $SE = 0.26$, $k = 1$).

In sum, therapists may want to explicitly address meaning in life because their clients explicitly ask meaning-oriented questions, and a sense of meaningfulness seems positively correlated with mental and physical health. An unfulfilled request for help with meaning-oriented questions may lead to higher levels of depression, lower quality of life, demoralization, suicidal ideation, physical disease, and shorter survival (Vos, 2016a, 2016b).

MEANING ACROSS THERAPIES

Because meaning is so closely aligned with positive, long-term well-being, it is understandable that many therapeutic schools pay attention to it. It may be argued that all effective therapists help individuals live a more meaningful life despite their emotional or existential struggles (Vos, 2018b). "Psychodynamic and humanistic therapy, clinical psychology, and counseling psychology as such, not a particular branch of them, are best understood as enterprises in search of meaning in life" (Metz, 2013, p. 405).

For example, cognitive behavior therapy may help to address unhelpful and unrealistic beliefs about meaning in life and explore how their sense of meaning, or lack thereof, may be the result of early-life maladaptive schemas (Masley et al., 2012); client changes during cognitive behavior therapy may be explained by their improved meaning-making skills (Marco et al., 2021). Motivational interviewing and Alcoholics Anonymous may help individuals transcend their addictions by focusing on social and larger types of meanings. Trauma-focused therapy may help individuals process their traumas that may have shattered their fundamental assumptions about life and reconstruct a sense of posttraumatic meaning (Steger & Park, 2012). Psychodynamic and transactional approaches may help individuals develop healthy ego functions, work with their defense mechanisms against intolerable feelings, and generate a sense of "I am okay" and "others are okay," which may enable them to explore the topic of meaning in a freer, less rigid way (Vos & van Rijn, in press). Jungian analysis has often been used to help individuals explore meaning, particularly in midlife, via individuation, active imagination, and exploring one's shadow. Carl Jung's concept of the shadow represents the hidden, unconscious aspects of an individual's personality that the conscious mind refuses to acknowledge. It often contains repressed ideas, weaknesses, desires, instincts, and shortcomings. Jung believed integrating the shadow into conscious awareness was crucial for psychological growth and self-realization, despite its potentially disturbing nature. Self-compassion therapy may help individuals follow what is meaningful with compassion for inevitable frustrations. Furthermore, research suggests that experiential and body work, such as mindfulness, somatic experiencing, and Gestalt therapy, may help clients become aware of their experiences and express, deepen, and consciously use these, which may help them listen better to what they intuit as the most meaningful (Vanhooren, 2019). In person-centered and relational therapies, meaning is often addressed in relational terms, such as *congruence*, based on the idea that congruence from the therapist can help the client to become more congruent with themselves, a concept which has received much empirical support (for an example, see Norcross & Lambert, 2019). These stereotypic sketches suggest that all different therapeutic approaches may have some relevance for their client's search for meaning. Based on an integrative attitude, EH therapists may use some of these therapeutic components, such as congruence, presence, working with resistance, reconstructing a sense of wholeness in the experiencing process, and experientially exploring the impact of one's attitudes and beliefs about life.

Whereas working with meaning may not be a central pillar of most of the aforementioned therapeutic approaches, meaning is central for EH therapists. For example, a global survey amongst existential therapists (including EH, existential–phenomenological, meaning-centered, and daseinsanalytical therapies) showed that they described explicitly and systematically addressing meaning in life as one of their four key competencies, alongside relational, existential, and school-specific skills (Correia et al., 2018).

Although meaning is also at the heart of EH therapies (Bugental & Bracke, 1992; Schneider, 2003), relatively few studies focus on meaning strictly from an EH perspective. Therefore, the following sections will allude to findings from other therapies, particularly meaning-centered therapies (Vos, 2016b, 2023c), as these are highly consistent with and easily integrated into EH therapy. There are 30 schools of meaning-oriented therapies that pay explicit and systematic attention to meaning in life. Their difference from EH approaches is that they explicitly focus on helping clients with meaning-oriented questions and have a relatively systematic way of examining meaning in life with their clients. For example, meaning-oriented therapists do not ask individuals random questions about what they find meaningful in life; instead, they systematically explore each possible pathway to meaning in life (logotherapists identify experiential, productive–creative and attitudinal pathways) or each type of meaning in life (see Vos, 2018b, 2023c). The conceptualization of the experience of meaning also seems more phenomenological and less reductionistic than in other therapeutic approaches.

Early Meaning-Oriented Therapies

The first meaning-oriented therapists to pay explicit attention to meaning in life were Alfred Adler and Karl Jaspers, who addressed meaning as a part of life's broader power and existential struggles. Jaspers (1925/2013) showed how questions about meaning could arise in situations of suffering, pain, or death, which he called

> boundary situations in life: at such inevitable crossroads, we can choose to sink into despair and resignation or take a leap of faith towards *transcendence*, that is transcending the situation in space and time, accepting our freedom to decide, and developing a larger, more authentic and meaningful perspective on life. (Vos, 2016b, p. 48, italics in original)

Like Soren Kierkegaard's religious stage of human development, Adler and Jaspers saw meaning as transcending the present, an awareness of one's time–location bound position as well as their potential in time and space. Inherent to many existential philosophies, this also includes being able to bear the duality of experiencing meaning in an often existentially frightening universe (Vos, 2015). Although these authors were mainly theoretical, they inspired practitioners. The transcendent nature of meaning can also be found in the work of Frankl and may explain why many existential therapists particularly address meaning in boundary situations in life.

Viktor Frankl

Self-transcendence is also at the heart of Viktor Frankl's (1946/1985) paradigm-shifting book, originally entitled *Saying Yes to Life in Spite of Everything* and later known as *Man's Search for Meaning*, about his experiences as an inmate in Nazi concentration camps. In this book, Frankl describes his observations of how the inmates' ability to identify meaning and imagine the future affected their longevity, as individuals seem to have a will to meaning, and how the inability to experience meaning can lead to a deterioration of mental and physical health such as hopelessness and fatalism. Frankl also describes how he believes that meaning in life can be found in every moment of living, even in suffering and death. Individuals have the freedom of will—even in concentration camps and other severe suffering—at least to choose how they respond to their life situation. Frankl's logotherapy ("logo" means "meaning") is based on these three pillars of will to meaning, freedom of will, and potential of meaning in all situations. In logotherapy, he applies ideas from Adler, Jaspers, and the philosopher Martin Heidegger. However, many of Frankl's assumptions seem to lack systematic empirical support or are fundamentally unverifiable, such as the will to meaning, freedom of will, the potential to find meaning in every situation, elaborated diagnostic models, and three pathways to meaning (experiential, creativity–productivity, and attitude; Van Dyck, 1987; Vos, 2016b). Consequently, Frankl has been criticized for having authoritarian overtones (May, 1978, Yalom, 1980) and basing himself on unvalidated assumptions and unalterable truths (Cooper, 2018). Early existential therapies like Frankl did not systematically address all types of meaning but instead addressed the therapist's personal preferences; trials suggest that therapies focusing on only a small number of meanings lead to smaller improvements than therapies that systematically address more meanings (Vos & Vitali, 2018). However, we may also want to see Frankl in his context and not unfairly judge him with the standards of our current research and therapeutic practice; he was very open to research and progress, and he told his students not to follow him blindly.

Frankl used a broad range of therapeutic techniques to help individuals live a more meaningful life, some of which are empirically supported (Vos, 2018b). For example, paradoxical intention means that clients are asked to practice or exaggerate a neurotic habit deliberately or in thought so that they stop avoidant, obsessive, or fighting behavior that could exacerbate their problems; this technique has proven particularly effective in anxiety disorders (K. A. Hill, 1987). De-reflection techniques can be used to stop hyperreflection and hyperintention, which are individuals' habits of reflecting so much on their problems or obsessing with curing their problems, respectively, that the problems become larger; similar defusion techniques have proven effective in acceptance and commitment therapy (Hayes et al., 2006). Frankl also helped clients develop a more positive and meaningful attitude toward their situation (Lukas, 2014), later operationalized and empirically supported as meaning-oriented coping styles and tertiary meaning-oriented coping (Park & Folkman, 1997). Although EH therapy tends to avoid techniques and highly structured interventions, many of Frankl's strategies, particularly helping clients develop a meaningful attitude toward difficult situations, are central to EH therapy.

Logotherapy and Existential Analysis

In line with Frankl's work, several meaning-oriented schools emerged such as logotherapy with key authors such as Elizabeth Lukas, Joseph Fabry, and Edward Marshall. Existential analysis integrates phenomenological and client-centered practices and helps individuals develop an authentic and responsible attitude toward their lives and situation so that they can experience themselves freely and say "yes" with an inner consent to (a) the world (i.e., feeling we exist), (b) life (i.e., feeling life is good and valuable), (c) self (i.e., feeling and showing authentic uniqueness), and (d) meaning. Thus, existential analysis helps clients to say, "Yes, I exist, my life is good, I can be myself, and I can achieve my goals" (Längle, 2019). The anthropology and treatment model from Frankl and the original logotherapeutic and existential–analytical schools have dominantly based themselves on philosophical reflections and rich clinical experience and less on systematic clinical research with today's scientific standards; there are few research studies on these therapies. Alfried Längle differs from some logotherapists and existential analysts with his accent on phenomenological, experiential, and relational skills, which seem in line with EH therapies.

Confrontational Existential Therapies

The first systematic therapy trials in which the topic of meaning was explicitly addressed were existential therapies, in which cancer patients were stimulated to express existential feelings as well as confront and accept life's limitations such as death, freedom, isolation, and meaninglessness (e.g., Spiegel et al., 1981). However, these early existential therapies did not systematically explore all possible types and subtypes of meaning. Meta-analyses of clinical trials indicate that these therapies had no or only small positive psychological effects, and some studies seemed biased with a risk of false positive results due to, for example, the lack of replicability of findings (Vos et al., 2015). The confrontational tone of these existential therapies seemed to be in line with the confrontational approach in workshops in the 1970s, where individuals would, for example, lie in a coffin hearing others give their eulogies so that they would be ultimately confronted with their mortality without the possibility of denial or avoidance. There are individual stories about clients becoming psychotic or suicidal in response to the therapist confronting them with life's limits and preventing them from grasping onto their sense of meaning, although they have been left out from several early studies without reporting it (several EH therapists and researchers have communicated this confidentially to me). Meta-analyses of working with meaning in therapies clearly show that the more one-dimensional confrontational an existential therapist is, the less effective they are, whereas therapists are more effective if they foster a dual attitude of facing life's limitations while trying to find a sense of meaning, self-compassion and therapeutic–relational safety in the present (Vos, 2015, 2018b; Vos & Vitali, 2018). EH therapies also seem to focus on this duality, facilitating clients to become aware of their resistances and struggles in supportive and self-compassionate ways and while in a safe relationship.

Second-Wave Positive Psychology (or Existential Positive Psychology)
The field of positive psychology pays explicit attention to meaning in life. For example, research indicates that positive well-being includes multiple aspects such as meaning, which have been summarized by the founding father Seligman (2005) in the PERMA model: positive emotion, engagement, positive relationships, meaning, and accomplishments or achievements. However, existential researchers have criticized the overly positive approach to meaning, as meaning cannot be artificially disentangled from negative and existential experiences such as our finitude (Batthyany & Russo-Netzer, 2014; Ivtzan et al., 2015; Kashdan & Biswas-Diener, 2014; Vos, 2015, Wong, 2012). Wong (2012) has proposed his own meaning therapy, which is a short, action-oriented therapeutic approach with specific exercises, based on the theoretical ABCDE model: helping clients (a) accept events in life, (b) believe in strengths and the possibility of change, (c) commit to actions, (d) discover hidden meanings, and (e) evaluate change and progress. While early positive psychology approaches may not easily fit with EH therapy, there are many opportunities for integration (Schneider, 2011).

New Developments
Since the turn of the millennium, many clinical trials have been conducted on brief, integrative, meaning-centered therapies for individuals at crossroads in life, such as cancer patients (Breitbart, 2016; Lee et al., 2004; van der Spek et al., 2014), grieving individuals (MacKinnon et al., 2013), and family therapy (Lantz, 2000; Schulenberg et al., 2010). The effectiveness of working with meaning in physical health care seems well-established, but there is less research on meaning in other populations including general mental health care (Vos, 2016b; Vos & Vitali, 2018).

At the same time, more research has emerged about the evolution of meaning across the lifespan and how therapists may offer different support at different life stages, showing how individuals experience meaning differently at different life stages (García-Alandete et al., 2019), even with different generations within the same family (Sahin & Kabasakal, 2023). Young individuals seem to dominantly follow the tradition, whereas in their twenties, they develop a more functionalistic and mechanistic approach to life, followed by a more phenomenological approach in midlife (Vos, 2023c). Young people seem to focus dominantly on materialistic, hedonistic, and self-oriented types (Bhattacharya, 2011; Vos, 2023a), although university students may also focus on social and sometimes larger types of meaning (C. E. Hill et al., 2013; Schankweiler, 2020). There seems to be a significant shift in the types and approaches to meaning around midlife, which may also be addressed by EH therapists (Guttmann, 2008). Older people focus more on social, larger, and existential–philosophical types of meaning (Vos, 2023a), and at the end of life, people seem to mainly struggle with a sense of meaninglessness due to losses and social isolation (Saarelainen et al., 2022). The presence of meaning has been shown to be an important aspect of well-being for older adults and may be an important focus when working with them, while both presence of and search for meaning may be more meaningful therapeutic therapy goals for younger adults (Battersby & Phillips, 2016). In response to the increasing awareness of age-specific, meaning-centered needs, specific therapies have been developed for students (Robatmili et al., 2015) and people around and beyond retirement (Edwards & Milton, 2014; Heisel, 2016; Mangione & Forti, 2018). In response to the silos that different therapists and researchers seem to be stuck in, as well as the frequently observed lack of systematic scientific basis for their meaning-centered therapies, Vos (2016a, 2016b, 2018b, 2023c) used the literature reviews and meta-analyses to develop and validate a generic 10-session Systematic Meaning in Life Therapy.

RESEARCH ON MEANING

This section will provide an overview of quantitative, qualitative, and mixed methods studies on the role of meaning in life in psychological therapies.

Quantitative Therapy Research

This section provides a general overview of quantitative research on working with meaning in therapies, particularly in EH therapy. In 2018, Vos and Vitali conducted a multilingual, systematic review and meta-analysis of all clinical trials on psychological therapies that focused on meaning in life. They found 60 trials with a combined sample of 3,713 individuals. Of the trials, 26 were randomized controlled trials ($n = 1,975$), 15 were nonrandomized controlled trials ($n = 709$), and 19 were nonrandomized noncontrolled trials with pre and post measurements ($n = 1,029$). Vos and Vitali found that clients experienced large improvements from pretreatment to immediate posttreatment and follow-up on quality of life ($g = 1.13$, $SE = 0.12$; $g = 0.99$, $SE = 0.20$) and psychological stress ($g = 1.21$, $SE = 0.10$; $g = 0.67$, $SE = 0.20$). Subsequently, the reviewers focused on the randomized controlled trials only and found that meaning therapies had large effect sizes compared with control groups, both immediate and at follow-up, on quality of life ($g = 1.02$, $SE = 0.06$; $g = 1.06$, $SE = 0.12$) and psychological stress ($g = 0.94$, $SE = 0.07$, $p < 0.01$; $g = 0.84$, $SE = 0.10$). The immediate effects were larger for general quality of life ($g = 1.37$, $SE = 0.12$) than for meaning in life ($g = 1.18$, $SE = 0.08$), hope and optimism ($g = 0.80$, $SE = 0.13$), self-efficacy ($g = 0.89$, $SE = 0.14$), and social well-being ($g = 0.81$, $SE = 13$). The homogeneity of these findings was validated by the lack of significance of moderators—such as type of sample—and alternative ways of selecting studies. Furthermore, the researchers conducted meta-regression analyses, which showed that an increase in the client's meaning in life predicted decreases in psychological stress ($\beta = -0.56$, $p < 0.001$), which seemed to confirm the assumption that the well-being of clients improved thanks to explicitly addressing meaning in life. Further analyses indicated that the more different types of meaning are addressed in therapy (e.g., discussing all six types of meaning in life instead of only discussing one type of meaning), the larger the effects are (Vos, 2021b; Vos & Vitali, 2018).

These positive findings for meaning-oriented therapies were in line with meta-analyses on all existential therapies, which showed that meaning-oriented therapies are more effective than other types of existential therapies, although there were relatively few trials on other existential therapeutic schools (Vos et al., 2015). These effect sizes were in line with effects that have been reported for other humanistic therapies (Elliott, 2002; Vos & van Rijn, 2022). Therefore, although further research would be beneficial in confirming that these benefits would include EH approaches, there is good evidence that this is relevant if EH therapists include a focus on meaning, particularly the different types of meaning.

Following these meta-analyses, Vos (2016b, 2018b) conducted a series of reviews of the therapeutic mechanisms and outcomes in meaning-centered therapies. These reviews indicate that meaning-oriented therapists aim to help clients live a meaningful and satisfying life despite life's challenges, which is consistent with the focus of EH therapy (Hoffman et al., 2015). There was a large variation in the number of therapy sessions, although most descriptions and manuals of therapy seem to have three general phases: assessment and introduction to the topic of meaning; systematically exploring different types of meaning, sometimes with the help of specific exercises and questionnaires; and applying meaning in daily life (Vos, 2016b). Analyses of treatment protocols and handbooks also show that therapists working with meaning strive toward these aims via five groups of therapeutic competencies. Each of these groups have multiple subcompetencies and are supported by much empirical evidence (see Vos, 2018b).

Assessment competencies help therapists evaluate clients' life situations, needs, preferences, and capacities regarding meaning in life in order to develop a specific meaning-related plan together with the clients to help them with the problems they are currently facing. Research confirms that in therapies in general, assessments, case formulations, and goal setting can improve therapy effectiveness (Tryon & Winograd, 2011; van Rijn, 2014).

Meaning-oriented competencies include explicating, systematically exploring, and improving meaningful aspects of the client's experiences. They include skills that have been shown to be effective in other therapies, such as

- providing psychoeducation;

- rephrasing or reframing the stories of the clients in terms of meaning;

- conducting guided exercises;

- connecting the topic of meaning with specific situations in everyday life (Cooper, 2008; Roth & Fonagy, 2013);

- unconditional positive regard and hope (Farber & Doolin, 2011);

- focusing on long-term meaning rather than short-term gratification and pleasure (Wong, 2012);

- life reviews (Westerhof et al., 2010);

- goal management, such as helping clients set concrete aims for their day-to-day lives, make a plan, experiment in daily life, evaluate and adjust the aims and method, and make long-term commitments (Lapierre et al., 2007); and

- balancing autonomy and connections: Meaning-oriented therapists often underline both their clients' autonomy, self-esteem, and self-discovery as well as being realistic and socially connected in their decision making; research indicates the effectiveness of balancing self and others in meaning in life (e.g., Batthyany & Russo-Netzer, 2014; Mikulincer et al., 2013; Schlegel et al., 2013; see also Mikulincer & Shaver, 2013).

Existential skills are about how to live a meaningful life despite life's inevitable challenges and existential givens such as being thrown into life, freedom of decision, responsibility, social connections, and mortality. Research indicates that existential challenges can give rise to existential moods such as death anxiety and boredom (e.g., Vos, 2018a; Vos, Cooper, Craig, & Cooper, 2015). Studies on terror management theory show how existential challenges—such as awareness of our mortality—can trigger existential anxiety. Individuals may respond to these with proximate and distal existential defense mechanisms, such as shifting their attention, denial, and avoiding reminders of existential givens or focusing on defending and conserving one's values (J. Greenberg et al., 2013). Although existential defense mechanisms may relieve short-term stress, they are associated with a lower long-term sense of meaning and fulfilment about life (Jim et al., 2006). However, studies on the effectiveness of addressing existential themes without simultaneously addressing meaning in life seem less effective, and therefore it has been recommended to address existential topics such as freedom and mortality simultaneously with meaning in life (Vos, Craig, & Cooper, 2015). This seems to assume a dual attitude of addressing meaning at the same time as existential topics (Vos, 2015) via flexible coping styles (Cheng et al., 2014) and meaning-oriented coping (Park & Folkman, 1997).

Relational competencies focus on "establishing an in-depth, authentic therapeutic relationship, along with reflection on and analysis of the relational encounter and combined with a phenomenological exploration of the client's experiences, which is particularly practiced by existential analysts" (Vos, 2016a, p. 49). Empirical research strongly supports the effectiveness of relational competencies in therapies (Norcross & Lambert, 2019), such as empathy, congruence, and the capacity to repair alliance ruptures, as discussed in other chapters in this volume as core EH practices.

Phenomenological and experiential competencies regard helping clients accept, explore, express, and deepen their phenomenological flow of experiences. Many EH therapists assume that individuals can become aware of their sense of meaning in life by tuning into their subjective flow of experiences. For example, therapists may stimulate clients (and themselves) to temporarily set aside all preexisting assumptions and biases (rule of epoche), neutrally describe the phenomena (rule of description), avoid placing any initial hierarchies of significance or importance upon the themes of description (rule of equalization), and identify the deeper sense of meaning that may arise from this process (eidetic reduction; e.g., Spinelli, 2005). Although using phenomenological therapeutic approaches without using other therapeutic competences seems relatively ineffective (Vos et al., 2015), specific techniques associated with the phenomenological approach are effective, such as the Socratic dialogue, which helps to elicit what the client already knows instead of pouring information into the client and is known for its moderate positive psychological effects (e.g., Overholser, 2010). Therapists may use other competencies and exercises to address the client's flow of experiencing; there is some evidence for the therapeutic helpfulness of mindfulness (Hofmann et al., 2010), art, drama, poetry, and drawing (Elliott, Greenberg, & Lietaer, 2004). A therapeutic process underlying these phenomenological and experiential competences seems to be the stimulation of experiential acceptance, such as fostering acceptance of world (e.g., accepting physical limitations of a disease), life (e.g., accepting your own experiences), self (e.g., accepting and showing who you are), and what clients experience as meaningful; other therapeutic approaches, such as acceptance and commitment therapy, seem to effectively help with experiential acceptance (Hayes et al., 2006).

In sum, EH therapists may help clients to live a meaningful and satisfying life despite life's challenges. Clients seem to experience such improvements thanks to the therapists explicitly and systematically using several evidence-based competencies: meaning-specific, assessment, relational, phenomenological, experiential, and existential therapeutic competencies. Although the clinical trials do not show different effects of meaning-oriented therapies in particular populations, it may be argued that meaning-oriented therapies may be best suited for boundary situations in life when individuals explicitly ask meaning-oriented questions such as confrontations with suffering, life-threatening and chronic physical disease, grief, and one's own finitude.

Qualitative Therapy Research

It is impossible to comprehensively review the sheer amount of qualitative research, case studies, and therapeutic studies on meaning in life. A quick literature search suggests that most qualitative studies on meaning-centered therapies focus on physically ill individuals, particularly cancer patients (for overviews, see Henoch & Danielson, 2009; Visser et al., 2010; Vos, 2016b). For example, focus groups with 23 cancer survivors showed that the participants wanted to discuss relationships, experiences, resilience, goals, leaving legacies, social roles, and uncertainties about the future (van der Spek et al., 2013). Cardoso and colleagues (2023) interviewed eight individuals who had received meaning therapy in palliative care and who described that the therapy addressed the themes of family, preservation of identity, life retrospection, clinical situa-tion, achievements, socioprofessional valorization, forgiveness, apology recon-ciliation, and saying goodbye. Similar findings were found in a study on integrative meaning therapy in cancer patients who described the themes of sense of stigma and loneliness, unjust and anticipatory guilt, reconsidering one's own life and nostalgia, rebirth, togetherness and gratitude, legacy, and acceptance (Grassi et al., 2022). In sum, these studies suggest that physically ill individuals experience various meaning-related needs, many of which may be addressed in therapy. A recurrent theme seems to be the meaning of relation-ships, reviewing one's life, and legacy.

There are similar studies on the role of meaning reconstruction in bereave-ment (Neimeyer, 2001). For example, Bogensperger and Lueger-Schuster (2014) discovered in interviews with parents the many ways how through therapy they tried to reconstruct meaning, for example, by trying to find per-sonal improvements and social actions. Few studies focus solely on the experi-ences of therapy on mental health, such as Zeng and colleagues (2021), who showed how depressed individuals describe the importance of accepting depression, appreciating work, embodying love and taking on responsibilities, and receiving spiritual comfort.

Few studies have examined therapeutic mechanisms and processes in meaning-centered therapies (Vos, 2023c), although meta-analyses suggest that the impact of meaning-centered therapies on mental health is most likely mediated by the improvement in the client's ability to experience meaning in life (Vos & Vitali, 2018). One qualitative study indicates that the effects of meaning-centered therapies on psychological well-being are mediated by an improved sense of meaning and peace (Rosenberg et al., 2018), although the precise mechanisms and causal relationship remain unclear.

These studies show how meaning can be relevant for many populations and how therapists may address their meaning-related needs. In line with aforementioned quantitative studies and meta-analyses, a metasynthesis of 12 meaning-centered therapy studies showed that a core component of all the interventions was the interpersonal client–therapist encounter, in which different types of meanings were explored and a sense of connectedness was reestablished. Individuals reported an improved sense of purpose in life, qual-ity of life, spiritual well-being, self-efficacy, optimism, and less distress, hope-lessness, anxiety, depression, and wish to hasten death (Guerrero-Torrelles et al., 2017).

Furthermore, interviews with existential therapists (C. E. Hill et al., 2017) showed that providing therapy helps them experience self-oriented meaning (e.g., feeling gratified, fulfilled, connected) and other-oriented meaning (e.g., helping others, making the world a better place). They believed that meaning is fundamental and underlies all human concerns. In contrast to the clients who had implicit meaning-related concerns, clients who explicitly presented meaning-related concerns were reported to have more interpersonal problems and physical problems but with similar amounts of psychological distress and loss or grief (C. E. Hill et al., 2017). Similar findings were found in counselors in Israel (Russo-Netzer, Sinai, & Zeevi, 2020). A replication study in China indicated some similarities (e.g., both seeing meaning as part of human existence and underlying most client's presenting concerns) and differences (e.g., Chinese therapists regarded meaning as involving a sense of responsibility to others whereas Western therapists did not mention this; Duan et al., 2022). These differences raise the question of how cultures may differ in how meaning is experienced and how therapists work with this.

MULTICULTURAL CONSIDERATIONS

Individuals do not experience meaning in a solipsistic vacuum but in an interactive coconstruction with their social context and broader society (Chao & Kesebir, 2013; Mikulincer & Shaver, 2014; Neimeyer, 2001; Stillman & Lambert, 2013). This chapter has shown so far how, across the globe, having a positive sense of meaning is positively related to mental and physical health, particularly if individuals focus mainly on social and larger types of meaning (Bhullar, 2019). Individuals seem to develop their sense of meaning at the intersection of multiple, continuously changing and often conflicting influences and identities, trying to balance in their experience among what they want and do not want, can and cannot do, and must and must not do (Vos, 2018b). Given the complex intrapsychic and interpersonal dynamics as well as the socioeconomic and political power structures within which meaning emerges, it is understandable that individuals may ask therapists for help. For example, individuals may struggle to accept and express the meaningfulness of their homosexual orientation in cultures, subcultures, or religions where they expect a negative response from others.

As society changes, people change in how they approach meaning and what meanings they find meaningful in life. For example, it is a historiological fallacy to assume that individuals in all eras have asked individual questions about their personal meaning in life; although philosophers may have written about meaning, ordinary citizens in Europe derived their sense of meaning from the position that they were relegated in the divine-cosmic-social order that the clergy and monarchs imposed onto them, and they only started asking questions about their personal meaning from the 16th century onward (Berman, 2009; Vos, 2018b, 2020, 2021a, 2023b). Globally, we can see the following trends in the types of meaning in life (Vos, 2020):

> Across cultures, individuals seem to report materialistic, hedonistic, self-oriented, social, larger, and existential–philosophical types of meaning. There do not seem to be cultural differences in the ability to see these as possible types of meaning. However, research indicates how individuals in different socioeconomic and political systems give different meaning-oriented answers. Meta-analyses of 107 studies with 45,710 individuals worldwide showed that the more capitalist a country is, the more individuals focus on materialist, hedonist, and self-oriented types of meaning and less on social and larger types of meaning. These

meta-analyses also showed that the more capitalist a country is, the lower the average mental health of its citizens; this seems to stem from the fact that these citizens focus more on materialist, hedonist, and self-oriented types of meaning. A Worldwide Survey of Meaning in Life of 1,281 participants in 49 countries also confirmed that the more capitalist a country is, the more its citizens focus on the unique capitalistic perspectives on meaning in life. This also showed that the national economic system influences how individuals experience meaning in life but does not completely determine their sense of meaning. Thus, regardless of their socioeconomic situation, individuals have some individual freedom to decide their own perspectives on life. In addition, the Worldwide Survey of Meaning in Life showed that socioeconomic circumstances can make individuals feel that they cannot fulfil their imagined meaning in life, and this lack of fulfilment can lead to psychological stress and lower quality of life. However, it seems that imagination is more important than the realization of meaning in life, possibly because it may be easier for individuals to change their imagination than their actual socioeconomic circumstances. (p. 161)

Following the social construction of our personal meaning, Vos (2020) has argued that there is no such thing as neutral economics and politics. All socioeconomic and political theories, models, and symbols explicitly or implicitly describe meaning. Vos (2020) describes how neoliberal countries seem dominated by the *capitalist life syndrome*, which he defines as that perspective on economics—albeit economics as a reality, symbol, or imagined model—that focuses on materialist, hedonist, and self-oriented types of meaning from a functionalist perspective. This perspective sees individuals and history as a functionalist process predominantly determined by materialist factors that make individuals feel unfree despite the capitalist imagination of freedom and that also lead to a crisis in the existential, psychological, and overall well-being of the capitalist life syndrome, and which can be reinforced by the techniques that manipulate the meanings of citizens and consumers. Vos also summarizes economic and sociological research showing a transition toward postmaterialist economies, such as the experience economy, moral economy, and meaning-oriented economy:

A Meaning-Oriented Economy has a predominantly nonfunctionalist approach towards social or larger meanings, seen from complex interaction between individuals and society, with a plurality of meanings; individuals with a meaning-oriented perspective on the economy have better existential, social, psychological, and physical well-being (Vos, 2020, p. 124).

EH therapists may want to critically reflect on the culture in which they provide therapy, their own cultural assumption about meaning, and the impact of society, culture, and traditions on their clients' meanings.

FUTURE RESEARCH NEEDS

Despite the large body of research literature, more replication and validation studies along with validated and reliable psychometric instruments are warranted. There needs to be particularly more research on diversity. That is, most studies have been conducted in Western countries on heterosexual cisgender people and particularly on individuals with a chronic or life-threatening disease. Therefore, less is known about the experiences of meaning, therapeutic mechanisms, and outcomes of working with meaning in life in other populations, such as underrepresented ethnic and neurodiverse groups. For example, research shows how lesbian, gay, bisexual, transgender, and queer or other individuals often have different life histories than cisgender heterosexual people, and they are more likely to have experienced rejection, discrimination, and oppression in life; it seems understandable that their histories will influence how they have developed a sense of meaning in life and lifestyle as well as how they experience different meaning-oriented questions than their cisgender straight counterparts (Vos et al., 2019). Furthermore, anecdotal experiences suggest that the approach to meaning in therapies is often intertwined with local religions and cultures, such as mixing meaning with Christian evangelical approaches in Africa; Islam in the Middle East; and with Confucianist, Buddhist, and Daoist ideas in Southeast Asia (professional experiences of the author). Although meta-analyses suggest that interventions with explicit religious or spiritual foci are less effective than religiously or spiritually neutral interventions, more studies are needed to confirm the effectiveness and accessibility of meaning-oriented treatments in religious or spiritual cultures (Vos & Vitali, 2018). Thus, more research is required to understand the experiences of meaning and meaning-oriented therapies in diverse populations. For example, future studies could examine how socioeconomic privileges—or a lack thereof—can influence meaning in life and how therapists can support individuals to live a meaningful and satisfying life despite life histories of multiple stressful life experiences and posttraumatic stress disorders (Fischer et al., 2020), such as structural injustice, moral injuries, and narcissistic abuse.

CONCLUSIONS

Meaning in life seems to be an important topic for many individuals, and their sense of meaningfulness is often intertwined with their mental and physical health. Many clients ask meaning-oriented questions in the therapy room. Therefore, many therapists address meaning. Clinical trials have shown that when therapists systematically and explicitly address meaning, their clients experience large improvements in psychological well-being and quality of life.

There seems to be a proliferation of well-intended attempts to include meaning in a broad range of psychological therapies. However, without proper background in the research on meaning, therapists may impose their preferences onto their clients, use ineffective therapeutic mechanisms, or use unsupported theories and models of meaning that may confuse or even harm clients. Clients seem to benefit the least from a functionalistic or mechanistic and traditional approach to life and from a dominant focus on materialistic, hedonistic, and self-oriented types of meaning, even though this approach and focus seems dominant in Western capitalistic countries. Instead, clients seem to benefit the most from systematically exploring all types of meaning in life with a phenomenological and relational approach, listening critically to their intuition and flow of experiencing. Therapists may help clients in this search for meaning; to do so, they may want to improve their assessment, meaning-specific, relational, phenomenological and experiential, and existential therapeutic competencies (for further reading, see Vos, 2016a, 2016b, 2018b, 2020, 2021c, 2023b).

REFERENCES

Andresen, R., Oades, L. G., & Caputi, P. (2011). *Psychological recovery.* John Wiley & Sons. https://doi.org/10.1002/9781119975182

Battersby, A., & Phillips, L. (2016). In the end it all makes sense: Meaning in life at either end of the adult lifespan. *International Journal of Aging & Human Development, 83*(2), 184–204. https://doi.org/10.1177/0091415016647731

Batthyany, A., & Russo-Netzer, P. (Eds.). (2014). *Meaning in positive and existential psychology.* Springer. https://doi.org/10.1007/978-1-4939-0308-5

Baumeister, R. F., Vohs, K. D., Aaker, J. L., & Garbinsky, E. N. (2013). Some key differences between a happy life and a meaningful life. *The Journal of Positive Psychology, 8*(6), 505–516. https://doi.org/10.1080/17439760.2013.830764

Bennett, B., Breeze, J., & Neilson, T. (2014). Applying the recovery model to physical rehabilitation. *Nursing Standard, 28*(23), 37–43. https://doi.org/10.7748/ns2014.02.28.23.37.e8292

Berman, M. (2009). *The politics of authenticity.* Verso.

Bhattacharya, A. (2011). Meaning in life: A qualitative inquiry into the life of young adults. *Psychological Studies, 56*(1), 280–288. https://doi.org/10.1007/s12646-011-0091-0

Bhullar, N. (2019). Beliefs about the meaning of life in American and Indian college students: Similar or different? *Psychological Studies, 64*(4), 420–428. https://doi.org/10.1007/s12646-019-00490-6

Bogensperger, J., & Lueger-Schuster, B. (2014). Losing a child: Finding meaning in bereavement. *European Journal of Psychotraumatology, 5*(1), 22910–22915. https://doi.org/10.3402/ejpt.v5.22910

Bower, J. E., Kemeny, M. E., Taylor, S. E., & Fahey, J. L. (2003). Finding positive meaning and its association with natural killer cell cytotoxicity among participants in a bereavement-related disclosure intervention. *Annals of Behavioral Medicine, 25*(2), 146–155. https://doi.org/10.1207/S15324796ABM2502_11

Brandstätter, M., Baumann, U., Borasio, G. D., & Fegg, M. J. (2012). Systematic review of meaning in life assessment instruments. *Psycho-Oncology, 21*(10), 1034–1052. https://doi.org/10.1002/pon.2113

Breitbart, W. S. (Ed.). (2016). *Meaning-centered psychotherapy in the cancer setting.* Oxford University Press.

Bugental, J. F. T., & Bracke, P. E. (1992). The future of existential–humanistic psychotherapy. *Psychotherapy, 29*(1), 28–33. https://doi.org/10.1037/0033-3204.29.1.28

Cardoso, A. R., Remondes-Costa, S., Veiga, E., Almeida, V., Rocha, J., Teixeira, R. J., Macedo, G., & Leite, M. (2023). Meaning of life therapy. *OMEGA—Journal of Death and Dying.* Advance online publication. https://doi.org/10.1177/00302228231209654

Chao, M. M., & Kesebir, P. (2013). *The experience of meaning in life.* Springer.

Cheng, C., Lau, H. P. B., & Chan, M. P. S. (2014). Coping flexibility and psychological adjustment to stressful life changes: A meta-analytic review. *Psychological Bulletin, 140*(6), 1582–1607. https://doi.org/10.1037/a0037913

Chu, S. T. W., & Mak, W. W. (2020). How mindfulness enhances meaning in life: A meta-analysis of correlational studies and randomized controlled trials. *Mindfulness, 11*(1), 177–193. https://doi.org/10.1007/s12671-019-01258-9

Cooper, M. (2008). *Essential research findings in counselling and psychotherapy*. Sage.

Cooper, M. (2015). *Existential psychotherapy and counselling*. Sage.

Duan, C., Hill, C. E., Jiang, G., Li, D., Li, Y., Zhang, S., Yan, Y., Yu, L., & Lu, T. (2022). Meaning in life: Perspectives of experienced Chinese psychotherapists. *Psychotherapy, 59*(1), 26–37. https://doi.org/10.1037/pst0000395

Dyck, M. J. (1987). Assessing logotherapeutic constructs: Conceptual and psychometric status of the purpose in life and seeking of noetic goals tests. *Clinical Psychology Review, 7*(4), 439–447. https://doi.org/10.1016/0272-7358(87)90021-3

Edwards, W., & Milton, M. (2014). Retirement therapy? Older people's experiences of existential therapy relating to their transition to retirement. *Counselling Psychology Review, 29*(2), 43–53. https://doi.org/10.53841/bpscpr.2014.29.2.43

Elliott, R. (2002). The effectiveness of humanistic therapies : A meta-analysis. In D. J. Cain (Ed.), *Humanistic psychotherapies* (pp. 57–81). American Psychological Association. https://doi.org/10.1037/10439-002

Elliott, R., Greenberg, L. S., & Lietaer, G. (2004). Research on experiential psychotherapies. In M. J. Lambert (Ed.), *Bergin and Garfield's handbook of psychotherapy and behavior change* (5th ed., pp. 493–539). John Wiley & Sons..

Eriksson, M. (2022). The sense of coherence: the concept and its relationship to health. In M. Eriksson (Ed.), *The handbook of salutogenesis* (pp. 61–68). Routledge.

Farber, B. A., & Doolin, E. M. (2011). Positive regard. *Psychotherapy, 48*(1), 58–64. https://doi.org/10.1037/a0022141

Fischer, I. C., Shanahan, M. L., Hirsh, A. T., Stewart, J. C., & Rand, K. L. (2020). The relationship between meaning in life and post-traumatic stress symptoms in US military personnel: A meta-analysis. *Journal of Affective Disorders, 277*, 658–670. https://doi.org/10.1016/j.jad.2020.08.063

Frankl, V. E. (1985). *Man's search for meaning*. Simon and Schuster. (Original work published 1946)

García-Alandete, J., Gallego Hernández de Tejada, B., Pérez Rodríguez, S., & Marco-Salvador, J. H. (2019). Meaning in life among adolescents: Factorial invariance of the purpose in life test and buffering effect on the relationship between emotional dysregulation and hopelessness. *Clinical Psychology & Psychotherapy, 26*(1), 24–34. https://doi.org/10.1002/cpp.2327

Grassi, L., Sabato, S., Caruso, R., Tiberto, E., Padova, S., Ruffilli, F., Folesani, F., Nanni, M. G., Martino, B. M., Zerbinati, L., & Testoni, I. (2022). Reflecting on meaning in an existential–reorientation group psychotherapy approach for cancer patients: A qualitative thematic analysis. *Palliative & Supportive Care, 20*(3), 313–320. https://doi.org/10.1017/S1478951521000936

Greenberg, J., Koole, S. L., & Pyszczynski, T. (Eds.). (2013). *Handbook of experimental existential psychology*. Guilford Press.

Greenberg, L. S., Elliott, R., & Lietaer, G. (1994). Research on experiential psychotherapies. In A. E. Bergin & S. L. Garfield (Eds.), *Handbook of psychotherapy and behavior change* (4th ed., pp. 509–539). John Wiley & Sons.

Guerrero-Torrelles, M., Monforte-Royo, C., Rodríguez-Prat, A., Porta-Sales, J., & Balaguer, A. (2017). Understanding meaning in life interventions in patients with advanced disease: A systematic review and realist synthesis. *Palliative Medicine, 31*(9), 798–813. https://doi.org/10.1177/0269216316685235

Guttmann, D. (2008). *Finding meaning in life, at midlife and beyond: Wisdom and spirit from logotherapy*. Bloomsbury. https://doi.org/10.5040/9798400651373

Hayes, S. C., Luoma, J. B., Bond, F. W., Masuda, A., & Lillis, J. (2006). Acceptance and commitment therapy: Model, processes and outcomes. *Behaviour Research and Therapy, 44*(1), 1–25. https://doi.org/10.1016/j.brat.2005.06.006

Heisel, M. J. (2016). Enhancing psychological resiliency in older men facing retirement with meaning-centered men's groups. *Logotherapy and Existential Analysis, 1*(1), 165–173. https://doi.org/10.1007/978-3-319-29424-7_15

Henoch, I., & Danielson, E. (2009). Existential concerns among patients with cancer and interventions to meet them: An integrative literature review. *Psycho-Oncology, 18*(3), 225–236. https://doi.org/10.1002/pon.1424

Hill, C. E., Bowers, G., Costello, A., England, J., Houston-Ludlam, A., Knowlton, G., May, M., Moraff, E., Pinto-Coelho, K., Rosenberg, L., Sauber, E., Crook-Lyon, R. E., & Thompson, B. J. (2013). What's it all about? A qualitative study of undergraduate students' beliefs about meaning of life. *Journal of Humanistic Psychology, 53*(3), 386–414. https://doi.org/10.1177/0022167813477733

Hill, C. E., Kanazawa, Y., Knox, S., Schauerman, I., Loureiro, D., James, D., Carter, I., King, S., Razzak, S., Scarff, M., & Moore, J. (2017). Meaning in life in psychotherapy: The perspective of experienced psychotherapists. *Psychotherapy Research, 27*(4), 381–396. https://doi.org/10.1080/10503307.2015.1110636

Hill, K. A. (1987). Meta-analysis of paradoxical interventions. *Psychotherapy, 24*(2), 266–270. https://doi.org/10.1037/h0085714

Hofmann, S. G., Sawyer, A. T., Witt, A. A., & Oh, D. (2010). The effect of mindfulness-based therapy on anxiety and depression: A meta-analytic review. *Journal of Consulting and Clinical Psychology, 78*(2), 169–183. https://doi.org/10.1037/a0018555

Hoffman, L., Vallejos, L., Cleare-Hoffman, H. P., & Rubin, S. (2015). Emotion, relationship, and meaning as core existential practice: Evidence-based foundations. *Journal of Contemporary Psychotherapy, 45*(1), 11–20. https://doi.org/10.1007/s10879-014-9277-9

Ivtzan, I., Lomas, T., Hefferon, K., & Worth, P. (2015). *Second wave positive psychology: Embracing the dark side of life.* Routledge.

Jaspers, K. (2013). *Psychologie der weltanschauungen* [Psychology of worldviews]. Springer. (Original work published 1925)

Jim, H. S., Purnell, J. Q., Richardson, S. A., Golden-Kreutz, D., & Andersen, B. L. (2006). Measuring meaning in life following cancer. *Quality of Life Research, 15*(8), 1355–1371. https://doi.org/10.1007/s11136-006-0028-6

Kashdan, T., & Biswas-Diener, R. (2014). *The upside of your dark side.* Penguin.

Kelso, K. C., Kashdan, T. B., Imamoğlu, A., & Ashraf, A. (2020). Meaning in life buffers the impact of experiential avoidance on anxiety. *Journal of Contextual Behavioral Science, 16*, 192–198. https://doi.org/10.1016/j.jcbs.2020.04.009

Kim, J., Holte, P., Martela, F., Shanahan, C., Li, Z., Zhang, H., Eisenbeck, N., Carreno, D. F., Schlegel, R. J., & Hicks, J. A. (2022). Experiential appreciation as a pathway to meaning in life. *Nature Human Behaviour, 6*(5), 677–690. https://doi.org/10.1038/s41562-021-01283-6

King, L. A., Hicks, J. A., Krull, J. L., & Del Gaiso, A. K. (2006). Positive affect and the experience of meaning in life. *Journal of Personality and Social Psychology, 90*(1), 179–196. https://doi.org/10.1037/0022-3514.90.1.179

Krause, N. (2004). Stressors arising in highly valued roles, meaning in life, and the physical health status of older adults. *The Journals of Gerontology Series B: Psychological Sciences and Social Sciences, 59*(5), S287–S297. https://doi.org/10.1093/geronb/59.5.S287

Längle, A. (2019). The history of logotherapy and existential analysis. In E. Van Deurzen, E. Craig, A. Längle, K. J. Schneider, D. Tantam, & S. du Plock (Eds.), *Wiley World handbook of existential therapy* (pp. 309–323). John Wiley & Sons.

Lantz, J. E. (2000). *Meaning-centered marital and family therapy: Learning to bear the beams of love.* Charles C.Thomas.

Lapierre, S., Dubé, M., Bouffard, L., & Alain, M. (2007). Addressing suicidal ideations through the realization of meaningful personal goals. *Crisis, 28*(1), 16–25. https://doi.org/10.1027/0227-5910.28.1.16

Lee, V., Cohen, S. R., Edgar, L., Laizner, A. M., & Gagnon, A. J. (2004). Clarifying "meaning" in the context of cancer research: A systematic literature review. *Palliative & Supportive Care, 2*(3), 291–303. https://doi.org/10.1017/S1478951504040386

Lukas, E. (2014). *Meaning in suffering* (2nd ed.). Institute of Logotherapy Press.

MacKinnon, C. J., Milman, E., Smith, N. G., Henry, M., Berish, M., Copeland, L. S., Körner, A., Chochinov, H. M., & Cohen, S. R. (2013). Means to meaning in cancer-related bereavement: Identifying clinical implications for counseling psychologists. *The Counseling Psychologist, 41*(2), 216–239. https://doi.org/10.1177/0011000012459969

Mangione, L., & Forti, R. (2018). Beyond midlife and before retirement: A short-term women's group. *International Journal of Group Psychotherapy, 68*(3), 314–336. https://doi.org/10.1080/00207284.2018.1429927

Marco, J. H., Alonso, S., & Baños, R. (2021). Meaning-making as a mediator of anxiety and depression reduction during cognitive behavioral therapy intervention in participants with adjustment disorders. *Clinical Psychology & Psychotherapy, 28*(2), 325–333. https://doi.org/10.1002/cpp.2506

Marshall, M., & Marshall, E. (2012). *Logotherapy revisited*. Create Space.

Masley, S. A., Gillanders, D. T., Simpson, S. G., & Taylor, M. A. (2012). A systematic review of the evidence base for schema therapy. *Cognitive Behaviour Therapy, 41*(3), 185–202. https://doi.org/10.1080/16506073.2011.614274

May, R. (1978). Response to Bulka's article. *Journal of Humanistic Psychology, 18*(4), 55. https://doi.org/10.1177/002216787801800407

May, R. (1981). *Freedom and destiny*. W. W. Norton & Company.

May, R. (1991). *The cry for myth*. W. W. Norton & Company.

Metz, T. (2013). Meaning in life as the aim of psychotherapy: A hypothesis. In T. Metz (Ed.), *The experience of meaning in life: Classical perspectives, emerging themes, and controversies* (pp. 405–417). Springer.

Mikulincer, M., & Shaver, P. R. (2013). Attachment orientations and meaning in life. In J. Hicks & C. Routledge (Eds.), *The experience of meaning in life: Classical perspectives, emerging themes, and controversies* (pp. 287–304). Springer. https://doi.org/10.1007/978-94-007-6527-6_22

Mikulincer, M., & Shaver, P. R. (2014). An attachment perspective on loneliness. In R. J. Coplan & J. C. Bowker (Eds.), *The handbook of solitude: Psychological perspectives on social isolation, social withdrawal, and being alone* (pp. 34–50). John Wiley & Sons

Neimeyer, R. A. (Ed.). (2001). *Meaning reconstruction and the experience of loss*. American Psychological Association. https://doi.org/10.1037/10397-000

Norcross, J. C., & Lambert, M. J. (Eds.). (2019). *Psychotherapy relationships that work*. Oxford University Press.

Ostafin, B. D., & Proulx, T. (2020). Meaning in life and resilience to stressors. *Anxiety, Stress, & Coping, 33*(6), 603–622. https://doi.org/10.1080/10615806.2020.1800655

Overholser, J. C. (2010). Psychotherapy according to the Socratic method: Integrating ancient philosophy with contemporary cognitive therapy. *Journal of Cognitive Psychotherapy, 24*(4), 354–363. https://doi.org/10.1891/0889-8391.24.4.354

Park, C. L. (2010). Making sense of the meaning literature: An integrative review of meaning making and its effects on adjustment to stressful life events. *Psychological Bulletin, 136*(2), 257–301. https://doi.org/10.1037/a0018301

Park, C. L., & Folkman, S. (1997). Meaning in the context of stress and coping. *Review of General Psychology, 1*(2), 115–144. https://doi.org/10.1037/1089-2680.1.2.115

Reker, G. T., & Chamberlain, K. (Eds.). (1999). *Exploring existential meaning: Optimizing human development across the life span*. Sage.

Reker, G. T., Peacock, E. J., & Wong, P. T. (1987). Meaning and purpose in life and well-being: A life-span perspective. *Journal of Gerontology, 42*(1), 44–49. https://doi.org/10.1093/geronj/42.1.44

Remmers, C., Topolinski, S., & Koole, S. L. (2016). Why being mindful may have more benefits than you realize: Mindfulness improves both explicit and implicit mood regulation. *Mindfulness, 7*(4), 829–837. https://doi.org/10.1007/s12671-016-0520-1

Robatmili, S., Sohrabi, F., Shahrak, M. A., Talepasand, S., Nokani, M., & Hasani, M. (2015). The effect of group logotherapy on meaning in life and depression levels of Iranian students. *International Journal for the Advancement of Counseling, 37*(1), 54–62. https://doi.org/10.1007/s10447-014-9225-0

Rosenberg, S. (2018). Dignity therapy. *American Journal of Psychiatry Residents' Journal, 13*(8), 6–7. https://doi.org/10.1176/appi.ajp-rj.2018.130803

Roth, A., & Fonagy, P. (2013). *What works for whom?* Guilford Press

Russo-Netzer, P., Sinai, M., & Zeevi, M. (2020). Meaning in life and work among counsellors: A qualitative exploration. *British Journal of Guidance & Counselling, 48*(2), 209–226. https://doi.org/10.1080/03069885.2019.1625026

Ryff, C. D., Dienberg Love, G., Urry, H. L., Muller, D., Rosenkranz, M. A., Friedman, E. M., Davidson, R. J., & Singer, B. (2006). Psychological well-being and ill-being: Do they have distinct or mirrored biological correlates? *Psychotherapy and Psychosomatics, 75*(2), 85–95. https://doi.org/10.1159/000090892

Ryff, C. D., Singer, B. H., & Dienberg Love, G. (2004). Positive health: Connecting well-being with biology. *Philosophical Transactions of the Royal Society of London Series B, Biological Sciences, 359*(1449), 1383–1394. https://doi.org/10.1098/rstb.2004.1521

Saarelainen, S. M., Mäki-Petäjä-Leinonen, A., & Pöyhiä, R. (2022). Relational aspects of meaning in life among older people: A group-interview gerontechnology study. *Ageing and Society, 42*(5), 1035–1053. https://doi.org/10.1017/S0144686X20001300

Sahin, S., & Kabasakal, Z. (2023). Viewing meaning in life in three generations. *Turkish Psychological Counseling and Guidance Journal, 13*(71), 409–428. https://ouci.dntb.gov.ua/en/works/7qYP8zB7/

Schankweiler, D. A. (2020). *What do we mean when we talk about meaning? A qualitative study on students' concepts and sources of meaning in life* [Bachelor's thesis, University of Twente]. University of Twente Student Theses. https://essay.utwente.nl/82037/

Schneider, K. (2011). Toward a humanistic positive psychology: Why can't we just get along? *Existential Analysis, 22*(1), 32–38. https://psycnet.apa.org/record/2011-05339-004

Schneider, K. J. (2003). Existential–humanistic psychotherapies. In S. B. Messer & A. S. Gurman (Eds.), *Essential psychotherapies: Theory and practice: Vol. 2* (pp. 149–181). The Guilford Press.

Schneider, K. J. (Ed.). (2011). *Existential–integrative psychotherapy: Guideposts to the core of practice.* Routledge. https://doi.org/10.4324/9780203941119

Schulenberg, S. E., Drescher, C. F., & Baczwaski, B. J. (2014). Perceived meaning and disaster mental health: A role for logotherapy in clinical-disaster psychology. In A. Batthyany & P. Russo-Netzer (Eds.), *Meaning in positive and existential psychology* (pp. 251–267). Springer. https://doi.org/10.1007/978-1-4939-0308-5_15

Schulenberg, S. E., Schnetzer, L. W., Winters, M. R., & Hutzell, R. R. (2010). Meaning-centered couples therapy: Logotherapy and intimate relationships. *Journal of Contemporary Psychotherapy, 40*, 95–102.

Shin, J. Y., & Steger, M. F. (2014). Promoting meaning and purpose in life. In A. C. Parks & S. Schueller (Eds.), *The Wiley Blackwell handbook of positive psychological interventions* (pp. 90–110). John Wiley & Sons. https://doi.org/10.1002/9781118315927.ch5

Spiegel, D., Bloom, J. R., & Yalom, I. (1981). Group support for patients with metastatic cancer: A randomized outcome study. *Archives of General Psychiatry, 38*(5), 527–533. https://doi.org/10.1001/archpsyc.1980.01780300039004

Spinelli, E. (2005). *The interpreted world.* Sage.

Steger, M. F. (2012). Experiencing meaning in life: Optimal functioning at the nexus of well-being, psychopathology, and spirituality. In P. T. P. Wong (Ed.), *The human quest for meaning: Theories, research, and applications* (2nd ed., pp. 165–184). Springer.

Steger, M. F., & Park, C. L. (2012). The creation of meaning following trauma. In R. A. McMackin, E. Newman, J. M. Fogler, & T. M. Keane (Eds.), *Trauma therapy in context* (pp. 171–191). American Psychological Association.

Stillman, T. F., & Lambert, N. M. (2013). The bidirectional relationship of meaning and belonging. In J. A. Hicks & C. Routledge (Eds.), *The experience of meaning in life: Classical perspectives, emerging themes, and controversies* (pp. 305–315). Springer. https://doi. org/10.1007/978-94-007-6527-6_23

Tryon, G. S., & Winograd, G. (2011). Goal consensus and collaboration. *Psychotherapy, 48*(1), 50–57. https://doi.org/10.1037/a0022061

van der Spek, N., Vos, J., van Uden-Kraan, C. F., Breitbart, W., Cuijpers, P., Knipscheer-Kuipers, K., Willemsen, V., Tollenaar, R. A., van Asperen, C. J., & Verdonck-de Leeuw, I. M. (2014). Effectiveness and cost-effectiveness of meaning-centered group psychotherapy in cancer survivors: Protocol of a randomized controlled trial. *BMC Psychiatry, 14*(1), 22. https://doi.org/10.1186/1471-244X-14-22

van der Spek, N., Vos, J., van Uden-Kraan, C. F., Breitbart, W., Tollenaar, R. A., Cuijpers, P., & Verdonck-de Leeuw, I. M. (2013). Meaning making in cancer survivors: A focus group study. *PLoS One, 8*(9), e76089. https://doi.org/10.1371/journal.pone.0076089

van Rijn, B. (2014). *Assessment and case formulation in counselling and psychotherapy.* Sage.

Vanhooren, S. (2019). Struggling with meaninglessness: A case study from an experiential–existential perspective. *Person-Centered and Experiential Psychotherapies, 18*(1), 1–21. https://doi.org/10.1080/14779757.2019.1572029

Vanhooren, S., Grosemans, A., & Breynaert, J. (2022). Focusing, the felt sense, and meaning in life. In *Person-Centered & Experiential Psychotherapies* (pp. 1–19). Advanced online publication. https://doi.org/10.1080/14779757.2022.2028660

Visser, A., Garssen, B., & Vingerhoets, A. (2010). Spirituality and well-being in cancer patients: A review. *Psycho-Oncology, 19*(6), 565–572. https://doi.org/10.1002/pon.1626

Vos, J. (2015). Meaning and existential givens in the lives of cancer patients: A philosophical perspective on psycho-oncology. *Palliative & Supportive Care, 13*(4), 885–900. https://doi.org/10.1017/S1478951514000790

Vos, J. (2016a). Working with meaning in life in chronic or life-threatening disease: A review of its relevance and the effectiveness of meaning-centred therapies. In P. Russo-Netzer, S. E. Schulenberg, & A. Batthyany (Eds.), *Clinical perspectives on meaning: Positive and existential psychotherapy* (pp. 171–200). Springer. https://doi.org/10. 1007/978-3-319-41397-6_9

Vos, J. (2016b). Working with meaning in life in mental health care: A systematic literature review of the practices and effectiveness of meaning-centered therapies. In P. Russo-Netzer, S. E. Schulenberg, & A. Batthyany (Eds.), *Clinical perspectives on meaning: Positive and existential psychotherapy* (pp. 59–87). Routledge. https://doi.org/10. 1007/978-3-319-41397-6_4

Vos, J. (2018a). Death in existential psychotherapies: A critical review. In R. E. Menzies, R. G. Menzies, & L. Iverach (Eds.), *Curing the dread of death: Theory, research, and practice* (pp. 145–166). Australian Academic Press.

Vos, J. (2018b). *Meaning in life: An evidence-based handbook for practitioners.* Macmillan.

Vos, J. (2020). *The economics of meaning in life: From capitalist life syndrome to meaning-oriented economy.* University Professors Press.

Vos, J. (2021a). Cardiovascular disease and meaning in life: A systematic literature review and conceptual model. *Palliative & Supportive Care, 19*(3), 367–376. https://doi. org/10.1017/S1478951520001261

Vos, J. (2021b). *The psychology of COVID-19.* Sage.

Vos, J. (2021c). Systematic pragmatic phenomenological analysis: Step-wise guidance for mixed methods research. *Counselling & Psychotherapy Research, 21*(1), 77–97. https:// doi.org/10.1002/capr.12366

Vos, J. (2023a). *Doing research in psychological therapies: A handbook and step-by-step guide.* Sage.

Vos, J. (2023b). The meaning sextet: A systematic literature review and further validation of a universal typology of meaning in life. *Journal of Constructivist Psychology, 36*(2), 204–231. https://doi.org/10.1080/10720537.2022.2068709

Vos, J. (2023c). *Systematic meaning in life psychotherapy: From systematic literature reviews to a systematic treatment manual.* PsyArXiv. Advance online publication. https://doi.org/10.31234/osf.io/xbk85

Vos, J. (in press). Three vital predictors of a beneficial meaningful life: Types, approaches, and quantity of realized meanings in life. *The Journal of Positive Psychology.*

Vos, J., Craig, M., & Cooper, M. (2015). Existential therapies: A meta-analysis of their effects on psychological outcomes. *Journal of Consulting and Clinical Psychology, 83*(1), 115–128. https://doi.org/10.1037/a0037167

Vos, J., Roberts, R., & Davies, J. (2019). *Mental health in crisis.* Sage.

Vos, J., & van Rijn, B. (2022). The effectiveness of transactional analysis treatments and their predictors: A systematic literature review and explorative meta-analysis. *Journal of Humanistic Psychology.* Advance online publication. https://doi.org/10.1177/00221678221117111

Vos, J. & van Rijn, B. (in press). *The handbook of transactional analysis psychotherapy: An evidence-based approach.* Sage.

Vos, J., & Vitali, D. (2018). The effects of psychological meaning-centered therapies on quality of life and psychological stress: A metaanalysis. *Palliative & Supportive Care, 16*(5), 608–632. https://doi.org/10.1017/S1478951517000931

Westerhof, G. J., Bohlmeijer, E., & Webster, J. D. (2010). Reminiscence and mental health: A review of recent progress in theory, research, and interventions. *Ageing and Society, 30*(4), 697–721. https://doi.org/10.1017/S0144686X09990328

Wong, P. T. (Ed.). (2012). *The human quest for meaning.* Routledge.

Yalom, I. D. (1980). *Existential psychotherapy.* Hachette.

Zeng, Y. Y., Long, A., Chiang, C. Y., Chiu, N. M., & Sun, F. K. (2021). Exploring the meaning of life from the perspective of patients with depression: A phenomenological study. *Archives of Psychiatric Nursing, 35*(5), 427–433. https://doi.org/10.1016/j.apnu.2021.06.004

10

Understanding Acceptance in Existential–Humanistic Psychotherapy

Roxanne Christensen and Aviva Vincent

Acceptance is a relational construct that refers to how a person internalizes their ability to be seen in a positive regard by others. It is also the other's experience of welcoming a person into relation. Because acceptance is bidirectional, it is often broken into two distinct facets: self-acceptance and acceptance of others. To refine the understanding of acceptance as an active choice, feeling, and emotion, other related constructs of warmth and empathy should be considered. However, this chapter considers acceptance specifically as a singular construct with a myriad of possible experiences.

The focus on acceptance in psychotherapy emerged from humanistic psychology (Hoffman et al., 2014). It is not surprising that existential–humanistic (EH) psychology uses the foundational works of Carl Rogers, Abraham Maslow, Clark Moustakas, and other colleagues to define the construct (for a discussion of Rogers and Maslow, see Pramanik & Khuntia, 2023). The EH variations discussed herein likely have similarities with practitioners who identify with Rogerian, client-centered, or humanistic (without identifying as existential–humanistic) modalities and pedagogies.

Acceptance is considered a determinant of psychological well-being (Pramanik & Khuntia, 2023) and can be considered an important aspect of EH therapy. This chapter begins by defining acceptance historically, contextually, and within the parameters of EH psychology. Next, we consider the research supporting the efficacy and effectiveness of acceptance in psychotherapy. Finally, we give consideration to how acceptance can be applied in multicultural contexts.

https://doi.org/10.1037/0000446-011
The Evidence-Based Foundations of Existential–Humanistic Therapy, L. Hoffman and V. Lac (Editors)

CONCEPTUALIZING ACCEPTANCE IN PSYCHOTHERAPY

The word "acceptance" is frequently used interchangeably with "positive regard" in psychotherapy. "Unconditional positive regard" is a term introduced by Rogers (1957) that became influential in large part through his article on the necessary and sufficient conditions of psychotherapy. We are using the term "acceptance" instead of "unconditional positive regard" or simply "positive regard" as it allows for more flexibility from Rogers's original conception, despite the obvious indebtedness to and overlap with Rogers's idea of unconditional positive regard. We are interested in both interpersonal acceptance (i.e., acceptance from another person) and self-acceptance; however, our primary focus is on the therapist's acceptance of the client. As will be discussed, one of the reasons that the therapist's acceptance is important is that it may help clients develop self-acceptance. The valuing and understanding of acceptance in psychotherapy emerged from humanistic psychology; therefore, we will focus primarily on humanistic psychology for an initial conceptualization of acceptance.

Acceptance is both an act and a way of being (Rogers, 1980). Rogers defines acceptance as a warm regard for another person no matter their condition, behavior, or feelings. Acceptance may also be a path toward deepening attachment to others. Williams and Lynn (2010) link attachment to acceptance through the concept of willingness. A willingness to accept others is an active choice to offer respect and connection with a person without being hindered or hinged upon their acting in a way that is desired or simply acceptable. As a result, both people experience a sense of enjoyment of offering, seeing, and feeling their whole self. A by-product of acceptance can be feelings of value and care, which is the starting point for self-exploration and developmental growth.

Acceptance is an essential element of relationship that acts as a conductor for the deepening of connection. When positively regarded, seen, and accepted as they are, a person is able to widen their capacity for self-reflection and reflexivity, vulnerability, and growth. Among therapeutic factors across modalities, it is the relationship between therapist and self, therapist and client, and eventually client and self-in-the-world, which significantly accounts for the process of therapeutic change and growth.

Acceptance in the Therapeutic Relationship

Acceptance is a core construct of the therapeutic alliance and engagement. For Moustakas (1995), acceptance was the precedent to connection, wherein he took delight in listening and sharing space and the client became part of the relational dynamic. Here, acceptance is moving into relation with another so that they are not being spoken at or even to, but rather are spoken with, and both learn through one another in a choreographed dialogue of reciprocity.

Acceptance is thus formed through an intrigue to know a person or oneself beyond any categorical notion of attributes and with absence of judgment (e.g., good and bad, shame and triumph). It is through acceptance that one can "feel really free to explore all the hidden nooks and frightening crannies of [one's] inner and often buried experience" (Moustakas, 1995, p. 34). Rogers explains that the benefit to clients is the shift toward self-acceptance: "Slowly [they] move toward taking the same attitude toward [them]self, accepting [them]self as [they are], and therefore ready to move forward in the process of becoming" (p. 63). The internalization of acceptance makes a pathway for increased feelings of self-worth and self-esteem (Pramanik & Khuntia, 2023).

Acceptance upends the notion that therapists are advice givers or the primary agents of change with an authoritative stance on knowing better than the client. Instead, the therapist is an expert in capacity building, brave space creation, and genuine caring in the process of therapy. Through the phenomenological process, the therapist upholds the safety and acceptance of the client, and the client can navigate the widened therapeutic environment toward self-directed healing. The inclination for a practitioner to avert or avoid the discussion of relationship between client and therapist or other interpersonal experiences in therapy is a disservice to the therapeutic relationship (Yalom, 2002).

An important aspect of acceptance is unconditional positive regard. Although unconditional positive regard is often valued in psychotherapy, it also poses a potential challenge. At the stage of acceptance, noticing the success of others is still subjective and posits that there is also room for criticism or rejection. As explained by Rogers (1995), "a positive evaluation is as threatening in the long run as a negative one, since to inform someone that [they are] good implies that you also have the right to tell [them they are] bad" (p. 55). Rogers highlights acceptance as a key ingredient to providing a climate for change in which therapeutic movement is more likely to occur. However, to maximize the positive impact of acceptance, therapists must be aware of its potential negative side. Therefore, acceptance is not as simple or binary as may be perceived. Therapists need to develop skills in how and when acceptance is utilized in therapy, including how to respond when clients experience it negatively or paradoxically.

Safety

In discussing safety, it is important to acknowledge that safety is rarely, if ever, absolute. In psychotherapy, the therapist helps the client strive toward greater degrees of experienced safety while recognizing that the client's experience of safety is always their subjective experience. The therapeutic relationship must build a foundation for connection, which is facilitated by the experience of acceptance. With this connection, the client can grow in their experience of safety in their authentic self, and they may be empowered to explore the therapeutic relationship with vulnerability. Acceptance provides the benefit of greater psychological safety, which opens space for creativity to envision oneself differently (Bernard, 2013). This could perhaps involve envisioning oneself as an idealized self who could develop the capacity for self-love or allowing for low-risk mistake making with opportunity for growth and learning rather than centering feelings of embarrassment or shame (Rogers, 1995). The therapeutic environment is the container where the client can experience greater safety while also taking risks to accept both themselves and the acceptance of the therapist (i.e., accepting their acceptance; see Tillich, 1952).

Yalom (2002) explores this in his discussion about engaging the client when they may be avoiding intimacy in the therapeutic engagement due to the belief that something about them is unacceptable: "The act of revealing oneself fully to another and still being accepted may be the major vehicle of therapeutic help" (p. 11). Clients who may be fearing exploitation, colonization, or abandonment can only engage in a relationship with their therapist within a container of felt safety, which then fosters a felt sense of safety within, leading to a corrective emotional experience. Yalom (2002) encourages space for clients to explore themselves, omitting character judgment failures, such that they may internalize and even memorialize the statements of the therapist and retain an embodied sense of the relationship. To believe in the absence of failures and the inherent strengths from within, the client must trust the safety established and the authenticity of the relationship (Hoffman et al., 2013, 2014). The therapeutic stance is to model life within the safety of the therapeutic environment, space, place, time, and persons.

Through acceptance, the client is empowered to reallocate energy once reserved for the potential of experiencing shame, exploitation, or abandonment, which allows them to engage in intimacy within themselves and between themselves and their therapist. As such, intimacy inherently exists in the meeting of two humans being. The outcome is that the client can begin to (carefully) seek other spaces where they believe they can experience acceptance while being authentic (Yalom, 2002).

Acceptance and Belonging

Different from passive resignation (i.e., "I guess this is just the way it is"), acceptance is a powerful action and behavioral decision. In the clinical relationship, acceptance is built from the therapist's ability to model physical and psychological safety, which then allows them to provide warmth and positive regard for the client. The client is likely to internalize safety, warmth, and positive regard as acceptance. Experiencing acceptance from a therapist opens the client to the possibility of self-acceptance. Self-acceptance facilitates opportunities for the acceptance of others, which promotes feelings of belonging. Thus, acceptance is experienced on the foundation of safety and on the precipice of belonging. This conceptual process tracks with the historical foundation set forth by Maslow (1991; see also Hoffman et al., 2014).

Allowing space for acceptance from others and moving into self-acceptance unshrouds the cloak of shame that keeps the exploration of the self unattainable; acceptance acts as a salve, easing out remorse, guilt, and perceived obligations to allow the human condition to heal. Consisting of feeling seen, being heard, and experiencing validation, acceptance represents the baseline standard of person-centered care. Best practice methods support a person-centered therapeutic alliance as being advantageous to clinical engagement to the extent that variations of mental health therapists (i.e., psychologists, social workers, counselors) center this approach in practice (Rice & Greenberg, 1992).

EH PERSPECTIVES ON ACCEPTANCE

As the focus on acceptance in psychotherapy emerged from humanistic psychology, it is not surprising that EH therapy bears many similarities to how acceptance has been discussed by Rogers, Moustakas, and others. However, there are also some important differences, even if these differences often are minor and a matter of degree. Many therapists who identify as Rogerian, client-centered, or humanistic (without identifying as existential–humanistic) would likely agree with the EH variations discussed in this section.

Rollo May (1982), in writing a short piece on Rogers, began a brief exchange on the topic of evil. In this article, May discusses Rogers's 1967 research project on client-centered therapists working with individuals diagnosed with schizophrenia. May (1982) notes that he was selected as a reviewer to observe and provide feedback on recordings of client-centered therapists recorded while working with these clients. He comments,

> While I felt the [client-centered] therapy was good on the whole, there was one glaring omission. This was that the client-centered therapists did not (or could not) deal with the angry, hostile, negative—that is, evil—feelings of the clients. (p. 15)

Part of May's concern was that in not accepting these negative feelings, the therapist was overidentifying with the client and, therefore, depriving the client of being experienced as a subject.

For May (1982), it is important to accept potential for evil in oneself and in clients: "Therapists need to be able to perceive and admit their own evil—hostility, aggression, anger—if they are to be able to see and accept these experiences in clients" (p. 17). There are two important takeaways here. First, authentic acceptance of clients must encompass acceptance of their negative potentials, urges, and actions. Acceptance does not mean condoning these when they are expressed in a hurtful or harmful manner. Instead, it is a deeper acceptance of the person including their "evil" thoughts and urges, which can allow a client to bring difficult and shameful aspects of themselves into the open where they can be explored and dealt with directly. It is through facing our potential for evil that we prevent it from taking hold. Similarly, Rogers posits that although one cannot always be unconditionally positively regarded given conditions that exist in the authenticity of the therapeutic relationship, the client is, inclusive of their ills and habits, nevertheless positively regarded as a whole and human person (Rogers, 1980).

Second, May (1982) recognizes that acceptance of the client begins with self-acceptance. This self-acceptance, too, must be inclusive of one's own potential for evil. Hoffman and colleagues (2013) similarly advocate that self-acceptance should be in the context of facing oneself, others, and the world directly. From an existential perspective, acceptance must be rooted in an honest facing of oneself, the world, and others.

Theoretically, Rogers (1957, 1995) agrees that acceptance, including self-acceptance, entails acceptance of the person including their negative behaviors or qualities. The difference between Rogers's client-centered approach and May's EH perspective pertains to how this is managed in psychotherapy. May feels that the client-centered therapists did not as readily welcome the angry, hostile, and negative feelings of the client, often resulting in the client not exploring them. In contrast, from an EH perspective, the therapist should shift between different therapeutic stances, which can allow for deeper exploration of these feelings (Schneider & Krug, 2017). This includes stances that welcome and explore feelings that May feels were discouraged by many client-centered therapists. Experiencing acceptance in the breadth of engagement through these different stances deepens the client's experience of acceptance.

In summary, EH approaches to acceptance agree with humanistic perspectives derived from Rogers; however, they go further by strongly emphasizing that acceptance must be rooted in an honest recognition of the other person, inclusive of negative thoughts, feelings, urges, and potentials. Although the acceptance of the client itself is healing, it also serves as a foundation for cultivating a relationship that invites a client to bring their full self into the therapy space. This allows for deeper exploration while enabling fuller acceptance of the client.

RESEARCH ON ACCEPTANCE

The empirical research on acceptance has generally supported the value of it in the context of psychotherapy. There are, however, different perspectives on how acceptance works in psychotherapy (i.e., being directly beneficial vs. primarily empowering other interventions). Despite this concept being prominent in literature for many years, there remains limited direct research on acceptance and the need for greater clarification. In this section, we begin by examining quantitative research and follow with a consideration of qualitative studies on acceptance.

Quantitative Research

Within the quantitative literature, there are different perspectives on acceptance. Acceptance has been viewed as a "universal character strength that ha[s] been overlooked" (Bernard, 2013, p. xiii) and it has been said that "there is little research evidence to understand the construct" of acceptance (Pramanik & Khuntia, 2023). Although philosophers, theorists, and practitioners have written about acceptance, there is limited empirical research to explore the mechanisms of change as experienced by clients. Acceptance is confounded with a multitude of other constructs (i.e., implied synonyms), such as unconditional positive self-regard, in empirical research (i.e., Murphy et al., 2020; see also Chamberlain & Haaga, 2001). As we have discussed, positive regard or unconditional positive regard can be viewed as an important aspect of acceptance. Even if there are some minor theoretical distinctions, it is unlikely that these constructs could be parsed in quantitative measures. Therefore, consideration of the research on positive regard is relevant to and supportive of the value of acceptance in psychotherapy.

Research about the specific feeling and impact of acceptance in isolation of other feelings and emotions remains sparse. In the environmental scan, a search in EBSCOhost, including all databases (all databases included in the search are available by request), using "acceptance," "existential–humanistic," and "psychology" with an open date range yielded nine sources. Five were relevant to the topic of discussion, with three in book format (Follette et al., 2016; Heery, 2020; Hoffman et al., 2014) and two in the form of peer-reviewed journals (Shahar, 2022; Strunk, 1970).

Predating the environmental scan findings, mental health education often includes the work of Rogers (1957, 1980) as the foundational context of therapeutic engagement with clients. Rogers is considered a pioneer for ascertaining the elements of client success and growth in the therapeutic process, inclusive of nonpossessive warmth, positive regard, and empathy as the qualities of connection to develop a therapeutic alignment and dynamic for change. The sentiment was echoed by Scherman (1981). Norcross and Wampold (2011) conducted a rigorous meta-analysis in which they identified that positive regard was vital to the mechanism of change.

Farber and colleagues centered their studies on the exploration of positive regard on therapeutic outcomes, though their study effects ranged from minimal to significant depending on client population (Farber & Doolin, 2011; Farber et al., 2018). The researchers completed a meta-analysis examining the relation between therapist positive regard and treatment outcome. Positive regard was discussed as a multifaceted experience inclusive of acceptance, validation, unconditional positive regard, nonpossessive warmth, and therapist affirmation. This work included clients across the lifespan (children through adulthood) and in the context of individual, group, and family sessions. Interestingly, the researchers found a higher effect when the type of treatment provided was psychoanalytic or psychodynamic, which they hypothesized was due to a scarcity of experiencing displays of support and positive regard in more traditional treatment (Farber & Doolin, 2011).

A later study by Farber and colleagues (2019) discusses the cautions of the ways in which positive regard becomes folded into therapeutic factors such as empathy and alliance. The limitations of their study were quantifying and explaining the subjectivity (i.e., felt sense) of acceptance in the client's experience. Yet there is an understanding that acceptance is imperative, in conjunction with warmth and positive regard. At the very least, dispassionate and neutral stances to the therapy relationship are not supported by research as being an effective standard for care (Farber et al., 2019).

Wampold (2007) finds that an effective component of psychotherapy was the internalized feelings of acceptance within the relationship created between the client and therapist. The felt sense of acceptance was identified as a robust variable predictor of outcome and potentially causal to the benefits of psychotherapy. This process is further supported by Norcross's (2002) similarly extensive meta-analyses of clinical elements of change. Priebe and colleagues (2011) provide a conceptual review of psychiatry practices that identifies the communication between practitioner and client as a pathway to healing wherein communication was defined by positive regard, respect, acceptance, and validation (Priebe et al., 2011).

Chamberlain and Haaga (2001) used the Unconditional Self-Acceptance Questionnaire to assess the impact of rational–emotive behavior therapy on the perception of self-acceptance. The research findings indicate that "people who were more unconditionally self-accepting tended to be lower in depression and anxiety and higher in happiness or general well-being" (p. 171). Though self-acceptance is a valid construct (Bernard, 2013), the findings must be interpreted cautiously as the Unconditional Self-Acceptance Questionnaire does not have consistently established psychometric properties; though iterations in non-English languages, such as Serbian and Portuguese, have been progressing (Faustino et al., 2024; Popov & Sokić, 2022). This study illuminates the status of empirical evidence regarding acceptance—evidence is still just emerging about this important construct of the therapeutic experience.

Qualitative Research

Although the qualitative research on acceptance is scant, there remains further support from this body of research. In two studies by Jayne and Ray (2015a, 2015b), acceptance and unconditional positive regard were considered together in the context of play therapy. In the first grounded theory study (Jayne & Ray, 2015b), which focused on the therapists' experience, they reported that therapists found "congruence, UPR [unconditional positive regard], and empathetic understanding are experienced and demonstrated in CCPT [client-centered play therapy] as dynamic, flowing process with overlapping, simultaneous dimensions" (p. 97). Furthermore, unconditional positive regard was most often expressed as acceptance, particularly during challenging times for the children. This points both to the relationship of acceptance and unconditional positive regard for these therapists as well as the complexity of the constructs.

In a second grounded theory study, Jayne and Ray (2015a) found a relationship between the therapist's self-acceptance and their ability to genuinely offer self-acceptance to their clients. Second, they found that other therapeutic interventions were less effective without genuine acceptance. Though this does not speak to the direct impact of acceptance, it supports that acceptance is foundational to the therapy process. In this study, unconditional positive regard was expressed both with positive (or actualizing) behaviors as well as negative (or self-limiting) behaviors. Although this is promising, an inherent limitation in this study was the lack of adequate ability to measure or report on the children's experience of acceptance.

Bigby and colleagues engaged in two studies that examine the culture in underperforming group homes (Bigby et al., 2012) and high-performing group homes (Bigby et al., 2015) for individuals with severe intellectual disability. In the first study, they found that the staff in underperforming group homes tended to view residents as being different or not like them (Bigby et al., 2012). Conversely, they found that in the high-performing group homes, a primary quality was a culture rooted in viewing residents with positive regard and as more "like us" (Bigby et al., 2015, p. 287). There is a limitation in that the residents' view of acceptance and positive regard was not measured, and likely there were other factors that contributed to the cultural difference in the group homes. Additionally, this research did not specifically measure change or effectiveness. The positive findings are similar to research by Kinniburgh-White and colleagues (2010) on the relationship between stepfathers and children in which acceptance was a primary factor associated with positive stepfather–stepchild relationships. Although the studies that Bigby and colleagues and Kinnibrugh-White and colleagues conducted are not in a therapy context, they do point to the role of acceptance in developing positive relationships, including in healing contexts.

Building on the theme of acceptance contributing to establishing positive relationships, Sackett and Cook (2022) used a hermeneutic phenomenological approach to examine meaningful experiences in family counseling. The first of three themes identified was "counseling sessions are a positive experience and something to look forward to" (p. 123). A subtheme that emerged from this first theme was the therapist demonstrating unconditional positive regard. Again, this does not look at specific outcomes, but the experience of unconditional positive regard was connected to better relationships and meaningful experiences in therapy.

Last, Traynor and colleagues (2011) conducted a qualitative study exploring therapists' perceptions of what therapeutic factors were helpful with clients experiencing psychotic symptoms. Though relational factors were consistently seen as important, unconditional positive regard was identified as particularly salient. An important limitation is that this study, again, examined only the therapist's perceptions. Though it would be problematic to draw too strong of a conclusion on the effectiveness of acceptance or positive regard from the scant qualitative research, this does provide some preliminary evidence suggesting that acceptance may contribute to therapy effectiveness.

MULTICULTURAL CONSIDERATIONS

Marginalized and underrepresented persons (i.e., persons of color, gender diverse individuals, and neurodiverse individuals) often engage in masking, camouflaging, and code switching to fit into mainstream culture. This form of self-preservation, which perpetuates fear of being found out, ostracized, and deemed unacceptable, has been associated with increased rates of self-harm and thwarted belonging (Chapman & Botha, 2023). The inverse is to experience acceptance, which is why representation of marginalized, underrepresented, and intersectional identities of therapists is ever more important.

Wampold (2007) poses the epistemological tightrope in which "psychotherapists use the language and research tools of medicine and science but employ treatment procedures that may depend on the same psychological machinery as religious, spiritual, and culturally indigenous interventions" (p. 861). He posits that psychotherapy consistently supports the change process through the relational context. The use of language and cultural meaning allows for the conveyance of information, influence of others, development of inferences of self and others, and capacity to build community (Wampold, 2007).

The majority of empirical research engages Western, White, adult, and cognitively able participants. Acceptance could be even more essential when more intentionally applied with minoritized, marginalized, and underrepresented clients—clients seeking validation and affirmation of their lived experiences. This can bridge the alliance between clients navigating societal shame, stigma, and self-doubt or judgment. Therapeutic guidelines provided by Farber and colleagues (2018) suggest the benefit of sharing positive regard to create the foundational elements on which change is built upon to effect positive change. The practitioner is encouraged to feel positively toward the client and share that feeling in an affirming manner to provide acceptance without an agenda. Importantly, acceptance is tailored to the needs and gains of the client rather than the satisfaction of the therapist—though the therapist may also feel the benefit of the therapeutic alliance formed.

The narrative of the *homeplace* (hooks, 1990) aids in establishing the importance of a safe space to challenge inhumane treatment, acknowledge grievances and limitations, and navigate resilience and agency. Homeplace is enacted through space and support to "acknowledge and embrace their varied and intersecting identities" (Vereen et al., 2017). Bell (1987) refers to homeplace as the decolonization of the mind via self-exploration and healing. Healing is a process that includes bearing witness to the systemic pain and suffering experienced by marginalized and underrepresented persons. Similarly, as Vereen and colleagues (2017) state, the nesting in "homeplace facilitates Black people's resistance to oppressive constructions of themselves, their communities, and the dismissal of their potential" (p. 80). Humanistic psychology is positioned to challenge the gatekeeping of the healing process.

Acceptance in the lens of Black existentialism provides an opportunity to confront racial and social inequity within clinical dialogue. In this regard, the whole human experience is valid, including intersectional identities that are often masked. Vereen and colleagues (2017) use homeplace in broad terms: "Humanistic thought through the lens of Black existentialism provides an opportunity to explore meaning making of lived humanity, resiliency of the individual, and perceptions of the Black collective" (p. 82).

Lemberger and Lemberger-Truelove (2016) identify that "social justice is a categorical imperative" (p. 3). The actualization of humanistic freedom presupposes that individuals and systems are not inherently equitable and that the histories of oppression and dehumanization continue to be perpetuated, necessitating witnessing, acknowledgment, and action. "Social justice praxis is never a passive endeavor, rather it requires the practitioner to seek out and confront injustices of all sorts" (Lemberger & Lemberger-Truelove, 2016, p. 3). Considerations in humanistic social justice praxis challenge all forms of injustice. To eradicate privilege and inequity, the voices of the oppressed must be amplified without the responsibility of education and effort on the shoulders of the marginalized. The practitioner is positioned at the juncture of the complexity of the injustice, the influence of the oppressor, and the needs of the oppressed. In this way, acceptance can be a homeplace.

Therapists must, however, recognize that acceptance can be experienced differently by different clients. For White therapists working primarily with White clients, they may have to adapt how they convey acceptance to different clients. Clients from marginalized and minoritized backgrounds may be weary of therapists' expressions of acceptance based upon prior experiences. For example, the client's experience of the therapist as culturally humble may be necessary and part of the client's experience of acceptance.

FUTURE RESEARCH

Though there is a body of research supporting the therapeutic value of acceptance, there remain gaps in the literature that would be important to address in future research. First, it is important to consider the opportunities to bring together empirical literature on this topic. At present, the keywords are not consistent. Thus, swaths of aligned research are easily missed because of the inability of databases to find the relevant works.

Second, it is advisable to research acceptance in the context of EH psychology specifically. To that end, it is imperative that researchers ensure an international methodology for the inclusion of diverse populations, diversity of thought, and diversity in healing and health perspectives and access in empirical studies. Psychometric properties of measures for specific populations must be considered, which may require revalidating the psychometric properties in studies.

Third, it is important to conduct more research examining the value of acceptance from the clients' perspective or experience of acceptance and positive regard. As noted by Traynor and colleagues (2011), most of the research on positive regard to date has relied on the therapist's perceptions, which may be different from the client's experience.

Fourth, a gap that could be addressed is considering how acceptance is conceptualized and experienced in different cultural contexts, both within and external to psychotherapy. Acceptance in a group upheld by seeing and valuing all of its members with interrelated investments for the whole of the group—such as is found in the African concepts of *ubuntu* and *sawubona* and similar collectivist or community-based ways of being—can yield a deeper understanding beyond the colonization of fitting a global concept into a homogeneically individualized model. Understanding various ways that acceptance is understood and experienced could serve as a basis to develop new or more complex measures of acceptance that can be used in future research while also helping therapists learn to adapt how they work with acceptance. Consistency of qualitative methods is also vital because literature on acceptance uses a robust lexicon that cannot be captured by quantitative measure alone. Mixed-methods research has the potential to inform culturally sensitive measures while deepening the field's understanding of acceptance. A specific research opportunity was identified by Farber and colleagues (2018), noting the opportunity to further explore the effects on symptom reduction and endurance using longitudinal methodology.

CONCLUSION

Acceptance in the context of psychotherapy is complex. Inconsistency in terminology and definitions along with overlap with similar concepts make it difficult to develop adequate measures in quantitative research and clear questions in qualitative research. Despite these limitations, there is sufficient research to suggest that acceptance is an important factor in psychotherapy. Although this is an important foundation, the therapist must be able to convey and work with acceptance in a skillful manner that adapts to individual and cultural differences and does not inadvertently discourage clients from delving deeper into some of the more negative aspects of themselves that they may personally find shameful or unacceptable. If these are not brought into the therapy experience, then the impact of acceptance may be limited. Therefore, although acceptance on the surface gives the appearance of something simple for the therapist to incorporate, it requires skill and nuance to effectively work with acceptance in psychotherapy.

REFERENCES

Bell, D. A. (1987). *And we are not saved: The elusive quest for racial justice*. Basic Books.

Bernard, M. E. (Ed.). (2013). *The strength of self-acceptance: Theory, practice and research*. Springer. https://doi.org/10.1007/978-1-4614-6806-6

Bigby, C., Knox, M., Beadle-Brown, J., & Clement, T. (2015). 'We just call them people': Positive regard as a dimension of culture in group homes for people with severe intellectual disability. *Journal of Applied Research in Intellectual Disabilities, 28*(4), 283–295. https://doi.org/10.1111/jar.12128

Bigby, C., Knox, M., Beadle-Brown, J., Clement, T., & Mansell, J. (2012). Uncovering dimensions of culture in underperforming group homes for people with severe intellectual disability. *Intellectual and Developmental Disabilities, 50*(6), 452–467. https://doi.org/10.1352/1934-9556-50.06.452

Chamberlain, J. M., & Haaga, D. A. (2001). Unconditional self-acceptance and psychological health. *Journal of Rational–Emotive & Cognitive-Behavior Therapy, 19*(3), 163–176. https://doi.org/10.1023/A:1011189416600

Chapman, R., & Botha, M. (2023). Neurodivergence-informed therapy. *Developmental Medicine and Child Neurology, 65*(3), 310–317. https://doi.org/10.1111/dmcn.15384

Farber, B. A., & Doolin, E. M. (2011). Positive regard. *Psychotherapy, 48*(1), 58–64. https://doi.org/10.1037/a0022141

Farber, B. A., Suzuki, J. Y., & Lynch, D. A. (2018). Positive regard and psychotherapy outcome: A meta-analytic review. *Psychotherapy, 55*(4), 411–423. https://doi.org/10.1037/pst0000171

Farber, B. A., Suzuki, J. Y., & Lynch, D. A. (2019). Positive regard and affirmation. In J. C. Norcross & M. J. Lambert (Eds.), *Psychotherapy relationships that work: Evidence-based therapist contributions* (3rd ed., pp. 288–322). Oxford University Press. https://doi.org/10.1093/med-psych/9780190843953.003.0008

Faustino, B., Vasco, A. B., Haaga, D. A. F., Chamberlain, J. M., Farinha-Fernandes, A., & Delgado, J. (2024). Exploring factor and correlational analysis of the Portuguese version of the Unconditional Self-Acceptance Questionnaire—Revised. *Journal of Rational–Emotive & Cognitive–Behavior Therapy, 42*(1), 98–109. https://doi.org/10.1007/s10942-022-00492-w

Follette, V. M., & Hazlett-Stevens, H. (2016). Mindfulness and acceptance theories. In J. C. Norcross, G. R. VandenBos, D. K. Freedheim, & B. O. Olatunji (Eds.), *APA handbook of clinical psychology: Theory and research* (pp. 273–302). American Psychological Association. https://doi.org/10.1037/14773-010

Heery, M. (2020). Global authenticity. In L. Hoffman, M. Yang, F. J. Kaklauskas, A. Chan, & M. Mansilla (Eds.), *Existential psychology East-West* (Vol. 1, Rev. ed., pp. 205–219). University Professors Press.

Hoffman, L., Lopez, A., & Moats, M. (2013). Humanistic psychology and self-acceptance. In M. Bernard (Ed.), *The strength of self-acceptance: Theory, research, and practice* (pp. 3–17). Springer. https://doi.org/10.1007/978-1-4614-6806-6_1

Hoffman, L., Lopez, A. J., & Moats, M. (2014). Humanistic psychology and self-acceptance. In M. Bernard (Ed.), *The strength of self-acceptance: Theory, research, and practice* (pp. 3–17). Springer. https://doi.org/10.1007/978-1-4614-6806-6_1

hooks, b. (1990). *Yearning: Race, gender and cultural politics.* South End Press.

Jayne, K. M., & Ray, D. C. (2015a). Play therapists' demonstration of attitudinal conditions in child-centered play therapy. *Person-Centered and Experiential Psychotherapies, 14*(2), 119–136. https://doi.org/10.1080/14779757.2014.952899

Jayne, K. M., & Ray, D. C. (2015b). Therapist-provided conditions in child-centered play therapy. *The Journal of Humanistic Counseling, 54*(2), 86–103. https://doi.org/10.1002/johc.12005

Kinniburgh-White, R., Cartwright, C., & Seymour, F. (2010). Young adults' narratives of relational development with stepfathers. *Journal of Social and Personal Relationships, 27*(7), 890–907. https://doi.org/10.1177/0265407510376252

Lemberger, M. E., & Lemberger-Truelove, T. L. (2016). Bases for a more socially just humanistic praxis. *Journal of Humanistic Psychology, 56*(6), 571–580. https://doi.org/10.1177/0022167816652750

Maslow, A. H. (1991). Critique of self-actualization theory. *The Journal of Humanistic Education and Development, 29*(3), 103–108. https://doi.org/10.1002/j.2164-4683.1991.tb00010.x

May, R. (1982). The problem of evil: An open letter to Carl Rogers. *Journal of Humanistic Psychology, 22*(3), 10–21. https://doi.org/10.1177/0022167882223003

Moustakas, C. E. (1995). *Being-in, being-for, being-with.* Jason Aronson, Inc.

Murphy, D., Joseph, S., Demetriou, E., & Karimi-Mofrad, P. (2020). Unconditional positive self-regard, intrinsic aspirations, and authenticity: Pathways to psychological well-being. *Journal of Humanistic Psychology*, 60(2), 258–279. https://doi.org/10.1177/0022167816688314

Norcross, J. C. (2002). *Psychotherapy relationships that work: Therapist contributions and responsiveness to patients.* Oxford Academic.

Norcross, J. C., & Wampold, B. E. (2011). Evidence-based therapy relationships: Research conclusions and clinical practices. *Psychotherapy*, 48(1), 98–102. https://doi.org/10.1037/a0022161

Popov, S., & Sokić, J. (2022). Psychometric characteristics of a Serbian translation of the Unconditional Self-Acceptance Questionnaire and the development of a short form. *Psihologija*, 55(1), 107–122. https://doi.org/10.2298/PSI200820005P

Pramanik, S., & Khuntia, R. (2023). Decoding unconditional self-acceptance: A qualitative report. *Journal of Rational–Emotive & Cognitive–Behavior Therapy*, 41(4), 932–949. https://doi.org/10.1007/s10942-023-00517-y

Priebe, S., Dimic, S., Wildgrube, C., Jankovic, J., Cushing, A., & McCabe, R. (2011). Good communication in psychiatry—A conceptual review. *European Psychiatry*, 26(7), 403–407. https://doi.org/10.1016/j.eurpsy.2010.07.010

Rice, L. N., & Greenberg, L. S. (1992). Humanistic approaches to psychotherapy. In D. K. Freedheim, H. J. Freudenberger, J. W. Kessler, S. B. Messer, D. R. Peterson, H. H. Strupp, & P. L. Wachtel (Eds.), *History of psychotherapy: A century of change* (pp. 197–224). American Psychological Association. https://doi.org/10.1037/10110-005

Rogers, C. R. (1957). The necessary and sufficient conditions of therapeutic personality change. *Journal of Consulting Psychology*, 21(2), 95–103. https://doi.org/10.1037/h0045357

Rogers, C. R. (1980). *A way of being.* Houghton Mifflin Harcourt.

Rogers, C. R. (1995). *On becoming a person: A therapist's view of psychotherapy.* Houghton Mifflin Harcourt.

Rogers, C. R., Gendlin, E., Kiesler, D., & Truax, C. (Eds.). (1967). *The therapeutic relationship and its impact: A study of psychotherapy with schizophrenics.* Univeristy of Wisconsin Press.

Sackett, C. R., & Cook, R. M. (2022). A phenomenological exploration of client meaningful experiences in family counseling. *Counseling Outcome Research and Evaluation*, 13(2), 116–133. https://doi.org/10.1080/21501378.2021.1922076

Scherman, A. (1981). *Reaching out: Interpersonal effectiveness and self-actualization.* Pearson.

Schneider, K. J., & Krug, O. T. (2017). *Existential–humanistic therapy* (2nd ed.). American Psychological Association. https://doi.org/10.1037/0000042-000

Shahar, G. (2022). Yalom, Strenger, and the psychodynamics of inner freedom: A contribution to existential psychoanalysis. *Psychoanalytic Psychology*, 39(1), 5–11. https://doi.org/10.1037/pap0000395

Strunk, O., Jr. (1970). Values move will: The problem of conceptualization. *Journal of the History of the Behavioral Sciences*, 6(1), 59–63.

Tillich, P. (1952). *The courage to be.* Yale University Press.

Traynor, W., Elliott, R., & Cooper, M. (2011). Helpful factors and outcomes in person-centered therapy with clients who experience psychotic processes: Therapists' perspectives. *Person-Centered and Experiential Psychotherapies*, 10(2), 89–104. https://doi.org/10.1080/14779757.2011.576557

Williams, J. C., & Lynn, S. J. (2010). Acceptance: An historical and conceptual review. *Imagination, Cognition and Personality*, 30(1), 5–56.

Vereen, L. G., Wines, L. A., Lemberger-Truelove, T., Hannon, M. D., Howard, N., & Burt, I. (2017). Black existentialism: Extending the discourse on meaning and existence. *The Journal of Humanistic Counseling*, 56(1), 72–84. https://doi.org/10.1002/johc.12045

Wampold, B. E. (2007). Psychotherapy: The humanistic (and effective) treatment. *American Psychologist*, 62(8), 857–873. https://doi.org/10.1037/0003-066X.62.8.857

Yalom, I. D. (2002). *The gift of therapy: An open letter to a new generation of therapists and their patients.* Harper Perennial.

11

Genuineness and the Real Relationship in Existential–Humanistic Psychotherapy

Zenobia Morrill

The therapeutic relationship has been a hallmark of existential–humanistic (EH) psychotherapy traditions. In Carl Rogers's (1951) client-centered therapy, the real relationship is deemed critical—the factor that vitalizes therapeutic change. Rogers's well-known facilitative conditions of psychotherapy include three essential conditions: empathy, unconditional positive regard, and genuineness. As his views evolved, Rogers (1962) attested that *genuineness* is the most fundamental of these essential attitudes in the ideal therapeutic relationship. Similarly, distinguished existential scholars, such as James Bugental (1987), emphasize presence and *Dasein*, or being there, as paramount to the development of mutual trust and transformation in therapy (Bugental, 1978; Geller & Greenberg, 2012; Schneider, 2008). From these perspectives, genuineness is a key feature of successful EH psychotherapy. Moreover, genuineness may be fundamental to the therapeutic relationship, known to be the vehicle of healing and positive therapy outcomes across theoretical orientations.

Robust empirical support underscores that the client–therapist relationship meaningfully and substantially contributes to outcome independent of the specific treatment approach (Elkins, 2009; Norcross & Lambert, 2018; van Hees et al., 2013; Wampold, 2009; Wampold & Imel, 2015). Yet there has been a history of its devaluation, evinced within clinical guidelines and evidence-based practices (Norcross & Lambert, 2018). Despite robust research on the significance of the client–therapist relationship, therapeutic interventions have been framed and studied apart from the relational elements that contextualize them.

https://doi.org/10.1037/0000446-012
The Evidence-Based Foundations of Existential–Humanistic Therapy, L. Hoffman and V. Lac (Editors)

The tendency to separate treatment techniques from their relational conditions has imitated biomedical approaches that view treatment as prescriptive and attendant to distinct symptomatology profiles (Norcross & Lambert, 2018). In contrast, core themes of EH psychotherapy have consistently upheld that the therapeutic relationship is instrumental (Angus et al., 2015; Cain, 2016; Elkins, 2016). Indeed, EH theory and practice depart from both a medicalized approach and a traditional psychoanalytic blank screen approach (Worth & Proctor, 2020) by privileging therapists' qualities, clients' unique experiences and preferences, and the relational bedrock which grounds them. EH theory has consistently proclaimed that the therapy relationship and in-session interventions are interdependent.

Genuineness and the real relationship have been advanced in EH psychology as distinctive features of the client–therapist relationship. Moreover, both constructs have garnered support and recognition through wider, transtheoretical efforts aimed at clarifying what works about the psychotherapeutic relationship and process more broadly (Flückiger et al., 2018; Norcross & Lambert, 2018; Wampold & Imel, 2015). For example, the Third Interdivisional American Psychological Association Task Force on Evidence-Based Relationships and Responsiveness concluded that Rogerian facilitative conditions (e.g., genuineness) are "core elements" of the therapeutic relationship (Norcross & Lambert, 2018, p. 304).

This chapter examines the research literature on genuineness and the real relationship with an emphasis on their EH origin, application, and contributions. The evidence clarifying and supporting genuineness and the real relationship in psychotherapy is summarized and presented. In addition, a critical lens is applied to examine limitations and taken-for-granted assumptions in EH psychotherapy as well as to investigate multicultural considerations and wider power dynamics that inform understanding the development, validation, and application of genuineness and the real relationship.

DEFINING GENUINENESS AND THE REAL RELATIONSHIP

Genuineness and the real relationship have been construed in myriad ways through both colloquial and field-specific discourses. In this chapter, EH definitions of genuineness and the real relationship are reviewed. This overview establishes the groundwork for the following sections, which feature examples of genuineness and the real relationship in EH psychotherapy. Then, the body of research that has empirically examined these constructs more broadly in the psychotherapy process and outcome literature are summarized.

Although genuineness is arguably most associated with Rogers's core conditions, the notion that realness is constructive and fruitful in psychotherapy has been traced back to existential philosophy (Bugental, 1965) as well as early psychoanalysis (Greenson, 1967; see also Gelso et al., 2018). Although different terms have been used to articulate the significance of a real relational presence in therapy, this underlying sentiment is shared across numerous theoretical orientations. That these concepts have endured and been reshaped across diverse subdisciplines in psychology (and the delivery of health services more generally; Wampold, 2021) demonstrates their overarching importance and essential application in good clinical practice.

Genuineness

Lambert (1992) proclaims that across most theoretical orientations, genuineness is considered to be "important for significant progress in psychotherapy, and, in fact, fundamental in the formation of a working alliance" (p. 104). Carl Rogers's (1957) definition of genuineness may be the most influential. He defines genuineness alongside congruence:

> The therapist should be, within the confines of this relationship, a congruent, genuine, integrated person. It means that within the relationship [they are] freely and deeply [themself], with [their] actual experience accurately represented by [their] awareness of [themself]. It is the opposite of presenting a façade, either knowingly or unknowingly. (p. 242)

As demonstrated here, genuineness and congruence have sometimes been used interchangeably, referring to both the therapist's authenticity with themself as well as their capacity to accurately represent themself in relationships rather than assuming a phony or distant presentation (Gelso, 2002). Genuineness presupposes that a person maintains a type of wholeness, security, and integration that enables them to be aware of—and able to discriminate between— their own experiences and another's. From this awareness, they can be present and open to relational encounters, where they express and represent their subjective experiences honestly, directly, and consistently as necessary (Barrett-Lennard, 2015). Barrett-Lennard (2015) wrote that unconditional positive regard may be a function of genuineness, which also contributes to setting "the upper limit, the degree to which empathic understanding of another is possible" (p. 12).

Overall, genuineness has been defined as multifaceted. It is composed of the therapist's self-awareness, presence, willingness to self-disclose, and emotional involvement in the client's story and the here-and-now interaction (Hill & Knox, 2002; Knox et al., 2001; Wyatt, 2001; Yalom, 2002). In order to attune to the client in this multidimensional way, the therapist is to invoke their whole personality and spirit rather than setting themselves aside or engaging in imitative performance. Following their extensive literature review of person-centered and experiential psychotherapies, Schnellbacher and Leijssen (2009) conclude that genuineness is "an inner attitude, a relational experience, and a dynamic process between client and therapist" (p. 208). However, these facets of genuineness, though linked, may represent distinct concepts.

For instance, authenticity and genuineness may be differentiated. In keeping with EH definitions, authenticity refers to the *intrapersonal* aspect that Rogers describes (e.g., honestly contending with and understanding oneself).

Consistent with this view, existential philosophers such as Nietzsche (1967), Heidegger (2008), and Sartre (1943) describe authenticity as a state of being, a personal quality or presence derived out of "[facing] up to the fundamental anxieties of living" (Thompson, 2004, p. 208). Authenticity may therefore describe an *individual* quality, bearing more relevance to therapists' effects (Castonguay & Hill, 2017) and the person of the therapist (McConnaughy, 1987), whereas genuineness manifests *interpersonally*. However, individual authenticity may enable genuineness interpersonally. Being authentic is instrumental in guiding the therapist's ability to engage sincerely, creatively, and spontaneously with clients. Authenticity also enables the therapist to practice openness to experience, including the capacity to be influenced by, and experience with, those they encounter. In these ways, authentically facing inner experiences may be a precursor to therapists' genuineness—including the capacity to be present, emotionally involved, and to engage in judicious self-disclosure in relationships.

As genuineness is interpersonal and pertains more directly to the therapeutic relationship, it includes the second part of Rogers's description that details how therapists represent themselves truthfully to the client. Importantly, Rogers (1951) specifies that genuineness is not the unfiltered, reckless disclosure of therapists' thoughts and feelings to clients. Rather, genuineness entails the therapist's commitment to avoid deception and withholding of salient or obvious feelings in the encounter. As Kolden and colleagues (2019) summarize, the therapist's "transparency is paramount but not unbridled" (p. 324). Therefore, although disclosing feelings with clients, supervisors, or colleagues may promote genuineness, it does not in and of itself demonstrate it. In EH therapy, for instance, therapists are more likely to take a conversational tone and may avoid using mystifying language that detaches them from everyday life (Hoffman & Granger, 2019).

Genuineness is assessed and determined by both parties, but the client's perception of genuineness is the deciding factor (e.g., Barrett-Lennard, 1962, 2015). Clients' evaluations of the relationship and of genuineness have been demonstrated to predict psychotherapy outcome more accurately (Kolden et al., 2011; Norcross & Lambert, 2018; Patterson, 1984). This distinct definition of genuineness as intersubjective and as an instrumental quality of mutual relational presence demonstrates that it can be cultivated, conveyed, and assessed intersubjectively, as it is cocreated and developed through the interactions between the client and therapist.

The Real Relationship

Since Rogers's (1951) mention of the real relationship, psychotherapy researchers have further developed and defined this construct. The real relationship has been defined by Gelso and Silberberg (2016) as follows:

> The personal or person-to-person relationship that exists between the psychotherapy participants from the moment of first contact, consisting of the extent to

which they perceive/experience each other in a way that befits who they are (termed realism) and respond to each other in an authentic, nonphony manner (termed genuineness). (p. 154)

Genuineness is one of the components of the real relationship that have been articulated (Greenson, 1967). Realism, the other component, refers to what is realistic in the relationship. In other words, it includes psychotherapy participants (i.e., the client and therapist) accurately perceiving and experiencing each other rather than distorting or transferring experiences from other situations, such as through transference and countertransference (Gelso et al., 2018).

The real relationship is considered to be applicable and effective across therapy orientations (Gelso et al., 2018; Gelso & Silberberg, 2016; Wampold & Budge, 2012). Scholars (Gelso, 2011; Greenson, 1967) understand the real relationship to be conceptually distinct from the working alliance. However, research has explored the substantial overlap between the two constructs (Horvath et al., 2011; Kelley et al., 2010; Marmarosh et al., 2009). For example, both the real relationship and the working alliance make up what is generally referred to as the therapeutic relationship. Greenson (1967) proposes that the overall therapeutic relationship is composed of three parts: (a) the working alliance, (b) the real relationship, and (c) transference and countertransference feelings. Despite their interrelatedness, there has been evidence to support that the real relationship is different from the working alliance and contributes unique variance to psychotherapy outcome (Fuertes et al., 2007; Kivlighan et al., 2016; Lo Coco et al., 2011; Marmarosh et al., 2009).

To explain further, although the real relationship and the working alliance are understood as "sister constructs" (Gelso, 2014, p. 125), the working alliance is separable from the real relationship in that it is more task oriented. It includes the extent to which the therapist and client have agreed upon the goals of therapy, the tasks that will facilitate those aims, and the bond between them (Bordin, 1979). The bond component of the Working Alliance Inventory (Horvath & Greenberg, 1989) overlaps most with the real relationship because it captures the personal and nonwork aspects of the relationship. For instance, when a client regards their therapist as a likable and competent professional, their fondness remains primarily contained within the expected roles of the working alliance. On the other hand, experiencing or perceiving genuine, person-to-person care within the relationship would represent an aspect of the real relationship more so than the working alliance (e.g., Gelso et al., 2018). However, the extent of the unique contributions of the real relationship distinct from the working alliance is still debated.

The strength of the real relationship can be measured by assessing both the magnitude and valence of genuineness and realism. Indeed, the strength of the real relationship is increased when therapy participants perceive the relationship to be more real and genuine and when participants regard the relationship with mostly positive feelings (Gelso et al., 2019). These distinctions across constructs also underscore the way that genuineness may be an essential component of the real relationship. Genuineness distinguishes the real relationship as a bond that is somewhat distinct from the working alliance. The influence of genuineness and the mutual encounter in EH theory is arguably intrinsic to the evolution and development of the real relationship construct and its positive effect on therapy outcome (Gelso et al., 2019; Lo Coco et al., 2011).

APPLICATIONS OF GENUINENESS AND THE REAL RELATIONSHIP IN EH PSYCHOTHERAPY

Often, the research on skills and methods that work in psychotherapy may be difficult to implement (Hill & Norcross, 2023). EH theory and practice clarify how genuineness and the real relationship may be applied in practice based upon moment-to-moment occurrences. In EH psychotherapy, building rapport is not merely adjunctive to implementing interventions; instead, it is viewed as the more central or primary practice that makes change happen. The relationship is the site for change. It also is the wellspring from which techniques such as immediacy or here-and-now interventions, self-disclosures, and reflections are successfully deployed. The real relationship in EH therapy fosters trust and durability, giving rise to the potency of these interventions and bolstering moments of rupture and repair. In turn, self-disclosure and exploration of what is happening regarding each participant's feelings in the here-and-now encounter can fructify the sanctity of the real relationship as it unfolds. Indeed, Irvin Yalom (2002) advocated for this type of genuine relating through both therapists' and clients' self-disclosures (e.g., "therapist disclosure begets patient disclosure," p. 29). Regarding genuineness in the therapy relationship, he writes, "Let your patients matter to you. . . . let them enter your mind, influence you, change you—and not conceal this from them" (p. 28).

When commonplace relationships and interactions tend to be shrouded in silences and taken-for-granted assumptions that foment disconnection, a genuine encounter can prove countercultural. Psychotherapy may serve as a site where other alternatives—other ways to be, participate in relationships, or approach the world—may be enacted. Arguably, the real relationship is a precursor to embodying such a novel experience. Psychotherapists are therefore cautioned against confusing genuineness with privileging a subtle type of avoidance, where conflict or honest reflection is bypassed to pacify clients' distress. The failure of the psychotherapy to faithfully represent important components of their experience in the relationship risks treating the client as fragile or minimizing the importance of their relationship to the client.

Put succinctly, cultivating real relationships may entail a genuine willingness to be known (Barrett-Lennard, 2015). Genuineness and the real relationship are undermined when the therapist is withholding or forecloses on an opportunity to reflect or inquire further about a pattern, inconsistency, or another aspect of the client or relationship dynamic, especially when it may be uncomfortable to do so. Genuineness demands that the therapist go there, particularly when social customs and quotidian relationships do not provide access to such opportunities. In the following sections, examples from EH psychotherapy cases are provided to illustrate EH application of genuineness and the real relationship. Included are (a) an existential case illustration followed by (b) a Rogerian client-centered example.

EH Therapy Case Example With Anastasia

This existential therapy case, written by Hoffman and Granger (2019), clarifies how self-disclosure can be harnessed by the therapist to model experiencing and expressing emotions genuinely in the therapy relationship. As a result, the therapeutic process was deepened. The client, "Anastasia," is a 34-year-old woman who is mourning the death of her 2-year-old daughter. The example includes honestly addressing a potential therapeutic rupture:

THERAPIST: I wanted to start off with something today. Last week it really seemed like you were mad at me.

ANASTASIA: No, I was a bit frustrated, but not mad.

THERAPIST: You looked mad. I'm a little unclear about the difference between being mad and being frustrated in your experience.

ANASTASIA: (long pause) I guess it is that I wasn't very upset, it wasn't a big deal.

THERAPIST: It doesn't feel very safe to be angry at me.

ANASTASIA: What do you mean? I wasn't angry. (slightly irritated)

THERAPIST: Okay, but would it be safe to be angry at me?

ANASTASIA: I guess . . . . I just really don't get angry.

THERAPIST: It is okay to get angry—everyone does sometimes. I wonder if it is hard for you to express it.

ANASTASIA: I guess, maybe.

THERAPIST: Maybe? Now that makes me angry. You're just blowing me off.

ANASTASIA: (surprised) I didn't mean to make you angry. I just meant I'm not sure. I'm not comfortable with anger . . . . I did have something I wanted to bring up today.

THERAPIST: Just wait, I think this is important.

ANASTASIA: I just don't want to talk about anger. You said I was in charge of what we talk about.

THERAPIST: You are, and if you really want to move on, we will. But I imagine this would still be on your mind—on both of our minds. I don't think either of us will really be able to focus on something else if this is sitting there unresolved.

ANASTASIA:	Alright. (look of disgust)
THERAPIST:	See, there, you seem angry again.
ANASTASIA:	Yeah, maybe, because you're trying to piss me off.
THERAPIST:	No, I'm not. I am trying to understand, and I may be wrong. I think it is necessary for us to be completely honest with each other.
ANASTASIA:	I never lied to you, what are you talking about?
THERAPIST:	I didn't think you lied. It just seemed like you may not be telling me everything, maybe not telling yourself everything. It seemed you were not acknowledging your anger.
ANASTASIA:	It doesn't feel safe. This is supposed to be a safe place.
THERAPIST:	I hope it is. But how can it truly be safe if you cannot be angry with me?
ANASTASIA:	(pause, Anastasia appeared to be considering this) I guess that makes sense. It's just that I was never allowed to get angry before. It was not okay in my family. If you got angry, then you were really going to get it.
THERAPIST:	And you're afraid I'm going to let you have it, too.
ANASTASIA:	Or you'll get rid of me.
THERAPIST:	(leaning in) I'm not getting rid of you. In fact, I feel quite close to you right now.
ANASTASIA:	(long pause) I do feel connected to you right now, too. I'm not sure what that means.
THERAPIST:	Maybe it means, in part, that this is something you needed to talk about in here. You can't get too close to someone when you're hiding something that needs to be talked about. (pp. 79–80)

In this example, the here-and-now of therapy is being explored alongside the therapist's modeling of experiencing and genuinely expressing anger. The therapist uses self-disclosure to directly express their internal experiences to the client. They do so by using a conversational tone rather than appearing distant or retreating behind a façade of therapeutic jargon. Notably, the therapist avoids psychological or medical labels, opting instead to (a) remain consistent with the type of language Anastasia uses, (b) root their observations within their genuine subjective experience, and (c) tentatively offer alternative language or possible explanations based upon Anastasia's response. In this process, collaborative exploration of what was happening between them in the moment was deepened. Had another approach been taken, one focused on labeling a problem rather than genuinely exploring their moment-to-moment experiences and understandings, damaging or unhelpful patterns from Anastasia's history may have been repeated. Instead, Anastasia was able to articulate and acknowledge the constraints she felt to experiencing anger. She then situated her experience within her relational and systemic contexts and history. The end of the exchange reveals a moment of mutual disclosure about connectedness, indicating that the genuineness of the encounter contributed to strengthening the real relationship.

The Barrett-Lennard Relational Inventory (Barrett-Lennard, 2015), a measure used to assess Rogerian conditions in psychotherapy, may be used to further understand this case illustration. Congruence (i.e., genuineness) items on the Barrett-Lennard Relational Inventory include the client endorsing the following: that their therapist "expresses exactly what they are feeling and thinking as [they] say it"; they "express their true impressions and feelings with me"; and that they do not "hide from [themself] anything that [they] feel with me." Alternatively, decreased feelings of genuineness are represented when clients endorse the following items about their therapist: "sometimes [they are] not at all comfortable but we go on, outwardly ignoring it"; "I believe that [they have] feelings [they] do not tell me about that are causing difficulty in our relationship"; and "there are times when I feel that [their] outward response to me is quite different from the way [they feel] underneath."

Similarly, Gelso and colleagues (2019) propound that the real relationship can be strengthened if the therapist shares aspects of themselves and their feelings with the client. This genuine sharing was demonstrated in the previous example. This existential therapy example also demonstrates the real relationship as it occurs at three levels in psychotherapy: (a) in the background of the client and therapist encounter, including during moments when the relationship is ruptured or threatened; (b) in the clients' and therapists' behaviors that more directly convey genuineness and realism; and (c) through all possible communications between the therapist and client (Gelso et al., 2019).

EH Therapy Case Example With Dione

Additionally, excerpts from Carl Rogers's 1977 therapy session (Brodley & Lietaer, 2003) were transcribed and are also presented here to illustrate a client-centered and phenomenological approach to genuineness and the real relationship. "Dione," a Black man in the United States, articulated his feelings of hurt and anger to Rogers in this therapy session. Dione, who presented with a diagnosis of leukemia, described that the pain of dismissive and derisive social messages and expectations imposed upon him interpersonally sometimes felt worse than the leukemia he had endured. Dione's experiences of hurt and anger became more salient in the session with Rogers, as demonstrated in the following excerpt:

DIONE: I don't know how you'd be angry in a productive way. . . . It's like now when I . . . if, if when you encounter people— whether it's in the street, whether it's in a professional situation

or whatever—if people send out certain messages . . . no matter
what they're saying or whatever . . . there are certain kinds of
messages that I'm getting, you know. They're saying that "hey,
you know . . . that isn't for me" kind of thing. . . . I'd like to work
with that . . . to try to communicate without alienating (Rogers:
Mmm.) people or whatever.

ROGERS: I get what you're saying, and I also feel quite strongly that I want
to say it's okay with me if you're angry *here*.

DIONE: (pause) But I don't, you know . . . it's hard to know how to be
angry, you know . . . hard to . . .

ROGERS: Sure, sure, I'm not saying you have to be. (Dione: Sure.) I'm just
saying it's okay with me.

DIONE: Mmm.

ROGERS: If you feel like being angry, you can be angry.

DIONE: You really believe that?

ROGERS: Damn right.

DIONE: (12 second pause) Well. (15 second pause, sigh) I'm not sure
how to respond to that at all, you know, because a part of that
anger is the . . . the hurt, and maybe if I'm . . . maybe what's happening is that if I'm . . . if I become angry and I really let it hang
out, that I really will see how hurt I am.

ROGERS: Mmm, mmm.

DIONE: And um, you know, that just came to me as you were talking.

ROGERS: Mmm, mmm.

DIONE: That, you know . . .

ROGERS: Perhaps at a deeper level you're afraid of the hurt that you may
experience if you let yourself experience the anger.

DIONE: For sure. (p. 88, ellipses added)

In this exchange, Dione is highlighting blocks he faces when feeling and
expressing his pain and anger. Rogers self-discloses his urge to share with Dione
that it would be okay if he expressed his anger in therapy. Dione then considers
that he may be afraid to authentically acknowledge his own hurt and also
seems reticent based upon his previous experience to express anger because he
risks alienating others. Later in this session, Rogers utilizes a here-and-now
process reflection to recognize and call attention to Dione's articulations of his
feelings:

ROGERS: So there are probably loads of people you wouldn't dare open up to on that, but I guess you're opening up to me to say, "Yes, but I have been really wounded, badly, by a lot of people."

DIONE: For sure. Mmm. I maybe think that you can understand that a little bit, in terms of about hurt and . . . you know, that I'm a person and uh, (pause) you know, I'm a person. And I don't really want that denied to me . . . (Rogers: Mmm.) you know, ever again.

ROGERS: Mmm, mmm.

DIONE: You know. I could really get angry.

ROGERS: Mmm. Mmm. (p. 98, ellipses added)

Throughout the session, Dione expresses his belief that Rogers may understand parts of the hurt he feels, but also that some things he could tell him might "blow [him] away" (p. 107). However, what is also at risk for Dione is to reexperience the hurt he has felt when basic aspects of his personhood have been rejected and denied to him, particularly in the context of 1970s racism in the United States. Dione explicitly shares that he wants to feel and express his experiences to Rogers but is unsure of how to do so. He fears he would not only "look horrible" (p. 103) to Rogers, but that the pain he accesses would exacerbate his own illness. Upon Dione sharing this, Rogers both recognizes and legitimizes Dione's process and then models expressing anger (e.g., "I realized I've used more profanity than you have"; "You'd like to just tell off the bastard" [p. 101]). This appears to offer levity to the session while also facilitating Dione's understanding of his own blocked feelings and vulnerabilities.

Dione begins to identify the increasing intensity of contacting his felt experience (e.g., "Whew! I'm getting warm" [p. 101]). Rogers continues to reflect and validate Dione's experiences, and Dione further clarifies the constraints and fears associated with this anger, hurt, and indignation:

DIONE: I feel so beaten. I think that if I show you how much I've been beaten or whatever, I'd probably, you know, become nothing in this chair, you know, just . . . (Rogers: Mmm, mmm.) You know? (laughs, long pause)

ROGERS: You might practically disappear if you really let me know how hurt and beaten and awful you feel.

DIONE: Mmm, for sure. For sure. You know, I could tell you some things that would just maybe blow you away, you know? (Rogers: Mmm.) . . . (sighs and appears on the edge of crying during a 20 second pause) It's really too much for me. Too much.

ROGERS: Too much. Mmm.

DIONE: I feel like it.

ROGERS: I, I think you feel as though, "I've gone about as far as I can go at this point".

DIONE: Yeah. Mmm, yeah, really. (laughs) When I start smiling, I know I am. (takes a sip of water)

ROGERS: Mmm. Taking a drink of water.

DIONE: For sure. (laughs) Well, you know, but I'm being truthful about it anyway.

ROGERS: Mmm, yeah. Yeah, I feel, I feel too. Uh, you've walked around that pit of hurt and pain and beatenness, and you've, you've felt some of it and uh, and perhaps that's as far as you can go right at this moment.

DIONE: Yeah.

ROGERS: Even though you know there's more there, you know that you're keeping some of it down. And to know those things may be helpful too.

DIONE: Yeah. You see, because I, I can talk about this leukemia and all this stuff and everything like that and . . . (Rogers: Mmm, mmm.) but, I guess it's you know . . .

ROGERS: Fascinating. And it's easier to talk about leukemia and the possibility of death and all that, than it is to talk about all the hurt and awfulness that you've suffered.

DIONE: Yeah. (sighs) Whew, oh, I really, whew, a lot, you know. (sighs) I have to stop. Okay?

ROGERS: Okay. All right, mmm. Gone about as far as you can go. (pp. 106–107, ellipses added)

Then the therapy session ends. This excerpt demonstrates a hallmark practice of client-centered therapy, which is following the client's pacing and wisdom regarding when and how to explore experiences. Importantly, however, Rogers did not refrain from being a genuine participant, offering Dione his own experiences, relevant observations, and tentative reflections—for instance, when he says, "I feel too . . . you've walked around that pit of hurt and pain . . . you've felt some of it. . . ." (p. 107). During this session, Dione expresses the ways in which he has been truthful, and at numerous times he appears to seek confirmation that Rogers understands how contacting his real experience may be too risky or too intense. He also expresses that he is unsure how to do it, or perhaps is questioning whether he, or their relationship, can withstand it. One of Rogers's comments about the session encapsulates both his own experiences of genuineness and the real relationship he felt with Dione: "As for me, I felt very present in the relationship, an understanding companion on this trip of exploration which seemed so potentially dangerous to him" (p. 109).

QUANTITATIVE EVIDENCE

In the past two decades, the real relationship has been examined in connection with psychotherapy outcomes. One of the first studies to examine the real relationship (Eugster & Wampold, 1996) utilized a scale that focused on assessing genuineness and was less focused on the realism component of the real relationship. Despite limitations of the measure, this study provided early evidence that therapists' and clients' assessment of the real relationship correlated with their ratings of session quality. According to Gelso and colleagues (2019), since 1996, most process and outcome studies on the real relationship have utilized the Real Relationship Inventory (RRI) instead, which measures both the realism and genuineness components. The RRI includes the client version (RRI-C; Kelley et al., 2010) and therapist version (RRI-T; Gelso et al., 2005). The empirical validation of these measures has supported the construct validity of the real relationship as well as its connection to other EH psychotherapeutic factors such as therapists' empathy (Fuertes et al., 2007).

Gelso and colleagues' (2019) meta-analysis examined the real relationship and psychotherapy outcome (i.e., pretest–posttest change), treatment progress, and session quality or outcome across 16 studies. There was a significant, moderate-sized association between the real relationship and outcomes across these indicators. In other words, the stronger the real relationship, the better the therapy outcomes. This association did not change when different outcome measures were used, and this was independent of the client or therapist rating of therapy relationship or outcomes. Moreover, the association between the real relationship and session outcomes was of a greater magnitude (moderate, $r = 0.38$) than that of the working alliance and session outcome (small, $r = 0.28$), as demonstrated by Horvath and colleagues' (2011) meta-analysis. Gelso and colleagues (2019) included several prior studies (Eugster & Wampold, 1996; Fuertes et al., 2007; Gelso et al., 2005; Lo Coco et al., 2011; Marmarosh et al., 2009), which established that the real relationship predicts outcome above and beyond what is accounted for by the working alliance. Moreover, some evidence from a non-U.S. sample suggested that therapists' genuineness, when rated by the client, significantly corresponded to outcomes (Lo Coco et al., 2011).

When it comes to fostering the real relationship in psychotherapy, Kivlighan and colleagues (2015) demonstrate that between-therapist differences are better predictors of treatment outcomes than between-client differences. In other words, therapists were seen to make a greater contribution to the real relationship as it manifested in the early stages of treatment, in its development throughout treatment, and as demonstrated by session evaluations rated by both parties. Some client qualities have been associated with the strength of the real relationship (Kelley et al., 2010). For instance, the client's ability to accurately observe themselves, attend to their feelings—compared with ignoring feelings, which was negatively associated—and the client's ability to form secure attachments (Moore & Gelso, 2011) all strengthened the real relationship.

Such evidence underscores the ways in which therapists might deliberately cultivate and strengthen the real relationship toward better outcomes and responsiveness to client factors. In particular, genuineness/congruence has been demonstrated to be significantly correlated (0.23) to therapy outcomes with a small-to-medium effect size of 0.46 (Kolden et al., 2018). Therefore, Kolden and colleagues (2018) put forward practice recommendations including that therapists strive for genuine and direct ways of relating with clients through acceptance, experiencing with, modeling, and encouraging clients' genuine expression. Given that the real relationship construct encapsulates genuineness as a fundamental component, Kolden and colleagues (2019) argue that research supporting the real relationship also serves to expand, amplify, and refine understandings of the role of genuineness/congruence as well. For instance, one study (i.e., Gullo et al., 2012) demonstrated that when compared with clients who terminated early in brief psychotherapy, clients who continued in therapy rated higher genuineness scores on the RRI. Their scores were also associated with greater treatment success. In addition, overall RRI scores (genuineness and realism summed) were also associated with treatment success, both when measured early and late in the therapy process. Such studies support genuineness as a cornerstone to the real relationship and corroborate that both positively contribute to treatment success.

Although the results of these studies and the meta-analytic reviews by Gelso and colleagues (2019) and Kolden and colleagues (2019) provide promising direction and indication that the real relationship and genuineness hold predictive validity in psychotherapy, there are limitations. For example, relatively few studies ($N = 7$) were included in Gelso and colleagues' (2019) meta-analysis. This scarcity contributes to low power and thus limits the interpretations that can be drawn about the real relationship and treatment outcome. Gelso and colleagues note that additional data are needed to determine the predictive validity of the strength of the real relationship on treatment outcome, particularly following termination and longer term follow-up. In addition, researcher allegiance biases may have influenced positive correlations for genuineness/congruence and outcome that were derived out of client-centered, eclectic, and interpersonal therapies (Kolden et al., 2018), despite the fact that the real relationship construct is not attached to any one theoretical orientation.

Neither of the meta-analyses by Gelso and colleagues (2019) and Kolden and colleagues (2019) on the real relationship and genuineness/congruence can claim causality. Nevertheless, longitudinal field studies (Gelso et al., 2012; Kivlighan et al., 2015; see also Gelso et al., 2019) provide a basis which supports that the real relationship plays a significant role in psychotherapy outcomes. Real relationship studies are important for further articulating the role of genuineness in psychotherapy as well, so that it is not entirely obscured or subsumed by overarching therapy relationship constructs (Kolden et al., 2018).

QUALITATIVE EVIDENCE

Relatively fewer qualitative studies have been conducted to examine genuineness and the real relationship in psychotherapy. This paucity is unfortunate, however, because qualitative inquiry is well-positioned to clarify nuanced application of clinical skills and to resolve conceptual discrepancies (Levitt et al., 2020; Levitt et al., 2024). Moreover, qualitative findings serve as a basis from which additional quantitative studies and meaningful inferences regarding causality may be pursued, but they also serve as empirical evidence in their own right to inform clinical practice principles, training, supervision, and application (Geller & Greenberg, 2012; Levitt et al., 2024).

As discussed in this chapter, genuineness and the real relationship are complex intersubjective phenomena. Both have important bearing on psychotherapy process and outcome. Qualitative inquiry can further articulate the lived experience of phenomena (e.g., how genuineness and the real relationship are experienced in psychotherapy, in moment-to-moment intervals) that might otherwise be difficult to explore. As Gelso and colleagues (2019) describe, "the real relationship (although it has been operationalized for research purposes) is something that must be experienced to be truly known" (p. 372). Qualitative inquiry offers nuanced examination of these EH constructs, particularly their experiential and relational aspects that are otherwise difficult to discern. For example, task analysis, case study, conversational analysis, interpersonal process recall, and other qualitative approaches may clarify when, how, with whom, and to what extent specific interventions contribute to strengthening genuineness and the real relationship amid the context-dependent nature of their success.

Despite the relative scarcity of qualitative empirical data, there are some studies that have explored the ways genuineness and the real relationship are experienced by participants in person-centered and experiential psychotherapies. For instance, Schnellbacher and Leijssen (2009) investigated the meaning and significance of therapists' genuineness from the client's perspective. This investigation also captured elements related to therapist self-disclosures. A multiple case study design ($N = 6$) was utilized to gather qualitative and quantitative data. Client participants included six women of Belgian nationality who participated in person-centered experiential therapies for an average duration of 16.2 months. Four of these six participants shared that they experienced acceptance, empathy, or focusing as the most crucial aspect of psychotherapy. Although this diverged from genuineness as the most crucial aspect of therapy, research suggests that genuineness may indirectly contribute to therapy outcomes by mediating factors such as acceptance, empathy, and concrete interventions (Klein et al., 2002).

Importantly, two of the six participants identified genuineness as the most crucial aspect. One highlighted their therapist's genuine emotional involvement and self-disclosures as facilitative of their ability to contact the relational here-and-now as well as their felt experiences and needs in a way that directly corresponded to their treatment goal. The second participant emphasized the "deeply human moments of encounter" (Schnellbacher & Leijssen, 2009, p. 218) as providing critical companionship for existential pain. These empirical data demonstrate that clients' experiencing of therapists' genuineness can be crucially informing of healing and desired change. Moreover, the authors concluded that individual clients determine whether and how genuineness represents a significant component of therapy to them.

Other qualitative research has similarly explored therapists' self-disclosure, finding that it may have positive effects on clients' perspectives of genuineness and the real relationship (Hill & Knox, 2002; Hill et al., 2018). One qualitative meta-analysis (Levitt et al., 2016) on clients' experiences in psychotherapy provided some support that genuineness and authentic care were important factors in the client–therapist relationship, providing a wellspring for clients' self-exploration and discovery. Another qualitative study (Burks & Robbins, 2011) examined authenticity in the therapeutic relationship. However, this interpretation of authenticity included the outer expression of the therapist's true inner experiences, fitting within the EH understanding of genuineness in this chapter. Therapist participants in this study shared that they experienced authenticity/genuineness as a reciprocal and circular process, defined by emotional involvement, realness, transparency, and honesty that increased their connectedness within the therapeutic relationship. Some therapist participants even shared that the reciprocity of this experience could further enhance their personal authentic development. Therapists' experiences of authenticity also included experiencing genuine care for their clients, serving to further support the interplay of these constructs.

Finally, a narrative analysis of clients' and therapists' experiences of significant events in time-limited person-centered therapy (Grafanaki & McLeod, 2002) more closely articulated experiences of congruence, a construct closely linked to genuineness (Kolden et al., 2018). To summarize, Grafanaki and McLeod (2002) found that therapists experienced congruence as (a) empathic attunement and experiential presence, (b) process directing and focusing, (c) covert use of resolved personal material, and (d) self-disclosure of personal material. Clients, however, experienced congruence as (a) sharing meaningful material about themselves, (b) reporting simple information about self and others, (c) momentary heightened awareness or realization, (d) process disclosure, (e) personal contact with the therapist, and (f) new ways of being or behaving. Conversely, incongruence manifested in therapists' experiences as including but not limited to disengagement, discomfort around professional competence and boundaries, and misdirection, and in clients' experiences as avoidance, deference, unwanted responsibility, and disorientation. These types of experiences illustrated the multifaceted ways that genuineness might also be perceived, weakened, and strengthened in psychotherapy.

MULTICULTURAL CONSIDERATIONS

The multicultural movement in psychology has challenged some of the individualistic assumptions within EH theory and practice that risk being universalized (Hoffman et al., 2019). Relying upon taken-for-granted assumptions of a

Western, individualistic self may contribute to reductive concepts of humanness that not only obscure the breadth and diversity of clients' experiences of health and suffering but also the cultural and political systems of power that shape them. These constraints have implications for psychotherapy when genuineness and the real relationship are construed as manifesting uniformly across relationships irrespective of setting, individuals' diverse intersecting identities, and other contextual factors. Honoring the intersubjective and contextual aspects of psychotherapy are vital to enacting genuineness and the types of real relationships that heal, as underscored in this chapter. Therefore, to consider cultural applications of genuineness and the real relationship requires critically examining the ways epistemic power has influenced the development, validation, and application of these constructs.

Although Rogers and other EH philosophers are appropriately celebrated for their important contributions to concepts of genuineness and the real relationship in psychotherapy, EH theory is invariably culture bound, predominantly in regard to Euro-American cultural assumptions and values (Hocoy, 2019). Western psychology has operated as an arbiter of what knowledge is considered legitimate in the psychotherapy process–outcome research literature. These power dynamics within the field not only marginalize other practices and ways of knowing that may contribute to an enriched understanding of what constitutes a real relationship but might also result in practices that do not fit the realities of people's lives.

An examination of how power dynamics have operated to restrict understandings of genuineness and the real relationship in psychology demonstrates the exclusion of Black psychology philosophy, Latine liberation psychologies, and other marginalized epistemologies. Indeed, techniques in psychotherapy process–outcome research have been conceptualized as separate from relationships and contexts (Norcross & Lambert, 2018). The devaluation of relational aspects in psychotherapy more broadly may represent Western emphasis and the value of hyperindividuality and atomism (i.e., the individual devoid of context). Moreover, collusion of Euro-American ideologies, such as neoliberal capitalism and hyperindividualism, promote a culture of efficiency and hedonism that may contribute to the idea that psychotherapy ought to be reducible to measurable components that can be applied to treat medical symptoms (see e.g., Morrill, 2021; Morrill & Levitt, 2021). In contrast, Black psychology and Latine community psychology are rooted in marginalized epistemologies that value collectivism, solidarity, and emancipation (Bryant-Davis & Comas-Díaz, 2016; Jackson, 2019). These approaches have represented the ways sociocontextual factors are inherent to conceptualizing and responding to suffering. In addition, by honoring individuals' interdependence, marginalized epistemologies also tend to underscore and reclaim the notion that relationships are crucial to healing, a value more conducive to understanding and enacting genuineness in psychotherapy relationships.

Marginalized theories and practices may corroborate the important role of genuine relating in psychotherapy, and they may also serve to enrich understanding of the real relationship. For example, analyzing the politics of power and privilege from the perspectives of those marginalized can shed light on the systemic and relational contexts that constrain opportunities for realism, genuineness, and affect clients' health overall (Morrill & Luiggi-Hernández, 2026). Double consciousness (Du Bois, 1903), for instance, provides a poignant articulation of the ways social oppression manifests as the simultaneous awareness of how one is being perceived by a hegemonic gaze—in this case, Black Americans' awareness of how they are perceived through the lens of a racist society. Does this perception facilitate or inhibit genuine expression in relationships? For instance, although Schneider's (2023) conceptualization of cosmic disintegration may be applied to Dione's presentation with Carl Rogers in the example provided, Frantz Fanon's (1952/2008) concepts of alienation and dehumanization also inform existential and phenomenological understandings of individuals' anger and pain as sociogenic, inseparable from social, historical, and structural factors.

Similarly, EH and feminist scholar Simone de Beauvoir (1997) highlights assumptions about authenticity and self-actualization in relation to gender oppression. She points out that when social oppression is not considered, the narrow focus on individuals' shortcomings is blaming and harmful. It can be risky, therefore, if EH constructs such as authenticity and self-actualization are used in ways that magnify individuals' qualities and deficits rather than understood as individuals' experiences within sociocultural, historical, and linguistic context to inform fostering genuine relating (Morrill & Luiggi-Hernández, 2026). It is in keeping with existential and phenomenological thought to resist polarities that divorce objects from subjects, individuals from context, and ethical principles from the unique situations in which they arise and must be applied (de Beauvoir, 1962). Incorporating these perspectives can enrich the application of the real relationship in psychotherapy. Cultural power confers a type of privilege that shapes how and whether individuals may readily access and express genuineness and realism. Such power may not be shared nor evenly distributed within and across relationships with the same therapist or client.

In addition to the epistemic constraints on conceptualizations of the real relationship, considerably less research has examined the real relationship in countries outside of the United States and the ways in which social identities and location influence the real relationship. The two studies conducted outside the United States included examination of real relationship on treatment in Italy (Lo Coco et al., 2011) and South Korea (see e.g., Gelso et al., 2019). Both support overall findings about the real relationship as a critical ingredient of change in psychotherapy.

Two studies have explored multicultural factors and their impact on the real relationship, however. The first study (Owen et al., 2011) examined client-rated working alliance, real relationship, and treatment outcomes. In addition, clients rated their therapist's multicultural orientation. Higher client ratings of the real relationship were associated with better treatment outcomes for White clients ($n = 95$) and clients with minoritized racial and ethnic identities ($n = 81$).

The more clients perceived their therapists as having a multicultural orientation (Davis et al., 2018), the stronger they experienced the real relationship to be. The second study (Kelley, 2015) explored the real relationship with lesbian ($n = 76$) and gay ($n = 40$) clients. They found that the real relationship predicted a significant variance in clients' positive feelings about their therapist. This relationship remained after accounting for the amount of time in therapy, therapists' interventions, and the working alliance. Both studies corroborated the association between the real relationship and treatment outcomes. When Gelso and colleagues (2019) conducted their review, no studies examining gender identity had been conducted, despite gender typically being featured as a variable in most studies.

FUTURE RESEARCH

Many aspects of genuineness and the real relationship can be further explored to aid in cultivating real therapeutic encounters across a diverse range of clients' experiences and in a way that is befitting of an ecological conceptualization in clinical practice. First, it is worth exploring the relationship between authenticity and genuineness, as the constructs have been defined within this chapter. Is it the case that psychotherapists who have nurtured their own self-awareness and authenticity tend to be more genuine and establish stronger real relationships across clients? And, given that client factors may contribute to or hinder real relationships, is it the case that clients who are more inclined toward authenticity are also more likely to accurately observe themselves and securely attach in ways conducive to genuineness? These questions connect to the second recommendation to pursue research that clarifies clients' and therapists' intersubjective contributions to genuineness and the real relationship. As previously described, qualitative research is well-positioned not only to develop rich descriptions of how these concepts are experienced and lived in psychotherapy interactions but also to highlight the situational contingencies which enable psychotherapists to skillfully recognize and respond to salient moments conducive to bolstering genuine encounters and good outcomes.

Third, more research is needed to establish the predictive validity of the real relationship on therapeutic outcomes. Although it is important to include epistemological diversity and ensure that EH research frameworks and methodologies are featured in future research studies, it also may be important to consider the ways researcher allegiance biases may risk overestimating the positive correlations found between genuineness and psychotherapy outcome. Fourth, given that some findings seem to point to the idea that genuineness is increased when honest and in-depth exploration is conducted alongside heightened instances of self-disclosure, it is worth exploring the possible implications of this connection (see also Chapter 12 of this volume). If it is the case that increased genuineness begets more accurate and in-depth disclosures on the part of the client, this knowledge can aid in understanding the necessary role of genuineness in crucial therapy moments that address shame and alienation as well as facilitate more accurate and ethical safety risk assessments. Fifth, and finally, there is a need to conduct more epistemologically and multiculturally diverse studies that articulate the nuances of genuineness across unique clients, contexts, and presentations. Given the dominance of Eurocentric epistemologies, methods, and samples, more studies may be conducted from outside of the United States and across the myriad differences that more closely represent the vast range of human diversity and social locations. Toward this aim, epistemological and methodological pluralism can be embraced, with a particular focus upon recentering marginalized perspectives to guide research processes.

CONCLUSION

EH theory has offered fundamental insights to the field's current understanding of genuineness—a facilitative factor in good psychotherapy. Importantly, genuineness and the real relationship are intersubjective phenomena, codeveloped and coassessed by the client and therapist. Therefore, cultivating genuineness in psychotherapy demands more than accumulating mere knowledge and technique as static, unchanging, and decontextualized practices. Rather, a genuine therapist seeking to cultivate real relationships with clients practices ongoing presence and honesty and contends meaningfully with self and others' experiences in order to faithfully represent themselves and their relational experiences with the client in psychotherapy. Keen perceptive skills are required to attune to and communicate within moment-to-moment relational processes in session. EH philosophy places authentic and honest exploration of the human condition and lived experiences at the heart of psychotherapy.

Within EH theory and practice, authentic self-understanding may powerfully support a capacity to genuinely relate. Moreover, EH therapists recognize the importance of following and facilitating clients' processes, as they occur uniquely and in relational and cultural contexts. Approaching psychotherapy with openness to the client's experiences enables the therapist to responsively tailor genuineness and real relating with each unique person. As with many psychotherapy processes and clients' experiences, genuineness and the real relationship are better understood as intersubjective and sociogenic in that they are informed by and occur within broader contexts. It aids the therapist to bring this critical lens to contextualizing their understanding of the clients' worldview as well as in-session relational dynamics. Taken together, a therapist who is interested in genuinely relating must also be willing to initiate and facilitate exploring together what is uniquely unfolding in session and—somewhat vulnerably—participate in this process by sharing how they, too, are experiencing it.

Although the real relationship has been a point of longstanding interest in psychotherapy since the inception of the talking cure, it has been a mainstay of EH practice. It is an ingredient that enables holistic change beyond already-existing measures of symptom reduction, honoring the clients' worldview and registers of meaning. Indeed, in EH therapy, genuine encounters form the real bond that animates healing and transformation.

REFERENCES

Angus, L., Watson, J. C., Elliott, R., Schneider, K., & Timulak, L. (2015). Humanistic psychotherapy research 1990–2015: From methodological innovation to evidence-supported treatment outcomes and beyond. *Psychotherapy Research, 25*(3), 330–347. https://doi.org/10.1080/10503307.2014.989290

Barrett-Lennard, G. T. (1962). Dimensions of therapist response as causal factors in therapeutic change. *Psychological Monographs: General and Applied, 76*(43), 1–36. https://doi.org/10.1037/h0093918

Barrett-Lennard, G. T. (2015). *The relationship inventory: A complete resource and guide.* John Wiley & Sons.

Bordin, E. S. (1979). The generalizability of the psychoanalytic concept of the working alliance. *Psychotherapy, 16*(3), 252–260. https://doi.org/10.1037/h0085885

Brodley, B. T. & Lietaer, G. (2003). Carl Rogers in the therapy room: A listing of session transcripts and a survey of publications referring to Rogers' sessions. *Person-Centered and Experiential Psychotherapies, 2*(4), 274–291. https://doi.org/10.1080/14779757.2003.9688320

Bryant-Davis, T., & Comas-Díaz, L. (Eds.). (2016). *Womanist and mujerista psychologies: Voices of fire, acts of courage.* American Psychological Association. https://doi.org/10.1037/14937-000

Bugental, J. F. (1965). The existential crisis in intensive psychotherapy. *Psychotherapy, 2*(1), 16–20. https://doi.org/10.1037/h0088602

Bugental, J. F. T. (1978). *Psychotherapy and process: The fundamentals of an existential–humanistic approach.* McGraw-Hill.

Bugental, J. F. T. (1987). *The art of the psychotherapist: How to develop the skills that take psychotherapy beyond science.* W. W. Norton & Company.

Burks, D. J., & Robbins, R. (2011). Are you analyzing me? A qualitative exploration of psychologists' individual and interpersonal experiences with authenticity. *The Humanistic Psychologist, 39*(4), 348–365. https://doi.org/10.1080/08873267.2011.620201

Cain, D. J. (2016). Toward a research-based integration of optimal practices of humanistic psychotherapies. In D. J. Cain, K. Keenan, & S. Rubin (Eds.), *Humanistic psychotherapies: Handbook of research and practice* (pp. 485–535). American Psychological Association. https://doi.org/10.1037/14775-016

Castonguay, L. G., & Hill, C. E. (Eds.). (2017). *How and why are some therapists better than others? Understanding therapist effects.* American Psychological Association. https://doi.org/10.1037/0000034-000

Davis, D. E., DeBlaere, C., Owen, J., Hook, J. N., Rivera, D. P., Choe, E., Van Tongeren, D. R., Worthington, E. L., Jr., & Placeres, V. (2018). The multicultural orientation framework: A narrative review. *Psychotherapy, 55*(1), 89–100. https://doi.org/10.1037/pst0000160

de Beauvoir, S. (1962). *The ethics of ambiguity* (B. Frechtman, Trans.). Citadel Press.

de Beauvoir, S. (1997). *The second sex* (H. M. Parshley, Trans.). Vintage. (Original work published 1949)

Du Bois, W. E. B. (1903). *The souls of Black folk: Essays and sketches.* Fawcett.

Elkins, D. N. (2009). *Humanistic psychology: A clinical manifesto. A critique of clinical psychology and the need for progressive alternatives.* University of the Rockies Press.

Elkins, D. N. (2016). *The human elements of psychotherapy: A nonmedical model of emotional healing.* American Psychological Association. https://doi.org/10.1037/14751-000

Eugster, S. L., & Wampold, B. E. (1996). Systematic effects of participant role on evaluation of the psychotherapy session. *Journal of Consulting and Clinical Psychology, 64*(5), 1020–1028. https://doi.org/10.1037/0022-006X.64.5.1020

Fanon, F. (2008). *Black skin, White masks* (R. Philcox, Trans.) Grove Press. (Original work published 1952)

Flückiger, C., Del Re, A. C., Wampold, B. E., & Horvath, A. O. (2018). The alliance in adult psychotherapy: A meta-analytic synthesis. *Psychotherapy, 55*(4), 316–340. https://doi.org/10.1037/pst0000172

Fuertes, J. N., Mislowack, A., Brown, S., Gur-Arie, S., Wilkinson, S., & Gelso, C. J. (2007). Correlates of the real relationship in psychotherapy: A study of dyads. *Psychotherapy Research, 17*(4), 423–430. https://doi.org/10.1080/10503300600789189

Geller, S. M., & Greenberg, L. S. (2012). *Therapeutic presence: A mindful approach to effective therapy*. American Psychological Association. https://doi.org/10.1037/13485-000

Gelso, C. (2014). A tripartite model of the therapeutic relationship: Theory, research, and practice. *Psychotherapy Research, 24*(2), 117–131. https://doi.org/10.1080/10503307.2013.845920

Gelso, C. J. (2002). Real relationship: The "something more" of psychotherapy. *Journal of Contemporary Psychotherapy, 32*(1), 35–40. https://doi.org/10.1023/A:1015531228504

Gelso, C. J. (2011). *The real relationship in psychotherapy: The hidden foundation of change*. American Psychological Association. https://doi.org/10.1037/12349-000

Gelso, C. J., Kelley, F. A., Fuertes, J. N., Marmarosh, C., Holmes, S. E., Costa, C., & Hancock, G. R. (2005). Measuring the real relationship in psychotherapy: Initial validation of the therapist form. *Journal of Counseling Psychology, 52*(4), 640–649. https://doi.org/10.1037/0022-0167.52.4.640

Gelso, C. J., Kivlighan, D. M., Jr., Busa-Knepp, J., Spiegel, E. B., Ain, S., Hummel, A. M., Yuehler, E. M., & Markin, R. D. (2012). The unfolding of the real relationship and the outcome of brief psychotherapy. *Journal of Counseling Psychology, 59*(4), 495. https://doi.org/10.1037/a0029838

Gelso, C. J., Kivlighan, D. M., Jr., & Markin, R. D. (2018). The real relationship and its role in psychotherapy outcome: A meta-analysis. *Psychotherapy, 55*(4), 434–444. https://doi.org/10.1037/pst0000183

Gelso, C. J., Kivlighan, D. M., Jr., & Markin, R. D. (2019). The real relationship. In J. C. Norcross & M. J. Lambert (Eds.), *Psychotherapy relationships that work: Evidence-based therapist contributions* (3rd ed., pp. 351–378). Oxford University Press.

Gelso, C. J., & Silberberg, A. (2016). Strengthening the real relationship: What is a psychotherapist to do? *Practice Innovations, 1*(3), 154–163. https://doi.org/10.1037/pri0000024

Grafanaki, S., & McLeod, J. (2002). Experiential congruence: Qualitative analysis of client and counsellor narrative accounts of significant events in time-limited person-centred therapy. *Counselling & Psychotherapy Research, 2*(1), 20–32. https://doi.org/10.1080/14733140212331384958

Greenson, R. R. (1967). *The technique and practice of psychoanalysis* (Vol. 1). International Universities Press.

Gullo, S., Lo Coco, G., & Gelso, C. (2012). Early and later predictors of outcome in brief therapy: The role of real relationship. *Journal of Clinical Psychology, 68*(6), 614–619. https://doi.org/10.1002/jclp.21860

Heidegger, M. (2008). *Being and time*. Harper Perennial.

Hill, C. E., & Knox, S. (2002). Self-disclosure. In J. C. Norcross (Ed.), *Psychotherapy relationships that work: Therapist contributions and responsiveness to patients* (pp. 255–265). Oxford University Press.

Hill, C. E., Knox, S., & Pinto-Coelho, K. G. (2018). Therapist self-disclosure and immediacy: A qualitative meta-analysis. *Psychotherapy, 55*(4), 445–460. https://doi.org/10.1037/pst0000182

Hill, C. E., & Norcross, J. C. (2023). Skills and methods that work in psychotherapy: Observations and conclusions from the special issue. *Psychotherapy, 60*(3), 407–416. https://doi.org/10.1037/pst0000487

Hocoy, D. (2019). The challenge of multiculturalism to humanistic psychology. In L. Hoffman, H. Cleare-Hoffman, N. Granger Jr., & D. S. John (Eds.), *Humanistic approaches to multiculturalism and diversity: Perspectives on existence and difference* (pp. 18–28). University Professors Press. https://doi.org/10.4324/9781351133357-3

Hoffman, L., Cleare-Hoffman, H., Granger, N., Jr., & St. John, D. (Eds.). (2019). *Humanistic approaches to multiculturalism and diversity: Perspectives on existence and difference.* Routledge. https://doi.org/10.4324/9781351133357

Hoffman, L., & Granger, N., Jr. (2019). An existential–humanistic psychotherapy case illustration. In L. Hoffman, M. Yang, F. J. Kaklauskas, A. Chan, & M. Mansilla (Eds.), *Existential psychology East–West* (Vol. 1, Rev. ed., pp. 73–93). University Professors Press.

Horvath, A. O., Del Re, A. C., Flückiger, C., & Symonds, D. (2011). Alliance in individual psychotherapy. *Psychotherapy, 48*(1), 9–16. https://doi.org/10.1037/a0022186

Horvath, A. O., & Greenberg, L. S. (1989). Development and validation of the Working Alliance Inventory. *Journal of Counseling Psychology, 36*(2), 223–233. https://doi.org/10.1037/0022-0167.36.2.223

Jackson, T. (2019). The history of Black psychology and humanistic psychology: Synergetic prospects. In L. Hoffman, H. Cleare-Hoffman, N. Granger Jr., & D. S. John (Eds.), *Humanistic approaches to multiculturalism and diversity* (pp. 29–44). Routledge. https://doi.org/10.4324/9781351133357-4

Kelley, F. A. (2015). The therapy relationship with lesbian and gay clients. *Psychotherapy, 52*(1), 113–118. https://doi.org/10.1037/a0037958

Kelley, F. A., Gelso, C. J., Fuertes, J. N., Marmarosh, C., & Lanier, S. H. (2010). The Real Relationship Inventory: Development and psychometric investigation of the client form. *Psychotherapy, 47*(4), 540–553. https://doi.org/10.1037/a0022082

Kivlighan, D. M., Jr., Gelso, C. J., Ain, S., Hummel, A. M., & Markin, R. D. (2015). The therapist, the client, and the real relationship: An actor–partner interdependence analysis of treatment outcome. *Journal of Counseling Psychology, 62*(2), 314–320. https://doi.org/10.1037/cou0000012

Kivlighan, D. M., Jr., Hill, C. E., Gelso, C. J., & Baumann, E. (2016). Working alliance, real relationship, session quality, and client improvement in psychodynamic psychotherapy: A longitudinal actor partner interdependence model. *Journal of Counseling Psychology, 63*(2), 149–161. https://doi.org/10.1037/cou0000134

Klein, M. H., Kolden, G. G., Michels, J. L., & Chisolm-Stockard, S. (2002). Congruence. In J. C. Norcross (Ed.), *Psychotherapy relationships that work: Therapist contributions and responsiveness to patients* (pp. 195–215). Oxford University Press.

Knox, S., Hess, S. A., Petersen, D. A., & Hill, C. E. (2001). A qualitative analysis of client perceptions of the effects of helpful therapist self-disclosure in long-term therapy. In C. E. Hill (Ed.), *Helping skills: The empirical foundation* (pp. 369–387). American Psychological Association. https://doi.org/10.1037/10412-022

Kolden, G. G., Klein, M. H., Wang, C.-C., & Austin, S. B. (2011). Congruence/genuineness. *Psychotherapy, 48*(1), 65–71. https://doi.org/10.1037/a0022064

Kolden, G. G., Wang, C.-C., Austin, S. B., Chang, Y., & Klein, M. H. (2018). Congruence/genuineness: A meta-analysis. *Psychotherapy, 55*(4), 424–433. https://doi.org/10.1037/pst0000162

Kolden, G. G., Wang, C. C., Austin, S. B., Chang, Y., & Klein, M. H. (2019). Congruence/genuineness. In J. C. Norcross & M. J. Lambert (Eds.), *Psychotherapy relationships that work: Evidence-based therapist contributions*, 3rd ed. (pp. 323–350). Oxford University Press.

Lambert, M. J. (1992). Psychotherapy outcome research: Implications for integrative and eclectical therapists. In J. C. Norcross & M. R. Goldfried (Eds.), *Handbook of psychotherapy integration* (pp. 94–129). Basic Books.

Levitt, H. M., Hamburger, A., Hill, C. E., McLeod, J., Pascual-Leone, A., Timulak, L., Buccholz, M., Frommer, J., Fuertes, J., Iwakabe, S., Martínez, C., Morrill, Z., Knox, S., Langer, P., Muran, J. C., Weie Oddli, H., Řiháček, T., Tomicic, A., & Tuval-Mashiach, R. (2024). Broadening the evidentiary basis for clinical guidance: Recommendations from qualitative psychotherapy researchers. *American Psychologist*. Advance online publication. https://doi.org/10.1037/amp0001363

Levitt, H. M., Morrill, Z., & Collins, K. M. (2020). Considering methodological integrity in counselling and psychotherapy research. *Counselling & Psychotherapy Research, 20*(3), 422–428. https://doi.org/10.1002/capr.12284

Levitt, H. M., Pomerville, A., & Surace, F. I. (2016). A qualitative meta-analysis examining clients' experiences of psychotherapy: A new agenda. *Psychological Bulletin, 142*(8), 801–830. https://doi.org/10.1037/bul0000079

Lo Coco, G., Gullo, S., Prestano, C., & Gelso, C. J. (2011). Relation of the real relationship and the working alliance to the outcome of brief psychotherapy. *Psychotherapy, 48*(4), 359–367. https://doi.org/10.1037/a0022426

Marmarosh, C. L., Gelso, C. J., Markin, R. D., Majors, R., Mallery, C., & Choi, J. (2009). The real relationship in psychotherapy: Relationships to adult attachments, working alliance, transference, and therapy outcome. *Journal of Counseling Psychology, 56*(3), 337–350. https://doi.org/10.1037/a0015169

McConnaughy, E. A. (1987). The person of the therapist in psychotherapeutic practice. *Psychotherapy, 24*(3), 303–314. https://doi.org/10.1037/h0085720

Moore, S. R., & Gelso, C. J. (2011). Recollections of a secure base in psychotherapy: Considerations of the real relationship. *Psychotherapy, 48*(4), 368–373. https://doi.org/10.1037/a0022421

Morrill, Z. (2021). *Power dynamics in psychotherapy: Eminent therapists' experiences navigating power from humanistic–existential and feminist–multicultural perspectives* [Unpublished doctoral dissertation]. University of Massachusetts Boston.

Morrill, Z., & Levitt, H. M. (2021). *Power dynamics in psychotherapy: Navigating power from humanistic-existential and feminist-multicultural perspectives* [Manuscript submitted for publication]. Department of Counseling and School Psychology, University of Massachusetts Boston.

Morrill, Z., & Luiggi-Hernández, J. G. (2026). Branches of humanistic and existential psychology. In L. Hoffman (Ed.), *APA handbook of humanistic and existential psychology: Vol. 1. History, research, philosophy, and theory* (pp. 47–70). American Psychological Association. https://doi.org/10.1037/000431-002

Nietzsche, F. (1967). *The will to power* (W. Kaufman & R. J. Hollingdale, Trans.). Random House.

Norcross, J. C., & Lambert, M. J. (2018). Psychotherapy relationships that work III. *Psychotherapy, 55*(4), 303–315. https://doi.org/10.1037/pst0000193

Owen, J. J., Tao, K., Leach, M. M., & Rodolfa, E. (2011). Clients' perceptions of their psychotherapists' multicultural orientation. *Psychotherapy, 48*(3), 274–282. https://doi.org/10.1037/a0022065

Patterson, C. H. (1984). Empathy, warmth, and genuineness in psychotherapy: A review of reviews. *Psychotherapy, 21*(4), 431–438. https://doi.org/10.1037/h0085985

Rogers, C. R. (1951). *Client-centered therapy*. Houghton Mifflin.

Rogers, C. R. (1957). The necessary and sufficient conditions of therapeutic personality change. *Journal of Consulting Psychology, 21*(2), 95–103. https://doi.org/10.1037/h0045357

Rogers, C. R. (1959). A theory of therapy, personality, and interpersonal relationships as developed in the client-centered framework. In S. Koch (Ed.), *Psychology: A study of a science: Vol. 3. Formulations of the person and the social context* (pp. 184–256). McGraw-Hill.

Rogers, C. R. (1962). The interpersonal relationship: The core of guidance. *Harvard Educational Review, 32*, 416–429.

Sartre, J. (1943). *Being and nothingness* (H. E. Barnes, Trans.). Routledge.

Schneider, K. J. (Ed.). (2008). *Existential integrative psychotherapy: Guideposts to the core of practice*. Routledge.

Schneider, K. J. (2023). *Life-enhancing anxiety: Key to a sane world*. University Professors Press.

Schnellbacher, J., & Leijssen, M. (2009). The significance of therapist genuineness from the client's perspective. *Journal of Humanistic Psychology, 49*(2), 207–228. https://doi.org/10.1177/0022167808323601

Thompson, M. (2004). Nietzsche and psychoanalysis: The fate of authenticity in a postmodernist world. *Existential Analysis, 15*, 203–217.

van Hees, M. L., Rotter, T., Ellermann, T., & Evers, S. M. (2013). The effectiveness of individual interpersonal psychotherapy as a treatment for major depressive disorder in adult outpatients: A systematic review. *BMC Psychiatry, 13*(1), 22. https://doi.org/10.1186/1471-244X-13-22

Wampold, B. E. (2009). Research evidence for the common factors models: A historically situated perspective. In B. L. Duncan, S. D. Miller, B. E. Wampold, & M. A. Hubble (Eds.), *The heart and soul of change: Delivering what works in therapy* (2nd ed., pp. 49–81). American Psychological Association.

Wampold, B. E. (2021). Healing in a social context: The importance of clinician and patient relationship. *Frontiers in Pain Research, 2*, 684768. https://doi.org/10.3389/fpain.2021.684768

Wampold, B. E., & Budge, S. L. (2012). The 2011 Leona Tyler Award address: The relationship—And its relationship to the common and specific factors of psychotherapy. *The Counseling Psychologist, 40*(4), 601–623. https://doi.org/10.1177/0011000011432709

Wampold, B. E., & Imel, Z. E. (2015). *The great psychotherapy debate: The evidence for what makes psychotherapy work*. Routledge. https://doi.org/10.4324/9780203582015

Worth, P., & Proctor, C. (2020). Congruence/incongruence (Rogers). In V. Zeigler-Hill & T. K. Shackelford (Eds.), *Encyclopedia of Personality and Individual Differences* (pp. 838–840). Springer. https://doi.org/10.1007/978-3-319-24612-3_1460

Wyatt, G. (2001). The multifaceted nature of congruence within the therapeutic relationship. In G. Wyatt (Ed.), *Rogers' therapeutic conditions: Evolution, theory and practice* (pp. 79–95). PCCS Books.

Yalom, I. (2002). *The gift of therapy. An open letter to a new generation of therapists and their patients*. Harper Collins.

12

Therapist Self-Disclosure in Existential–Humanistic Psychotherapy

Derrick Sebree Jr., and Vanessa Brown

Self-disclosure has historically been thought of as a risky endeavor for a therapist to engage in. Freud wrote, "The physician should be impenetrable to the patient, and like a mirror, reflect nothing but what is shown to him [*sic*]" (1912, as cited in Peterson, 2002, p. 21). Thus, self-disclosure remained in a negative light until the civil rights movement and the third force of behavioral science, existential–humanistic (EH) psychology. Interestingly, Freud was known to share personal details with his patients, demonstrating that even blank-slate therapists still saw the value in building an authentic relationship with the client (Farber, 2006). Yet EH therapists remain more likely to self-disclose than psychoanalytic therapists (Farber, 2006).

Early humanistic psychologist Sidney Jourard (1959) introduced the term "self-disclosure" to psychological discourse during a time when many other EH therapists were talking about similar concepts (e.g., transparency, genuineness, congruence, authenticity). As Farber (2006) notes, Jourard and the EH therapists intended self-disclosure to be a process of connection and identity exploration, "We trust, we disclose, we are disclosed to, we feel closer to another, we open ourselves up more to explore self and other" (pp. 12–13), which develops an I-thou relationship as Buber describes it. On the heels of EH theorists, feminist therapists advocated for the explicit use of self-disclosure as a means of reducing power dynamics (Danzer & Andresen, 2019a), noting in the power differentials subsection of the *Feminist Therapy Institute Code of Ethics* that "a feminist therapist discloses information to the client that facilitates the therapeutic process, including information communicated to others. The therapist is responsible for using

https://doi.org/10.1037/0000446-013
The Evidence-Based Foundations of Existential–Humanistic Therapy, L. Hoffman and V. Lac (Editors)

self-disclosure only with purpose and discretion and in the interest of the client" (Feminist Therapy Institute, 1999, p. 4). It can be argued that Indigenous and Black American healing professionals were long practicing these tenets based on a foundation of community, collective trauma, and shared meaning (Watkins & Shulman, 2008). Despite the longstanding use of self-disclosure to foster connection and exploration, the negative connotations about self-disclosure that were established in the early 1900s remain. Therapists continue to be warned that self-disclosure is an ethical misstep that blurs therapeutic boundaries, even though studies indicate that up to 90% of therapists acknowledge "intentionally disclosing to clients at least some of the time" (Danzer, 2019). From an ethical standpoint, beneficence can easily be argued based on evidence that therapist self-disclosure "conveys the humanity of the therapist, helps to develop rapport with clients, and permits a level of authenticity that may contribute to the formation of a positive relationship, roundly understood to be central to therapeutic healing and growth" (Danzer, 2019, p. 9).

In EH circles, appropriate self-disclosure has long been understood as the basis for developing the qualities between therapist and client necessary for a positive therapeutic outcome. In Rogers's (1961) assessment of behavioral therapies, he notes that the therapist's goal was to identify problematic behaviors, explore the reason for the behavior, and provide reeducation on more adaptive behaviors all whilst aiming to be impersonal: to withhold one's personal self from the therapy in hopes of emphasizing only the client's behavior change. Rogers (1961) notes that clients who underwent this method of therapy often ended up worse off than clients who had no therapy. Upon further examination, it was found that clients who underwent client-centered therapy (which focuses more on the benefits of self-disclosure) had "the greatest amount of positive change . . . with lasting improvement" (p. 47). These findings have remained steady over the years (Wampold, 2015), as we will discuss further on in this chapter. The following section details a case example that demonstrates the efficacy of therapist self-disclosure in the case of a client with anxiety.

CASE EXAMPLE

Liam was a 29-year-old Black American male presenting to therapy with anxiety occurring at the onset of becoming a father.[1] He initiated therapy with Dr. Hill, a White American female specializing in EH interventions.

Liam was nervous to share with Dr. Hill his concerns about parenting. He felt ashamed of not knowing how to calm his infant daughter and resenting her for the sleepless nights. He assumed that his therapist would judge him for not having the answers. Dr. Hill could sense the relational distance and said in a humorous tone, "I remember when my son was that age, and I was ready to

---

[1]The case of Liam has been modified to disguise the client's identity and protect their confidentiality.

lock him away just so I could sleep! How are you doing?" This shared experience between therapist and client allowed an opportunity for Liam to feel jointly human. The energy shifted and Liam chuckled, "Yeah, I basically don't know what I'm doing." Matching his laughter, Dr. Hill related, "None of us do, I was so lost . . . and still am with mine being 15 now!" Opening the dialogue further, Liam shared a story about being so tired that he fell asleep while holding his daughter. He shared the self-deprecating statements and worst-case scenarios that raced through his mind. Knowing that an important intervention in relieving parenting anxiety is to connect with other parents about expectations, Dr. Hill shared that many of those thoughts had run through her mind as well. Her willingness to be transparent about her own anxieties surrounding parenthood provided an opportunity to bridge into potential interventions that might offer relief to Liam.

DEFINING SELF-DISCLOSURE

Self-disclosure in the clinical realm was initially understood as "any reference to self" by the therapist but has come to be understood as a set of specific interventions involving the therapist strategically sharing personal information (Hill et al., 2018, p. 446). While a client can gather significant personal information from nonverbal statements such as a therapist's wedding ring, choice of books, family photos, or inclusive insignia, *therapist self-disclosure* (TSD) encapsulates intentional statements by the therapist that share personal information about the therapist's life and experience (Danzer, 2019; Hill & Knox, 2001; Hill et al., 2018; Ziv-Beiman & Shahar, 2016). TSDs are often in regard to the therapist's experience outside of the therapy room, such as sharing a personal experience with the proposed intervention or revealing that the therapist has a shared trait in common with the client. Therapist self-disclosure often pertains to the therapist's personal experiences, values, and struggles. When reflecting on a client's review of posting on social media about their sexual assault, a therapist might disclose by saying, "So many of us have MeToo stories. I think getting to see that we aren't alone is the part I've experienced as most healing." This statement reveals a shared experience that can lead to a deeper level of relational connection and rapport. It also raises potential interventions and coping strategies (e.g., relational empathy and interpersonal support), which can be built on in therapeutic work.

This is in contrast to self-disclosure about the therapist's experience of the therapy session, referred to as *immediacy* or *self-involving* responses (see also Chapter 9 of this volume). Immediacy can be defined as the therapist's process of disclosing their personal feelings, thoughts, or experiences about the client, the therapy process, or the therapeutic relationship (Hill, 2020; Mayotte-Blum et al., 2012; Ziv-Beiman et al., 2017). For example, during a session in which a typically reserved client is sharing more openly, a therapist might reveal "I find myself really enjoying this session today. I normally am so curious about what you might be holding back, but I don't want to push you to open up, either. I've really appreciated hearing more from you." In this particular example, the disclosure models emotional sharing and transparency while also reinforcing the potential growth that has occurred in the session.

Therapist self-disclosure and immediacy are not always used as a means of connecting with a client but can also feel disconnecting and still remain effective in their use. Take the example of a cisgender heterosexual therapist trying to convey understanding of a gay client's reference to their coming out experience. Rather than using reflective statements or making an attempt at empathy (thus lacking cultural empathy), it could prove beneficial for the therapist to acknowledge the cultural differences in their experiences. As Comas-Diaz (2016) notes, "culturally competent clinicians subscribe to a position of 'knowing they do not know'" (p. 164). The therapist might disclose, "As a straight person, I'm realizing it's a privileged position for me not to know what coming out is like. If you're up to it, I want to hear more about your experience of that." In this example, there is a disclosure that highlights a difference or possible area of misunderstanding, possibly even uncovering the therapist's potential to be an oppressor (or at the very least, certainly possessing a privileged status that the client does not hold). If the therapist finds it appropriate, they might even bring these components into their work with the client. Without this disclosure acknowledging individual differences, the therapist increases the chance of causing harm based on cultural influence that biases even empathic responses (Hoffman et al., 2019).

CONTEXTUALIZING SELF-DISCLOSURE IN AN EH CONTEXT

Therapist self-disclosure and immediacy have long been understood within the EH and person-centered orientations as basic tenets of an effective therapeutic relationship, yet under different terminology. Truax and Carkhuff (1965) cite numerous authors—including Rogers (1957), Jourard (1959), Snyder & Snyder (1961), and many others—who focused on the importance of therapist transparency and congruence (or genuineness; see also Chapter 11 of this volume). From an EH perspective, transparency is the therapist's willingness to allow the client to get to know the therapist as a person (Lietaer, 1993). While this often involves therapist self-disclosure and immediacy, it is also experienced in the therapist's unique personality, mannerisms, and way of relating to the client. Yalom distinguishes between professional and personal transparency. Professional transparency reveals the therapist's process of therapy, such as what guides the chosen intervention (Berman, 2019). A professional transparency might include "I am noticing your shoulders are tense. Let's breathe into that area." Personal transparency is a sharing of the therapist's experience, such as "I feel like the energy just got sucked from the room." Yalom asserts that therapist transparency serves to build a more accurate representation of the therapist so as to minimize transference and also to serve as a model for interpersonal sharing (Berman, 2019). "How can we as therapists expect transparency in clients when we ourselves are not open and real in the relationship?" (Truax & Carkhuff, 1965). Transparency is the willingness of the therapist to be seen as a fellow human. Yet for effective transparency to occur, it requires a level of congruence.

Rogers (1961) coined the term congruence to mean that "the feelings the therapist is experiencing are available [and they are] able to communicate them if appropriate" (p. 61). A congruent therapist is "accessible, approachable, and sincere rather than obscured behind stereotypical roles or hidden behind protective facades" (Kolden et al., 2018, p. 425). Although congruence often involves self-disclosure, or transparency, the therapist must be self-aware and intentional for congruence to occur. Therefore, congruence involves an intra-personal element of mindfulness, awareness, and authenticity. Rather than being avoidant or fearful of openly sharing these personal experiences and dis-coveries, person-centered therapists with a high level of congruence embrace transparency through "curiosity about the encounter, a willingness to engage, and the capacity to reciprocally and respectfully share" (Kolden et al., 2018, p. 425). Rogers (1961) encourages therapist self-exploration, noting that thera-pists who are more aware of themselves can be more genuine in their relation-ships with clients. On the other hand, if a therapist is unable or unwilling to be genuine, the client may experience the therapist as fake, playing a role, or incongruent. Gendlin (1962) adds to the concept of congruence, noting the importance of congruence being an interpersonal process (self-disclosure) and for therapists to show their humanness even if that means not appearing in a good light. In short, "the more genuine and congruent the therapist in the rela-tionship, the more probability there is that change in the personality in the client will occur" (Rogers, 1961, p. 62).

Self-disclosure is foundational to the practice of EH therapy as a means of conveying congruence, genuineness, and transparency. Rather than justifying its use as what it serves in therapy (a transactional understanding), EH thera-pists understand qualities such as congruence, transparency, and genuineness to be the basis of authentic human relationships. Research has established that the therapeutic relationship is integral for therapeutic change (Wampold, 2015). Though there is risk of the therapist imposing on the client when self-disclosing, there is equal risk of failing to develop a close therapeutic rela-tionship when choosing not to self-disclose (Lietaer, 1993).

According to McCarthy Veach (2011), common reasons that therapists might decide to limit their use of self-disclosure include to

- avoid blurring boundaries,

- stay focused on client,

- prevent concern about clinician welfare,

- prevent merging,

- prevent premature closure,

- avoid information overload and confusion,

- prevent client feeling burdened by clinician problems,

- avoid interfering with transference,

- prevent client demoralization by clinician successes or failures,

- avoid giving client information to manipulate clinician, and

- avoid clinician discomfort. (p. 352)

Yet many of these can be avoided with appropriate and effective self-disclosure, and other reasons in this list reflect elements of behavioral and psychodynamic approaches (such as transference interference and staying focused on the client). However, it is not without risk; all aspects of treatment and relationship involve potential benefits and risks. In reflecting on the risks and benefits of congruence and transparency, Rogers writes,

> Since this concept is liable to misunderstanding, let me state that it does not mean that the therapist burdens his [sic] client with overt expression of all his feelings. Nor does it mean that the therapist discloses his total self to his client. It does mean, however, that the therapist denies to himself none of the feelings he is experiencing and that he is willing to experience transparently any persistent feelings that exist in the relationship and to let these be known to his client. (1966, as cited in Lietaer, 1993, p. 17)

Weiner (1978) notes that self-disclosure in the context of EH therapy aims to reduce client objectification through choosing an I-thou relationship rather than an I-it relationship. Buber (1923/1958) contends that an I-thou relationship occurs when one participates as a whole self, though this is a fleeting occurrence. While self-disclosure can be an integral part of working toward the I-thou relationship with a client, therapists also risk manipulative self-disclosure, which would then establish an I-it objectified relationship instead (Weiner, 1978). An example might be a therapist disclosing how helpful antidepressant medication has been to the therapist in an attempt to manipulate the client to seek psychiatric care. Instead, this reiterates the client as an object in the relationship (a "consumer" as community mental health organizations often say), which creates distance in the relationship. When professionals view clients as objects, there is a risk of dehumanization. Within an EH context, therapists examine the being-in-relationship and might employ self-disclosure to add depth and genuineness. Self-reflection is a core intervention of EH psychotherapy. Consideration for best practices must include aspects such as appropriate timing and identifying the goal of the therapist self-disclosure. As part of best practices, contemporary research data demonstrate support for the use of therapist self-disclosure.

RESEARCH ON SELF-DISCLOSURE

Research on therapist use of self-disclosure has continued to grow, both from quantitative and qualitative methodologies. As an EH clinical practitioner, remaining present and making use of process comments in a here-and-now context corresponds to the use of immediacy within therapy. Therapist self-disclosures can serve to deepen the therapeutic relationship. In this section, contemporary research on therapist self-disclosure and immediacy is reviewed.

Quantitative Research

Pinto-Coelho and colleagues (2016) note that there is a growing body of naturalistic therapy studies revealing that the positive aspects of TSD outweigh the negative. Quantitative measures consisting of random clinical trials, multi-modal analysis, mixed methods designs, and analysis of variance designs have been utilized to conduct detailed research on the impacts of TSD on therapeutic processes and outcomes (Levitt et al., 2016; Pinto-Coelho et al., 2016; Ziv-Beiman et al., 2017). In a meta-analysis of 53 quantitative studies, Henretty and colleagues (2014) found that overall self-disclosure has a favorable impact on clients. When examining various quantitative studies, a deeper understanding of this impact can be gained.

In Levitt and colleagues' (2016) study, a collection of 52 recordings of therapist–client dyads were coded for instances of self-disclosure, type of self-disclosure, and treatment outcome. They found that most therapists self-disclosed at some point during the work and that the type of therapist self-disclosure mediated treatment outcome. Specifically, it was discovered that therapists self-disclosed with a variety of goals in mind: encouragement, treatment direction, care, humanizing, empathy, therapy mechanics, and relationship repairs. However, disclosures that were asides to the therapy discourse (i.e., personal opinions or experiences not at all related to the therapy content), that conveyed similarity to the client, were neutral (rather than conveying positive or negative emotionality), and those that humanized the therapist were found to be correlated to a decrease in clinical symptoms or depression and anxiety. Additionally, the researchers found that interpersonal problems (such as relational conflict and feelings of loneliness) improved the most with disclosures that were either neutral or positive and conveyed similarity to the client.

Barrett and Berman (2001) surveyed 36 clients across 18 therapists regarding the effects of increasing and decreasing therapist disclosure on therapy outcomes. In the increasing self-disclosure group, therapists were provided reasons to support the use of self-disclosure in therapy and given instruction on how to do so. In the decreasing self-disclosure group, therapists were provided arguments against the use of self-disclosure in treatment and instructed to restrict self-disclosure and maintain the focus on the client. Client symptoms were measured using the Hopkins Symptom Checklist before the initiation of treatment and then subsequently after each session. Sessions were recorded and observed for frequency of self-disclosure. An analysis of the data found that "clients in the increased disclosure condition reported less symptom distress and indicated that they liked their therapist more" (p. 601). It was also noted that even when told to increase self-disclosure, therapists disclosed infrequently and briefly, where "the mean number of therapist self-disclosures in the increased disclosure condition was less than 5 per therapy session, and these disclosures averaged less than 15 s [seconds] in length" (p. 602). The brief nature of self-disclosures was also supported by other studies.

Pinto-Coelho and colleagues (2016) reviewed 185 therapist self-disclosure events (immediacy instances were not included in the data set) and found verbal therapist self-disclosure to have a favorable impact on client's engagement and perception of the therapeutic and working alliance. Additionally, they found therapist self-disclosure to be brief in nature, averaging 11 seconds. This allowed the therapist to maintain the therapeutic frame and not shift the focus of the session to their disclosure. Less intimate disclosures, such as those regarding information about a therapist's education or professional background, were rated with lower client ratings of the therapeutic relationship. Meanwhile, disclosures of feeling and insight corresponded with higher client ratings of the therapeutic relationship. This further supports person-centered conditions such as authenticity, congruency, and transparency as being central thematic elements to the therapeutic relationship, and they are illuminated by continuing research.

Subsequent studies into TSD have undertaken empirical methods, such as the randomized clinical trial by Ziv-Beiman and colleagues (2017). The researchers randomly divided 86 clients experiencing mild to moderate distress among 22 therapists. Therapists were told the intent of the study was to examine the effect of therapeutic skill on outcome and were assigned to one of four treatment conditions:

- training and told to use immediacy (i.e., to share feelings about the patient, therapy, or relationship),

- training and told to use TSD (i.e., to share personal details about the therapist's life),

- training and told not to self-disclose, and

- no training and told to not self-disclose.

During the training portion, therapist participants were informed about brief psychotherapy and Hill and Knox's (2009) psychotherapy model of exploration, insight, and action. Therapist participants were asked to use techniques based on Hill's work, such as approval and reassurance, closed and open questions, restatements, reflection of feelings, challenges, interpretations, information, and direct guidance. Client participants completed a symptom inventory prior to the start of the study and upon completion of 12 therapy sessions. This study represents the first ecologically valid study comparing two types of self-disclosure treatment to a non-self-disclosure modality. Individuals reporting distressing psychiatric symptoms prior to treatment reported a greater reduction postsession when immediacy was implemented via an integrative model (McCormic et al., 2019). Additionally, the clients and therapists viewed the therapists more favorably when the treatment included immediacy. The authors noted that a favorable view of the therapist could be a potential moderating variable, motivating the therapeutic process.

Jowers and colleagues (2019) conducted research on the impacts of trainee therapist personal traits on their use of immediacy and self-disclosure with clients. Their thoughts and feelings related to these sessions were then queried. A multitrait, multimethod approach allowed researchers to investigate an array of trainee characteristics across 33 Master of Science in Clinical Psychology students: "The volunteer patient group (n = 33) was 67% female, 39% European American, 36% African American, 15% Asian American, 6% Hispanic, and 3% other. The mean age of the group was 20.55 years (SD = 4.03)" (Jowers et al., 2019, p. 159). Trainees often reported utilizing self-disclosure to create a supportive environment. Most trainee self-disclosures were similar to disclosures of feeling (e.g., "I would feel this way in your shoes") or similarities (e.g., "I too have struggled with anxiety"). Of the trainees, 13 utilized immediacy in the first and second sessions, and the results were longer exchanges discussing deeper and more meaningful topics than when self-disclosure was used (Jowers et al., 2019).

Moderate levels of immediate disclosure, or disclosure relegated to the therapy here-and-now process, have been shown to be favorable by clients, trainees, and therapists compared with no immediate disclosures (Hill, 2020; Jowers et al., 2019; Kasper et al., 2008; Ziv-Beiman et al., 2017). The working relationship and the dynamic element of it are what EH theorists are intimately familiar with, rooted in the traditions of Rogers, Moustakas, Bugental, Buhler, and so forth. Next, this section will review qualitative inquiries on the impacts and roles of TSD and immediacy within psychotherapy.

Qualitative Research

The qualitative inquiries into the experiences of therapist self-disclosure and immediacy have been well-documented. Hill and colleagues (2018) conducted a meta-analysis of 21 studies with a total sample of 184 cases. The method for the qualitative meta-analysis involved a thematic process of bracketing the various findings from the selection of qualitative (and three quantitative) studies. The themes that emerged most often were

- enhanced therapy relationship,

- improved client mental functioning,

- client gained insight, and

- overall helpful for client.

Wasil and colleagues (2019) conducted a series of semistructured interviews with 13 clients diagnosed with eating disorders. Of the participants, 11 spontaneously reported that hearing recovery stories of their therapists' own eating disorder recovery positively impacted their motivation to recover. TSD and immediacy are both nuanced interventions that have the ability to invite relationship depth and openness of the therapeutic experience; however, TSD must also be used with caution (Fuertes et al., 2019; Hill et al., 2018; Jowers et al., 2019). Immediacy is largely seen by some scholars as an integral part of repairing and furthering the therapeutic relationship (Hill et al., 2018, 2019; Jowers et al., 2019).

Kasper and colleagues (2008) conducted a case study design employing qualitative and quantitative methods. Among a series of 12 sessions, the researchers found that when the therapist (Dr. N) utilized immediacy, the client (Lily) was immediate in her responses more often. The emergent themes of Dr. N's self-disclosures were that they

- drew parallels between external and therapy relationships;

- encouraged expression of immediate feelings;

- processed termination;

- felt disappointed, sad, or hurt;

- inquired about Lily's reactions;

- inquired about Dr. N's impact on Lily;

- expressed caring;

- felt close;

- wanted to connect; and

- felt proud.

During debriefing and reviewing of the psychotherapy experience with the client, further qualitative data were gathered (Kasper et al., 2008). The client noted that the frequent questions and inquiries related to immediacy were somewhat difficult to address at times:

> Hence, from these statements in the final session, Lily found immediacy helpful because it got her talking about relationship issues that she would not have otherwise discussed. On the other hand, Lily felt a little put off by the immediacy because she did not always understand the reason for it. She also indicated that immediacy was difficult and that she engaged in it mostly out of deference because it was expected of her. (Kasper et al., 2008, p. 292)

Kasper and colleagues (2008) found that the rate of the client's use of immediate statements was highest (79%) when preceded by therapist immediate disclosures; the numbers remained at 20% without therapist immediacy preceding the client immediacy. Dr. N used immediacy in most instances to help Lily draw parallels from the external world to the therapy relationship. For example, when Lily revealed fear about connecting to people, Dr. N asked, "How might that happen here?" When Lily attempted to return to external events, Dr. N brought them back to the immediate moment to reflect on the therapeutic relationship. Although the data collected from this case study indicated that the client's symptoms became worse between pretreatment and posttreatment in terms of clinical distress, the client self-reported an improved understanding of self. In postsession debriefings, the client indicated that she often applied things learned in therapy to other relationships. Immediacy continues to have a growing body of research, often involving mixed-methods research, much like TSD.

Hill and colleagues (2008) conducted a 17-session case study of brief psychotherapy with a 20-year-old Black American woman who identified as part of the lesbian, gay, bisexual, transgender, and queer (LGBTQ+) community. The therapist (Dr. W) identified as a 55-year-old heterosexual White male. Dr. W reported identifying first with psychodynamic theory followed by humanistic theory. With a humanistic–psychodynamic frame of therapy, Dr. W reported that he felt the therapeutic relationship was genuine. The judges rated 56 immediacy events through the course of the brief therapy. The most frequent types of immediacy were the following (Hill et al., 2008):

- reinforcing the client for in-session behavior,

- encouraging the client to collaborate,

- inquiring about the client's reactions to therapy, and

- reminding the client that it was okay to disagree.

The use of immediacy in a psychotherapy encounter must also be with awareness of context and power dynamics within the room (Lee, 2014). As therapists, our context and bias are part of the self we bring to therapy authentically. In a follow-up case study, Hill and colleagues (2008) conducted a mixed-method analysis of 17 sessions. The three most emergent themes were that the therapist (a) reinforced the client for something she did in the session, (b) wanted to collaborate with client in working out her difficulties, and (c) inquired about client's reaction to therapy. Postsession analysis of content revealed that immediacy had four main impacts: (a) immediacy allowed the therapist and the client to negotiate their relationship and establish boundaries; (b) the therapist's expression of real caring—or in the EH perspective, empathy and genuineness—enabled the client to be genuine and authentic; (c) immediacy allowed for exploration of shame-based topics; and (d) immediacy provided the client with a corrective relational experience. The ability to be immediate or attend to the here-and-now process is an essential component of EH psychotherapy (see Chapter 9 of this volume). As EH practitioners, we must model to our clients how to address such challenges.

Not all studies found self-disclosure to be solely beneficial. Berg and colleagues (2016) interviewed 12 psychotherapists about their views on sharing personal experiences with clients. All but one of the participants indicated that they had self-disclosed with clients and most participants indicated that they self-disclosed in response to a client's story. For example, a therapist might reveal also coming from a dysfunctional family to normalize a client who shared about their own dysfunctional family. Many of the therapists provided examples of self-disclosure being instrumental in maintaining the therapeutic relationship, such as when a participant had ruptured the therapeutic relationship due to being distracted with a personal crisis. After the therapist shared the personal crisis, the client was able to understand that the distraction was a natural reaction and not about the client or their relationship. However, some therapists also provided examples of when self-disclosure was detrimental to the therapeutic work. This typically occurred when a therapist shared a negative emotional experience that was "too emotionally intense for the patient to handle" (p. 255). One therapist shared the wisdom that therapists should attend to the dosage or level of self-disclosure when choosing this as an intervention.

In EH therapy, the therapeutic relationship is the main vehicle of healing, meaning that there must be intent given to this here-and-now process of relating. Self-disclosure within this space is seen as essential to conveying therapist transparency to deepen the therapeutic encounter (Vinogradov & Yalom, 1990). Yalom refers to this as *therapist transparency*. For TSD, the use of the self as therapist to model and facilitate client exploration follows a different process (Hill et al., 2018, 2019). In the therapist's experience of the client, the client also experiences the therapist. It is our imperative as therapists to make sure that experience is authentic, genuine, and unconditional. Given that TSD is a nuanced intervention that involves a depth of engagement by the therapist and client, it is important to consider the cultural and interpersonal contexts and impacts of conducting these interventions, including when they are contraindicated.

MULTICULTURAL CONSIDERATIONS

Lee (2014) notes,

> In order to closely examine and make use of TSD in cross-cultural encounters, it is crucial to clarify how the therapist's personal, professional, or cultural values are disclosed and used in therapy and how the client responds to the therapist's explicit and implicit self-disclosure. (p. 21)

Therapist self-disclosure can be contraindicated when the therapist has little understanding of themselves as a sociocultural being in a therapeutic relationship where they hold a great deal of power. EH therapists must consider how others view their disclosure from that person's context (Hill et al., 2019). The use of immediacy is important as a conjunctive intervention, as the manifestation of the here-and-now process will require repairing in order to grow amidst cultural ruptures. Maintaining a position of curiosity and cultural humility are key when employing TSD and immediacy as interventions.

Calling attention to cultural processes, as depicted by intrapersonal and interpersonal phenomena, must be centered on the client and their context. The epistemological views of EH therapy can allow clients to grow into their potential; however, this requires the divestment of colonial, supremacist notions of therapist as expert:

> In order to make the multiple voices (within the client and/or between the client and therapist) synthesized and meaningful, it is crucial to take a position of "not knowing" and engage dialogues in openly exploring the process. . . . We observed a negative shift in the therapeutic relationship after the therapists' self-disclosure of culturally embedded ideas. (Lee, 2014, p. 22)

Cultural discourse is an integral aspect of EH therapy given the vastly specific cultural contexts that are intrinsic to human existence on this earth (Hoffman et al., 2019).

As Farber (2006) points out, there is a significant lack of culturally specific research pertaining to therapist self-disclosure, and much of the research includes White or European clients and therapists. A study of 444 undergraduate students who rated the Counselor Disclosure Scale after imagining their therapist's ethnic background found that when there is a mismatch in racial identity between therapist and client (i.e., if the therapist is Black and the client is White), "clients indicate a stronger preference for self-disclosure regarding the counselor's personal relationships and personal and professional successes and failures" (Cashwell et al., 2003 p. 198). In a study of 62 East Asian clients who rated the helpfulness of self-disclosures from a White American therapist with European ancestry, it was found that clients found it more helpful when the therapist disclosed strategies and insights rather than facts, approval, or feelings (Kim et al., 2003). While culturally specific studies regarding self-disclosure are limited, the data suggests that some clients may benefit more from certain types of self-disclosure. Rather than asking whether self-disclosure is helpful for clients of particular cultural backgrounds, therapists are encouraged to explore how self-disclosure looks different within the client's cultural context and modify the type and level of self-disclosure used within therapy.

A population that has undergone considerable research related to TSD is the LGBTQ+ community. Specifically, as clients discuss and navigate their own coming out process, therapist self-disclosure can moderate a sense of visibility surrounding sexual orientation and gender identity (Gibson, 2012). Where race and gender expression might be nonexplicit forms of self-disclosure gathered through visual data, issues of sexuality are often considered taboo for therapists to disclose in the context of a professional relationship. Therapists who identify with the LGBTQ+ community take inherent risks based on sociocultural norms. For example, a therapist using she/her pronouns and the term "wife" to describe her spouse is coming out to her client. Gibson (2012) notes that such self-disclosures are often viewed as too much or are sexualized where straight therapists discussing their partners would not experience similar pushback or risk.

Another consideration is when therapist self-disclosure has the ability to harm the client–therapist relationship, such as when a therapist shares about their own religious identity (or lack thereof) without first assessing the impact on the client. Magaldi and Trub (2018) conducted a qualitative study consisting of semistructured interviews. The researchers discovered that in some cultural contexts involving disclosure of religion or spirituality by therapists to participants, therapists chose to not self-disclose in service of the client while others noted personal discomfort (Magaldi & Trub, 2018). In these 21 interviews, therapists often noted their own uneasiness towards discussing spiritual, religious, or non-religious culture. Rather, therapists were more likely to lead a conversation toward avoidance; systemic influences; implicit or explicit disclosure of one's spiritual, religious, or nonreligious culture; or focus on race and ethnicity. In this context, the therapist is unwelcoming of the client's interest in spiritual, religious, or nonreligious dialogue. These represent situations of leading, where the therapist guides the client in therapy. From the EH perspective, the client's ability to navigate their own growth is crucial. Much of the research regarding therapist self-disclosure and immediacy has yet to explore the contextual variances of the experience. It is evident that continued research on the impacts of therapist self-disclosure and immediacy from an EH perspective is needed.

FUTURE RESEARCH

Future research must elucidate the various processes that underlie therapist self-disclosure and immediacy. There is a critical need for further insight into how various forms of self-disclosure impact the therapeutic relationship in addition to how immediacy impacts common factors, such as the therapeutic relationship or working alliance. The various studies highlighted throughout this chapter employ a variety of practices, such as mixed-method studies. However, much of the research is within the discipline of psychodynamic theory and cognitive behavior therapy. Although a portion involves integrative therapy, there is little research from an EH perspective. The research that exists, highlighting the potential for depth and insight facilitated by therapist self-disclosure, would benefit from being expanded.

Additionally, there is a lack of population-specific research. For example, is self-disclosure as effective with a cisgender heterosexual White man as it is with a two-spirit Indigenous person? This is difficult to parse out because although studies collected demographic information regarding gender and ethnicity (but not sexual orientation), the data did not seem to be included in the analysis. More research is needed to understand the role self-disclosure might play in facilitating rapport and therapeutic outcome for identity-specific concerns. If a therapist comes out as gay to a gay client or if a White therapist reflects openly about having a Black son when a Black mother shares her fears about raising a Black son, will that self-disclosure increase rapport and does that translate to improved outcomes?

CONCLUSION

Self-disclosure and immediacy are both foundational to EH therapy because of their role in developing and deepening an authentic client–therapist relationship. Without authenticity, there is a risk of a loss of human connection and relationship that is necessary for therapeutic change to occur. This is especially true when therapists weigh the risks and benefits of self-disclosure. While it is important for the therapist to hold congruence within themselves, it is not always necessary to verbalize those thoughts to the client. Rather, self-disclosure is most effective when it is brief, relates to the client's context, and when the goal is to improve the therapeutic relationship. Additionally, to practice from a multicultural inclusive lens with the goal of operating from a person-centered and culturally specific praxis, it is necessary to identify self in relation to other. The therapist must have a willingness to bring their own identity into the room to understand how that identity influences the client. Self-disclosure and immediacy can help therapists and clients realize the genuine qualities of relating to another cultural being.

REFERENCES

Barrett, M. S., & Berman, J. S. (2001). Is psychotherapy more effective when therapists disclose information about themselves? *Journal of Consulting and Clinical Psychology, 69*(4), 597–603. https://doi.org/10.1037/0022-006X.69.4.597

Berg, H., Antonsen, P., & Binder, P. (2016). Sediments and vistas in the relational matrix of the unfolding "I": A qualitative study of therapists' experiences with self-disclosure in psychotherapy. *Journal of Psychotherapy Integration, 26*(3), 248–258. https://doi.org/10.1037/a0040051

Berman, J. (2019). *Writing the talking cure: Irvin D. Yalom and the literature of psychotherapy.* State University of New York Press. https://doi.org/10.1353/book65936

Buber, M. (1958). *I and thou* (R. G. Smith, Trans.; 2nd ed.). T & T. Clark Ltd. (Original work published 1923)

Cashwell, C. S., Shcherbakova, J., & Cashwell, T. H. (2003). Effect of client and counselor ethnicity on preference for counselor disclosure. *Journal of Counseling and Development, 81*(2), 196–201. https://doi.org/10.1002/j.1556-6678.2003.tb00242.x

Comas-Diaz, L. (2016). Multicultural therapy. In H. S. Friedman (Ed.), *Encyclopedia of mental health* (2nd ed., pp. 163–168). Academic Press. https://doi.org/10.1016/B978-0-12-397045-9.00184-1

Danzer, G. (2019). Introduction. In G. Danzer (Ed.), *Therapist self-disclosure: An evidence-based guide for practitioners* (pp. 3–8). Routledge.

Danzer, G., & Andresen, K. (2019a). The different types of self-disclosure. In G. Danzer (Ed.), *Therapist self-disclosure: An evidence-based guide for practitioners* (pp. 39–46). Routledge.

Danzer, G., & Andresen, K. (2019b). Theoretical and clinical perspectives. In G. Danzer (Ed.), *Therapist self-disclosure: An evidence-based guide for practitioners* (pp. 16–23. Routledge.

Farber, B. A. (2006). *Self-disclosure in psychotherapy.* Guilford Press.

Feminist Therapy Institute. (1999). *Feminist Therapy Institute code of ethics.*

Fuertes, J. N., Moore, M., & Ganley, J. (2019). Therapists' and clients' ratings of real relationship, attachment, therapist self-disclosure, and treatment progress. *Psychotherapy Research, 29*(5), 594–606. https://doi.org/10.1080/10503307.2018.1425929

Gendlin, E. T. (1962). Client-centered developments and work with schizophrenics. *Journal of Counseling Psychology, 9*(3), 205.

Gibson, M. F. (2012). Opening up: Therapist self-disclosure in theory, research, and practice. *Clinical Social Work Journal, 40*(3), 287–296. https://doi.org/10.1007/s10615-012-0391-4

Henretty, J. R., Currier, J. M., Berman, J. S., & Levitt, H. M. (2014). The impact of counselor self-disclosure on clients: A meta-analytic review of experimental and quasi-experimental research. *Journal of Counseling Psychology, 61*(2), 191–207. https://doi.org/10.1037/a0036189

Hill, C. E. (2020). *Helping skills: Facilitating exploration, insight, and action* (5th ed.). American Psychological Association. https://doi.org/10.1037/0000147-000

Hill, C. E., & Knox, S. (2001). Self-disclosure. *Psychotherapy: Theory, Research, Practice, Training, 38*(4), 413–417. https://doi.org/10.1037/0033-3204.38.4.413

Hill, C. E., & Knox, S. (2009). Processing the therapeutic relationship. *Psychotherapy Research, 19*(1), 13–29. https://doi.org/10.1080/10503300802621206

Hill, C. E., Knox, S., & Pinto-Coelho, K. (2018). Therapist self-disclosure and immediacy: A qualitative meta-analysis. *Psychotherapy, 55*(4), 445–460. https://doi.org/10.1037/pst0000182

Hill, C. E., Knox, S., & Pinto-Coelho, K. G. (2019). Self-disclosure and immediacy. In J. C. Norcross & M. J. Lambert (Eds.), *Psychotherapy relationships that work* (3rd ed., pp. 379–420). Oxford University Press. https://doi.org/10.1093/med-psych/9780190843953.003.0011

Hill, C. E., Sim, W., Spangler, P., Stahl, J., Sullivan, C., & Teyber, E. (2008). Therapist immediacy in brief psychotherapy: Case study II. *Psychotherapy, 45*(3), 298–315. https://doi.org/10.1037/a0013306

Hoffman, L., Cleare-Hoffman, H., Granger, N., Jr., & St. John, D. (Eds.). (2019). *Humanistic approaches to multiculturalism and diversity: Perspectives on existence and difference.* Routledge. https://doi.org/10.4324/9781351133357

Jourard, S. M. (1959). I–thou relationship versus manipulation in counseling and psychotherapy. *Journal of Individual Psychology, 15*(2), 174–179.

Jowers, C. E., Cain, L. A., Hoffman, Z. T., Perkey, H., Stein, M. B., Widner, S. C., & Slavin-Mulford, J. (2019). The relationship between trainee therapist traits with the use of self-disclosure and immediacy in psychotherapy. *Psychotherapy, 56*(2), 157–169. https://doi.org/10.1037/pst0000225

Kasper, L. B., Hill, C. E., & Kivlighan, D. M. (2008). Therapist immediacy in brief psychotherapy: Case study I. *Psychotherapy, 45*(3), 281–297. https://doi.org/10.1037/a0013305

Kim, B. S. K., Hill, C. E., Gelso, C. J., Goates, M. K., Asay, P. A., & Harbin, J. M. (2003). Counselor self-disclosure, East Asian American client adherence to Asian cultural values, and counseling process. *Journal of Counseling Psychology, 50*(3), 324–332. https://doi.org/10.1037/0022-0167.50.3.324

Kolden, G. G., Wang, C. C., Austin, S. B., Chang, Y., & Klein, M. H. (2018). Congruence/genuineness: A meta-analysis. *Psychotherapy, 55*(4), 424–433.

Lee, E. (2014). A therapist's self-disclosure and its impact on the therapy process in cross-cultural encounters: Disclosure of personal self, professional self, and/or cultural self? *Families in Society, 95*(1), 15–23. https://doi.org/10.1606/1044-3894.2014.95.3

Levitt, H. M., Minami, T., Greenspan, S. B., Puckett, J. A., Henretty, J. R., Reich, C. M., & Berman, J. S. (2016). How therapist self-disclosure relates to alliance and outcomes: A naturalistic study. *Counselling Psychology Quarterly, 29*(1), 7–28. https://doi.org/10.1080/09515070.2015.1090396

Lietaer, G. (1993). Authenticity, congruence and transparency. In D. Brazier (Ed.), *Beyond Carl Rogers* (pp. 17–46). Constable and Company.

Magaldi, D., & Trub, L. (2018). (What) do you believe?: Therapist spiritual/religious/non-religious self-disclosure. *Psychotherapy Research, 28*(3), 484–498. https://doi.org/10.1080/10503307.2016.1233365

Mayotte-Blum, J., Slavin-Mulford, J., Lehmann, M., Pesale, F., Becker-Matero, N., & Hilsenroth, M. (2012). Therapeutic immediacy across long-term psychodynamic psychotherapy: An evidence-based case study. *Journal of Counseling Psychology, 59*(1), 27–40.

McCarthy Veach, P. (2011). Reflections on the meaning of clinician self-reference: Are we speaking the same language? *Psychotherapy, 48*(4), 349–358.

McCormic, R. W., Pomerantz, A. M., Ro, E., & Segrist, D. J. (2019). The "me too" decision: An analog study of therapist self-disclosure of psychological problems. *Journal of Clinical Psychology, 75*(4), 794–800. https://doi.org/10.1002/jclp.22736

Peterson, Z. D. (2002). More than a mirror: The ethics of therapist self-disclosure. *Psychotherapy, 39*(1), 21–31. https://doi.org/10.1037/0033-3204.39.1.21

Pinto-Coelho, K. G., Hill, C. E., & Kivlighan, D. M., Jr. (2016). Therapist self-disclosure in psychodynamic psychotherapy: A mixed methods investigation [Retracted article]. *Counselling Psychology Quarterly, 29*(1), 29–52. https://doi.org/10.1080/09515070.2015.1072496

Rogers, C. R. (1957). The necessary and sufficient conditions of therapeutic personality change. *Journal of Consulting Psychology, 21*(2), 95–103.

Rogers, C. R. (1961). The process equation of psychotherapy. *American Journal of Psychotherapy, 15*(1), 27–45.

Snyder, W. U., & Snyder, B. J. (1961). The psychotherapy relationship. *The Journal of Nervous and Mental Disease, 133*(4), 355–356.

Truax, C. B., & Carkhuff, R. R. (1965). Client and therapist transparency in the psychotherapeutic encounter. *Journal of Counseling Psychology, 12*(1), 3–9. https://doi.org/10.1037/h0021928

Vinogradov, S., & Yalom, I. D. (1990). Self-disclosure in group psychotherapy. In G. Stricker & M. Fisher (Eds.), *Self-disclosure in the therapeutic relationship* (pp. 191–204). Springer. https://doi.org/10.1007/978-1-4899-3582-3_13

Wampold, B. E. (2015). How important are the common factors in psychotherapy? An update. *World Psychiatry, 14*(3), 270–277. https://doi.org/10.1002/wps.20238

Wasil, A., Venturo-Conerly, K., Shingleton, R., & Weisz, J. (2019). The motivating role of recovery self-disclosures from therapists and peers in eating disorder recovery: Perspectives of recovered women. *Psychotherapy, 56*(2), 170–180. https://doi.org/10.1037/pst0000214

Watkins, M., & Shulman, H. (2008). *Toward psychologies of liberation.* Palgrave Macmillan.

Weiner, J. L. (1978). On a problem of Chen, Willmore, et al. *Indiana University Mathematics Journal, 27*(1), 19–35.

Ziv-Beiman, S., Keinan, G., Livneh, E., Malone, P. S., & Shahar, G. (2017). Immediate therapist self-disclosure bolsters the effect of brief integrative psychotherapy on psychiatric symptoms and the perceptions of therapists: A randomized clinical trial. *Psychotherapy Research, 27*(5), 558–570. https://doi.org/10.1080/10503307.2016.1138334

Ziv-Beiman, S., & Shahar, G. (2016). Therapeutic self-disclosure in integrative psychotherapy: When is this a clinical error? *Psychotherapy, 53*(3), 273–277. https://doi.org/10.1037/pst0000077

13

The Self in Existential–Humanistic Psychotherapy

Anne Y. J. Hsu

The self is a subject matter that is both central yet paradoxically often conveniently assumed and neglected in general psychology. This is in part due to both its broad use in psychology and

> the totality of the individual, consisting of all characteristic attributes, conscious and unconscious, mental, and physical. Apart from its basic reference to personal identity, being, and experience, the term's use in psychology is wide-ranging. (American Psychological Association [APA], n.d.)

Psychology professor and poet Tom Greening, commenting on how psychologists have struggled to more narrowly define the self, writes, "We never seem to find ourselves agreeing on what it is that constitutes our Being [sic]" (n.d.).

An examination of the etymology of psychology, with its root word *psyche*, shows that this Greek word first showed up in Sanskrit as *babhasti*, meaning "to move," "to breathe," or "to blow" (Bradford, 2020). In Christianity, breath is humankind's source of life, first breathed into Adam by God. In Latin, *spirare* ("to breathe") is the root for the words "inspire," "aspire," and "expire." Similarly, in Asia, "breath" or "wind" is *chi* or *prana*. Relatedly, in Greek, "wind" is *anemos*, the basis for "anima," meaning motion or living. Meanwhile, in Sanskrit, "soul," or *atman*, entered European languages as *atmos*—like in "atmosphere." This consideration alludes to how existential–humanistic (EH) therapists may appreciate the self and not treat the psyche as a concrete, stable, patterned, individualistic, neuro-bio-chemical-physiological concept. Instead, EH therapists recognize the ontological nature of self as intertwined with one's context and potentiation.

https://doi.org/10.1037/0000446-014
The Evidence-Based Foundations of Existential–Humanistic Therapy, L. Hoffman and V. Lac (Editors)

This chapter presents shared viewpoints of the self and its applications in psychology and EH psychology. First, a discussion on epistemology and an overview of theoretical antecedents to EH psychology is necessary to compare general and clinical definitions of the self to EH therapy's definition of the self. Second, the ontological nature of the self is described in a contextualized EH case illustration. Third, some research on the self in EH context is highlighted. Critical multicultural considerations in EH therapy then follow. Finally, future research needs and recommendations are presented.

DEFINING THE SELF

A basic EBSCO search using the keyword "the self" in the title and "psychology research" or "psychotherapy studies" as the subject in peer reviewed articles yields a plethora of work, mostly with hyphenated titles like self-efficacy, self-esteem, self-regulation, and self-care, rather than the self as such. The abundant literature on hyphenated applied self-concepts is a product of treating general psychology as a science, thereby force-fitting concrete and measurable qualities to abstract, complex, and fluid constructs. The lack of empirical investigation of the self as such, or an assumption that the self is self-explanatory or even self-evident in the field of psychology, is the result of a mismatch between subject matter and epistemology: "According to Husserl, in our everyday practices and routines, we are in a certain attitude (he calls it 'the natural attitude') towards things toward the world, and somehow this is a state of self-forgetfulness" (Moran, 2018, p. 82). Unfortunately, if one begins with the environment and objectifies things, then one assumes the self and doesn't begin with an interrogation for clarification of what the self is. This has contributed to an absence of the self in our current day psychology as a discipline (Polkinghorne, 2015). Nevertheless, psychotherapists must work with the self, and EH therapists must participate in bringing the EH self to light. Thus, in this chapter, readers will find supporting research on the self to include hyphenated concepts that consider the self.

General psychologists share an overall attitude of treating psychology as a natural science, despite little reflection on its implications. They also tend to operate on the assumptions that the self is real and reducible, therefore definable in a stable, patterned, individualistic, neuro-bio-chemical-physiological manner (Bradford, 2020). Interestingly, neuroscience evidence supports EH therapy's position that the self as a concrete notion does not exist (Letheby & Gerrans, 2017). In addition, the implications of naming aspects of being or treating beings as mechanistic objects, though convenient, is problematic.

Unlike nonpractitioners, most psychotherapists do share some objections to treating psychology as a natural science, as what concerns them in therapy often eludes what researchers uncover in lab settings (Giorgi, 1970). Those who espouse EH views tend to critique this naturalistic and mechanistic understanding and treatment of the self as objectifying, dehumanizing, and inauthentic (Polkinghorne, 2015). Yet research on the self does have utility in communicating and understanding clients.

The Self in General Therapy

Personal growth is an umbrella concept that encompasses most of the positive hyphenated applied self-concepts used among psychotherapists. Self-efficacy, self-regulation, self-acceptance, and self-worth, among others, are often seen as the by-products or defining characteristics of personal growth. It also connotes better handling of whatever psychopathologies one experiences. Self-help books often focus on these terms. Likewise, clients enter therapy seeking to obtain self-growth. Correspondingly, as demonstrated in the literature, the consensus among the experts with different approaches was that they each viewed therapy as a process to facilitate a client's personal growth in some form (Aafjes-van Doorn et al., 2020). A review of later integrated therapies, such as motivational interviewing, mindfulness dialectical behavioral therapy, and acceptance and commitment therapy, seems to task the therapists with accessing the client's natural desire to grow. Therapy can then be understood as a deliberate journey efforted to become more congruent and authentic to one's purpose and values, thereby strengthening one's agency, autonomy, and acceptance. For therapists who engage in therapy regularly for self-growth, it is also assumed they will be able to enjoy better therapeutic effectiveness (Wilson et al., 2015, as cited in Aafjes-van Doorn et al., 2020).

Personal growth in this light resembles that of EH concepts of authenticity and self-actualization, though the emphasis on strengthening associated self-concepts and empowering clients differs from EH appreciation for Buddhist concepts of detachment and no-self (Bradford, 2021). An even greater distinction is how personal growth is not evaluated centrally on the improvement of diagnostic qualifiers because the focus was never on symptomology and symptom reduction. Instead, clients are viewed as growth potentials and treated via therapeutic relationships, the ultimate tool EH therapists use to facilitate clients' becoming and knowing oneself (Schneider, 2016).

EH Therapy's Definition of Self

An overview of the theoretical antecedents to EH therapy's definition of the self is presented here. The emergence of postmodernism and EH psychology as a human science lays the foundation. As there are many views of the self among different therapeutic modalities and within EH therapy's definition of self, Spinelli's (2005) reference to the three grand theories will be reviewed. Further, although various influences are acknowledged, emphasis is drawn to Martin Heidegger's being-in-the-world, the Eastern influence of Buddhism's sense of no-self, and American EH therapists' concepts of self. Note that although differences exist between humanistic psychology and existential psychology, as well as between European and American EH therapy, the aim in this chapter is to generally define EH therapy's conception of the self.

Both postmodernism and EH psychology embrace plurality, value diversity, and are skeptical of singular concepts and objective ways of knowing. Instead, through discourse, subjective representations of signifiers (or what positivism calls "reality") are called into question. Postmodernism posits that the self is socially constructed as a product of socio-cultural-political-economic influences whose representations take the form of narratives. A common postmodern view of the self is not one with the isolated characteristics of a singular, concrete, autonomous being (Hoffman et al., 2015; Sleeth, 2006, 2007). Rather, the self is a construction that occurs in relationships and contexts and is embedded in constructivism, contextualism, and perspectivism.

Relatedly, human science also embraces various approaches of research to understand beings in and of their worlds. Giorgi (1970) urges the importance of the development and maturity of psychology as a human science in a manner that recognizes natural science's inadequacy for psychology without relegating it to a topic that can only be approached through philosophy—thus creating the option of a middle ground. He suggests taking into consideration other social sciences while cautioning that the natural attitude of natural science must be bracketed. Further, Giorgi advocates for studying humans on a phenomenal level that utilizes presence, reflectivity, and relatedness between the phenomenon and the researcher, allowing for a truer exploration of beings' lived experiences, intentionality, and constructs within their human contexts.

EH therapy has historical foundations in phenomenology with variations in definition among EH psychologists. An overview of Spinelli's "Three Grand Theories" (2005) is provided here and compared with philosopher Zahavi's (2008) three concepts of the self. The first grand theory views "human beings as a subjectively distinct and separate being" (Spinelli, 2005, p. 305). This Cartesian view of the self is only accessible by the very individuals where the subject of experience is the self (Zahavi, 2008). The Western cultural notion of individuality aligns with this conception of the distinct constant identity. Put simply, "self" can be equated to "I" and "others" can be conceptualized as "you." General psychology and psychotherapy's definitions align with this and thus aim to strengthen the self by way of increasing ego strength, self-confidence, self-respect, self-worth, self-efficacy, self-regulation, self-care, and self-compassion while reducing self-harm, self-hate, and self-sabotage. Overall, the assumption appears to be that a stronger self is better and less pathological.

The second grand theory corresponds with Zahavi's (2008) hermeneutical self, and it embraces subjectivity and intersubjectivity (Spinelli, 2005). The identification of mirror neurons—a type of neural activity in one person when they observe another engaging in an action that would correspond with the same neural activity (Ferrari & Coudé, 2018; Trieu et al., 2019)—supports this view, which challenges individualism and argues that the self exists in "I and you." Many EH therapists align their definitions of self with this grand theory in that it is fluid and evolving. This is a narrative selfhood that stems from a

Latin word for identity, *ipse*, meaning the question of self-understanding and meaning. The process of questioning and understanding requires language to answer who one is. To behold oneself, the narrative self must engage the hermeneutic loop of perpetuating the parts and whole of investigating and making meaning through interpretation. The goal focuses on the development of self-awareness, self-understanding, personal myth, and personal significance.

The third grand theory corresponds with Zahavi's (2008) phenomenological self that considers relatedness, the inter-ness of beings, intersubjectivity, relational being, singular wholes, and interconnected parts (Spinelli, 2005). This phenomenological radical turn may be a foundation of EH therapy. This view rejects the individualistic perspective of the self but supplements the hermeneutical self, as there needs to be an integratedness to the hermeneutical elements. By doing so, a more holistic view is available. The integratedness or relatedness can be better explained by tracing it to Husserl's concept of life-world and Heidegger's being-in-the-world (Zahavi, 2008). Both refer to the condition of an interconnected, unitary, dynamic phenomenon that links the observer and the observed experience. This entails a nonfragmented worldview, as the connectivity is inseparable and there are no finite boundaries between the being and the world. Ashworth (2003) breaks down the contingencies of Husserl's life-world into fractions: selfhood, sociality, embodiment, spatiality, temporality, and project or intentionality. Existence then is concurrently a dynamic, temporal, becoming process of being and the world. This theory of self also concerns a self-development or evolvement through self-in-the-world awareness and engagement.

Heidegger's (2007) Dasein and being-in-the-world is one of the most influential European theoretical foundations of existential psychology's understanding of self and selfhood. Dasein literally translates to "being there" or "existence"; its Chinese translation is "herein" (此在) or "here-being." In roll call, one would respond in Chinese with "being" (在) when referring to physical presence; likewise, when engaging in something, 在 denotes a present verb tense. As such, it does not merely have a temporal quality but also a spatial one. Dasein thus is the being who already presents openness to engage in various modes of being. As a self, Dasein holds a sense of being as an identity, one that is embedded in a curious, dynamic, transcendental, nonlinear, temporal–spatial, coconstitutional world. The practice involves distinguishing between they, or the one-self, and I, the authentic self. It also involves navigating the tension between the one-self and the authentic self through integrating the two, coexisting among the two, or continuously teasing out the social, cultural, economic, and political influences of they-self. In practice, Husserl's phenomenology serves the primary task of apprehending lived experiences in subjective and intersubjective contexts for one in the process of EH therapy (Churchill & Wertz, 2015).

It is unclear how much Eastern influence Zen Buddhism had on Heidegger, but Buddhism's concept of the self, or rather no-self, bears resemblance to the openness Dasein presents in the world. Buddhist psychology is based on Siddhartha Gautama's enlightened experience after long periods of nonverbal meditation practice. The teaching can be accessed through Yogacara or Vijnana-vada (Mosig, 2006). The Buddhist path to enlightenment is a Dao (i.e., a philosophy, way of knowing, or understanding) to see through the illusions in life and arrive at the truth or as-it-is-ness. The illusions in life include that of believing that the self is a real entity, thus leading to seeds of suffering in the form of ego, desire, attachment, and selfishness. Taken to a larger context, the pursuit of a self leads to individual, interpersonal, and global suffering and wrongdoing.

The self is illusory as a standalone entity, as it cannot exist without the interconnectedness, relatedness, and embeddedness of others and the world. Its true existence is fundamentally in a state of gestalt. Thus, its existential truth is that of impermanence. The world in which this no-self resides is opened through five essential, interconnected *skandhas*: form, feelings, perceptions, impulses, and consciousness (Mosig, 2006). The self, along with each of the aggregates, requires that of the others to exist—they are connected and birth the other. There is an Appalachian folk song where the lyrics whimsically and circularly begin with a tree in the woods in the ground with grass all around and progressively add each of the elements: limb, branch, nest, egg, and bird. It ends with the bird in the egg, in the nest, on the branch, on the limb, on the tree, in the ground with green grass all around. Indeed, what is a tree without limbs and branches? To dissolve the illusion of the self paradoxically also expands oneself as one becomes enlightened to the true nature of boundaries, leading to compassion for one and all.

Schneider's (1999) paradoxical principle of constriction and expansion as the nature within oneself is focused on a process of opening and closing, centering, and facing or confronting. The paradoxical self offers a framework from which to view human conditions. Dread for one tension or tendency may lead to dysfunction, whereas confrontation of the dread may facilitate centering and well-being. In this view, the self is a process, and its paradoxical pulls are also embedded in a process. When one can reach the extent of great expansion and at the same time behold focus and acuity, one reaches a higher stage of consciousness involving the integration of one's subjective and objective self (May, 1958). Bugental (1978) also concurs in treating the I-concept as a possibility and process and therapy as a growth process embedded in transitoriness and nothingness. This way of working with the self evokes dread among other existential limitations and calls on courage and confrontations to assist the process of the tendency for growth, authenticity, or actualization (Polkinghorne, 2015). In summary, EH therapy's conception of the self is a fluid, relational, dialectical, hermeneutical, transcendental, experiential process that is embedded, coconstituted, and inseparable from other individuals, processes, and contexts.

SITUATING THE SELF IN AN EH CONTEXT

Rollo May (1953, 1981) synthesized the existential or *ex-stere* (Latin; to become) and the Greek origin of humanism (knowing thyself) in EH therapy to a process of freeing clients from the dialectics of their existential givens in the world through facilitating clients' "knowing and becoming oneself" (Schneider & Krug, 2017). This section concerns how the self is understood and used in EH therapy. First, I delineate how, as a therapist providing the context of therapy, I create a world and show up to the sessions with my presence, clearing, or being-in-the-world to clients (Amari, 2021). Then, through a de-identified case illustration, I will elaborate on how the self is understood and used in EH therapy.

As an EH therapist, I serve as the first point of using the self for the therapeutic relationship. I, a being-in-the-world—with my lived experiences as a cisgender female immigrant of color with history, life choices, and practice preferences—already present in a non–blank slate context to clients. My sociocultural, political, and economic influences give away my world. Likewise, my accent, voice, choice of words, and use of tone also indirectly elicit different reactions or give different impressions to clients. As therapeutic relationships develop and I become more transparent with clients (Amari, 2021; Friedman, 2015), I become a part of my clients' worlds. This phenomenon is paved partially by relational depth, where a bidirectional self-expansion takes place (Cooper, 2012). Therapists and clients contribute to one another's worlds, and these influences flow into contexts beyond that of the therapy setting (Friedman, 2015). This is the nature of the process of a being-in-the-world interacting with another being-in-the-world on an intimate and regular, trusting basis (Buber, 1990). In particular, the work or the responsibility of an EH therapist involves actively using themselves as clearings for clients, thereby serving as a therapy tool in actively making clients aware of their present patterns.

A case illustration can help illuminate some of these points. Hue Juan is a 30-year-old second-generation Vietnamese Chinese American who succinctly introduced herself as a list of psychopathological diagnoses with a historical and current regimen of psychopharmaceutical prescriptions when she first left me a voice message seeking therapy.[1] Though informative, an EH therapist is more concerned with who the client is as a person and how their diagnoses and medications are viewed in their eyes and in their world. Per May's (1975) EH assumption, one's lived experiences are how one forms or creates a sense of self. Also of an EH therapist's interest is clients' awareness of their existential predicaments objectively and subjectively (May, 1958). Thus, we focused on what it meant to be her in her context: who she was, what gave her personal significance, and how her struggles were impacting her functioning in her current world, including with her relationships. A detailed intake was guided by Hoffman and Cleare-Hoffman's (2025) EH case formulation template. Overall, I observed that she was polite yet nervous and focused on information, which gave away her hyperconstriction of self (Schneider, 1999). I would, in time, offer my reaction to her multiple voice messages as information about her way

---

[1]Though the details of this case example were modified to protect the identity of the client whom this was based on, the client's permission to have their case shared was still obtained.

of being. This is one of the processes of drawing the therapists' experience or reaction to the clients' awareness, as what takes place within the session often shows up as a pattern beyond the therapy space.

Hue Juan described a potent existential theme of an alienated self—from her culture, community, and creativity. As a child, she struggled with her cultural identity when her parents enrolled her in a prestigious Chinese school where she experienced rejection from wealthy Chinese kids who exhibited anti-Vietnamese sentiments and marked her as Vietnamese. Later, she attended a public school and found friendship among other creative peers. Though she continued to face bullying, she was invested in her creativity and recognized her parents' joy and pride in her. She was a slender, secure, and talented artist. However, that old self now felt dead and unfamiliar. She didn't recognize her body, she second guessed her perception and judgment, and creativity became so painfully foreign. This was her current state of nonbeing, an existential slow death. This state is marked by lethargy, boredom, indecisiveness, and grief. Clinically, her symptoms have long been recognized as depression and medically treated with various selective serotonin reuptake inhibitors, but the result was a perpetual contraction of her being. Hue Juan feared she was behind in life's markers of an independent adult at her age. Overwhelmed with her dread of facing the adult world, she felt inadequate; comparing herself with her parents who were survivors of war, she felt ashamed and had suicidal ideations.

Due to Hue Juan's sensitive ability to narrate her lived experiences, a rich EH case conceptualization and approach was possible. Her alienation from her world and herself became a point of access from which to set fundamental EH therapy goals. This often involves releasing clients from their sense of thrownness (Schneider & Krug, 2017). Ultimately, the release would result in an exercise of freedom and responsibilities—a freedom from her feeling trapped, debilitated, and alienated by her world; a freedom to engage in relationships with herself and her community; and a sense of agency when exercising in expansion or constriction of her paradoxical natural tendencies (Schneider, 1999).

Although early on in our therapy I noted a misdiagnosis, I waited to bring this to her awareness. Being in private practice and not bound by insurance in her case, I addressed her diagnoses after we established an understanding of the meaning, pragmatics, and the construction of psychiatric verdicts. This way of prioritizing by bringing her fluid process as a being-in-the-world to her awareness before examining her diagnoses speaks to the importance of valuing herself as having the potential to grow, construct, and recreate instead of having the view of self as being a client with static and determined challenges.

The therapy process that unfolded involved continually collecting traces of the more abstract and transient aspects of her experiences of self. This was to allow the development and nurturance of a self-expansioning and (paradoxically) a self-integration practice by engaging in living her potential in her world again. We attended to her fantastical dreams and enjoyment of arts; graduated to mindfully attuning to bodily tension and sensations in various states; and eventually broached fragmented poetry, sketches, self-portraits, and personal myths. The work was arduous but had rewarding moments even after she found her voice, confronted her bullies, established friendships with old acquaintances, and found ways to honor her parents' best interests while asserting her position in her exploration of work and management of physical health. There were still moments of breakdowns and phases of doubt where destructive, dreaded, dysfunctional tendencies would revisit her way of being, but the experience of becoming is not a linear path, and she began to recognize herself and find ways to face her world again.

RESEARCH SUPPORT

EH therapy's view of the self is complex and not easy to directly research. Nonetheless, there is research relevant to the way the EH self is conceived and approached in EH therapy, which is reviewed in this section. I begin with providing an overview of the quantitative research and then address the qualitative research.

Quantitative Research

One of the most prominent contributions of EH psychology is from one of the founding humanistic psychologists, Abraham Maslow. His model on the hierarchy of needs involves the highest strata being self-actualization. Whereas Maslow's hierarchy was initially proposed in the 1950s, more recently Kaufman (2023) developed a 30 item Characteristics of Self-Actualization Scale (CSAS). In his study, 522 participants were recruited to establish the scale's norms. Scale validation demonstrated 10 key characteristics: continued freshness of appreciation, acceptance, authenticity, equanimity, purpose, efficient perception of reality, humanitarianism, peak experiences, good moral intuition, and creative spirit. As support for EH's approach to the self, those reporting greater characteristics of self-actualization on the CSAS had greater sense of well-being, including self-acceptance, personal growth, autonomy, purpose, and self-transcendental experiences.

   In an applied study, Lewis and colleagues (2022) examined how mindfulness, particularly nonattachment to self, can aid athletes in self-actualization. This correlational study involved 223 semi-elite to elite athletes completing athlete mindfulness questionnaires, nonattachment to self-scale, and the CSAS. They focused on three factors, one from each variable, as indicators in their analysis. They found that although both mindfulness and nonattachment to self predicted self-actualization scores in these athletes, mindfulness was a stronger mediator variable to nonattachment to self's effect on self-actualization than nonattachment to self was to mindfulness's effect on self-actualization.

   Authenticity is also central to EH psychology (see also Chapter 7 of this volume). An authentic self has explored and come to a better understanding of oneself—including one's freedom and responsibility—and would live in a self-motivated way, engaging their world congruently and meaningfully. Efforts to study the authentic self can be traced to Bugental's (1952) study. He devised a method to assess self and not-self attitudes. Although the following applied study does not specifically use this method, its procedure does in part utilize the self rater's sense of self and not-self attitudes. Schlegel and colleagues (2009) systematically conducted five studies that employed the idea of how cognitively accessible one's self-concepts or schemas are and hypothesized that the accessibility and behavior based on these schemas can predict one's sense of life's meaning. They divided the studies into trait focused and action focused, and they examined how one's privately acknowledged self and publicly expressed self impacted one's sense of meaning. The authors concluded based on their results that the integrity of one's self through the cognitive accessibility of these traits enhances one's meaning in life.

The EH approach promotes self-awareness, which is involved in both authenticity and actualization (see also Chapter 7). Self-awareness is also an aspect of mindfulness that is easier than other aspects of mindfulness, like being present, to describe and implement. In a mixed method study examining the effects of self-awareness, Sutton (2016) first held a focus group, then reduced items generated from the focus group into a 38 item self-awareness outcome questionnaire. There were four factors, of which the first three were deemed positive and the last one negative (i.e., reflective self-development, acceptance, proactivity, and costs). Regression analysis revealed aspects of self-awareness in our day-to-day lives that lead to various positive outcomes (i.e., reflective self-development, acceptance, and proactivity) and one negative outcome (i.e., costs).

In terms of physiological awareness, biofeedback is an older but well-studied technique that supports the benefits of practicing self-awareness. As biofeedback takes place in real time, it allows a faster look at how physiological and, more subtly, psychological changes can be influenced or regulated by oneself (Shaffer & Moss, 2006). In more recent years, with the popularity of smart technology, individuals are able to log aspects of their lives with ease and provide lifelog data. In applying lifelog objective data to assist subjective self-awareness, Li and colleagues (2021) examined four topics: sleep quality prediction, personality detection, mood detection and prediction, and depression detections. Their studies on real data showed promising correlations between daily activity records and the prediction and detection of these four topics. Most meaningfully, the objective data are another source from which to fine tune daily self-awareness.

Self as context (SAC) is one of the six core processes of acceptance and commitment therapy. SAC provides guidance for self-awareness, introspection, and personal growth. Prior literature on SAC suggests "five conceptual subcomponents . . . awareness of a distinct, transcendent, enduring, perspective-taking, and observing self" (Godbee & Kangas, 2020, p. 918). Departing from viewing the self as content, or products of one's experiences, SAC guides individuals to observe and recognize their ability to sharpen their own awareness. The aware-ness serves to defuse personal narratives and transcends from the thoughts or feelings one experiences. SAC was systematically reviewed by Godbee and Kangas (2020), where they qualified 20 experimental and quasi-experimental studies to further examine. The methodologies of these studies varied and had mostly nonclinical participants. Nonetheless, the results yielded support for SAC as a promising effectual independent process for acceptance and commit-ment therapy, with limitations.

Self-transcendence is another important concept in EH lineage. In discussing the varieties of religious experiences, James (2004) describes how transcenden-tal experiences may appear differently cross-culturally but are still valued and richly meaningful to individuals. Though it is difficult to define (Yaden et al., 2017), Huang and Yang (2022) operationally defined self-transcendence as benefiting the society, whereas self-enhancement is benefiting oneself. The aim of Huang and Yang's (2022) seven studies was to compare the roles of self-transcendence with self-enhancement in participants' sense of meaning and in work, life, and relationships, as well as in happiness. They found that self-transcendence outweighed meaning in jobs, lives, and advice giving. Yet benefits to the self weighted slightly more when it came to happiness. They also found that benefit to the self had a stronger role in personally rated meaning than meaning rated by others. Thus, the results suggest a stronger relationship between self-transcendence and meaning making than between self-transcendence and happiness.

Although neuroscience studies on psychedelic microdosing do not stem from a shared point of view on the self, participants' self-reported experience of ego dissolution being a catalyst to psychotherapeutic benefits serves as evidence supporting EH therapy's definition and approach to the self (Lebedev et al., 2015). An area where change was found to be significant was a disrupted inter-play between medial temporal lobe and neocortex. Mason and colleagues' (2020) study further confirmed specifically the decoupling of these regions. They inferred that the disruption of these regions was associated with semantic autobiographical information that challenged one's sense of identity. This was correlated with participants' reports of a positive ego dissolution experience, described as almost mystical or transcendental. In sum, if psychotherapeutic benefits of microdosing psilocybin is in part attributed to the subjective experi-ence of one's ego dissolution (Lebedev et al., 2015), then detaching oneself from preconceived concrete notions of self or self as content as in EH therapy's approach to becoming is a route to well-being.

Qualitative Research

The qualitative research on the self is sparser; however, some relevant studies are discussed in this section. Considering self-awareness in the context of adult development, a systematic literature review by Carden and colleagues (2022) used a qualitative, inductive thematic coding analysis approach. They sifted through over 400,000 papers to extract their themes from the final list of 31 peer-reviewed articles. Their findings can be grouped into intra- and interpersonal components. The practical applications include how to be self-aware (such as with self-evaluation), understanding the process and attention required in self-awareness, and the purpose of understanding oneself and understanding the impact one's actions have on others. Considering self-awareness in the context of mindfulness, Mathews and Anderson (2021) conducted a longitudinal descriptive phenomenological study on mindfulness. They conducted interviews and focus groups with chronically ill patients for their lived experience and meaning with learning mindfulness and used life-world fractions (Ashworth, 2003) to aid in the analysis. Aligned with EH's definition of the self, this study found that participants are not passive individuals being instilled with a modality but instead are intentional agents in shaping the lived experience of acquiring a new attentional approach. Some participants' lived experience was an embodied integrated mindfulness, whereas others' lived experience was learning a stress management tool. Further, in embodied mindfulness, participants expressed challenges relating to fear, disturbance, and vulnerability, calling for much courage. The lived experiences unveiled in this study bear resemblance to EH therapy's approach to self: Our clients' intentionality and courage are key since they are active participants in their world and EH's approach to self involves being awe-provoking.

In a small qualitative descriptive study, Smith and colleagues (2016) investigated the self-concept of five EH therapists. The study aimed to explore how these therapists conceptualized their professional identities and their relationship to the philosophical underpinnings of EH therapy. One of the primary themes that emerged from the data was that the therapists did not perceive their theoretical orientation as distinct from their personal identity; rather, they viewed it as an integral expression of their self-concept. Subthemes that emerged within this theme included (a) a shared worldview between the therapists and the EH philosophy; (b) an evolving commitment to the philosophy over time; and (c) a continued, personal, and meaningful engagement with the philosophical principles. The second major theme centered on the therapists' conceptual positioning, which emphasized a deeper integration of personal and professional practices. Subthemes within this theme highlighted (a) a growing appreciation for the subjective over the objective, (b) a shift toward valuing the tentative over the certain, and (c) an increased focus on experience rather than theory. These findings suggest a dynamic and evolving relationship between therapists' personal identities and their professional practice within the EH framework. While this was a small study, the overarching themes serve as clear evidence of EH's sense of self.

In a grounded theory study on self-transcendent experiences, 15 healthy adults provided their narratives (Garcia-Romeu et al., 2015). Their phenomenological qualities of self-transcendence involved somatic manifestations including embodied sensations, perceptual alterations (including self-boundaries and contextual boundaries with time and space), and cognitive affective shifts (including the sense of vulnerability and paradox). Although not defined as self-transcendence, subjective reports of ego dissolution in a positive manner by healthy participants undergoing microdosing of psychedelics appear to describe a similar phenomenon (Mason et al., 2020). Both the narrative of transcendent experiences and ego dissolution seem to involve an element of broadening or flexibility of the sense of self that coincides with EH's definition of self. Moreover, Rogers (1989, 2021) noted that therapists should be willing to engage, explore, and expand along with their clients at a relational depth. One case study examined how self-expansion develops in a therapeutic relationship and enters a depth that allows for therapeutic change (Adamczyk, 2018). Self-expansion as a result of bidirectional encounters is a catalyst for clients' therapeutic growth (Cooper, 2012).

The timing of COVID-19 lockdowns paved the way for an interesting phenomenon for many individuals experiencing solitude as an avenue to the transformation of self. Paterson and Park (2023) were interested in how millennials who self-reported the solitude as positive viewed solitude and how it may have transformed them. Eight millennials served as participants undergoing semistructured interviews and provided their accounts of personal experience of solitude imposed by COVID-19 lockdowns and how it changed their sense of solitude and self. Interpretative phenomenological analysis was used for thematic analysis. Three main themes emerged. First, participants found a self-discovery involving exploring personal incongruence between public lives and private beliefs and desires. The inauthenticity sensed and the autonomy discovery mirrors a starting process of EH therapy. The subsequent theme was cultivating a more congruent, authentic self through introspection, self-awareness, and meaning making. This aspect also resembles the iterative process of EH therapy. The third theme was a perceived transformation encompassing freedom and integrity, not unlike EH therapy's central goal. This qualitative study not only demonstrated the value of positive solitude but also revealed an interesting process seemingly analogous to EH therapy's direction with the self.

MULTICULTURAL CONSIDERATIONS

The psychology of an individual cannot be devoid of one's world. The American Psychological Association's (APA; 2017) *Multicultural Guidelines* espouse Bronfenbrenner's (1977) ecological model. The EH approach values an even more critical consideration by finding ways to not only understand and facilitate clients' own awareness and relationship to their five concentric circles (i.e., the microsystem, mesosystem, ecosystem, macrosystem, and chronosystem) but to also possibly seek ways to impact the societal forces and the laws and governmental influences outside of the therapy setting. In this section, the issues surrounding sociopolitical power differentials and identity politics within the ever-developing therapeutic relationship pave the foundation to a critical, multiculturally sensitive therapeutic environment. Correspondingly, some of the modes of engaging in the therapeutic dynamic such as authenticity are considered through this critical lens. Finally, the importance of client cultural identity congruent therapies is suggested through a discussion on the limitations of language.

Power Differential

EH therapy approaches a view of an authentic self that is an ongoing relational identity with one's temporal, social–cultural climates where the therapist is aware that they exist in relationship with clients (Amari, 2021; Friedman, 2015). As such, there is a recognition that the therapy context as well as who we are in the relationship with the client all contribute to the individual who emerges to the therapist. This means EH therapists will not only apply an ecological contextualized case formulation (Felder & Robbins, 2021). Especially for relationships where social–cultural identity or issues are focal for the clients, it is integral that therapists practice reflexivity on who they are as an organized self (Hermans, 2016), as guided by APA's (2017) Multicultural Guideline 5, and practice attending to one's social position and relationship to the world (van Deurzen, 2007).

As the therapeutic relationship encounters and grows, the therapist will facilitate dialogues and a receptiveness to disclose and reflect with the clients on their cultural–political attitudes, as well as potential similarities and differences of values from their clients. This will be done ethically, reflexively, and relationally (Amari, 2021). This means that even outside of the therapy room, the therapist will continue to actively learn the history and maintain awareness of historical, social, political, and economic power differentials. In addition, EH therapists are inclined to act on addressing issues of power, privilege, and inequities in ways that they can as individuals with social positions. This includes bringing attention to inequities in our society that hinder human rights or cast barriers to one's pursuit and use of their potential. This goes beyond what takes place within the context of therapy or even issues of mental health to also include institutional issues of administration, criminal justice, and education access, among other factors.

In short, the EH therapeutic relationship is not just about meeting the clients, being culturally sensitive of where the therapists come from, and recognizing differences within the relationship, but it also entails being open and willing to engage in these dialogues with the clients in sessions as well as act with multicultural ethics on the issues in the real world beyond the therapy context.

Authenticity

With the foundation of an EH therapeutic relationship in place, the pursuit of ecologically aware authentic sociocultural self continues. This applies both to the therapist as well as the client. APA's (2017) Multicultural Guideline 4 encourages the therapist to educate themselves continually about their clients' cultures. EH therapists should also endeavor to further understand their own cultures, including the cultural historical dynamics between the therapists' and the clients' cultures. Yalom and Leszcz (2005) also suggest that therapists check in with how much the clients identify with their sociocultural influences or identities. This often involves recognizing the multicultural and specific generational worldviews and challenges clients are met with. This is not intended to categorize clients but to recognize from which point of social and cultural forces the clients may aspire to transcend (Maslow, 1968). Transcending from is not departing from; it is congruent with Foucault and Heidegger's authentic self being a becoming, as an ongoing process of individuation and connectedness to the worldly context of social, cultural, historical, political, and economic climate.

EH therapists also recognize that authenticity presents differently cross-culturally and plays different roles in one's experience of well-being. Slabu and colleagues (2014) found that cognitive style plays a role in authenticity in that Western cultures demonstrate less interdependence and more of an analytic cognitive style, whereas Eastern cultures tend to have a more holistic cognitive style. A Sri Lankan study that used the Authenticity Scale (Wood et al., 2008) found that female students tend to show higher authenticity than male students (De Zoysa, 2021). Another quantitative study that used the Authenticity Scale found that authenticity completely mediated well-being in the Chinese sample while it only partially mediated well-being in other populations (Chen & Murphy, 2019). This study also suggested that the person-centered therapy, which is humanistic in its foundations, has the value of helping clients become more aware of themselves and their cultural values by nonjudging and by reflecting observations to the clients. EH therapists recognize that identity is nonstatic as maturation and life transitions take place in an evolving sociocultural context, and in turn, this interacts with one's worldview and sense of identity (Hoffman et al., 2015). As the clients evolve in their becoming, the EH therapists' experience of the relational depth shall too evolve.

Cultural Congruent Therapies

EH therapists advocate for cultural congruent therapies as a recognition that the traditional Western talk therapy may not be the best fit for individuals who hold non-Western-centric cultural identities. Multicultural research increasingly has found that most therapies' effectiveness is culturally and linguistically bound (Maraldi & Krippner, 2019). In a meta-analysis study of 76 studies, Griner and Smith (2006) did find noteworthy indication that culturally adapting mental health modalities is worthwhile, especially when the tailored at the ethnic group level. However, challenges still present for clients of higher chronological age. Although EH therapists and psychologists in general have become better at acknowledging Indigenous modalities and referring their clients to therapists with similar cultural–lingual backgrounds, many regulatory barriers under the APA and jurisdictional guidelines still prevent some of these culturally sensitive practices from actualizing (APA Division 32 Task Force on Indigenous Psychology, n.d.). Nonetheless, APA's (2017) *Multicultural Guidelines* do recognize the limitations of language, and EH therapists recognize the assumptions, impressions, and limitations of the cultural signifiers of traditional Western talk therapy on a client's sense of cultural identity. To illustrate, Taiwanese scholar Hwang (Shiah & Hwang, 2019) warned the psychology community of Taiwan to not blindly import Western psychotherapy practices at the expense of neglecting what Confucian wisdom has to offer.

An example concept that does not translate well from Western culture to Chinese and Taiwanese culture is shame. Shame is deemed a trait emotion in the West leading to the felt sense of a shamed self (Collardeau et al., 2022). In China and Taiwan, however, shame is an integral aspect of an evolving reflexive self (Bedford & Hwang, 2003). With over 150 words related to shame identified in the Chinese lexicon, shame in Chinese promotes bettering oneself or becoming one's best possible self. Shame in this context can be instrumental to self-transformation. Arguably, this may also be true in other populations based on my clinical work. My clients who are neither Chinese nor identifying with European American cultures have had in-depth conversations with me on how shame is felt or sensed regularly and experienced not as a stigma but rather as an instrument to better oneself. This is similar to Rollo May's (1958) conception of guilt, including existential guilt, that recognizes its potential to help people grow.

Self-cultivation is an inherent cultural practice in Chinese and Taiwanese heritage. This practice can be traced to the idea of a Confucian self, a self that is embedded in community and seeks to live ethically in harmony and to do so responsibly through ongoing self-reflection and cultivation (Shiah & Hwang, 2019). Valuing reflection is a sentiment that can be compared to humanistic actualization and existential authenticity. Also, a nonfixed but impermanent, potentially ever-changing Confucian self resembles the EH definition of self. When an EH therapist approaches a client who does not identify with the Western culture or the Western definition of self, orienting to the EH mindset of self may involve embracing a multitheoretical mindset and may provide a safer space for clients to navigate the many nuanced and intricate thoughts and emotions, such as shame, that may not be adequately appreciated otherwise.

FUTURE RESEARCH NEEDS

The topic of the self has been more philosophically discussed than empirically researched. Future research is called for to better understand the EH self. It would be beneficial to first examine some of these concepts qualitatively and, wherever possible, cross-culturally. Where appropriate, more structured or elaborated models may also be extended, as they may be useful to create applications by way of constructing surveys and instruments. This would lend opportunities for quantitative, clinical, and cross-cultural studies to be conducted in many creative ways.

There are many aspects of the EH self that can be approached, such as Rogerian unconditional positive self-regard, Maslow's actualizing self, Foucault's relational self, Schneider's paradoxical self, and May's "I am." If one considers concepts related to the EH therapy process of assisting the clients' becoming, then applied topics like how to use the self or how to examine the I-thou relationship would also be of value. Likewise, language and nuanced emotions closely related to trait or being states like shame can benefit from a greater cross-cultural frame. Finally, from a critical multicultural lens, the lived experience of the self-identified where the subjective experience of "I am" differs from what one recognizes as the objective experience of "them," especially in a cultural or subcultural context, is also worthy of investigation.

Qualitative research approaches and methodologies including phenomenology, narrative studies, and clinical case studies may be a good vantage point from which to examine some of the conceptual ideas of the EH self and aspects related to the EH self. Revealing the constituents and themes of the various conditions, ingredients, or processes of the self may allow therapists to have more insight into their process. Some directions can include the phenomenology of ego dissolution and fluidity of self-concepts. But if principles and models can be better articulated, instruments may be devised for later quantitative studies. For example, Rogers's theory of authenticity formed a basis for Wood and colleagues' (2008) Authenticity Scale. Maslow's self-actualization theory was foundational in the development of CSAS (Lewis et al., 2022). Still, instruments like this one and hopefully future EH instruments can be further normed and translated for comparative and cross-cultural studies. In addition to developing models and instruments via traditional qualitative and quantitative psychological research means, comparative psycholinguistic studies would be an invaluable means to better appreciate concepts that do not readily translate.

CONCLUSION

This chapter was an earnest attempt to overview EH therapy's conceptions of the self. Still, at the conclusion of this writing, I have only broached the surface of relevant research to include in this chapter. A comparison was first laid out between the general and clinical definitions of the self to that of EH's notion of self. Then, EH therapy's approach to self was illustrated with a case study. Research and critical multicultural considerations followed. Finally, future research needs and recommendations were suggested.

The view of the self in American academic psychology as a science tends to be one of a reducible, individualistic, neuro-bio-chemical-physiological, concrete, autonomous entity. This differs from EH therapy's conception of self as a narrative dialectical selfhood between subjectivity and intersubjectivity; it is fluid, relational, transcendental, experiential, and inseparable from others and contexts. EH therapy's approach to the self involves a culturally sensitive, mindfully guided journey involving questioning self-understanding and meaning and integrating one's paradoxical tendencies. The focus is on a process of becoming a self capable of exercising authenticity, freedom, and responsibility in one's relationships with oneself, that which includes one's world.

The dimension of relationships to one's world is particularly meaningful in a critical multicultural context. EH therapists weigh the historical, geopolitical, and power dynamics in the therapeutic relationship and in the collective social justice context. They remain open to multiple worldviews and continually evolving definitions and meaning of authenticity to clients' identities. They are also appreciative of culturally congruent modalities and mindful of cultural linguistic nuances. In sum, although EH therapy's approach and conceptions of the self have a rich foundation in various philosophical and multicultural roots, the evidence-based practices of EH therapy's conception of self in psychotherapy and psychology merit more research.

REFERENCES

Aafjes-van Doorn, K., Garay, C., Etchebarne, I., Kamsteeg, C., & Roussos, A. (2020). Psychotherapy for personal growth? A multicultural and multitheoretical exploration. *Journal of Clinical Psychology, 76*(7), 1255–1266. https://doi.org/10.1002/jclp.22942

Adamczyk, K. S. (2018). The impact of expanding the self on the ability to work at relational depth. *Counselling Psychology Review, 33*(2), 47–54. https://doi.org/10.53841/bpscpr.2018.33.2.47

Amari, N. (2021). The use of self in counseling psychology and Buber's "turning." *The Humanistic Psychologist, 49*(4), 543–554. https://doi.org/10.1037/hum0000174

American Psychological Association. (n.d.). Self. In *APA dictionary of psychology*. Retrieved October 4, 2021, from https://dictionary.apa.org/self

American Psychological Association. (2017). *Multicultural guidelines: An ecological approach to context, identity, and intersectionality*. http://www.apa.org/about/policy/multicultural-guidelines.pdf

American Psychological Association Division 32 Task Force on Indigenous Psychology. (n.d.). *"Home."* Retrieved October 4, 2021. https://indigenouspsych.org/

Ashworth, P. (2003). An approach to phenomenological psychology: The contingencies of the lifeworld. *Journal of Phenomenological Psychology, 34*(2), 145–156. https://doi.org/10.1163/156916203322847119

Bedford, O., & Hwang, K. (2003). Guilt and shame in Chinese culture: A cross-cultural framework from the perspective of morality and identity. *Journal for the Theory of Social Behaviour, 33*(2), 127–144. https://doi.org/10.1111/1468-5914.00210

Bradford, K. (2020). The subject matter of psychology: Psyche, Dasein, non-self. *Existential Analysis, 31*(2), 336–350.

Bradford, K. (2021). Non-self psychology: The Buddhist phenomenology of self experience. *Existential Analysis, 32*(1), 101–112.

Bronfenbrenner, U. (1977). Toward an experimental ecology of human development. *American Psychologist, 32*(7), 513–531. https://doi.org/10.1037/0003-066X.32.7.513

Buber, M. (1990). *A believing humanism* (M. Friedman, Trans.). Prometheus Books.

Bugental, J. F. T. (1952). A method for assessing self and not-self attitudes during the therapeutic series. *Journal of Consulting Psychology, 16*(6), 435–439. https://doi.org/10.1037/h0055727

Bugental, J. F. T. (1978). *Psychotherapy and processes: The fundamentals of an existential–humanistic approach*. Random House.

Carden, J., Jones, R. J., & Passmore, J. (2022). Defining self-awareness in the context of adult development: A systematic literature review. *Journal of Management Education, 46*(1), 140–177. https://doi.org/10.1177/1052562921990065

Chen, S., & Murphy, D. (2019). The mediating role of authenticity on mindfulness and wellbeing: A cross cultural analysis. *Asia Pacific Journal of Counselling and Psychotherapy, 10*(1), 40–55. https://doi.org/10.1080/21507686.2018.1556171

Churchill, S. D., & Wertz, F. J. (2015). An introduction to phenomenological research in psychology: Historical, conceptual, and methodological foundations. In K. Schneider, J. F. T. Bugental, & J. F. Pierson (Eds.), *The handbook of humanistic psychology: Theory, research, and practice* (2nd ed., pp. 275–295). Sage.

Collardeau, F., Dupuis, H. E., & Woodin, E. (2022). The role of culture and social threats in constructing shame: Moving beyond a Western lens. *Canadian Psychology, 64*(2), 132–143. https://doi.org/10.1037/cap0000329

Cooper, M. (2012). Experiencing relational depth in therapy: What we know so far. In R. Knox (Ed.), *Relational depth: New perspectives and developments* (pp. 62–76). Palgrave Macmillan.

De Zoysa, P., Kumar, S., Amarasuriya, S. D., & Mendis, N. S. R. (2021). Being yourself: An assessment of authenticity in undergraduates of a university in Sri Lanka. *Asia Pacific Journal of Counselling and Psychotherapy, 12*(2), 138–153. https://doi.org/10.1080/21507686.2021.1924810

Felder, A. J., & Robbins, B. D. (2021). Approaching mindful multicultural case formulation: Rogers, Yalom, and existential phenomenology. *Person-Centered and Experiential Psychotherapies, 20*(1), 1–20. https://doi.org/10.1080/14779757.2020.1748697

Ferrari, P. F., & Coudé, G. (2018). Mirror neurons, embodied emotions, and empathy. In K. Z. Meyza & E. Knapska (Eds.), *Neuronal correlates of empathy: From rodent to human* (pp. 67–77). Elsevier Academic Press. https://doi.org/10.1016/B978-0-12-805397-3.00006-1

Friedman, M. (2015). Therapy as an I–thou encounter. In K.J. Schneider, J. F. T. Bugental & J. F. Pierson (Eds.), *The handbook of humanistic psychology: Leading edges in theory, research and practice* (pp. 451–472). Sage.

Garcia-Romeu, A., Himelstein, S. P., & Kaminker, J. (2015). Self-transcendent experience: A grounded theory study. *Qualitative Research, 15*(5), 633–654. https://doi.org/10.1177/1468794114550679

Giorgi, A. (1970). *Psychology as a human science: A phenomenologically based approach*. Harper & Row.

Godbee, M., & Kangas, M. (2020). The relationship between flexible perspective taking and emotional well-being: A systematic review of the "self-as-context" component of acceptance and commitment therapy. *Behavior Therapy, 51*(6), 917–932. https://doi.org/10.1016/j.beth.2019.12.010

Greening, T. (n.d.). *My (failed) search for authenticity*. Mindfreedom.org. Retrieved February 13, 2024, from https://mindfreedom.org/front-page/selection-on-psychology-and-other-pathologies-by-greening/

Griner, D., & Smith, T. B. (2006). Culturally adapted mental health intervention: A meta-analytic review. *Psychotherapy, 43*(4), 531–548. https://doi.org/10.1037/0033-3204.43.4.531

Heidegger, M. (2007). *Being and time* (J. Macquarrie & E. Robinson, Trans.). Harper Perennial Modern Classics.

Hermans, H. (Ed.). (2016). *Assessing and stimulating a dialogical self in groups, teams, cultures, and organizations*. Springer.

Hoffman, L., & Cleare-Hoffman, H. (2025). *Case formulation in existential–humanistic therapy*. American Psychological Association. https://doi.org/10.1037/0000464-000

Hoffman, L., Stewart, S., Warren, D., & Meek, L. (2015). Toward a sustainable myth of self: An existential response to the postmodern condition. In K. J. Schneider, J. F. T. Bugental, & J. F. Pierson (Eds.), *The handbook of humanistic psychology: Leading edges in theory, research and practice* (2nd ed., pp. 105–134). Sage. https://doi.org/10.4135/9781483387864.n9

Huang, M., & Yang, F. (2022). Self-transcendence or self-enhancement: People's perceptions of meaning and happiness in relation to the self. *Journal of Experimental Psychology: General, 152*(2), 590–610. https://doi.org/10.1037/xge0001297

James, W. (2004). *The varieties of religious experience: A study in human nature* (H. H. Rowntree, Ed.). Modern Library.

Kaufman, S. B. (2023). Self-actualizing people in the 21st century: Integration with contemporary theory and research on personality and well-being. *Journal of Humanistic Psychology, 63*(1), 51–83. https://doi.org/10.1177/0022167818809187

Lebedev, A. V., Lövdén, M., Rosenthal, G., Feilding, A., Nutt, D. J., & Carhart-Harris, R. L. (2015). Finding the self by losing the self: Neural correlates of ego-dissolution under psilocybin. *Human Brain Mapping, 36*(8), 3137–3153. https://doi.org/10.1002/hbm.22833

Letheby, C., & Gerrans, P. (2017). Self unbound: Ego dissolution in psychedelic experience. *Neuroscience of Consciousness, 2017*(1). https://doi.org/10.1093/nc/nix016

Lewis, K. J., Walton, C. C., Slemp, G. R., & Osborne, M. S. (2022). Mindfulness and nonattachment-to-self in athletes: Can letting go build well-being and self-actualization? *Mindfulness, 13*(11), 2738–2750. https://doi.org/10.1007/s12671-022-01990-9

Li, J., Ma, W., Zhang, M., Wang, P., Liu, Y., & Ma, S. (2021). Know yourself: Physical and psychological self-awareness with lifelog. *Frontiers in Digital Health, 3*, 676824. https://doi.org/10.3389/fdgth.2021.676824

Maraldi, E. O., & Krippner, S. (2019). Cross-cultural research on anomalous experiences: Theoretical issues and methodological challenges. *Psychology of Consciousness: Theory, Research, and Practice, 6*(3), 306–319. https://doi.org/10.1037/cns0000188

Maslow, A. H. (1968). *Toward a psychology of being* (2nd ed.). D. Van Nostrand.

Mason, N. L., Kuypers, K. P. C., Müller, F., Reckweg, J., Tse, D. H. Y., Toennes, S. W., Hutten, N. R. P. W., Jansen, J. F. A., Stiers, P., Feilding, A., & Ramaekers, J. G. (2020). Me, myself, bye: Regional alterations in glutamate and the experience of ego dissolution with psilocybin. *Neuropsychopharmacolology, 45*, 2003–2011.

Mathews, G., & Anderson, C. (2021). The lived experience of learning mindfulness as perceived by people living with long-term conditions: A community-based, longitudinal, phenomenological study. *Qualitative Health Research, 31*(7), 1209–1221. https://doi.org/10.1177/1049732321997130

May, R. (1953). *Man's search for himself*. W. W. Norton & Company.

May, R. (1958). Contributions of existential psychotherapy. In R. May, E. Angel, & H. F. Ellenberger (Eds.), *Existence* (pp. 37–91). Jason Aronson.

May, R. (1975). *The courage to create*. W. W. Norton & Company.

May, R. (1981). *Freedom and destiny*. W. W. Norton & Company.

Moran, D. (2018). The phenomenological approach. In G. Stanghellini, M. Broome, A. Raballo, A. V. Fernandez, P. Fusar-Poli, & R. Rosfort (Eds.), *The Oxford handbook of phenomenological psychopathology* (pp. 205–215). Oxford Academic Books.

Mosig, Y. D. (2006). Conceptions of the self in Western and Eastern psychology. *Journal of Theoretical and Philosophical Psychology, 26*(1–2), 39–50. https://doi.org/10.1037/h0091266

Paterson, J., & Park, M. S.-A. (2023). "It's allowed me to be a lot kinder to myself": Exploration of the self-transformative properties of solitude during COVID-19 lockdowns. *Journal of Humanistic Psychology*. Advance online publication. https://doi.org/10.1177/00221678231157796

Polkinghorne, D. (2015). The self and humanistic psychology. In K. J. Schneider, J. F. T. Bugental, & J. F. Pierson (Eds.), *The handbook of humanistic psychology: Leading edges in theory, research and practice* (pp. 87–104). Sage. https://doi.org/10.4135/9781483387864.n8

Rogers, C. R. (1989). A theory of therapy, personality, and interpersonal relationships, as developed in the client-centered framework. In H. Kirschenbaum & V. L. Henderson (Eds.), *The Carl Rogers reader* (pp. 236–257). Constable.

Rogers, C. R. (2021). *Client-centered therapy: Its current practice, implications, and theory*. Robinson.

Schlegel, R. J., Hicks, J. A., Arndt, J., & King, L. A. (2009). Thine own self: True self-concept accessibility and meaning in life. *Journal of Personality and Social Psychology, 96*(2), 473–490. https://doi.org/10.1037/a0014060

Schneider, K. J. (1999). *The paradoxical self: Toward an understanding of our contradictory nature*. Humanity Books.

Schneider, K. J. (2016). Existential–integrative therapy: Foundational implications for integrative practice. *Journal of Psychotherapy Integration, 26*(1), 49–55. https://doi.org/10.1037/a0039632

Schneider, K. J., & Krug, O. (2017). *Existential–humanistic therapy* (2nd ed.). American Psychological Association., https://doi.org/10.1037/0000042-000

Shaffer, F., & Moss, D. (2006). Biofeedback. In C.-S. Yuan, E. J. Bieber, & B. A. Bauer (Eds.), *Textbook of complementary and alternative medicine* (2nd ed., pp. 1–22). Informa Healthcare.

Shiah, Y.-J., & Hwang, K.-K. (2019). Developing self-cultivation counseling psychology theories and empirical studies based on the Chinese cultural traditions of Confucianism, Buddhism and Taoism: Towards self-enlightenment psychotherapy. *Chinese Journal of Guidance & Counseling, 54*, 1–20.

Slabu, L., Lenton, A. P., Sedikides, C., & Bruder, M. (2014). Trait and state authenticity across cultures. *Journal of Cross-Cultural Psychology, 45*(9), 1347–1373. https://doi.org/10.1177/0022022114543520

Sleeth, D. B. (2006). The self and the integral interface: Toward a new understanding of the whole person. *The Humanistic Psychologist, 34*(3), 243–261. https://doi.org/10.1207/s15473333thp3403_3

Sleeth, D. B. (2007). The self system: Toward a new understanding of the whole person (part 2). *The Humanistic Psychologist, 35*(1), 27–43. https://doi.org/10.1080/08873260709336695

Smith, V., Leeming, D., & Burr, V. (2016). Philosophy and identity: The relationship between choice of existential orientation and therapists' sense of self. *Existential Analysis, 27*(2), 287–302.

Spinelli, E. (2005). *The interpreted world: An introduction to phenomenological psychology* (2nd ed.). Sage.

Sutton, A. (2016). Measuring the effects of self-awareness: Construction of the Self-Awareness Outcomes Questionnaire. *Europe's Journal of Psychology, 12*(4), 645–658. https://doi.org/10.5964/ejop.v12i4.1178

Trieu, M., Foster, A. E., Yaseen, Z. S., Beaubian, C., & Calati, R. (2019). Neurobiology of empathy. In A. E. Foster & Z. S. Yaseen (Eds.), *Teaching empathy in healthcare* (pp. 17–39). Springer. https://doi.org/10.1007/978-3-030-29876-0_2

van Deurzen, E. (2007). Existential therapy. In W. Dryden (Ed.), *Dryden's handbook of individual therapy* (5th ed., pp. 195–226). Sage.

Wood, A. M., Linley, P. A., Maltby, J., Baliousis, M., & Joseph, S. (2008). The authentic personality: A theoretical and empirical conceptualization and the development of the Authenticity Scale. *Journal of Counseling Psychology, 55*(3), 385–399. https://doi.org/10.1037/0022-0167.55.3.385

Yaden, D. B., Haidt, J., Hood, R. W., Jr., Vago, D. R., & Newberg, A. B. (2017). The varieties of self-transcendent experience. *Review of General Psychology, 21*(2), 143–160. https://doi.org/10.1037/gpr0000102

Yalom, I., & Leszcz, M. (2005). *The theory and practice of group psychotherapy* (5th ed.). Basic Books.

Zahavi, D. (2008). *Subjectivity and selfhood: Investigating the first-person perspective*. Michigan Institute of Technology Press.

III

INTEGRATIVE STRATEGIES IN EXISTENTIAL–HUMANISTIC PSYCHOTHERAPY

14

Integrative Considerations of Mindfulness in Existential–Humanistic Psychotherapy

Donna Rockwell, O'Dell O. Johnson, and Shea Scharding

Mindfulness has become a trendy and somewhat revered health care application as an integrative consideration in psychotherapy, stress reduction programs, relaxation techniques for self-care, awareness and insight development, and other interventions to enhance well-being. Mindfulness is here to stay. There are studies that question the broad brush with which mindfulness is applied to almost every personal or societal ill; however, there is some agreement that mindfulness's ability to calm one's sometimes hair-trigger fight-flight-freeze reaction to daily stressors is a meaningful skill to master, as it supports greater prefrontal cortex activation and central nervous system homeostasis and thus more personal agency. Increasing mindfulness may allow individuals to respond instead of reacting and also express wisdom rather than engaging in ruminative fretting, often a mental default and habit of mind.

This chapter explores the concept of mindfulness and the evidence-based use of mindfulness contemporarily in the field of existential–humanistic (EH) psychology and psychotherapy. The chapter surveys how mindfulness informs the human experience of existential suffering and examines how this approach can extend into an effective multicultural application of mindfulness in EH therapy. Finally, the chapter provides a future vision for research that can translate into multicultural and intersectional integration of mindfulness in EH psychotherapy.

https://doi.org/10.1037/0000446-015
The Evidence-Based Foundations of Existential–Humanistic Therapy, L. Hoffman and V. Lac (Editors)

DEFINING MINDFULNESS

Mindfulness is being integrated into society across its entire spectrum, from childhood education to corporate culture to psychotherapy, even while its definition remains elusive. Today's mindfulness bears similarities and differences to Buddhist contemplative practice (Anālayo, 2019). Individuals can participate in nonclinical mindfulness programs at community centers, schools, workplaces, and on cell phone applications (Eby et al., 2019; Sommers-Spijkerman et al., 2021). Mindfulness training is provided at nearly 80% of U.S. medical schools (Phan-Le et al., 2022). Lam and colleagues (2023) found that nearly half of the study participants ($n = 953$) indicated they had meditated at some point in their lifetime, and a third had practiced within the last year. Mindfulness can appear prolific and ubiquitous. While mindfulness as a brand is part of our current nomenclature, there is much confusion and misunderstanding about its meaning.

Within the medical and psychotherapeutic community, mindfulness is "the awareness that arises by paying attention, on purpose, in the present moment, and non-judgmentally" (Kabat-Zinn, 2013, p. 19). A more condensed definition is provided by Germer and colleagues (2005): "(1) awareness, (2) of present experience, (3) with acceptance" (p. 7). However, another definition derived through a review of mindfulness and psychotherapy literature defines mindfulness as "the non-judgmental observation of the ongoing stream of internal and external stimuli as they arise" (Baer, 2003, p. 125). Bishop and colleagues (2004) add, "adopting an orientation of curiosity, openness, and acceptance toward current experience" (p. 6).

It is important to understand and define the experience of mindfulness in the general populace. The definitions provided by Kabat-Zinn (2013), Germer and colleagues (2005), Baer (2003), and Bishop and colleagues (2004) are frequently found in academic and clinical discussions of mindfulness. Alvear and colleagues (2022) conducted a study to understand how meditators define mindfulness. From a sample of 326 meditators, they found multiple themes, including attention and awareness, nonjudgmental attitude, and the presence of psychospiritual states. They concluded that the definitions generally aligned with a scientific rather than a Buddhism-based definition. There is evidence that mindfulness understandings vary generationally (Van Doren et al., 2022). In a study of American college-aged adults, Van Doren and colleagues (2022) found consensus among the participants that mindfulness evolved from Buddhism, is spiritual while secular, reduces suffering, provides a competitive advantage, and is practiced more by liberal females than conservative males. More importantly, they found consensus among participants that mindfulness can be learned. In a study by Haddock and colleagues (2022) on how mindfulness is perceived, participants identified mindful individuals as thoughtful and having empathetic qualities such as caring and kindness.

Mindfulness is, at its essence, a unique experience for each person. Individuals can develop mindfulness through meditation; people often use the terms interchangeably, though they are different activities and skills (Sutcliffe et al., 2016). While one person's practice may be formal sitting meditation, another may practice mindfulness by gardening, playing the piano, or rock climbing. Mindfulness is a lived experience that is uniquely felt and expressed and innately human.

History of Mindfulness

While most Western accounts of mindfulness trace its origination to the Buddha's time, this is a misnomer. Mindfulness is best understood as finding its human origins in Ancient Egypt and by human ancestors who discovered the spiritual value of silence in mindfulness, accessed through simply sitting in stillness, as insight and wisdom poured forth in that quieted and sacred space (Najovits, 2003). Anālayo (2022a) identified the Indian *tetralemma*, a four-part schema for logical arguments, as contributing to the Buddhist view of nondualistic thought. The quietude of a still and present-centered mind has been appreciated through eons, perhaps since the beginning of human presence on Earth.

The threads of mindfulness weave back to a time of deep humanistic inquiry, to the Buddha from the 5th to the 3rd century B.C.E. (Anālayo, 2019, 2022b). The Buddha's teachings described mindfulness as awareness of life's Four Noble Truths, a framework to achieve liberation from suffering's emotional hold (Anālayo, 2022c). These truths state that (a) life naturally contains suffering or stress, (b) there is a cause of the stress, (c) there is a way to eradicate the negative effects of stress, and (d) there is a clear path elucidated to do so, and this path is available to everyone (Anālayo, 2022c).

Three Buddhist concepts align with mindfulness: suffering, impermanence, and non-self (Schmid & Taylor Aiken, 2021). Buddhist philosophy, however, distinguishes "right mindfulness" as mindfulness that supports humanity and wholesome intentions and "wrong mindfulness" as using the quality of awareness for personal gain (Rowe, 2017, p. 48). Mindfulness and meditation offer a means to transform existential resentment into gratitude and appreciation (Rowe, 2017, 2024). Cultivating appreciation, according to the theory of Buddhist teacher Chogyam Trungpa Rinpoche, creates psychological space for improved social relations and increased humanity (Rowe, 2017). In this way, meditation becomes a solution to the fear and vulnerability created by "systemic dominations like colonialism, capitalist exploitation, White supremacy, and hetero-patriarchy" (Rowe, 2017, p. 63).

Mindfulness practitioners were primarily in the East until the late 1960s (Nehring & Frawley, 2020). Once introduced into Western culture, interest in mindfulness grew exponentially, primarily through the New Age and Human Potential movements (Nehring & Frawley, 2020; Wrenn, 2022). Jon Kabat-Zinn, a leader in clinical mindfulness, adapted mindfulness as a psychological and self-help intervention without a direct spiritual or religious connection (Kabat-Zinn, 2003; Nehring & Frawley, 2020). Kabat-Zinn's mindfulness-based stress reduction (MBSR) program became the first of many clinical applications of mindfulness in psychotherapy.

CONTEXTUALIZING MINDFULNESS IN EH PSYCHOTHERAPY

Mindfulness and EH psychotherapy share several common threads. When woven together, these threads create a vibrant tapestry of integrated modalities unique to the therapist and client. Various components and outcomes of mindfulness and EH therapies are related conceptually, including meaning, emotional regulation, and relationships (Hoffman et al., 2015). Mindfulness has developed a strong evidence base supporting its use and therapeutic integration with EH applications.

History of Mindfulness and EH Therapy

Early existentialists utilized processes that bear similarity to aspects of mindfulness. Albert Camus, Søren Kierkegaard, Friedrich Nietzsche, and others used mindful precision and depth of inquiry to cut through the religious zeitgeist of the time to reveal a deeper, more raw connection to lived experience. After all, embodying one's lived world is itself a contemplation on how to face the reality of the present moment while holding one's eventual death as an unavoidable existential truth, all the while busying oneself with the painstaking construction of a life replete with its existential meaning (Becker, 2020; Frankl et al., 1946/2019). The phenomenology movement introduced Martin Heidegger's *Dasein* (being there) to exploring lived experience by investigating a person's understanding of being in the world as an ontological experience (Heidegger, 2008). This phenomenological view rejected the Cartesian notion of duality in a subject–object sense and moved toward developing a more integrative and unitary consciousness. As Schneider and Krug (2017) described,

> EH therapy amalgamates European humanistic and existential philosophy and American humanistic psychology. Consolidated in the early 1960s, EH therapy welds the European heritage of self-inquiry, struggle, and responsibility with the American tradition of spontaneity, optimism, and practicality. Brought together, EH therapy forms a dynamic and timely stew. (p. 232)

Mindfulness in the Context of EH Therapy

EH therapists used the components of mindfulness, such as present moment awareness or a nonjudgmental attitude, without formally integrating mindfulness practices (Felder & Robbins, 2021). Felder and Robbins argue that sociocultural attunement from the therapist can create person-centered themes, or what they call "experiential restructuring" and "sociocultural self-actualization" (p. 1). In this way, mindfulness can bridge meditation and sociocultural personhood from the phenomenological perspective of lived experience (Felder & Robbins, 2016). Niemiec and colleagues (2010) found that the client's trait mindfulness can reduce defensive responses to existential themes as trait mindfulness supports conscious decision making in response to threats.

Mindfulness and EH therapy share many commonalities that allow for a smooth integration of the two modalities in therapeutic settings. Hoffman and colleagues (2015) reviewed the evidence base for EH psychology practices and found empirical evidence for three core tenets: relationships, emotional awareness, and meaning. With its focus on present moment awareness and nonjudgmental acceptance, mindfulness allows for exploring these EH concepts within the individual and their lived experience. The synergy between mindfulness and EH therapy extends beyond the core elements to include how mindfulness's outcomes and personal impacts can create a more profound understanding for both the therapist and the client of the individual, their search for meaning, and their cultural influences.

The necessity for such focused introspection was noted by Bugental (1992):

> Each person must in some way answer the basic questions life puts to us all: "Who and what am I? What is this world in which I live?" We answer these questions with our lives, with how we identify ourselves, how we use our powers, how we relate to others, how we face all the possibilities and limitations of being human. (p. 6)

Bugental (1992) insists that the EH therapist plays an active role in the client's growth process: "Life-changing therapy gives primary attention to the patient's subjective experiencing and does so by making the therapist's own subjective experiencing central to the work" (p. 5). The therapeutic alliance then plumbs the depths available for insight, transformation, and actualization (Maslow, 1993).

Mindfulness bears similarities to the core foundations of EH therapy. The goal of mindfulness is to pay bare attention to the present moment rather than dwelling on past or future thinking. By doing so, the participant sees present reality more clearly for what it is: an honest, intentional portrayal absent the use of mental filters, experiential avoidance, and dysfunctional coping mechanisms to make the experience more palatable. The participant is emotionally, mentally, physically, or spiritually distanced from the experience. Instead of inauthenticity, mindfulness and EH ways of being in the world emphasize working directly with emotions, cultivating present moment awareness, and expressing ourselves authentically in our lived world as self-aware beings while practicing genuine positive regard toward self and others (Rogers, 1980). By developing empathy, exchanging self for others, or walking a mile in another person's shoes, we can reflexively examine our lived world as it is being experienced in real time (Perls, 1971). In this way, mindful awareness shines a penetrating light on our individual and collective lives as they become examined and, according to Socrates, worth living. In a parallel sense, in EH psychotherapy, feeling a sense of awe and worthiness can be transformational in service to experiencing an authentic embodiment that is holistically encountered and meaningfully celebrated (Schneider & Krug, 2017). A sense of meaning may then spontaneously arise from the reverent and existential state of I and thou, extending from self-awareness, self-compassion, and self-affiliation and moving outward with an engaged heart to the whole wide world (Buber & Smith, 2010; Salzberg, 2011).

RESEARCH ON MINDFULNESS

Integrating an EH approach with mindfulness can result in positive therapeutic outcomes supported by empirical studies. Through neuropsychophysiology, mindfulness can be used to restructure the brain. The research identified many outcomes of mindfulness, criticisms, and even adverse effects. Such studies supported therapists in better evaluating if, when, and how mindfulness should be incorporated. Clinical mindfulness programs were studied to evaluate the efficacy and acceptability of mindfulness to multiple therapeutic outcomes. Empirical support for the use of mindfulness in EH therapy also exists. Quantitative and qualitative research explored these outcomes and the efficacy of a combined approach in various contexts. The following sections review these topics and the associated research.

The Neuropsychophysiology of Mindfulness

Mindfulness is a state of consciousness that impacts an individual's brain, body, and behavior (Tang, 2017). Within an individual, mindfulness can exist as both a state and a trait (Sutcliffe et al., 2016). Trait mindfulness, often called dispositional mindfulness, represents an individual's overall level of mindfulness, whereas state mindfulness refers to the state of consciousness in a specific moment, such as right after meditating (Karl & Fischer, 2022; Qu et al., 2022; Sutcliffe et al., 2016). Mindfulness is effective with as little as 10 minutes per day of practice and has been shown to produce positive outcomes even when self-guided or digitally delivered (Creswell, 2017; Fincham et al., 2023; Taylor et al., 2021). The efficacy of mindfulness is a product of its neuropsychophysiology, which produces meaningful changes in the central and peripheral nervous and endocrine systems (Tang, 2017).

Neuroscientific studies have shown both structural and functional changes in the brain due to mindfulness practice (Kang & Falk, 2020; B. Liu et al., 2017). According to Tang (2017), mindfulness comprises enhanced attentional control, improved emotional regulation, and modified self-awareness. Each of these elements corresponds to select structures within the brain. Mindfulness has increased cortical folding, thickness, brain volume, gray matter, and cerebral blood flow (Bremer et al., 2022; Rahrig et al., 2022; Tang, 2017). Mindfulness can also increase brain-derived neurotrophic factor production, further enhancing overall neuroplasticity (Yang et al., 2020).

Valk and colleagues (2017) showed changes in the brain's socio-affective and cognitive areas in response to mindfulness training. The attention training increased cortical thickness in prefrontal regions, whereas the socio-affective training resulted in structural plasticity and changes to the temporal cortices. Findings such as Valk and colleagues support the argument that mindfulness can enhance social understanding. When practiced and used relationally, mindfulness can foster enhanced well-being, authenticity, willingness to change, increased ethical behavior, reduced bias, and awareness of social systems and politics (Johnson et al., 2020; Kang & Falk, 2020; S. Liu et al., 2020; Schuh et al., 2019).

Physiologically, mindfulness may be interpreted as taking part in any activity that calms the brain's sympathetic nervous system in the face of stress and activates the parasympathetic nervous system with its sensations of ease, centeredness, and present moment awareness (Tang, 2017). The sympathetic nervous system releases stress hormones, such as cortisol, that alter the body's homeostasis or allostatic load (McEwen, 2000). In small doses, these hormones are protective. As the levels of hormones rise, the body compensates for the new allostatic load by adapting a new baseline equilibrium (Schoenberg & Gonzalez, 2023). Over time, increased stress hormones can result in inflammatory diseases and chronic illness (McEwen, 2000). The body plays an essential and grounding role in mindfulness, such as in a body scan meditation or mindful breathing. Tang (2017) elegantly stated,

> Stress has two types: (1) somatic stress in the body, e.g., a racing heart, indigestion, or the jitters; and (2) stress in mental cognitive stress, e.g., worrisome thoughts that keep one up at night or that continually intrude into one's attention during the day. Most importantly, stress from body and mind work together and interact. Research indicates that there is no single best way to erase cognitive or somatic anxiety, including meditation and yoga. Not everyone will benefit from a body-focused method, just as meditation may not be the best way to fight stress for each person. *However, a body-mind technique that can help you relax your body and calm your mind seems a promising choice and is worth the effort.* (p. 27; italics in original)

Individual differences in psychological and biological resources, such as personal resilience, heart rate variability, cardiac vagal tone, and oxytocin levels, for example, may compound the effects for some people while delaying the effects for others (Barczak-Scarboro et al., 2021; Buric et al., 2022; Ferreira-Garcia et al., 2021). Several studies found that the quality and type of the mindfulness or meditation practice (such as loving kindness, body scan, or walking meditations) impacted the strength of the individual outcomes, suggesting that the practitioner's intentionality is a component of the achieved outcomes (Day et al., 2023; Palmer et al., 2023; Rahrig et al., 2022; Zeng et al., 2023).

Outcomes of Mindfulness Practices

The personal benefits of mindfulness activities are considerable, as is the evidence base supporting the practice (Baminiwatta & Solangaarachchi, 2021; Creswell, 2017; Schlechta Portella et al., 2021). Mindfulness practice improves mental and physical health, enhances cognition, improves well-being, and reduces stress (Althammer et al., 2021; Eby et al., 2019). In a review of mindfulness interventions, Creswell (2017) reported multiple individual physical and mental health outcomes as areas of improved health, including chronic pain, immunity, health behaviors, and clinical symptoms. Psychologically, mindfulness is an evidence-based treatment for depression and anxiety symptoms, addiction and substance use, relapse, and posttraumatic stress disorder (Creswell, 2017).

The research community has yet to fully establish if mindfulness is effective in all populations (Eichel et al., 2021). Mindfulness practice may lead to adverse effects for some participants (Buric et al., 2022; Farias et al., 2020; Hanssen et al., 2021; Pauly et al., 2022). Farias and colleagues (2020) systematically reviewed 83 meditation studies and found that adverse effects occur in approximately 8.3% of participants. The most frequently cited adverse effects consisted of anxiety, depression, and cognitive issues (Farias et al., 2020). The adverse effects of mindfulness-based interventions (MBIs) are not always harmful to the individual experiencing them. Many participants view them as a necessary part of the therapeutic process (Hanssen et al., 2021). In an international cross-sectional study, Pauly and colleagues (2022) found that 3.1% of MBI participants needed countermeasures, and less than 1% experienced lasting consequences. There is no indication that the adverse effects of meditation are dissimilar to other psychological interventions (Britton et al., 2021).

Mindfulness may contribute to a healthy workplace (Eby et al., 2019; Michaelsen et al., 2023). In an analysis of mindfulness training in the workplace, Johnson and colleagues (2020) found 51 unique outcomes of mindfulness training at the individual, workplace, and organizational levels. Workplace outcomes included employee engagement, job performance, productivity, and work–life balance, whereas group and team outcomes included less conflict, increased cooperation, and group cohesion. On the organizational level, mindfulness training resulted in increased leader procedural justice enactment, workplace culture, and organizational climate. Michaelsen and colleagues (2023) conducted a systematic review and metaregression analysis of 91 randomized controlled trials ($N = 4,927$) on MBIs in the workplace. They found significant changes with smaller effect sizes in mindfulness, well-being, mental health, stress, resilience, physical health, and work-related factors.

Criticisms of Mindfulness

As the popularity of mindfulness has increased, so have criticisms of the modernized practice (Nehring & Frawley, 2020; Pagis, 2019). Researchers and practitioners have voiced concerns that removing the spiritual components of mindfulness appropriates cultural practices, eliminating the most meaningful aspects (Nehring & Frawley, 2020). By presenting mindfulness as a clinical healing method, Kabat-Zinn frames mindfulness as part of the medicalization of everyday life and the therapy–disease cycle (Carvalho, 2021; Kołodziejska & Paliński, 2023; Pagis, 2019). Kołodziejska and Paliński (2023) conducted a qualitative analysis of *Headspace* blog posts that showed the app framed mindfulness as scientific and medical and described their services in medical or therapeutic terms to monitor health and well-being. Medicalized mindfulness is typically presented in secular formats, focusing on self-improvement over collective improvement. According to Wrenn (2022), "Neoliberalism teaches through the socialization process that each individual should be accountable to herself [*sic*], and in so doing, it also leads to the erosion of each individual's responsibility to others and to the community as a whole" (p. 158).

Another prominent criticism, dubbed "McMindfulness," argues that the commercialization of mindfulness is antithetical to its original Buddhist goals (du Plessis & Just, 2022; Hyland, 2017; Nehring & Frawley, 2020; Pagis, 2019). For example, the use of mindfulness by military forces as a means of preparing for battle is both anti-Buddhist and anti-humanist (Segall, 2021; Wrenn, 2022). Similarly, critics have accused organizations providing mindfulness in the workplace of appropriating the concept for profit, productivity, and neoliberal goals (Pagis, 2019; Schmid & Taylor Aiken, 2021; Wrenn, 2022). In this way, mindfulness is used for behavior modification or to support capitalism instead of as a means of liberation from and critical analysis of social systems and structures (Leggett, 2021; Wrenn, 2022). For example, acceptance of the current circumstances can be understood as approval of the status quo rather than a problem to be solved (Choi et al., 2021). Nonjudgmental acceptance can be interpreted in marginalized communities as the need to accept oppressive conditions (Choi et al., 2021; Leggett, 2021; Pagis, 2019; Schmid & Taylor Aiken, 2021).

There are legitimate concerns about the diversity and composition of the mindfulness movement (Pagis, 2019), particularly given the cultural appropriation of mindfulness practices. American meditation practitioners are overwhelmingly White, middle- and upper-class, and highly educated (Pagis, 2019). The skew in demographic representation extends to research on mindfulness interventions (Eichel et al., 2021). Underrepresenting minoritized populations in mindfulness research or not reporting those statistics perpetuates systemic racism and other forms of discrimination that have led to existing inequalities (Eichel et al., 2021). The value of increasing diversity within mindfulness research extends beyond scientific generalization. The United States' diversifying population means that it will become a majority-minority country within a decade (Frey, 2020). Marginalized communities are increasingly likely to experience environments that negatively impact health, behavior, and quality of life outcomes than majority White communities (Healthy People 2030, n.d.). The existential nature of this population shift can be addressed in psychotherapy by integrating mindfulness into an EH therapeutic approach.

Clinical Mindfulness Programs

There is a narrative thread in clinical psychology that mindfulness training was introduced into health care as the third wave of cognitive behavior therapy, with robust research highlighting positive patient transformations (Hayes & Hofmann, 2017). Several contemporary clinical applications of mindfulness include psychotherapeutic approaches intended to deal with significant mental health challenges, such as MBSR, acceptance and commitment therapy (ACT), mindfulness-based cognitive therapy (MBCT), and mindfulness-based relapse prevention (MBRP). Mindfulness-based approaches have been evaluated in multiple studies and meta-analyses since their introduction. They continue to be investigated for applicability to specific physical and mental health and wellness needs. For example, Gloster and colleagues (2020) reviewed 20 meta-analyses of ACT ($N = 12,477$) and found the therapy efficacious for anxiety, depression, substance use, pain, and transdiagnostic groups. In this review, ACT was generally superior to control conditions, including inactive controls, treatment as usual, and active interventions (Gloster et al., 2020).

Similarly, Ramadas and colleagues (2021) conducted a systematic review of the effectiveness of MBRP in individuals with substance use disorders, which showed overall efficacy and specifically reduced cravings, frequency of use, and depressive symptoms. The evidence base supporting the use of MBSR and MBCT for health and well-being in nonclinical populations was analyzed by Querstret and colleagues (2020). They reviewed 49 studies of MBSR and MBCT in nonclinical populations ($N = 4,733$) and found a significant reduction of worry, stress, depression, and anxiety, as well as improved well-being. Although clinical mindfulness programs center on mindfulness training and practice, they include other therapeutic components that support the intended therapeutic use. Mindfulness's effects on the mind and body make it a valuable addition to any integrative psychotherapy approach.

Quantitative Research on Mindfulness and EH Therapy Core Concepts

Several quantitative research studies have explored the outcomes of a therapeutic integration of mindfulness and EH psychotherapy. One of the most direct examinations of the integrated therapeutic approach was done through a randomized controlled trial known as the EXMIND study (Akase et al., 2020; Kawano et al., 2021; Sakai et al., 2019). Sakai and colleagues (2019) wanted to determine if the sequential combination of the two treatments would produce improved outcomes for healthy patients. The EXMIND intervention consisted of a 4 week MBI followed by a 4 week existential approach ($n = 69$) and was compared with an 8 week MBI group ($n = 68$) and a wait-list control group ($n = 31$; Sakai et al., 2019). Sakai and colleagues published the original study's results to determine if the sequential combination of the two treatments would produce improved outcomes for healthy patients. The initial study confirmed the cooperative nature of the treatments and found that although both interventions increased self-compassion, the EXMIND group results were more robust.

The second EXMIND study, published by Akase and colleagues (2020), sought to identify the factors that predicted the changes in self-compassion observed in the original study. Using the baseline, 4 week, and 8 week self-compassion scores, they conducted multiple regression analyses and calculated Pearson's correlation coefficients based on several other baseline scales. The analysis suggested that purpose in life was significantly and positively associated with self-compassion scores. At the same time, novelty seeking was significantly and negatively associated with the change in self-compassion from the intervention.

Kawano and colleagues (2021), in a secondary analysis of the EXMIND data, sought to identify the predictors that led to the EXMIND results. Participants were grouped based on their change in response pattern to the Self-Compassion Scale: a positive response to the MBI and a negative response to the existential approach (n = 15), a negative response to the MBI and a positive response to the existential approach (n = 23), a positive response to both interventions (n = 20), and a negative response to both interventions (n = 2). They found that the participants who reacted positively to both interventions identified as having more maternal overprotectiveness in childhood than those in the other groups, suggesting that a combined approach might work best for clients who experienced childhood maternal overprotectiveness.

While the EXMIND studies directly examined the relationship between mindfulness and EH therapy, other studies have identified outcomes that provide evidential support for an integrated approach. Krieger and colleagues (2019) conducted a randomized controlled trial on an internet-based compassion intervention for individuals with high levels of self-criticism. The participants completed the Self-Compassion Scale, the Comprehensive Inventory of Mindfulness Experience, and a subscale (to measure existential shame) of the Multifarious Expressions of Shame survey. Krieger and colleagues found that the intervention could be used transdiagnostically and adjunctively to decrease self-criticism, as often seen in individuals with depression and anxiety. Palitsky and colleagues (2022) conducted several studies that explored whether religious worldview impacted the acceptability of an MBI by examining scriptural literalism and existential flexibility. Palitsky and colleagues stated, "MBI framing, as well as participants' religious and existential perspectives, may influence MBI acceptability and implementation" (2022, p. 1). These studies support tailoring integrated interventions to the client's desired outcomes and worldview.

Qualitative Research on Mindfulness and EH Therapy Core Concepts

Qualitative research on mindfulness and EH therapy provides insights into patient experiences in these areas. Bellin (2017) conducted a narrative investigation of individuals who identify with marginalized groups within the United States. Bellin's research identified five critical humanistic skills in exploring how humanistic psychotherapy can help clients alleviate meaning and frustration driven by oppression. These included providing a safe therapeutic container, providing unconditional positive regard, providing context, aiding the client in taking responsibility for their feelings and actions, and helping the client overcome frustration while acknowledging the reality of oppressive forces.

In addition to examining the therapeutic relationship between mindfulness and EH therapy, studies have also examined the relationship between mindfulness and EH therapists (Bonner et al., 2021; Ivers & Johnson, 2022). Ivers and

Johnson (2022) explored the relationship between mindfulness and multicultural counseling competence among various mental health practitioners. The qualitative results of the study indicate that mindfulness practices could enhance a practitioner's awareness and acceptance of their own cultural biases while not imposing their views on the client (Ivers & Johnson, 2022). In a 3-year mixed-methods study of clinical psychology students, Rockwell (2019) found that mindfulness provided therapists in training the courage to "directly face" their personal and professional experiences (p. 193). Although the existential nature of marginalization and the ability of mindfulness to calm the nervous system make an integrated approach appealing, care must be taken to adopt the practices to multicultural audiences.

MULTICULTURAL CONSIDERATIONS

EH perspectives, coupled with the benefits of mindfulness, can serve as tools for personal and collective transformation, provided they can be adapted to diverse, multicultural audiences. Hoffman, Granger, and colleagues (2016) examined the Black Lives Matter movement from the EH perspective. They found that the movement creatively harnessed pain, anger, and suffering as a platform for cultural change and increased human dignity. The natural alignment of social justice and humanistic values provides fertile grounds for EH therapy and mindfulness to support multicultural objectives. This section reviews the intersectional history of EH therapy, mindfulness, and multiculturalism; proposes a framework for integrating these concepts; and concludes with methods for identifying and integrating cultural adaptations that can enhance the value and efficacy of mindfulness and associated therapeutic modalities.

When integrating mindfulness into EH therapy, multiculturalism should be one of the most salient points to consider, and it has been largely missing in past approaches. Before multiculturalism in mindfulness can become realized, EH psychology must recognize the physical, psychological, and spiritual harm that still premediates in multicultural groups' subconsciousness. If not, multiculturalism in mindfulness cannot become fully actualized.

An experiential example of how multicultural mindfulness can be applied within EH therapy was demonstrated to the participants of Hoover Treatment Center's inpatient recovery and rehabilitation program. The program, known as the Soul of Healing Community Day Program, was designed as part of unpublished research by coauthor of this chapter O'Dell Johnson, founder of the Research Institute for Social Equity. This organization helps those who experience addiction, the criminal justice system, and reentry through holistic mind-body-soul integration. Johnson incorporated best practices, including Chopra and Simon's (2004) soul of healing immersion training; Engel's (1977) biopsychosocial model that incorporates the biological, psychological, and social environment of daily life; and Kuhn's (1962) structure of scientific revolutions paradigm shift model. The goal was to help participants understand how they are intimately connected to the world in multiplicity and how that way of knowing can metamotivate personal empowerment. The participants, based on their pre- and poststudy evaluations, showed that the introduction to mindfulness practices changed the way they looked at the world as well as their struggle with addiction. The group desired to learn more about applying mindfulness daily as they recovered.

In another instance, multicultural mindfulness adaptations played a significant role in addressing stress, anxiety, and depression cross-culturally on a global scale in the wake of George Floyd's murder (Ao, 2021). Community-based organizations began to offer MBSR in cities and rural communities across the United States. In these spaces, community members work through their emotions related to structural racism and discrimination in a familiar environment where they can speak openly, share, and learn from each other's lived experiences (Ao, 2021). Additionally, multicultural considerations for Asian Americans are important because mindfulness-based therapy disparities continue to exist for this population (Hall et al., 2011). The development of effective treatments for both Black and Asian Americans is vital because psychological treatment disparities persist between persons of color and White Americans of European descent (Hall et al., 2011). The mindfulness disparities among Asian Americans are complex given that mindfulness concepts and techniques were developed in South Asian cultures and appropriated from them. In working with these disparities, it will be important to decolonize them, which might include acknowledging the appropriation of mindfulness and supporting Indigenous practitioners in reintegrating the spiritual and cultural aspects that have been removed. Multicultural adaptations include the integration of relevant cultural considerations and factors, such as interdependence and spirituality, into practice (Hall et al., 2011). Therefore, a culturally syntonic approach that accentuates specific components of mindfulness and acceptance psychotherapies is needed to adapt other components of mindfulness-based approaches to be more consistent with both ethnic group and cultural values.

Cross-Cultural Adaptation Models

Proper cultural adaptation requires communicating with the population and truly understanding their needs. Many frameworks for cultural adaptation exist and can be used to ensure the cultural appropriateness of a treatment or intervention (Domenech Rodríguez & Bernal, 2012). Bernal and colleagues (2009) proposed one example: the ecological validity framework. The framework comprises eight categories: language, persons, metaphors, content, concepts, goals, methods, and context (Bernal et al., 2009). The categories of adaptation address cultural alignment among the therapist, client, and treatment. For example, adaptations within the persons category might include modifying components such as therapeutic alliance, ethnic match, and client expectations.

Adapting MBIs by tailoring the content and context to incorporate attributes specific to the audience's culture is acceptable and effective (Castellanos et al.,

2020; Eichel et al., 2021). Adaptations are made primarily to increase engagement rather than for efficacy reasons and aim to align treatment with the client's culture and perspective (Castellanos et al., 2020). When adaptations are made, they are typically superficial to the material, such as using the participants' native language (Castellanos et al., 2020). In their review of MBIs for Hispanic populations, Castellanos and colleagues (2020), using the Bernal and colleagues' (2009) framework, found that language and person adaptations were by far the most prevalent in the reviewed studies, with 90% and 80% including these adaptations, respectively. Conversely, concept adaptations, such as how treatment is explained to the client, were not used in any study, and goal adaptations were only used in 1% of the studies reviewed. The remaining categories of adaptations were seen in 10%–30% of the reviewed studies. No study addressed cultural considerations in all eight categories.

There are, however, indications that intergroup differences may result in differences in efficacy. For example, Greenfield and colleagues (2018) found that race, ethnicity, and racial group composition moderated the effectiveness of MBRP. In the study, participants had improved outcomes from MBRP when their race or ethnicity was reflected in the group composition (Greenfield et al., 2018). However, differences in efficacy between groups were also found. MBRP was more effective for alcohol use among White populations, whereas among marginalized populations, MBRP was more effective at preventing drug use relapse (Greenfield et al., 2018).

Spears (2019) provides several suggestions for adaptations, including (a) discussing key terms like mindfulness and meditation with participants, (b) warning participants of potential adverse impacts and mitigation strategies such as leaving their eyes open or shortening the length of the intervention, and (c) directly addressing any barriers participants may encounter with their practice. Spears also discussed the importance of religion and empowerment, noting specifically the difference between mindful acceptance and resignation. Proulx and colleagues (2018) similarly proposed that when working with marginalized American communities, care should be taken to be inclusive and to respect and appreciate the culture's strengths. Ultimately, Proulx and colleagues recommended that the very facets of mindfulness itself be brought to every cultural encounter: "trust, gratitude, patience, beginner's mind, curiosity, non-judging acceptance, and non-attachment" (p. 369).

FUTURE RESEARCH NEEDS

Additional research will be required to strengthen the connections among EH therapy, mindfulness, and multiculturalism. Specifically, four areas are ripe for qualitative and quantitative inquiry: education and training on multicultural mindfulness, increased adaptation of MBIs for cultural coherence, comparative efficacy of spiritual and nonspiritual mindfulness, and an exploration of how collective mindfulness, social psychology, and EH concepts can support social justice movements.

Several authors have identified sampling problems within mindfulness research. Eichel and colleagues (2021) conducted a retrospective systematic review of mindfulness research from 2000 to 2016 to examine demographic diversity. Eichel and colleagues found that of 94 randomized controlled trials, 79% of research participants were White and 70% were female. Additionally, participants were predominantly middle-aged and highly educated. These demographics do not parallel U.S. census demographic statistics. Researchers found that White individuals were sampled at an almost 20% higher rate than the U.S. population (Spears, 2019). This lack of diversity extends to sexuality- and gender-diverse groups as well. Sun and colleagues (2021) conducted a systematic review of MBIs for sexuality- and gender-diverse groups, identifying that population as particularly vulnerable to psychological and behavioral health issues that mindfulness may aid. Less than 2% of 769 reviewed studies reported sexuality and gender samples and results for MBIs (Sun et al., 2021). Education and training on cultural adaptations, including language translations and train-the-trainer programs for facilitators from the community or population serviced, would aid in integrating mindfulness practices into diverse communities.

Research on the efficacy of mindfulness and EH therapy within specific populations is important and necessary. However, there is a growing need for intersectional solutions and research that can address multicultural needs more robustly. In addition to considerations for intersectionality, research should establish what types of cultural adaptations are most effective for specific populations. Due to the rising awareness of systematic inequity and structural racism, researchers may now be encouraged to report the race, sex, gender, age, and socioeconomic status of research participants (Eichel et al., 2021). Thus, though intersectionality has been challenging to track in research, improved reporting requirements may shed light on this topic through future research and regression analysis.

Qualitative and quantitative research may also illuminate a better understanding of the importance of spirituality in mindfulness and how that may vary between clinical applications of mindfulness and everyday use by nonclinical populations. Comparative efficacy of spiritual and nonspiritual mindfulness may illuminate critical insights into the mechanisms of mindfulness and the mind-body-soul relationship.

Finally, future research on collective mindfulness and social psychology may provide insights into applying EH therapeutic concepts to public mental health initiatives. Despite being a primarily internal process, mindfulness training often occurs in social spaces. Research has shown that collective mindfulness results in more robust experiences and a greater sense of spirituality (Pagis, 2019). In relationships, mindfulness is related to decreased anger and increased compassion and people feeling less dependent on their significant others (Pagis, 2019).

Hoffman (2021) discusses the impacts on the mental health field from the COVID-19 pandemic and how EH therapy can assist. Hoffman notes that EH practices can help populations deal with "existential guilt, existential shattering, existential anxiety, and existential perspectives on self-care" (p. 33). Citing presence, a core concept of mindfulness, as a critical relational component of trauma recovery, Hoffman argues that short-term strategies incorporating mindfulness and somatic components were appropriate counterparts to EH therapy. Mindfulness can promote posttraumatic growth as a potential alternative outcome to posttraumatic stress disorder (Tedeschi s, 2018). For example, worldwide events, such as the COVID-19 pandemic and climate change acceleration, increase the potential for research studies investigating EH therapy and mindfulness as a healing modality for these existential challenges (Vos, 2023).

CONCLUSION

There is strong evidence for the effectiveness of mindfulness with many clients and its effectiveness outside of psychotherapy. There is also strong evidential support for EH therapy, as discussed in this book. There is emerging evidence for using mindfulness in EH therapy. Existential and humanistic principles, including valuing empathy, compassion, and human dignity, are as important when applied collectively as when they are applied to an individual. Hoffman, Granger, and Mansilla (2016) note that criticism of EH psychotherapy includes concerns that the field encourages acceptance of current circumstances or focuses on individual behavior modification rather than liberation or critical analysis of social systems and structures. To make this connection effective, social movements could strategically use mindfulness and meditation in ways that support and develop more than just awareness and acceptance of the present moment. More deeply appreciating the heart-centered aspects of mindfulness, such as compassion, empathy, and gratitude—components shared with EH principles—is a critical step in moving from awareness and reflection into an engaged, mindfulness-in-action that can genuinely change the world. Jon Kabat-Zinn (2021b) has written about mindfulness's liberating power as a transformation tool. According to Kabat-Zinn (2021a), mindfulness

> begins a journey toward realizing who we really are and living our lives as if they really mattered. . . . And not just for ourselves. In little but far from insignificant ways, our lives and our embodied practice matter for the world as well as for ourselves. (p. 791)

REFERENCES

Akase, M., Terao, T., Kawano, N., Sakai, A., Hatano, K., Shirahama, M., Hirakawa, H., Kohno, K., & Ishii, N. (2020). More purpose in life and less novelty seeking predict improvements in self-compassion during a mindfulness-based intervention: The EXMIND study. *Frontiers in Psychiatry, 11*, 252. https://doi.org/10.3389/fpsyt.2020.00252

Althammer, S. E., Reis, D., van der Beek, S., Beck, L., & Michel, A. (2021). A mindfulness intervention promoting work–life balance: How segmentation preference affects changes in detachment, well-being, and work–life balance. *Journal of Occupational and Organizational Psychology, 94*(2), 282–308. https://doi.org/10.1111/joop.12346

Alvear, D., Soler, J., & Cebolla, A. (2022). Meditators' non-academic definition of mindfulness. *Mindfulness, 13*(6), 1544–1554. https://doi.org/10.1007/s12671-022-01899-3

Anālayo, B. (2019). Adding historical depth to definitions of mindfulness. *Current Opinion in Psychology, 28,* 11–14. https://doi.org/10.1016/j.copsyc.2018.09.013

Anālayo, B. (2022a). Beyond the limitations of binary thinking: Mindfulness and the Tetralemma. *Mindfulness, 13*(6), 1410–1417. https://doi.org/10.1007/s12671-021-01678-6

Anālayo, B. (2022b). Situating mindfulness, part 1: Early Buddhism and scientific research in psychology. *Mindfulness, 13*(3), 577–583. https://doi.org/10.1007/s12671-021-01673-x

Anālayo, B. (2022c). Situating mindfulness, part 2: Early Buddhist soteriology. *Mindfulness, 13*(4), 855–862. https://doi.org/10.1007/s12671-021-01680-y

Ao, B. (2021, April 21). How mindfulness and meditation have helped Philadelphians of color cope with stress. *Philadelphia Inquirer.* https://www.inquirer.com/health/mindfulness-meditation-people-of-color-racism-philadelphia-penn-20210421.html

Baer, R. A. (2003). Mindfulness training as a clinical intervention: A conceptual and empirical review. *Clinical Psychology: Science and Practice, 10*(2), 125–143. https://doi.org/10.1093/clipsy.bpg015

Baminiwatta, A., & Solangaarachchi, I. (2021). Trends and developments in mindfulness research over 55 years: A bibliometric analysis of publications indexed in Web of Science. *Mindfulness, 12*(9), 2099–2116. https://doi.org/10.1007/s12671-021-01681-x

Barczak-Scarboro, N. E., Van Cappellen, P., & Fredrickson, B. L. (2021). For whom do meditation interventions improve mental health symptoms? Looking at the roles of psychological and biological resources over time. *Mindfulness, 12*(11), 2781–2793. https://doi.org/10.1007/s12671-021-01742-1

Becker, E. (2020). *The denial of death.* Profile Books Ltd.

Bellin, Z. J. (2017). Attending to meaning in life in the lives of marginalized individuals. *The Journal of Humanistic Counseling, 56*(3), 211–227. https://doi.org/10.1002/johc.12054

Bernal, G., Jiménez-Chafey, M. I., & Domenech Rodríguez, M. M. (2009). Cultural adaptation of treatments: A resource for considering culture in evidence-based practice. *Professional Psychology: Research and Practice, 40*(4), 361–368. https://doi.org/10.1037/a0016401

Bishop, S. R., Lau, M., Shapiro, S., Carlson, L., Anderson, N. D., Carmody, J., Segal, Z. V., Abbey, S., Speca, M., Velting, D., & Devins, G. (2004). Mindfulness: A proposed operational definition. *Clinical Psychology: Science and Practice, 11*(3), 230–241. https://doi.org/10.1093/clipsy.bph077

Bonner, M. W., Ford, D. J., Jr., Ferguson, A. L., Nadrich, T., Branch, C. J., Hannon, M. D., & Vereen, L. G. (2021). Creating homeplace for Black male counselor educators: A heuristic inquiry. *The Journal of Humanistic Counseling, 60*(3), 215–236. https://doi.org/10.1002/johc.12166

Bremer, B., Wu, Q., Mora Álvarez, M. G., Hölzel, B. K., Wilhelm, M., Hell, E., Tavacioglu, E. E., Torske, A., & Koch, K. (2022). Mindfulness meditation increases default mode, salience, and central executive network connectivity. *Scientific Reports, 12*(1), 13219. https://doi.org/10.1038/s41598-022-17325-6

Britton, W. B., Lindahl, J. R., Cooper, D. J., Canby, N. K., & Palitsky, R. (2021). Defining and measuring meditation-related adverse effects in mindfulness-based programs. *Clinical Psychological Science, 9*(6), 1185–1204. https://doi.org/10.1177/2167702621996340

Buber, M., & Smith, R. G. (2010). *I and thou.* Martino Publishing.

Bugental, J. F. T. (1992). *The art of the psychotherapist: How to develop the skills that take psychotherapy beyond science.* W. W. Norton & Company.

Buric, I., Farias, M., Driessen, J. M. A., & Brazil, I. A. (2022). Individual differences in meditation interventions: A meta-analytic study. *British Journal of Health Psychology, 27*(3), 1043–1076. https://doi.org/10.1111/bjhp.12589

Carvalho, A. (2021). Rethinking the politics of meditation: Practice, affect and ontology. *The Sociological Review, 69*(6), 1260–1276. https://doi.org/10.1177/00380261211029457

Castellanos, R., Yildiz Spinel, M., Phan, V., Orengo-Aguayo, R., Humphreys, K. L., & Flory, K. (2020). A systematic review and meta-analysis of cultural adaptations of mindfulness-based interventions for Hispanic populations. *Mindfulness, 11*(2), 317–332. https://doi.org/10.1007/s12671-019-01210-x

Choi, E., Farb, N., Pogrebtsova, E., Gruman, J., & Grossmann, I. (2021). What do people mean when they talk about mindfulness? *Clinical Psychology Review, 89,* 102085. https://doi.org/10.1016/j.cpr.2021.102085

Chopra, D., & Simon, D. (2004). *The seven spiritual laws of yoga: A practical guide to healing body, mind, and spirit.* John Wiley & Sons.

Creswell, J. D. (2017). Mindfulness interventions. *Annual Review of Psychology, 68*(1), 491–516. https://doi.org/10.1146/annurev-psych-042716-051139

Day, M. A., Matthews, N., Davies, J. N., Walker, C., Bray, N., Kim, J., & Jensen, M. P. (2023). Outcome expectancies, effects, and mechanisms of brief training in mindfulness meditation vs. loving-kindness meditation vs a control condition for pain management: A randomized pilot study. *Journal of Pain & Palliative Care Pharmacotherapy.* Advance online publication. https://doi.org/10.1080/15360288.2022.2141944

Domenech Rodríguez, M. M., & Bernal, G. (2012). Frameworks, models, and guidelines for cultural adaptation. In G. Bernal & M. M. Domenech Rodríguez (Eds.), *Cultural adaptations: Tools for evidence-based practice with diverse populations* (pp. 23–44). American Psychological Association. https://doi.org/10.1037/13752-002

du Plessis, E. M., & Just, S. N. (2022). Mindfulness—It's not what you think: Toward critical reconciliation with progressive self-development practices. *Organization, 29*(1), 209–221. https://doi.org/10.1177/1350508421995755

Eby, L. T., Allen, T. D., Conley, K. M., Williamson, R. L., Henderson, T. G., & Mancini, V. S. (2019). Mindfulness-based training interventions for employees: A qualitative review of the literature. *Human Resource Management Review, 29*(2), 156–178. https://doi.org/10.1016/j.hrmr.2017.03.004

Eichel, K., Gawande, R., Acabchuk, R. L., Palitsky, R., Chau, S., Pham, A., Cheaito, A., Yam, D., Lipsky, J., Dumais, T., Zhu, Z., King, J., Fulwiler, C., Schuman-Olivier, Z., Moitra, E., Proulx, J., Alejandre-Lara, A., & Britton, W. (2021). A retrospective systematic review of diversity variables in mindfulness research, 2000–2016. *Mindfulness, 12*(11), 2573–2592. https://doi.org/10.1007/s12671-021-01715-4

Engel, G. L. (1977). The need for a new medical model: A challenge for biomedicine. *Science, 196*(4286), 129–136. https://doi.org/10.1126/science.847460

Farias, M., Maraldi, E., Wallenkampf, K. C., & Lucchetti, G. (2020). Adverse events in meditation practices and meditation-based therapies: A systematic review. *Acta Psychiatrica Scandinavica, 142*(5), 374–393. https://doi.org/10.1111/acps.13225

Felder, A. J., & Robbins, B. D. (2016). The integrated heart of cultural and mindfulness meditation practice in existential phenomenology and humanistic psychotherapy. *The Humanistic Psychologist, 44*(2), 105–126. https://doi.org/10.1037/hum0000021

Felder, A. J., & Robbins, B. D. (2021). Approaching mindful multicultural case formulation: Rogers, Yalom, and existential phenomenology. *Person-Centered and Experiential Psychotherapies, 20*(1), 1–20. https://doi.org/10.1080/14779757.2020.1748697

Ferreira-Garcia, R., Costa, M. A., Gonçalves, F. G., de Nonohay, R. G., Nardi, A. E., Freire, R. C. D. R., & Manfro, G. G. (2021). Heart rate variability: A biomarker of selective response to mindfulness-based treatment versus fluoxetine in generalized anxiety disorder. *Journal of Affective Disorders, 295,* 1087–1092. https://doi.org/10.1016/j.jad. 2021.08.121

Fincham, G. W., Mavor, K., & Dritschel, B. (2023). Effects of mindfulness meditation duration and type on well-being: An online dose-ranging randomized controlled trial. *Mindfulness, 14*(5), 1171–1182. https://doi.org/10.1007/s12671-023-02119-2

Frankl, V. E. (2019). *Man's search for meaning.* Beacon Press. (Original work published 1946)

Frey, W. H. (2020). The nation is diversifying even faster than predicted, according to new census data. *The Brookings Institute.* https://www.brookings.edu/research/new-census-data-shows-the-nation-is-diversifying-even-faster-than-predicted/

Germer, C. K., Siegel, R., & Fulton, P. R. (2005). *Mindfulness and psychotherapy.* Guilford Press.

Gloster, A. T., Walder, N., Levin, M. E., Twohig, M. P., & Karekla, M. (2020). The empirical status of acceptance and commitment therapy: A review of meta-analyses. *Journal of Contextual Behavioral Science, 18,* 181–192. https://doi.org/10.1016/j.jcbs.2020. 09.009

Greenfield, B. L., Roos, C., Hagler, K. J., Stein, E., Bowen, S., & Witkiewitz, K. A. (2018). Race/ethnicity and racial group composition moderate the effectiveness of mindfulness-based relapse prevention for substance use disorder. *Addictive Behaviors, 81,* 96–103. https://doi.org/10.1016/j.addbeh.2018.02.010

Haddock, G., Foad, C. M. G., & Thorne, S. (2022). How do people conceptualize mindfulness? *Royal Society Open Science, 9*(3), 211366. https://doi.org/10.1098/rsos.211366

Hall, G. C. N., Hong, J. J., Zane, N. W. S., & Meyer, O. L. (2011). Culturally competent treatments for Asian Americans: The relevance of mindfulness and acceptance-based psychotherapies. *Clinical Psychology: Science and Practice, 18*(3), 215–231. https://doi.org/10.1111/j.1468-2850.2011.01253.x

Hanssen, I., Scheepbouwer, V., Huijbers, M., Regeer, E., Lochmann van Bennekom, M., Kupka, R., & Speckens, A. (2021). Adverse or therapeutic? A mixed-methods study investigating adverse effects of mindfulness-based cognitive therapy in bipolar disorder. *PLoS One, 16*(11), e0259167. https://doi.org/10.1371/journal.pone.0259167

Hayes, S. C., & Hofmann, S. G. (2017). The third wave of cognitive behavioral therapy and the rise of process-based care. *World Psychiatry, 16*(3), 245–246. https://doi.org/10.1002/wps.20442

Healthy People 2030. (n.d.). *Healthy People 2030: Building a healthier future for all.* https://health.gov/healthypeople

Heidegger, M. (2008). *Basic writings* (D. F. Krell, Ed.). Harper Perennial Modern Thought.

Hoffman, L. (2021). Existential–humanistic therapy and disaster response: Lessons from the COVID-19 pandemic. *Journal of Humanistic Psychology, 61*(1), 33–54. https://doi.org/10.1177/0022167820931987

Hoffman, L., Granger, N., & Mansilla, M. (2016). Multiculturalism and meaning in existential and positive psychology. In P. Russo-Netzer, S. E. Schulenberg, & A. Batthyany (Eds.), *Clinical perspectives on meaning* (pp. 111–130). Springer International Publishing. https://doi.org/10.1007/978-3-319-41397-6_6

Hoffman, L., Granger, N., Jr., Vallejos, L., & Moats, M. (2016). An existential–humanistic perspective on Black Lives Matter and contemporary protest movements. *Journal of Humanistic Psychology, 56*(6), 595–611. https://doi.org/10.1177/0022167816652273

Hoffman, L., Vallejos, L., Cleare-Hoffman, H. P., & Rubin, S. (2015). Emotion, relationship, and meaning as core existential practice: Evidence-based foundations. *Journal of Contemporary Psychotherapy, 45*(1), 11–20. https://doi.org/10.1007/s10879-014-9277-9

Hyland, T. (2017). McDonaldizing spirituality: Mindfulness, education, and consumerism. *Journal of Transformative Education, 15*(4), 334–356. https://doi.org/10.1177/1541344617696972

Ivers, N. N., & Johnson, D. A. (2022). The relationship between mindfulness and multi-cultural counseling competence among mental health practitioners. *The Journal of Humanistic Counseling, 61*(1), 43–57. https://doi.org/10.1002/johc.12170

Johnson, K. R., Park, S., & Chaudhuri, S. (2020). Mindfulness training in the workplace: Exploring its scope and outcomes. *European Journal of Training and Development, 44*(4–5), 341–354. https://doi.org/10.1108/EJTD-09-2019-0156

Kabat-Zinn, J. (2003). Mindfulness-based interventions in context: Past, present, and future. *Clinical Psychology: Science and Practice, 10*(2), 144–156. https://doi.org/10.1093/clipsy.bpg016

Kabat-Zinn, J. (2013). *Full catastrophe living: How to cope with stress, pain and illness using mindfulness* (Rev. ed.). Hachette Book Group.

Kabat-Zinn, J. (2021a). The challenge of a life's time—And a lifetime. *Mindfulness, 12*(3), 788–794. https://doi.org/10.1007/s12671-020-01588-z

Kabat-Zinn, J. (2021b). The liberative potential of mindfulness. *Mindfulness, 12*(6), 1555–1563. https://doi.org/10.1007/s12671-021-01608-6

Kang, Y., & Falk, E. B. (2020). Neural mechanisms of attitude change toward stigmatized individuals: Temporoparietal junction activity predicts bias reduction. *Mindfulness, 11*(6), 1378–1389. https://doi.org/10.1007/s12671-020-01357-y

Karl, J. A., & Fischer, R. (2022). The state of dispositional mindfulness research. *Mindfulness, 13*(6), 1357–1372. https://doi.org/10.1007/s12671-022-01853-3

Kawano, N., Terao, T., Sakai, A., Akase, M., Hatano, K., Shirahama, M., Hirakawa, H., Kohno, K., & Ishii, N. (2021). Maternal overprotection predicts consistent improvement of self-compassion during mindfulness-based intervention and existential approach: A secondary analysis of the EXMIND study. *BMC Psychology, 9*(1), 20. https://doi.org/10.1186/s40359-021-00521-w

Kołodziejska, M., & Paliński, M. (2023). "Train your mind for a healthy life." The medicalization of mediatized mindfulness in the West. *Current Psychology, 42*(18), 15210–15222. https://doi.org/10.1007/s12144-022-02814-8

Krieger, T., Reber, F., von Glutz, B., Urech, A., Moser, C. T., Schulz, A., & Berger, T. (2019). An internet-based compassion-focused intervention for increased self-criticism: A randomized controlled trial. *Behavior Therapy, 50*(2), 430–445. https://doi.org/10.1016/j.beth.2018.08.003

Kuhn, T. S. (1962). *The structure of scientific revolutions*. University of Chicago Press.

Lam, S. U., Riordan, K. M., Simonsson, O., Davidson, R. J., & Goldberg, S. B. (2023). Who sticks with meditation? Rates and predictors of persistence in a population-based sample in the USA. *Mindfulness, 14*(1), 66–78. https://doi.org/10.1007/s12671-022-02061-9

Leggett, W. (2021). Can mindfulness really change the world? The political character of meditative practices. *Critical Policy Studies, 16*(3), 261–278). https://doi.org/10.1080/19460171.2021.1932541

Liu, B., Liu, J., Wang, M., Zhang, Y., & Li, L. (2017). From serotonin to neuroplasticity: Evolvement of theories for major depressive disorder. *Frontiers in Cellular Neuroscience, 11*, 305. https://doi.org/10.3389/fncel.2017.00305

Liu, S., Xin, H., Shen, L., He, J., & Liu, J. (2020). The influence of individual and team mindfulness on work engagement. *Frontiers in Psychology, 10*, 1–8. https://doi.org/10.3389/fpsyg.2019.02928

Maslow, A. H. (1993). *The farther reaches of human nature*. Penguin Compass.

McEwen, B. S. (2000). Allostasis and allostatic load: Implications for neuropsychopharmacology. *Neuropsychopharmacology, 22*(2), 108–124. https://doi.org/10.1016/S0893-133X(99)00129-3

Michaelsen, M. M., Graser, J., Onescheit, M., Tuma, M. P., Werdecker, L., Pieper, D., & Esch, T. (2023). Mindfulness-based and mindfulness-informed interventions at the workplace: A systematic review and meta-regression analysis of RCTs. *Mindfulness, 14*, 1271–1304. https://doi.org/10.1007/s12671-023-02130-7

Najovits, S. (2003). *Egypt, trunk of the tree: A modern survey of an ancient land* (Vols. 1 & 2). Algora Publishing.

Nehring, D., & Frawley, A. (2020). Mindfulness and the 'psychological imagination.' *Sociology of Health & Illness, 42*(5), 1184–1201. https://doi.org/10.1111/1467-9566.13093

Niemiec, C. P., Brown, K. W., Kashdan, T. B., Cozzolino, P. J., Breen, W. E., Levesque-Bristol, C., & Ryan, R. M. (2010). Being present in the face of existential threat: The role of trait mindfulness in reducing defensive responses to mortality salience. *Journal of Personality and Social Psychology, 99*(2), 344–365. https://doi.org/10.1037/a0019388

Pagis, M. (2019). The sociology of meditation. In M. Farias, D. Brazier, & M. Lalljee (Eds.), *The Oxford handbook of meditation*. Oxford University Press. https://doi.org/10.1093/oxfordhb/9780198808640.013.50

Palitsky, R., Kaplan, D. M., Brener, S. A., Mascaro, J. S., Mehl, M. R., & Sullivan, D. (2022). Do worldviews matter for implementation-relevant responses to mindfulness-based interventions? An empirical investigation of existential and religious perspectives. *Mindfulness, 13*(12), 2952–2967. https://doi.org/10.1007/s12671-022-02010-6

Palmer, R., Roos, C., Vafaie, N., & Kober, H. (2023). The effect of ten versus twenty minutes of mindfulness meditation on state mindfulness and affect. *Scientific Reports, 13*(1), 20646. https://doi.org/10.1038/s41598-023-46578-y

Pauly, L., Bergmann, N., Hahne, I., Pux, S., Hahn, E., Ta, T. M. T., Rapp, M., & Böge, K. (2022). Prevalence, predictors and types of unpleasant and adverse effects of meditation in regular meditators: International cross-sectional study. *BJPsych Open, 8*(1), e11. https://doi.org/10.1192/bjo.2021.1066

Perls, F. (1971). *Gestalt therapy verbatim*. Random House Publishing Group.

Phan-Le, N. T., Brennan, L., & Parker, L. (2022). The search for scientific meaning in mindfulness research: Insights from a scoping review. *PLoS One, 17*(5), e0264924. https://doi.org/10.1371/journal.pone.0264924

Proulx, J., Croff, R., Oken, B., Aldwin, C. M., Fleming, C., Bergen-Cico, D., Le, T., & Noorani, M. (2018). Considerations for research and development of culturally relevant mindfulness interventions in American minority communities. *Mindfulness, 9*(2), 361–370. https://doi.org/10.1007/s12671-017-0785-z

Qu, Y., Todorova, G., & Dasborough, M. T. (2022). Someone must be mindful: Trait mindfulness as a boundary condition for paradoxical leader behaviors. *Journal of Leadership & Organizational Studies, 29*(4), 486–499. https://doi.org/10.1177/15480518221115487

Querstret, D., Morison, L., Dickinson, S., Cropley, M., & John, M. (2020). Mindfulness-based stress reduction and mindfulness-based cognitive therapy for psychological health and well-being in non-clinical samples: A systematic review and meta-analysis. *International Journal of Stress Management, 27*(4), 394–411. https://doi.org/10.1037/str0000165

Rahrig, H., Vago, D. R., Passarelli, M. A., Auten, A., Lynn, N. A., & Brown, K. W. (2022). Meta-analytic evidence that mindfulness training alters resting state default mode network connectivity. *Scientific Reports, 12*(1), 12260. https://doi.org/10.1038/s41598-022-15195-6

Ramadas, E., Lima, M. P., Caetano, T., Lopes, J., & Dixe, M. D. A. (2021). Effectiveness of mindfulness-based relapse prevention in individuals with substance use disorders: A systematic review. *Behavioral Sciences, 11*(10), 133. https://doi.org/10.3390/bs11100133

Rockwell, D. (2019). Mindfulness and courage: Lifelong training in clinical psychology: Implications and applications of a three-year study. In L. Hoffman, M. Yang, M. Mansilla, J. Dias, M. Moats, & T. Claypool (Eds.), *Existential psychology East–West* (Vol. 2, pp. 175–196). University Professors Press.

Rogers, C. (1980). *A way of being*. Houghton Mifflin.

Rowe, J. K. (2017). Georges Bataille, Chogyam Trungpa, and radical transformation: Theorizing the political value of mindfulness. *The Arrow: A Journal of Wakeful Society, Culture, and Politics, 4*(2), 47–69.

Rowe, J. K. (2024). *Radical mindfulness: Why transforming fear of death is politically vital.* Routledge.

Sakai, A., Terao, T., Kawano, N., Akase, M., Hatano, K., Shirahama, M., Hirakawa, H., Kohno, K., Inoue, A., & Ishii, N. (2019). Existential and mindfulness-based intervention to increase self-compassion in apparently healthy subjects (the EXMIND Study): A randomized controlled trial. *Frontiers in Psychiatry, 10,* 538. https://doi.org/10.3389/fpsyt.2019.00538

Salzberg, S. (2011). Mindfulness and loving-kindness. *Contemporary Buddhism, 12*(1), 177–182. https://doi.org/10.1080/14639947.2011.564837

Schlechta Portella, C. F., Ghelman, R., Abdala, V., Schveitzer, M. C., & Afonso, R. F. (2021). Meditation: Evidence map of systematic reviews. *Frontiers in Public Health, 9,* 742715. https://doi.org/10.3389/fpubh.2021.742715

Schmid, B., & Taylor Aiken, G. (2021). Transformative mindfulness: The role of mind-body practices in community-based activism. *Cultural Geographies, 28*(1), 3–17. https://doi.org/10.1177/1474474020918888

Schneider, K. J., & Krug, O. T. (2017). *Existential–humanistic therapy* (2nd ed.). American Psychological Association. https://doi.org/10.1037/0000042-000

Schoenberg, P. L. A., & Gonzalez, K. M. (2023). Allostatic mechanism of mind-body medicine for neuroinflammation. *OBM Integrative and Complimentary Medicine, 8*(1). https://doi.org/10.21926/obm.icm.2301005

Schuh, S. C., Zheng, M. X., Xin, K. R., & Fernandez, J. A. (2019). The interpersonal benefits of leader mindfulness: A serial mediation model linking leader mindfulness, leader procedural justice enactment, and employee exhaustion and performance. *Journal of Business Ethics, 156*(4), 1007–1025. https://doi.org/10.1007/s10551-017-3610-7

Segall, S. Z. (2021). Mindfulness in and out of the context of Western Buddhist modernism. *The Humanistic Psychologist, 49*(1), 40–55. https://doi.org/10.1037/hum0000159

Sommers-Spijkerman, M., Austin, J., Bohlmeijer, E., & Pots, W. (2021). New evidence in the booming field of online mindfulness: An updated meta-analysis of randomized controlled trials. *JMIR Mental Health, 8*(7), e28168. https://doi.org/10.2196/28168

Spears, C. A. (2019). Mindfulness-based interventions for addictions among diverse and underserved populations. *Current Opinion in Psychology, 30,* 11–16. https://doi.org/10.1016/j.copsyc.2018.12.012

Sun, Y., Wong, S. Y. S., Zhang, D., Chen, C. H. J., & Yip, B. H. K. (2021). Behavioral activation with mindfulness in treating subthreshold depression in primary care: A cost-utility and cost-effectiveness analysis alongside a randomized controlled trial. *Journal of Psychiatric Research, 132,* 111–115. https://doi.org/10.1016/j.jpsychires.2020.10.006

Sutcliffe, K. M., Vogus, T. J., & Dane, E. (2016). Mindfulness in organizations: A cross-level review. *Annual Review of Organizational Psychology and Organizational Behavior, 3*(1), 55–81. https://doi.org/10.1146/annurev-orgpsych-041015-062531

Tang, Y.-Y. (2017). *The neuroscience of mindfulness meditation: How the body and mind work together to change our behaviour.* Springer. https://doi.org/10.1007/978-3-319-46322-3

Taylor, H., Strauss, C., & Cavanagh, K. (2021). Can a little bit of mindfulness do you good? A systematic review and meta-analyses of unguided mindfulness-based self-help interventions. *Clinical Psychology Review, 89,* 102078. https://doi.org/10.1016/j.cpr.2021.102078

Tedeschi, R. G., Shakespeare-Finch, J., Taku, K., & Calhoun, L. G. (2018). *Posttraumatic growth: Theory, research, and applications.* Routledge. https://doi.org/10.4324/9781315527451

Valk, S. L., Bernhardt, B. C., Trautwein, F.-M., Böckler, A., Kanske, P., Guizard, N., Collins, D. L., & Singer, T. (2017). Structural plasticity of the social brain: Differential change after socio-affective and cognitive mental training. *Science Advances, 3*(10), e1700489. https://doi.org/10.1126/sciadv.1700489

Van Doren, N., Oravecz, Z., Soto, J. A., & Roeser, R. W. (2022). Examining the cultural consensus on beliefs about mindfulness among US college-attending young adults. *Mindfulness, 13*, 2420–2433. https://doi.org/10.1007/s12671-022-01956-x

Vos, J. (2023). Existential psychological therapies: An overview of empirical research. *Pratiques Psychologiques, 29*(4), 211–229. https://doi.org/10.1016/j.prps.2023.06.001

Wrenn, M. V. (2022). Corporate mindfulness culture and neoliberalism. *The Review of Radical Political Economics, 54*(2), 153–170. https://doi.org/10.1177/04866134211063521

Yang, T., Nie, Z., Shu, H., Kuang, Y., Chen, X., Cheng, J., Yu, S., & Liu, H. (2020). The role of BDNF on neural plasticity in depression. *Frontiers in Cellular Neuroscience*. Advance online publication. https://doi.org/10.3389/fncel.2020.00082

Zeng, X., Zheng, Y., Gu, X., Wang, R., & Oei, T. P. (2023). Meditation quality matters: Effects of loving-kindness and compassion meditations on subjective well-being are associated with meditation quality. *Journal of Happiness Studies, 24*(1), 211–229. https://doi.org/10.1007/s10902-022-00582-7

15

The Creative and Expressive Arts Therapies and Existential–Humanistic Psychotherapy

Ilene A. Serlin, Rainbow Tin Hung Ho, Fulya Kurter Musnitsky, and J. Ryan Kennedy

Imagine a soldier returning from war unable to tell of the horrors they witnessed or a community suffering from flooding and devastation trying to make sense of what happened. Western therapies that rely on verbal interventions emphasizing cognitive and behavioral approaches are the typical treatments offered, but frequently they are inadequate in reaching certain individuals who may not be able to initially process trauma well verbally and cognitively (Herman, 1992; Malchiodi, 2020). However, one of the primary reasons that verbal cognitive and behavioral approaches are recommended in such circumstances is that they are outcome oriented, thereby rendering them more justifiable by many third-party payment sources. In contrast, existential–humanistic (EH), artistic, systemic, social justice, and postmodern approaches are generally more process based. Therefore, they are harder to demonstrate as being evidence based and may be overlooked, even though they may be equally effective (Norcross, 2011). As Rollo May (1975) stated, "Creative courage . . . is the discovering of new forms, new symbols, new patterns on which a new society can be built. . . . But those who present directly and immediately the new forms and symbols are the artists" (p. 15).

What's important to note, though, is that the creative and expressive arts therapies offer a potent alternative to verbal cognitive and behavioral approaches and are consistent with the principles of other evidence-based practices in psychology. The American Psychological Association Presidential Task Force on Evidence-Based Practice (2006) defines evidence-based practice in psychology as "the integration of the best available research with clinical

https://doi.org/10.1037/0000446-016
The Evidence-Based Foundations of Existential–Humanistic Therapy, L. Hoffman and V. Lac (Editors)

expertise in the context of patient characteristics, culture, and preferences" (p. 273). This means that within the context of a strong therapeutic relationship, the mental health professional will integrate best practices from research with sound clinical judgment and that these two things will be tempered by the cultural and linguistic context of the client.

This is something that creative and expressive arts therapists are already doing, bolstered by both the training programs and professional associations that support them. The fact that creative and expressive arts therapists are often more focused on process-based therapeutic work rather than outcome-based research on their modalities doesn't diminish the fact that creative and expressive arts therapies are effective, but it does often obfuscate the perception of them by medical and educational establishments (Bella & Serlin, 2013). This results in training new psychologists in a very narrow band of psychological tools and deprives many of help. To address this situation, this chapter focuses on describing what creative and expressive arts therapies are, their EH perspective, and how they access and integrate key concepts from evidence-based practice into outcome evaluations.

To begin, general definitions of creative and expressive arts therapies are provided, and their central distinctions are highlighted. This is followed by a brief overview of each of the creative arts therapies: (a) art therapy, (b) dance/movement therapy, (c) music therapy, (d) drama therapy, (e) psychodrama, and (f) poetry therapy. Locating creative and expressive arts therapies within the framework of an EH context is featured in the subsequent section of the chapter. This is important because it illustrates how so many practices associated with creative and expressive arts therapies support and even invigorate the theoretical and phenomenological intentions of existential and humanistic therapy. The chapter then presents an overview of a variety of research studies pointing to the clinical efficacy of creative and expressive arts therapies across a wide range of demographic and diagnostic populations. These include quantitative, qualitative, and arts-based research findings. To conclude, several multicultural considerations are brought forth for discussion, both from a historical perspective as well as from a more contemporaneous viewpoint.

DEFINING AND CONCEPTUALIZING CREATIVE AND EXPRESSIVE ARTS THERAPIES

What are creative and expressive arts therapies, why are they effective, and how do they align with the principles of evidence-based practice? Although creative and expressive arts therapies are often used interchangeably and share many aspects in common, they are distinct and different professions. Each has its own training programs with levels of credentialing, codes of ethics, standards of practice, scholarly journals, and professional conferences. Although the creative arts themselves have a long history in ancient and indigenous healing practices from around the world (Aristotle, 1961; Jung, 1966), they have only recently been established and recognized as having a part in psychotherapeutic professions. Indeed, all the individual creative arts therapies professional associations have collaborated in creating a field known as creative arts therapies, which is held within the National Coalition of Creative Arts Therapies Association (NCCATA). This organization is made up of delegates from the governing leadership of each of the individual creatives arts therapies associations represented within the association (NCCATA, n.d.).

By contrast, expressive arts therapies use all the arts in an intermodal manner rather than focusing on any single one. They assist clients in tracking psychological issues through the expression of symbols and metaphors that emerge and develop vis-à-vis all the forms of expressive arts media. Expressive arts therapies have their own professional association as well, with national and international training programs and credentialing (International Expressive Arts Therapy Association, n.d.). All expressive arts therapists are mental health professionals with advanced degrees and clinical training. Increasingly, they partner with interdisciplinary teams to meet serious crises and traumas (Bella & Serlin, 2013).

What do creative and expressive arts therapies have in common? Both fields claim their origins in the impulse to create and tell stories from early human history, and some have called these early shamanic healers "humankind's first psychotherapists" (Katz, 2017; Serlin, 1993). All creative arts therapies are based in the power of creativity and creative expression, something the great EH psychologist Rollo May called "the most basic manifestation of a man or woman fulfilling his or her own being in the world" (1975, p. 40). Both creative and expressive arts therapies also rely on the force of the human imagination and work with images to help reveal truths of human existence and bring them into embodied form (Feder & Feder, 1998). The role of the body and embodied cognition are also central aspects of arts therapies (Merleau-Ponty, 1945/1962), supported by more recent understandings in neuroscience and somatic therapies that the mind and body are interrelated (van der Kolk, 2015). Shaping inner subjective and raw experiences into an outer form in a safe-enough environment that is contained and supported by a creative or expressive arts therapist can bring perspective, reflection, and meaning to life (Brooke, 2006).

What makes creative and expressive arts therapies effective? First, creative and expressive arts therapies rely on symbolic and somatic forms of communication that do not require words and are often more indirect, safer forms of expression than verbal approaches. They give form to the invisible and voice to the unspeakable (Brooke, 2006). Second, they can work on the individual, interpersonal, and collective levels. They can address themes such as cultural loss, social injustice, and community healing rituals (Franklin, 2017). Third, they are culturally sensitive and responsive, using both universal archetypal forms of expression and exploration as well as local and indigenous cultural forms (Brooke & Myers, 2015; Katz, 2017).

What Are the Individual Creative Arts Therapies?

The NCCATA includes art therapy, dance/movement therapy, music therapy, drama therapy, psychodrama, and poetry therapy as the primary creative arts therapies (NCCATA, n.d.). Creative arts therapists are trained and credentialed according to their distinct profession, and each creative arts therapy field is governed by a separate professional association with a unique scope of practice. There are more than 15,000 creative arts therapists practicing in the United States and around the world. The following sections include a brief description of each.

Art Therapy
Art therapy can be defined as "an integrative mental health and human services profession that enriches the lives of individuals, families, and communities through active art-making, creative process, applied psychological theory, and human experience within a psychotherapeutic relationship" (American Art Therapy Association, n.d.). The American Art Therapy Association was founded in 1969, and at the time of writing there are 37 master's degree programs in art therapy accredited by the Commission on Accreditation of Allied Health Education Programs (https://caahep-public-site-5be3d9.webflow.io/) and five master's degree programs approved by the American Art Therapy Association, all in the United States. There are three levels of credentialing in art therapy available through the Art Therapy Credentials Board (https://atcb.org/). The first is the registered art therapist for those who have met basic standards in education, experience, and supervision. The second level is the board-certified registered art therapist for those who have earned the registered art therapist certification and further completed a national examination demonstrating the integration of both knowledge and skill. Finally, there is a credential specific to art therapy supervisors called art therapy certified supervisor for board-certified registered art therapists wishing to supervise.

Dance/Movement Therapy
The American Dance Therapy Association defines dance/movement therapy as the psychotherapeutic use of movement to promote emotional, social, cognitive, and physical integration of the individual for the purpose of improving health and well-being (American Dance Therapy Association, n.d.) Although the profession of dance/movement therapy began officially in the United States in 1966 with the founding of the American Dance Therapy Association, its origins are found in ancient and indigenous healing practices (Serlin, 1993). Dance/movement therapists are trained in verbal psychotherapy techniques, but it is also "one of the few modalities offering practitioners such a complete vehicle for bringing body-based, movement-oriented assessment and intervention tools directly into their psychotherapeutic work" (Serlin & Kennedy, 2020, p. 62). At the time of writing, there are seven U.S.-based master's level programs approved by the American Dance Therapy Association. The Dance/Movement Therapy

Certification Board (https://www.adta.org/dmtcb) provides two levels of credentialing. The entry-level credential is the registered dance/movement therapist for those who have completed the foundational requirements in education, experience, and supervision. The board-certified dance/movement therapist is the advanced credential that requires additional supervised hours along with submission of a paper outlining the practitioner's theoretical orientation along with an accompanying paper highlighting how that theoretical orientation is demonstrated in a practical dance/movement therapy session.

Music Therapy

As a modern profession, the American Music Therapy Association (AMTA) defines music therapy as

> the clinical and evidence-based use of music interventions to accomplish individualized goals within a therapeutic relationship by a credentialed professional who has completed an approved music therapy program. Music therapy interventions can address a variety of health care and educational goals. (2005, What Is Music Therapy section)

Some of the many therapeutic objectives of music therapy include promoting wellness, managing stress, alleviating pain, expressing feelings, enhancing memory, improving communication, and promoting physical rehabilitation (AMTA, 2005; Bruscia, 1998). In the United States, music as therapy began in 1832 at the Perkins School for the Blind in Boston, Massachusetts and expanded in 1840 to the American Asylum for the Deaf in New York. In 1950, the National Association for Music Therapy was founded. As of 2022, there were 90 AMTA-approved schools listed on their website in the United States and none abroad. The only professional credential for music therapists is the music therapist board certified offered through the Certification Board for Music Therapists (https://www.cbmt.org/).

Drama Therapy

Drama therapy is the intentional use of drama or theater processes to achieve therapeutic goals (Landy, 2007). The North American Drama Therapy Association defines drama therapy as

> an embodied practice that is active and experiential. This approach can provide the context for participants to tell their stories, set goals and solve problems, express feelings, or achieve catharsis. Through drama, the depth and breadth of inner experience can be actively explored and interpersonal relationship skills can be enhanced. (n.d., para. 2)

The North American Drama Therapy Association was founded in 1979 by pioneers in the field, such as Eleanor Irwin, David Read Johnson, and others. In 2022, there were five master's programs in the United States and one in Canada accredited by the North American Drama Therapy Association. The registered drama therapist is the entry-level credential available for qualified drama therapists, and the board-certified trainer is available for advanced practitioners.

Psychodrama

Psychodrama employs guided dramatic action to examine issues (American Society of Group Psychotherapy and Psychodrama, n.d.). Conceived and developed by Jacob L. Moreno in 1921, psychodrama employs guided dramatic action to examine problems or issues raised by an individual (i.e., psychodrama) or a group (i.e., sociodrama; Moreno, 1947). Using a variety of experiential methods such as sociometry, role theory, and group dynamics, psychodrama facilitates insight, personal growth, and integration on cognitive, affective, and behavioral levels. It can also clarify issues, increase physical and emotional well-being, enhance learning, and develop new skills. The American Society of Group Psychotherapy and Psychodrama was founded in 1942 by Jacob Moreno. In 2022, there were no specific training programs approved by the American Society of Group Psychotherapy and Psychodrama though many individual courses at numerous universities were listed on their website, but many institute-based training programs are currently available. There are two credentials available through the American Board of Examiners in Psychodrama, Sociometry, and Group Psychotherapy (https://psychodramacertification.org/): the certified psychodramatist at the entry level and the trainer, educator, and practitioner at the advanced level.

Poetry Therapy

Poetry therapy is the use of language, symbols, and stories in therapeutic, education, growth, and community-building capacities (Alschuler, 2006). It relies upon the use of poems, stories, song lyrics, imagery, and metaphor to facilitate personal growth, healing, and greater self-awareness. Bibliotherapy, narrative, journal writing, metaphor, storytelling, and ritual are all within the realm of poetry therapy (National Association for Poetry Therapy, n.d.). In 1969, the American Association for Poetry Therapy became the National Association for Poetry Therapy. The association offers two levels of credentialing: certified poetry therapist and registered poetry therapists. Currently, there are no academic programs in the United States that offer a full master's degree in poetry therapy, but there are individual courses available at a variety of institutions, and training can also be done individually through private mentorship with a certified or registered poetry therapist.

CONTEXTUALIZING CREATIVE AND EXPRESSIVE ARTS IN AN EH THERAPY CONTEXT

Professional psychology has been increasingly focused on short-term symptom reduction techniques. Driven by insurance companies and a focus on higher profits, the common human condition is becoming pathologized, requiring diagnoses and medication. Common emotions like shyness and sadness are seen as problems to be fixed. Pain and suffering are to be avoided if possible. Psychological services are becoming more anonymous and impersonal. With telehealth and videoconferencing platforms, the world seems to be becoming more two-dimensional.

What's potentially lost in all of this is the connection to the body, an orientation to a tactile reality, and a relationship to nature and the outside world. Correspondingly, the language of psychology and psychotherapy, in particular, runs the risk of becoming overly clinical, sterile, biological, and technological. Where is the language of the soul in this landscape? Many people who seek psychological support do so because of difficulty finding meaning in their work, feelings of disempowerment, and a sense of inauthenticity. In addition, more systemic problems such as climate change, migration and dislocation, breakdown of communities, cultural loss, and widespread trauma seem to be adding to a sense of existential dread that underlies the individual presenting problems of so many clients (Yalom, 1980) and is resulting in skyrocketing incidences of teenage suicide.

Existential and humanistic psychology provide a path to skillfully contend with the fundamental issues of human life, including the realities of change, loss, and death. They help people name and negotiate the four ultimate concerns or existential challenges identified by Irvin Yalom (1980) as foundational and recurring themes in existential psychology. These ultimate concerns are (a) death and nonbeing, (b) isolation and loneliness, (c) meaninglessness, and (d) the weight of responsibility attached to the freedom of choice. With the support of an existentially oriented mental health professional in a safe-enough environment, clients can find the courage to explore some of these core themes and begin to find their own identity, meaning, and sense of connection within the relationships they choose to have (Schneider & May, 1994).

Rollo May, writing after World War II and living in the United States during a time when the country was preoccupied with threats of nuclear war from the Soviet Union, was one of the first mental health professionals to acknowledge the importance and gravity of existential anxiety. His books became popular as he named this dread and urged people living in the United States not to numb themselves with addictions, medications, or denial (May, 1977). Instead, he importantly noted that anxiety could be harnessed to transform fear into action.

May (1975) explicitly valued the role of the arts in the practice of EH therapy. Besides being a practicing artist himself, he viewed the creation of a life well-lived as an artistic process. He scorned the language of technological psychology and the overuse of pathologizing diagnoses. May understood life as a blank canvas, with the human-as-artist having to find the courage to create even in the face of the great void. All artists experience the terror of the blank page or the unformed movement, but they can follow May's (1975) advice in his book *The Courage to Create* and commit themselves to living more deeply (Serlin, 2009). Indeed, in *The Courage to Create*, May (1975) emphasizes that "we express our being by creating" (p. 8). May believed that the ultimate creativity is a life well-lived and that the role of the mental health professional is to help clients find their own voices and, in so doing, find their own well-lived lives. As this happens, therapists and clients can see the beauty and the personal and universal patterns of all human experience; indeed, art can clarify, deepen, and ennoble this endeavor.

Humanistic psychology brings a lighter touch to existential darkness by emphasizing joy, creativity, play, freedom, and improvisation. Early pioneers of humanistic psychology balanced the mind of Freud and cognitive psychology with the addition of a focus on embodiment and the present moment. The zeitgeist during the 1950s to 1980s saw a resurgence of interest in freedom, the body, and spirituality (Hoffman, 2004). During the early 1970s, the Association for Humanistic Psychology was the first professional organization in the United States to embrace the mind and body disciplines. Somatic psychology, first developed by Thomas Hanna (1988), built on the subjective awareness of one's own sensory–motor condition and provided processes to help heal trauma in the body. Other early humanistic pioneers included Moshé Feldenkrais, Ida Rolf, Eleanor Criswell, Ilana Rubenfeld, Charlotte Selver, Alexander Lowen, and Anna Halprin. Laura Perls (1992) brought in the whole person—mind and body—through Gestalt therapy, and Eugene Gendlin developed the practice of focusing. Sidney Jourard contributed the concept of transparency of the self (Jourard, 1971), Charles Moustakas brought in the element of play, and many used story and narrative to help clients express themselves. Abraham Maslow encouraged the process of self-actualization (Maslow, 1962), and Carl Rogers emphasized unconditional positive regard, genuineness, and accurate empathy as important ingredients in the creative process of psychotherapy (Rogers, 1961). In her book *Composing a Life*, Mary Catherine Bateson (1989), daughter of noted cultural anthropologist Margaret Mead and social scientist and cyberneticist Gregory Bateson, used a musical metaphor of jazz to describe how to create a life. James Bugental (1992), a student of Rollo May and an important figure in the history of EH psychology in the United States, explicitly talked about therapy as an artistic process. He argued that psychology, as both a science and an art, had neglected the art in favor of "physics envy." In his work, he emphasized the art of psychology as an intuitive and open-ended process not unlike a description of composing a life. In this process, the client and therapist cocreate shared meaning by finding the structure in the chaos, tolerating uncertainty, respecting images and emotions, and creating an authentic life of meaning.

Although the creative and expressive arts therapies use certain vocabularies and traditions that are specific to their historical artistic roots and contemporary therapeutic disciplines, most nevertheless have strong threads connecting them to the psychological frameworks found in existential and humanistic perspectives. For example, they are rooted in congruence among the body, mind, and spirit and build on the inner strengths, resilience, and creativity of the client. They believe in the innate capacity of the human for self-actualization (Maslow, 1962) and the key roles of authenticity and genuineness (Bugental, 1992). The therapist starts where the client is at, practices positive regard, and uses kinesthetic empathy (Hawkins, 1964) to attune, mirror, reflect, and dialogue with the client. Sessions generally unfold in a process-focused manner, with the therapist helping contain, clarify, and support emerging imagery and creative process.

One art therapist who specifically identifies as an existential art therapist is Bruce Moon. He defines existential art therapy as

> a dynamic approach to the therapeutic use of arts processes and imagery that focuses attention on the ultimate concerns of human existence. . . . In existential art therapy, the art process is a powerful medicine that evolves through stages of creation and contemplation. (1990, pp. xviii–xix)

He claims, quoting Shaun McNiff, that "all art is existential" by helping clients restore meaning and purpose in their lives (Moon, 1990, p. xvii). By focusing on the process of art as well as the product, art therapy can help clients become authors of their own lives. Like other existential and humanistic therapists, Moon calls his patients "clients," indicating a nonpathologizing, mutually respectful, and cocreative therapeutic process. The role of the therapist is not to analyze the work of art, but instead to focus on doing with, being open to, and honoring pain. The art therapist shares the journey with the client, accepting all forms of expression, not avoiding pain. The therapist is transparent and interactive, with therapy as a "mutual exchange of self-discovery between client and therapist" (Moon, 1990, p. 98).

Ilene Serlin similarly describes existential dance/movement therapy as a process in which the inner subjective experience is felt, shaped, and communicated with the help of a witnessing therapist. Through a process she calls Kin-Aesthetic Imagining (Serlin, 1996), sensations and expressions arising from bodily felt movement become a nonverbal expressive text like poetry, or "action poesis," and verbal imagery, which, like poetry, moves away from the rational and linear to creative, symbolic writing and speaking (Sartre, 1972).

Through movement, participants can explore existential themes such as the fear of death, the loss of identity, and the seeming randomness of many life events, perhaps discovering the choice to live a life of greater meaning (Frankl, 1946/1959; Kurter et al., 2016). Using movements of strength and commitment, each person can feel the existential moment of choosing life, committing to change, and experiencing breakthroughs. Through mirroring, attunement, and shared rhythms, a group can address existential issues of loneliness and connection. The life of a group goes through stages of existential responsibility; confrontation with mortality, freedom, and fate; and even death and rebirth. Likewise, each individual in the group goes through existential choices such as commitment to the group, meaning derived from the experience, and being alone versus being together with others. The ability to tolerate ambiguity as the group process emerges in movement and the ability to find a balance between the polarities of individual and community, limits and freedom, death and rebirth, and meaning and meaninglessness is a sign of psychological health. Finding congruence between verbal and nonverbal expression or between thoughts, emotions, and actions allows participants to discover and integrate parts of themselves into an authentic expression of self in relation to others and the world (Serlin & Liu, 2020). Creative and expressive arts therapies groups allow for an expression of existential despair and death anxiety while also building hope, hardiness (Maddi, 1999), and optimism and resilience (Serlin & Cannon, 2004). Symbolic expression can cross cultures and has been effective in international trauma situations (Figley et al, 2023; Serlin, 2023; Serlin et al., 2019).

RESEARCH SUPPORT

Creative and expressive arts therapies are only beginning to produce a body of research supporting their effectiveness, having been historically limited by the lack of large grants and pools of research participants. In addition, outcome measures have been difficult to define and measure since the arts therapies are, by definition, not manualized, one-size-fits-all replicable treatment modalities (Karkou & Sanderson, 2006). Therefore, most research in the creative and expressive arts therapies has steered away from quantitative methods and has been more qualitative in nature, such as narrative, anecdotal, and interviews-based methodologies. However, with the contemporary pressure to produce outcome research, the arts therapies have started completing more outcome-oriented measures. For instance, the publication of the large-scale review conducted by the World Health Organization (Fancourt & Finn, 2019) in Europe on the impacts of arts on health and well-being highlighted the central role the arts can play in the prevention of illness, the promotion of health, and the treatment of disease and dysfunction across the lifespan.

Further, Wampold and Imel (2015) urge that the most important variable in the therapeutic process is the relationship between therapist and client, not the technique or theoretical perspective. In that sense, both EH and arts-based therapies can provide evidence of their effectiveness. Nevertheless, most research studies in the field have not been specific to existential and humanistic approaches. A meta-analytic study on the therapeutic mechanisms of change in creative arts therapies (de Witte et al., 2021) denoted that empathy, warmth, positive regard, and congruence, which are all important components in EH psychology, were the common therapeutic factors across all creative and expressive arts therapies.

Quantitative Research

Creative and expressive arts therapies need a common language to communicate with mainstream health care professionals in order to extend and expand their utilization for the public as practices that can be used consistent with evidence-based practice. To that end, randomized controlled trials (RCTs), which are sometimes touted as the gold standard in research in mainstream medicine due to their rigorous design and implementation, have been adopted in research studies on creative and expressive arts therapies. More recently, systematic reviews and meta-analyses that integrate the findings from different

RCTs and mixed-method studies have become available. Due to the funding resources and availability of participants, some populations, such as people with cancer, chronic illnesses, and age-related illnesses, are better studied than other populations.

For example, in the field of oncology, some countries like Canada have already established guidelines for using creative and expressive arts therapies as complementary treatments for cancer survivors (Canadian Cancer Society, n.d.). Some of the benefits documented by their use include relieving anxiety, depression, and distress while improving the quality of life of patients with cancer (Puetz et al., 2013). Creative arts therapies used in oncology settings include music therapy (Köhler et al., 2020), art therapy (Bosman et al., 2021), and dance/movement therapy (Goodill, 2018). Apart from improving symptoms and psychosocial well-being, music therapy and dance/movement therapy have also been shown to improve patients' subjective perception of pain (Bradt et al., 2015), pain severity, and pain tolerance (Ho et al., 2016). Additionally, art therapy has been found to promote the well-being of children undergoing cancer treatment (Derman & Deatrick, 2016).

Creative and expressive arts therapies have also been used with older adults to support healthy aging. Research in neuroscience has shown strong support for the benefits of the arts to maintain brain plasticity and address symptoms of other neurological or degenerative diseases such as stroke and Parkinson's disease (Elkis-Abuhoff & Gaydos, 2018). A systematic review of studies on creative arts therapies for older adults with depression confirmed their effects in reducing depression, regardless of the art modality being used (Dunphy et al., 2019). Cowl and Gaugler (2014) integrated 112 published research reports showing that creative arts therapy is effective in supporting older people with Alzheimer's disease and dementia. Ho and colleagues (2020) demonstrated in an RCT that dance/movement therapy could help older individuals with mild dementia reduce depression, negative mood, and loneliness. Physical benefits, as indicated by the capacity to maintain daily functioning, and physiological benefits, as shown in a diurnal cortisol slope, were also evident and lasted for a year. Cognitive improvement was observed immediately after the intervention, though extended effects might require a longer duration of therapy (Ho et al., 2020).

Working with children using verbal therapy is not always easy due to their limited cognitive and verbal abilities. Creative and expressive arts therapies that rely less on verbal communication may therefore have advantages. After reviewing six studies and two ongoing RCTs, Moula and colleagues (2020) concluded that art therapy improves schoolchildren's quality of life, self-concept, problem-solving skills, and attitudes toward school while decreasing anxiety along with emotional and behavioral difficulties. Wigham and colleagues reviewed 16 studies on using arts-based intervention on children and youth with chronic health conditions (Wigham et al., 2020). They found that arts-based therapies helped improve the quality of life, coping behaviors, anxiety, self-concept, and mood in the study participants, who were mostly children diagnosed with cancer.

Qualitative Research

The role of the therapist and the active participation of the client in therapy are key to success in the creative and expressive arts therapies. Qualitative research that focuses on the subjective experiences of the participants has been the major research method to capture these data points in the field. Although unpacking the experiences of the participants can also help uncover the process and mechanism of change during these therapies, the small sample sizes in most of the qualitative studies and the diverse presentation of diagnostic and demographic profiles make it difficult to have a comprehensive view of the impacts. Fortunately, metasynthesis of qualitative studies helps aggregate the small samples into larger sample sizes and then integrate their diverse findings into representative themes. This can help with understanding the depth and breadth of the impacts that creative and expressive arts therapies have been producing in a variety of populations (Leavy, 2015; Wertz et al., 2011).

Raybin and colleagues (2020) reviewed seven studies on creative arts therapy for children with cancer. They aggregated the results from 162 participants and found that creative arts therapy helped children cope, connect with other people, communicate with others, and establish continuity. The authors suggested promoting creative arts therapy to improve the symptoms of children with cancer. Saunders and colleagues (2019) revealed the potential benefits of arts-based intervention to support people with gender-related identity issues, deepen reflections on their cancer diagnosis, and construct a new gender identity postcancer.

Creative arts therapies have been applied in crisis situations for trauma survivors (van Westrhenen & Fritz, 2014) as well as for those who care for the survivors (Havsteen-Franklin et al., 2020). Although reviews conducted in the 1970s as well as later ones that had a small sample size and methodological issues (van Westrhenen & Fritz, 2014) did not come to a conclusion about creative arts therapy's impact, a 2020 review by Havsteen-Franklin and colleagues demonstrated some benefits. By synthesizing the works from six studies, they showed that arts-based therapies supported the role of caregivers' adaptation, growth, and recovery after a crisis. They also played an important role in reducing the symptoms of trauma and stress while utilizing the community for healing resources.

With an increasing global aging population, age-related neurological and degenerative issues have become more and more important. The nonpharmacological and interactive process of creative and expressive arts therapies makes them acceptable to most older people. In a systematic review on the efficacy of creative arts therapy in the treatment of Alzheimer's disease and dementia conducted by Cowl and Gaugler (2014), 62 out of 112 studies reported qualitative results, and all the studies reported at least one positive outcome. Other common themes elucidated from these studies included improved socialization, amelioration of behavioral symptoms, emotional improvements, self-expression, and benefits for caregivers and families. In another review of 75 articles that included quantitative and qualitative studies related to the use of creative arts in older adults with depression, Dunphy and colleagues (2019) concluded that interventions led by creative arts therapists produced promising results, both quantitative and qualitative. Lo and colleagues (2019) identified the themes mentioned in 11 qualitative studies on creative arts therapies with stroke survivors as functional restoration, psychological support, social engagement, and spiritual experience. Participants in some of these studies also mentioned the shortcomings and barriers to participation in creative arts therapies.

Most available qualitative research in the creative and expressive arts therapies, therefore, demonstrates some benefits that might not be captured in quantitative studies. Although scientific research emphasizes the replicability of research procedures and the generalizability of the outcomes, humanistic person-centered creative and expressive arts therapy does not follow a fixed protocol and therefore cannot be replicated at will. Qualitative research thus becomes crucial to understand the unique experience of these therapies for different individuals and populations. In the past decades, increased mixed-method studies have been conducted using both quantitative and qualitative approaches, demonstrating the increased concern for and understanding of not only the outcomes of creative and expressive arts therapies but also the process of change and mechanism of the approaches (de Witte et al., 2021; Dunphy et al., 2019).

Arts-Based Research

Some creative and expressive arts therapists have written about the need for the arts therapies to have their own language and their own research methodology that is congruent with the flowing process of the arts (Hervey, 2000; Leavy, 2015; McNiff, 1998). McNiff (1998) argues that the arts need their own unique kind of research method as a third alternative to quantitative and qualitative methods, one that understands, honors, and respects the image as a form of data and the imagination as a valid way of knowing. He posits that arts-based research can maintain standards of ethics and rigor not as a set of rules but as a methodical, disciplined process. Since the arts involve dimensions of emotion and meaning that are difficult to quantify, qualitative descriptions are needed to capture the nuances of felt experience (Wertz et al., 2011). And because this experience is sometimes beyond words, it needs symbols to capture its depth (Politsky, 1995). Arts-based approaches and research can help address and document the unique qualities of each experience, document change over time, and communicate findings in active and embodied ways.

In arts-based research, all stages of the research process are permeated with art. In the process called artistic inquiry, the three parts are (a) data gathering, (b) data analysis, and (c) presentation of data (Hervey, 2000). The research question might be explored in the form of a dance. For example, if the research question is, "What is the experience of loss?" dancers could explore the question as a process of inquiry and learn about their unique experience of loss. Descriptions could be gathered through interviews, videos, journals, or drawings. Then the data could be aggregated and presented. In traditional research, it would be in a published article with graphs and numbers. In arts-based research, on the other hand, the results might be performed. Some case studies can be performed, and other data show up as art curated or performed in a gallery. The presentation of data can be one more way in which each layer of narrative recontextualizes and adds a new dimension of understanding and truth about the experience.

Arts-based research presents new ethical challenges (Feder & Feder, 1998). Chief among them is whether the representation is accurate, trustworthy, and "conveys the qualitative experience, including the emotions of the participants, while still maintaining its integrity as a whole" (Hervey, 2000, p. 125). Does it contribute to positive ends? Are the participants clear that they will go through a process of transformation in which the forms of documentation will be shared with others? Ensuring informed consent and supporting a cocreative process with multiple check-in points helps meet these ethical challenges.

Arts-based research approaches the necessary questions of reliability and validity by challenging the prevailing Western notion of truth. In positivist research, truth must be either individual or universal, whereas in artistic inquiry, truth can be both. Knowledge is both personal and universal (Polanyi, 1958), subjective and objective. The concept of validity in positivist research can be met with the concept of authenticity in artistic inquiry (McNiff, 1998). Another check on reliability and validity is trustworthiness. Patricia Leavy (2015) identifies basic guidelines for this goal. One is the insight that disciplined inquiry is a kind of craft, like learning to play the piano. Leavy supports the feminist stance of recognizing the validity of emotions as data and suggests that poetic criteria are acceptable. She also argues against the need for an objective observer. By maintaining that the subjectivity of the researcher, as well as the research participant, is a valid source of data, Leavy advances the idea that research can—and perhaps should—be transformative for the researcher as well as the participant.

MULTICULTURAL CONSIDERATIONS

As with all the other mental health disciplines, the necessity and importance of adequately addressing multicultural themes, as well as those of appreciating diversity, striving for equity, and committing to inclusion, fall squarely into the purview of both creative and expressive arts therapies as well as EH psychotherapy (Stewart et al., 2017). Not only do multicultural considerations need to be integrated into the clinical practice of these psychotherapeutic approaches, but they need to be embedded into all aspects of research, supervision, education, and clinical training associated with these fields.

Of particular concern to both creative and expressive arts therapists and EH psychotherapists is a keen understanding of the cultural psychological concepts of emic and etic perspectives (Kashima, 2019). The emic viewpoint comes from within a culture and prioritizes the beliefs, values, and customs of a particular group of people while attempting to understand those phenomena from that culture's vantage point. In doing so, there is a tendency to derive unique meanings from various situations that don't necessarily cut across cultures. By contrast, the etic viewpoint elevates the host culture's beliefs, values, and customs because it attempts to look at the cultural phenomena of a particular group or culture from outside that group's context, often with a scientific or supposed neutral perspective. As a result, the etic approach often generates broad theories that tend to be generalized across cultures and frequently are described as universal to human experience. Both approaches have their place in trying to understand the complexities of the human experience, though it behooves the committed practitioner from one cultural orientation to be duly cautious about ascribing global attributions to people, practices, and products from another culture that may be inaccurate, incomplete, or outright incompetent in their understanding of the other culture.

Because the creative and expressive arts work with artistic media such as color, shape, texture, sound, rhythm, and configuration, as well as cultural artifacts such as symbols, images, myths, stories, songs, postures, and gestures, there can and has been a trend to view those things through Western, educated, industrialized, affluent, and democratic (Henrich et al., 2010) models of understanding that fail to recognize that those models are themselves located within a particular cultural backdrop or milieu. This can lead to projecting universal meaning onto those uniquely derived artistic media and cultural artifacts that potentially discount, diminish, and perhaps even delete the possibility of other truths or realities being possible. Likewise, because EH psychotherapists work with constructs such as human development, personal growth, and meaning seeking, they too need to be mindful of emic and etic perspectives within all of these themes so that they remain open and curious to different cultural interpretations of the human experience while also appreciating that there may be some common or universal themes that cut across cultures (Corley, 2019).

To more skillfully navigate the myriad cultural complexities that mental health professionals of all backgrounds encounter each day, mental health professionals not only are being asked to gain some degree of competence, but they are also being asked to be more culturally humble, aware, sensitive, and responsive. Multicultural competencies are increasingly viewed as a crucial skill for practicing psychotherapists (Vallejos & Johnson, 2019), though this term can be somewhat problematic in that it may inadvertently infer arrival at or completion of a multicultural learning process, when actually the process never ends. Three domains to assess and cultivate multicultural competency, offered by Arthur and Collins (2010), include cultural self-awareness, awareness of client cultural identities, and a culturally sensitive working alliance. Murray-García and Tervalon (2014) extend the notion of cultural competence to that of cultural humility and an awareness of power dynamics in the therapeutic relationship.

Cultural humility means that therapists engage in an ongoing critical self-reflection of their own identity, assumptions, and biases and make efforts to be transparent and transcend them when working with someone from a different culture. Murray-García and Tervalon (2014) offer four principles that promote cultural humility: (a) a lifelong process of critical self-reflection and self-critique,

(b) redressing the power imbalances in the patient–provider relationship, (c) developing mutually beneficial partnerships with communities on behalf of individuals and defined populations, and (d) advocating and maintaining institutional accountability that parallels the three previous principles. The principle of cultural humility was extended to the arts therapies by Louvenia Jackson (2020). In addition, creative and expressive arts therapists are also encouraged to go through their own artistic embodied process to experience their own vulnerabilities and continue to grow in understanding of self and others (Brooke & Myers, 2015).

As the fields of creative and expressive arts develop around the globe, increasing complications arise due to issues of quality control. As was noted in this article, the primary dance/movement therapy professional model used in the world at this time is from the American Dance Therapy Association. Its language and practices of dance tend to be Western. Evaluation systems, cultural norms of normal and abnormal movement styles, and use of indigenous dance forms are rooted in specific cultures, and non-Western cultures are forming their own versions of the creative and expressive arts therapies with their own norms, training systems, and professional organizations (Kwong et al, 2019). This cultural complexity is further compounded by the embeddedness of the creative arts therapies within the larger mental health structure. How are creative and expressive arts funded? Where do they fit into the psychiatric and psychology hierarchies? What is the experience and policy for using medications versus holistic healing?

For example, major training programs and associations are being developed in India, South Africa (Speiser et al., 2024), China (Serlin 2023), Australia, Japan, and Hong Kong (Ho et al, 2020). Through careful documentation and research, creative and expressive arts therapists are finding their own unique voices.

In sum, although creative and expressive arts are historically located in all the world's cultures, therapists must be careful to practice cultural humility, resist using an etic perspective that reduces or invalidates an emic experience, and continuously engage in a process of ongoing self-reflection. The increase in cultural sensitivity and competence helps creative and expressive arts therapists derive clinical meaning and therapeutic direction from their work with clients whose social locations and intersectional identities differ from theirs.

FUTURE RESEARCH

As the fields of humanistic and expressive arts therapies are growing rapidly around the globe, future research is recommended to solidify the scientific foundations and increase international collaborations (Chang, 2016). It would be of benefit to include diverse research methodologies that give voices to multicultural communities, including arts-based, phenomenological, dialogical, heuristic, narrative, feminist, and womanist methods. In addition, including physiological measures of change during the course of arts-based therapy would be beneficial. Interest in artificial intelligence and brain scans offer new avenues of measuring the therapeutic process in and between individuals and groups and could be incorporated into future research. Last, it would be productive to include outcome research on arts-based therapy as integrated into EH therapy. Although EH expressive arts therapies know that a smile or image is worth a thousand words, having strong research helps the field better communicate its methods and findings with other colleagues around the world.

CONCLUSION

The aim of this chapter was to specifically consider the place of creative and expressive arts therapies—including art, dance/movement, music, drama, psychodrama, and poetry therapies—within the contemporary framework of EH psychology and, more generally, within the field of professional psychology and psychotherapy. Given that so much emphasis in psychology and psychotherapy has been placed on the utilization of treatment modalities that are evidence based, the question of whether creative and expressive arts therapies can be, in fact, practiced consistent with evidence-based principles is explored within this chapter. The chapter noted that creative and expressive arts therapies have historically been excluded from lists of effective psychotherapies, variously labeled, because verbal treatments that rely heavily on cognitive and behavioral interventions are much more amenable to meeting the quantitative protocols required for demonstrating the outcomes needed for a modality or approach to be deemed effective or even as a promising practice.

In conclusion, we encourage creative and expressive arts therapists to integrate evidence-based practice foundations into their therapeutic work by weaving together the best parts of both quantitative and qualitative ways of working, celebrating both inductive and deductive ways of knowing and working, and making appropriate cultural adaptations. Creative and expressive arts therapies can contribute a symbolic, nonverbal form of communication to support the culturally sensitive, aware, and responsive practices needed by today's practitioners. Practiced within a respectful, dialogical encounter, creative and expressive arts therapies can bring the art back into the art and science of psychology. Creative and expressive interventions such as creative process work, active imagination, self-expression, improvisational exploration, and play can help clients address ultimate existential concerns that are central to EH therapy (e.g., nonbeing, isolation, meaninglessness, freedom; Yalom, 1980). Because evidence-based practice doesn't eliminate key therapeutic ingredients such as intuition, creative process, and therapeutic alliance, creative and expressive arts therapists can bring the strengths of their humanistic and existential roots into a potent dialogue with today's need for practicing consistent with evidence-based principles. Fortunately, creative and expressive arts therapists are well situated for doing just this because they are masters at cross-cultural communication and healing.

REFERENCES

Alschuler, M. (2006). Poetry, the healing pen. In S. L. Brooke (Ed.), *Creative arts therapies manual: A guide to the history, theoretical approaches, assessment, and work with special populations of art, play, dance, music, drama, and poetry therapies* (pp. 253–262). Charles C. Thomas.

American Art Therapy Association. (n.d.). *The profession*. https://arttherapy.org/about-art-therapy/

American Dance Therapy Association. (n.d.). *What is dance/movement therapy?* https://adta.memberclicks.net/what-is-dancemovement-therapy

American Music Therapy Association. (2005). *What is music therapy?* https://www.musictherapy.org/about/musictherapy/

American Society of Group Psychotherapy and Psychodrama. (n.d.). *What is psychodrama?* https://asgpp.org/what-is-psychodrama/

American Psychological Association Presidential Task Force on Evidence-Based Practice. (2006). Evidence-based practice in psychology. *American Psychologist, 61*(4), 271–285. https://doi.org/10.1037/0003-066X.61.4.271

Aristotle. (1961). *Poetics* (S. H. Butcher, Trans.). Hill and Wang.

Arthur, N., & Collins, S. (Eds.). (2010). *Culture-infused counselling* (2nd ed.). Counselling Concepts.

Bateson, M. C. (1989). *Composing a life*. Atlantic Monthly Press.

Bella, K. A., & Serlin, I. A. (2013). Expressive and creative arts therapies. In H. L. Friedman & G. Hartelius (Eds.), *The Wiley-Blackwell handbook of transpersonal psychology* (pp. 529–543). John Wiley & Sons. https://doi.org/10.1002/9781118591277.ch29

Bosman, J. T., Bood, Z. M., Scherer-Rath, M., Dörr, H., Christophe, N., Sprangers, M. A. G., & van Laarhoven, H. W. M. (2021). The effects of art therapy on anxiety, depression, and quality of life in adults with cancer: A systematic literature review. *Supportive Care in Cancer, 29*(5), 2289–2298. https://doi.org/10.1007/s00520-020-05869-0

Bradt, J., Shim, M., & Goodill, S. W. (2015). Dance/movement therapy for improving psychological and physical outcomes in cancer patients. *Cochrane Database of Systematic Reviews*. https://doi.org/10.1002/14651858.CD007103.pub3

Brooke, S. L. (Ed.). (2006). *Creative arts therapies manual: A guide to the history, theoretical approaches, assessment, and work with special populations of art, play, dance, music, drama, and poetry therapies*. Charles C. Thomas.

Brooke, S. L., & Myers, C. E. (Eds.). (2015). *Therapists creating a cultural tapestry: Using the creative therapies across cultures*. Charles C. Thomas.

Bruscia, K. E. (1998). *Defining music therapy* (2nd ed.). Barcelona Publishers.

Bugental, J. F. T. (1992). *The art of the psychotherapist: How to develop the skills that take psychotherapy beyond science*. W. W. Norton & Company.

Canadian Cancer Society. (n.d.). *Complementary therapies*. https://cancer.ca/en/treatments/complementary-therapies

Chang, M. H. (2016). Cultural consciousness and the global context of dance/movement therapy. In S. Chaiklin (Ed.), *The art and science of dance/movement therapy: Life is a dance* (2nd ed., pp. 317–334). Routledge.

Corley, N. A. (2019). Using poetry to re-present the narratives of Black students and Black single mothers. *Journal of Poetry Therapy, 32*(3), 156–163. https://doi.org/10.1080/08893675.2019.1625148

Cowl, A. L., & Gaugler, J. E. (2014). Efficacy of creative arts therapy in treatment of Alzheimer's disease and dementia: A systematic literature review. *Activities, Adaptation and Aging, 38*(4), 281–330. https://doi.org/10.1080/01924788.2014.966547

Derman, Y. E., & Deatrick, J. A. (2016). Promotion of well-being during treatment for childhood cancer: A literature review of art interventions as a coping strategy. *Cancer Nursing, 39*(6), E1–E16. https://doi.org/10.1097/NCC.0000000000000318

de Witte, M., Orkibi, H., Zarate, R., Karkou, V., Sajnani, N., Malhotra, B., Ho, R. T. H., Kaimal, G., Baker, F. A., & Koch, S. C. (2021). From therapeutic factors to mechanisms of change in the creative arts therapies: A scoping review. *Frontiers in Psychology, 12.* https://doi.org/10.3389/fpsyg.2021.678397

Dunphy, K., Baker, F. A., Dumaresq, E., Carroll-Haskins, K., Eickholt, J., Ercole, M., Kaimal, G., Meyer, K., Sajnani, N., Shamir, O. Y., & Wosch, T. (2019). Creative arts interventions to address depression in older adults: A systematic review of outcomes, processes, and mechanisms. *Frontiers in Psychology, 9.* https://doi.org/10.3389/fpsyg.2018.02655

Elkis-Abuhoff, D. L., & Gaydos, M. (2018). Medical art therapy research moves forward: A Review of clay manipulation with Parkinson's Disease. *Art Therapy: Journal of the American Art Therapy Association, 35*(2), 68–76. https://doi.org/10.1080/07421656.2018.1483162

Fancourt, D., & Finn, S. (2019). *What is the evidence on the role of the arts in improving health and well-being? A scoping review.* World Health Organization Regional Office for Europe. https://apps.who.int/iris/handle/10665/329834

Feder, E., & Feder, B. (1998). *The art and science of evaluation in the arts therapies: How do you know what's working?* Charles C. Thomas.

Figley, C., Walker, L., & Serlin, I. (Eds.). (2023). *Pandemic providers: Psychologists respond to Covid.* Springer. https://doi.org/10.1007/978-3-031-27580-7

Frankl, V. E. (1959). *Man's search for meaning: An introduction to logotherapy.* Washington Square Press. (Original work published 1946)

Franklin, M. A. (2017). *Art as contemplative practice: Expressive pathways to the self.* SUNY Press.

Goodill, S. W. (2018). Accumulating evidence for dance/movement therapy in cancer care. *Frontiers in Psychology, 9.* https://doi.org/10.3389/fpsyg.2018.01778

Hanna, T. L. (1988). *Somatics: Reawakening the mind's control of movement, flexibility, and health.* Da Capo Press.

Havsteen-Franklin, D., Tjasink, M., Kottler, J. W., Grant, C., & Kumari, V. (2020). Arts-based interventions for professionals in caring roles during and after crisis: A systematic review of the literature. *Frontiers in Psychology, 9.* https://doi.org/10.3389/fpsyg.2020.589744

Hawkins, A. M. (1964). *Creating through dance.* Prentice-Hall.

Henrich, J., Heine, S. J., & Norenzayan, A. (2010). The weirdest people in the world? *Behavioral and Brain Sciences, 33*(2–3), 61–83. https://doi.org/10.1017/S0140525X0999152X

Herman, J. L. (1992). *Trauma and recovery: The aftermath of violence—From domestic abuse to political terror.* BasicBooks.

Hervey, L. W. (2000). *Artistic inquiry in dance/movement therapy: Creative alternatives for research.* Charles C Thomas.

Ho, R. T. H., Fong, T. C. T., Chan, W. C., Kwan, J. S. K., Chiu, P. K. C., Yau, J. C. Y., & Lam, L. C. W. (2020). Psychophysiological effects of dance movement therapy and physical exercise on older adults with mild dementia: A randomized controlled trial. *The Journals of Gerontology. Series B, Psychological Sciences and Social Sciences, 75*(3), 560–570. https://doi.org/10.1093/geronb/gby145

Ho, R. T. H., Fong, T. C. T., Cheung, I. K. M., Yip, P. S. F., & Luk, M. Y. (2016). Effects of a short-term dance movement therapy program on symptoms and stress in patients with breast cancer undergoing radiotherapy: A randomized, controlled, single-blind trial. *Journal of Pain and Symptom Management, 51*(5), 824–831. https://doi.org/10.1016/j.jpainsymman.2015.12.332

Hoffman, H. H. (2004). *Connections and parallels between humanistic psychology and modern dance at Jacob's Pillow.* Mellen Press.

International Expressive Arts Therapy Association. (n.d.). *Who we are.* https://www.ieata.org/who-we-are

Jackson, L. (2020). *Cultural humility in art therapy: Applications for practice, research, social justice, self-care, and pedagogy*. Jessica Kingsley Publishers.

Jourard, S. M. (1971). *The transparent self* (Rev. ed.). Van Nostrand Reinhold.

Jung, C. G. (1966). *Collected works of C. G. Jung: Vol 15. Spirit in man, art, and literature* (G. Adler & R. F. C. Hull, Eds.). Princeton University Press.

Karkou, V., & Sanderson, P. (Eds.). (2006). *Arts therapies: A research-based map of the field*. Elsevier. https://doi.org/10.1016/B978-0-443-07256-7.X5001-3

Kashima, Y. (2019). A history of cultural psychology: Cultural psychology as a tradition and a movement. In D. Cohen & S. Kitayama (Eds.), *Handbook of cultural psychology* (2nd ed., pp. 53–78). Guilford Press.

Katz, R. (2017). *Indigenous healing psychology: Honoring the wisdom of the First Peoples*. Healing Arts Press.

Köhler, F., Martin, Z.-S., Hertrampf, R.-S., Gäbel, C., Kessler, J., Ditzen, B., & Warth, M. (2020). Corrigendum: Music therapy in the psychosocial treatment of adult cancer patients: A systematic review and meta-analysis. *Frontiers in Psychology, 9*. https://doi.org/10.3389/fpsyg.2020.02095

Kurter, F., Bicer, E., Aysoy, E., & Serlin, I. (2016). Life, death, and transformation: Keep moving. *Journal of Applied Arts & Health, 7*(1), 107–116. https://doi.org/10.1386/jaah.7.1.107_1

Kwong, M. K., Ho, R. T. H., & Huang, Y. T. (2019). A creative pathway to a meaningful life: An existential expressive arts group therapy for people living with HIV in Hong Kong. *The Arts in Psychotherapy, 63*, 9–17. https://doi.org/10.1016/j.aip.2019.05.004

Landy, R. (2007). Drama therapy: Past, present and future. In I. A. Serlin (Ed.), *Whole person healthcare: Vol. 3. The arts and health* (pp. 143–165). Praeger.

Leavy, P. (2015). *Method meets art: Arts-based research practice* (2nd ed.). Guilford Press.

Lo, T. L. T., Lee, J. L. C., & Ho, R. T. H. (2019). Creative arts-based therapies for stroke survivors: A qualitative systematic review. *Frontiers in Psychology, 10*. https://doi.org/10.3389/fpsyg.2019.01538

Maddi, S. R. (1999). The personality construct of hardiness: Effects on experiencing, coping, and strain. *Consulting Psychology Journal, 51*(2), 83–94. https://doi.org/10.1037/1061-4087.51.2.83

Malchiodi, C. A. (2020). *Trauma and expressive arts therapy: Brain, body, and imagination in the healing process*. Guilford Press.

Maslow, A. (1962). *Toward a psychology of being*. Van Nostrand. https://doi.org/10.1037/10793-000

May, R. (1975). *The courage to create*. Bantam Books.

May, R. (1977). *The meaning of anxiety*. W. W. Norton & Company.

McNiff, S. (1998). *Art-based research*. Jessica Kingsley Publishers.

Merleau-Ponty, M. (1962). *Phenomenology of perception* (C. Smith, Trans.). Routledge and Kegan Paul. (Original work published 1945)

Moon, B. L. (1990). *Existential art therapy: The canvas mirror*. Charles C. Thomas.

Moreno, J. L. (1947). *The theater of spontaneity*. Beacon House.

Moula, Z., Aithal, S., Karkou, V., & Powell, J. (2020). A systematic review of child-focused outcomes and assessments of arts therapies delivered in primary mainstream schools. *Children and Youth Services Review, 112*. https://doi.org/10.1016/j.childyouth.2020.104928

Murray-García, J., & Tervalon, M. (2014). The concept of cultural humility. *Health Affairs, 33*(7), 1303–1303. https://doi.org/10.1377/hlthaff.2014.0564

National Association for Poetry Therapy. (n.d.). *The National Association for Poetry Therapy mission*. https://poetrytherapy.org/Mission

National Coalition of Creative Arts Therapies Associations. (n.d.). *About NCCATA*. https://www.nccata.org/aboutnccata

Norcross, J. C. (2011). *Psychotherapy relationships that work: Evidence-based responsiveness* (3rd ed.). Oxford University Press. https://doi.org/10.1093/acprof:oso/9780199737208.001.0001

North American Drama Therapy Association. (n.d.). *What is drama therapy?* https://www.nadta.org/what-is-dramatherapy-

Perls, L. (1992). *Living at the boundary* (J. Wysong, Ed.). The Gestalt Journal Press.

Polanyi, M. (1958). *Personal knowledge: Towards a post-critical philosophy*. University of Chicago Press.

Politsky, R. H. (1995). Toward a typology of research in the creative arts therapies. *The Arts in Psychotherapy, 22*(4), 307–314. https://doi.org/10.1016/0197-4556(95)00016-X

Puetz, T. W., Morley, C. A., & Herring, M. P. (2013). Effects of creative arts therapies on psychological symptoms and quality of life in patients with cancer. *JAMA Internal Medicine, 173*(11), 960–969. https://doi.org/10.1001/jamainternmed.2013.836

Raybin, J. L., Barr, E., Krajicek, M., & Jones, J. (2020). How does creative arts therapy reduce distress for children with cancer? A metasynthesis of extant qualitative literature. *Journal of Pediatric Oncology Nursing, 37*(2), 91–104. https://doi.org/10.1177/1043454219888807

Rogers, C. (1961). *On becoming a person*. Houghton Mifflin Company.

Sartre, J. P. (1972). *The psychology of imagination*. The Citadel Press.

Saunders, S., Hammond, C., & Thomas, R. (2019). Exploring gender-related experiences of cancer survivors through creative arts: A scoping review. *Qualitative Health Research, 29*(1), 135–148. https://doi.org/10.1177/1049732318771870

Schneider, K. J., & May, M. (1994). *The psychology of existence: An integrative, clinical perspective*. McGraw-Hill.

Serlin, I. A. (1993). Root images of healing in dance therapy. *American Journal of Dance Therapy, 15*(2), 65–76. https://doi.org/10.1007/BF00844028

Serlin, I. A. (1996). Kinesthetic imagining. *Journal of Humanistic Psychology, 36*(2), 25–33. https://doi.org/10.1177/00221678960362005

Serlin, I. A. (2009). A tribute to Rollo May and the arts. *Journal of Humanistic Psychology, 49*(4), 486–489. https://doi.org/10.1177/0022167809341747

Serlin, I. A. (2023). Dance movement therapy with Chinese counselors. *Journal of Alternative, Complementary & Integrative Medicine, 9*(2), 1. https://doi.org/10.24966/ACIM-7562/100327

Serlin, I. A., & Cannon, J. (2004). A humanistic approach to the psychology of trauma. In D. Knafo (Ed.), *Living with terror, working with trauma: A clinician's handbook* (pp. 313–331). Jason Aronson.

Serlin, I. A., & Kennedy, J. R. (2020). Dance/movement as a holistic treatment: Using creative, imaginal, and embodied expression in healing, growth, and therapy. In C. L. Fracasso, S. Krippner, & H. L. Friedman (Eds.), *Holistic treatment in mental health: A handbook of practitioners' perspectives* (pp. 61–75). McFarland and Company.

Serlin, I. A., Krippner, S., & Rockefeller, K. (Eds.). (2019). *Integrated care for the traumatized: A whole-person approach*. Rowman and Littlefield.

Serlin, I. A., & Liu, C. (2020). An existential–humanistic approach to movement: An East/West dialogue. *Creative Arts Education and Therapy, 6*(1), 85–96. https://doi.org/10.15212/CAET/2020/6/10

Speiser, P., Speiser, V. M., Saner, R., Saner Yiu, L., Robelot-Timtchenko, N., Kalmanowitz, D., & Llyod, B. (2024). Using the arts to work with refugees and displaced persons in times of crisis and war. *South African Journal of Arts Therapies, 2*(1), 82–95. https://doi.org/10.36615/j37y0w48

Stewart, S. L., Moodley, R., & Hyatt, A. (Eds.). (2017). *Indigenous cultures and mental health counseling: Four directions for integration with counseling psychology*. Routledge.

Vallejos, L., & Johnson, Z. (2019). Multicultural competencies in humanistic psychology. In L. Hoffman, H. Cleare-Hoffman, N. Granger, Jr., & D. St. John (Eds.), *Humanistic approaches to multiculturalism and diversity: Perspectives on existence and difference* (63–75). Taylor and Francis/Routledge. https://doi.org/10.4324/9781351133357-6

van der Kolk, B. (2015). *The body keeps the score: Brain, mind, and body in the healing of trauma*. Penguin Books.

van Westrhenen, N., & Fritz, E. (2014). Creative arts therapy as treatment for child trauma: An overview. *The Arts in Psychotherapy, 41*(5), 527–534. https://doi.org/10.1016/j.aip.2014.10.004

Wampold, B. E., & Imel, Z. E. (2015). *The great psychotherapy debate: The evidence for what makes psychotherapy work* (2nd ed.). Routledge. https://doi.org/10.4324/9780203582015

Wertz, F. J., Charmaz, K., McMullen, L. M., Josselson, R., Anderson, R., & McSpadden, E. (2011). *Five ways of doing qualitative analysis: Phenomenological psychology, grounded theory, discourse analysis, narrative research, and intuitive inquiry*. Guilford Press.

Wigham, S., Watts, P., Zubala, A., Jandial, S., Bourne, J., & Hackett, S. (2020). Using arts-based therapies to improve mental health for children and young people with physical health long-term conditions: A systematic review of effectiveness. *Frontiers in Psychology, 11*. https://doi.org/10.3389/fpsyg.2020.01771

Yalom, I. D. (1980). *Existential psychotherapy*. Basic Books.

16

Experiential Techniques in Existential–Humanistic Psychotherapy

Trey Cole

Eugene Gendlin (1982), as part of a dialogue on pluralism within phenomenology, noted that when "we formulate experience, that is by no means the first-time [*sic*] experience and language have met! Experience is the living process in the cultural world. . . . Therefore, they are also part of our bodily feelings, and can re-emerge from them" (p. 322). Highlighting this inseparable dynamic between what is implicitly felt or known in the body—what some have referred to as that which is palpable (Madison & Gendlin, 2012)—and how that and other experiences are captured through language, Gendlin draws attention to an oft-neglected aspect of psychotherapy: that which has not yet been given language. Psychotherapy, often referred to as the talking cure, has historically placed primary emphasis on what is said, whether internally or verbally; however, understanding the whole person presenting to psychotherapy requires exploration and acknowledgment of both what is and is not yet linguistically formulated. Just as existential and humanistic theories have challenged historic subject and object bifurcations in favor of viewing humans as *being-in-the-world*—inseparably interrelated—so too must caution be maintained in conceiving of individuals as containing essence-laden entities within (e.g., preontological and ontological, prereflective and reflective), lest what possibilities emerge in the process of *being-as-becoming* be lost to the rigidification of language alone.

This chapter focuses on integrating experiential therapy techniques within existential–humanistic (EH) practice as a pragmatic resource for those interested in expanding the horizon of their clinical work. In doing so, it seeks to address

https://doi.org/10.1037/0000446-017
The Evidence-Based Foundations of Existential–Humanistic Therapy, L. Hoffman and V. Lac (Editors)

challenges posed by Gendlin and others to view the person in the fullness of their experiencing. To do this, the initial section will define what is meant by experiential techniques, considering general definitions and delineating points of comparison and divergence from EH theory. Following, these techniques will be contextualized within EH therapy, wherein illustrations and examples will be used to supplement and illuminate areas of integration. Finally, an in-depth review of relevant qualitative and quantitative literature as well as important multicultural considerations will be elucidated, alongside future research needs.

As a brief caveat, despite this chapter's focus on experiential techniques, it is by no means a recipe book for clinicians to apply haphazardly or in a one-size-fits-all approach. Echoing the cautions of Minuchin and Fishman (1981), at the end of the day, "the therapist should be a healer: a human being concerned with engaging other human beings therapeutically around areas and issues that cause them pain. . . . The goal, in other words, is to transcend technique" (p. 1). Stated differently, a consistent artifact in all psychotherapy research remains that the person of the therapist cannot be abstracted from the treatment; therefore, how and in what context the therapist applies a technique, alongside the context from which they have emerged, is of equal or perhaps greater importance than the specific technique. As such, the content of this chapter should serve as one of many guides rather than the only guide for integrating experiential techniques under the guise of EH theory and therapy.

DEFINING EXPERIENTIAL TECHNIQUES

Although some disagreement remains regarding whether experiential psychotherapies may be broadly characterized as a subcomponent in the tradition or as one of many expressions of existential and humanistic psychology, they nevertheless share some theoretical and practical similarities (Schneider et al., 2014). Within the purview of experiential therapies, one may further delineate more specific approaches such as person-centered, focusing-oriented, emotion-focused, Gestalt, process–experiential, expressive, and body-oriented therapies (Elliott et al., 2013). As such, in order to better illuminate what experiential techniques are and how they may be used, it is useful to consider the theoretical and practical underpinnings from which they arise.

At the theoretical level, both experiential and EH therapies, to some degree, take a view of human nature as inherently good, growth-oriented, and choiceful (Elliott et al., 2004). Characteristically, they both place primary emphasis on the development of strong therapeutic bonds, use of the phenomenological method, in vivo experiencing, and meaning making. Specific to this chapter, both therapies view human existence as *embodied*, meaning that individuals can understand and experience themselves both through and as their own body. As discussed previously, at a pre-reflective (i.e., nonconceptual) level, embodiment may be felt as a diffuse bodily experience; once reflected, embodiment may be expressed as an interplay of mutually affected cognition, emotion, and behavior (Madison, 2014a).

Despite many areas of overlap, some nuances between the characteristics of these therapies do exist. One distinction may be in how each modality understands humans as inherently good and growth oriented. Experiential therapies have tended to embrace these traditionally humanistic values that promote humans as consistently moving towards self-actualization and betterment (Rogers, 1961, 1980); however, EH therapies, especially those focused more existentially, tend to critique this view of human nature as limiting, preferring a more neutral view that can better encapsulate and flexibly understand experiences deemed less desirable or negative (Buber et al., 1997). Stated differently, EH theory understands meaning making—that is, the way humans organize their experience—as ontological but does not place valuation on what that meaning may be. In contrast, terms like "betterment" or "goodness" have clear value-laden implications (Hoffman et al., 2015).

Another distinction arises in how one understands the use of the phenomenological method and horizontalization (e.g., rank-ordering, valuation) of experience. Though both therapies place great importance on attunement and making certain the client feels heard, how they do this requires some clarification. Experiential therapies frequently reference experiences that are deeper or create distinctions between emotions that are primary versus secondary (Elliott & Greenberg, 2007). As Elliott and colleagues (2004) discuss, the process–experiential approach aims to "maintain a creative tension between the client-centered emphasis on creating a genuinely empathic and prizing therapeutic relationship, and a more active, task-focused process-directive style of engagement that promotes deeper experiencing" (p. 2). Further, how an emotion emerges and whether it is viewed as adaptive, reactive, or maladaptive requires different response patterns of either following or guiding depending on how the therapist labels it (Elliott & Greenberg, 2007). These differentiations between depth and order of emotional experiences, however, are not as readily accepted within the EH understanding of the phenomenological method. As DuBose (2015) describes,

> If care is "best" when well matching the uniqueness of one's way of being-in-the-world, then the genericity of the word, "standard," must give way to a relativity of diverse ways of being-in-the-world that are neither better nor worse than each other on rank-ordered scales of measurement, but simply "are," as different. (p. 34)

Phenomenologically, the effort to maintain pace with the client's existence as it presents itself is always just that—an aim, never an achievement. When the therapist labels experiences, either directionally (i.e., deeper or superficial) or evaluatively (i.e., adaptive and maladaptive or primary and secondary), or takes as their task to guide toward something, there will always be a consistent risk of directing client towards the therapist's preferred version of health or well-being (E. Spinelli, personal communication, 2020; Wade, 1996). By extension, this also includes the developmental context of their foundational theory, which for many were versions shaped by predominantly White male theorists.

CONTEXTUALIZING EXPERIENTIAL TECHNIQUES WITHIN EH THERAPY

Despite some of the theoretical differences between experiential and EH therapies, therapists should not immediately assume that experiential techniques
are ill-fitting to EH practice. As a framework, consider the metaphor of different
psychotherapeutic modalities as houses in the same neighborhood, wherein
the foundations are made up of the philosophical grounding, the houses' structures contain the core psychological principles, and the interior décor and
design are made up of methods or techniques regarding how those core principles are expressed. If one were to conduct a real estate assessment, however,
aspects of each home may be more or less comparable or changeable. The philosophical foundations, for example, are the least flexibly comparative (i.e.,
individuals as free vs. determined). The structure of the homes are not as mal-
leable as the décor and are still often sturdy and structurally would require
great work to change (i.e., classical vs. relational psychoanalysis). The interior
décor and design, therefore, make up methods or techniques and are the most
fluid and exchangeable. This last point is why identifying a therapist's orientation through their interaction or technique alone can be difficult, even if their
stated theoretical goals differ (Norcross & Wampold, 2019a, 2019b).

As noted previously, EH therapy has historically "viewed the language of
technique with suspicion because it . . . stands firm against mechanized, linear,
reductionist, and manualized approaches to therapy" (Hoffman, 2009, p. 27);
however, as an approach that seeks to engage phenomenologically, many
experiential techniques may serve a valuable purpose in helping therapists
both connect with and enrich descriptions of their clients' experiences, especially in how those experiences are embodied and given felt meaning. Viewed
in this manner, applying experiential techniques contextually and idiosyncrati-
cally may support a particular way of being with a client, rather than merely
doing something to them.

Providing a comprehensive overview of all experiential techniques is beyond
the scope of this chapter, and some practitioners may note that certain techniques either do not belong solely to any one experiential therapy or that others are not covered; however, with some discretion, it is nonetheless important
to contextualize and provide examples of techniques from dominant experiential therapies to illustrate their goodness of fit within EH practice. Specifically,
in the following sections, Gestalt, process–experiential, focusing and body-
oriented, and guided imagery and visualization techniques will be highlighted
and described.

Gestalt Techniques

From a Gestalt perspective, techniques are often referred to as experiments and
may be used to help clients increase self-awareness and acceptance (Yontef &
Jacobs, 2008). As Paruzel-Czachura and Konieczniak (2020) note,

> A very important assumption of the Gestalt approach is that people solve their life problems properly if they are able to use their energy and abilities. . . . The therapist's task is to help the clients increase their self-awareness and to re-assimilate the energy they expend on behaviors that limit their stream of consciousness. (p. 15)

Fond of theater, Fritz and Laura Perls utilized the concept of *enactment* to highlight how the therapeutic dyad may experientially play out different roles in the client's life via the statement of certain words or expression of emotions (Serlin & Shane, 1999). In this way, relational patterns are both disclosed and intervened in through the therapeutic relationship as performative rather than merely reported. This technique fits squarely into EH practice, especially pertinent to what theorists have referred to as the relational mode or here-and-now (Hoffman, 2009; Yalom, 1980; see also Chapter 8 of this volume). The past, present, and future are understood as mutually influencing each other in a given moment (i.e., past-as-currently-lived and future-as-currently-lived), allowing the therapist to explore problems as they are currently lived as opposed to something that happened then and there, wherein the therapy would have no experiential access.

Process–Experiential Techniques

Developed primarily through the efforts of Elliott and Greenberg (2007), process–experiential (sometimes referred to as emotion-focused) therapy gives precedence to "emotions as a source of meaning, direction and growth" (p. 241). Through this approach, emotions are viewed as primarily organizing and adaptive, providing the basic building blocks through which different worldview constructions and behavioral reactions are formed (Greenberg, 2002). Paralleling EH theory, emotions are not sought after to be changed so much as to be contextually understood and experienced differently (Hoffman et al., 2015). Those working from a process–experiential lens view the therapeutic relationship as a creative dialectic wherein the therapist acts as process consultant, seeking both to follow and guide the client toward a preferred outcome together. Therein, Elliott and colleagues (2004) identify six *modes of engagement* that can be worked through in the immediate encounter to experientially process the client's conflict, including attending, experiential search, active expression, interpersonal contact, self-reflection, and action-planning.

Focusing and Body-Oriented Techniques

Though a resurgence in the psychotherapeutic community today might seem to be a novelty, focusing and body-oriented approaches have a rich history across several domains of inquiry (Gendlin, 1969; Heller, 2012; Merleau-Ponty, 1962). So much overlap exists between these and EH approaches that some refer to focusing and body-orientation as palpable existentialism (Madison, 2014b) or operating from the immediate mode (Hoffman, 2009). According to

Madison (2014b), this approach "prioritises the client's bodily experiences over therapeutic concepts, manualised expectations or logical inference" (p. 25), and it involves attending to what felt sensations might be occurring in the immediate moment of interaction through which meaning constructs may arise. Importantly, in addition to attending to the client's perceptions, the therapist is implicated in the moment-to-moment creation of the felt relational space with their client, which, whether disclosed or not, may be used as a reference point from which to attune what is present in the interaction.

Guided Imagery and Visualization Techniques

As techniques, guided imagery and visualization have also been used in a wide array of settings, ranging from sports performance and executive coaching to pain management and learning methods (Bigham et al., 2014; Utay & Miller, 2006; Van Kuiken, 2004). Indeed, some have even contended that the basis of classical psychoanalytic and behavioral techniques is based in guided imagery (Schoettle, 1980). Related to psychotherapy generally, guided imagery has been used for autonomic downregulation, along with increasing motivation through imagining possible future outcomes (Sandu, 2020); related to EH therapies in particular, these techniques create more possibilities for enhanced and multilayered descriptive clarifications available to the therapist and client through metaphoric attunement (Spinelli, 2014b).

According to Spinelli (2014a), use of guided imagery and visualization through metaphor may help clarify "how statements of disturbance . . . can be expressed through various analogies or comparisons with objects, conditions or events that initially would be unrelated to what is being expressed," which allows a "linking up between the client's often abstract of intangible statements of disorder with specified figures of speech or tangible objects" (p. 21). The specific metaphor used is only important insofar as it collaboratively connects with and illuminates the client's experience. How one describes oneself is already an expression, through the concretizing properties of language, of the boundaries of self-experience. Utilizing such imagery and visualization, then, allows clients to understand themselves more flexibly within the constricted bounds of their self-conception. Once the client can metaphorically extend their problem and self-conception beyond the bounds of previous understanding, so too may novel alternatives or ways of navigating such self-experiences concurrently arise.

RESEARCH SUPPORT

As with any approach to evaluating the evidence base of a given psychotherapeutic framework, a cohesive set of operational definitions and parameters must be established from which to guide the research. As may be apparent in both the present chapter and the book, defining the foundations and common themes across existential and humanistic therapies remains quite the challenge, as important distinctions exist between practitioners and geographic locations (Cooper, 2003). Add to that the nuance of integrating experiential techniques from other approaches, and the task can appear daunting; however, as Hoffman and colleagues (2015) have discussed in line with many common approaches to psychotherapy research, EH therapy connects strongly to the very foundations known as effective change agents. Further, when applied thoughtfully and appropriately, the flexibility within the approach opens it to valuable contributions from other approaches and techniques (Schneider, 2008). As EH and experiential therapies have their own evidence bases, sometimes separate from one another, it would be next to impossible to explicate the full extent of available research. However, I would draw your attention to the influential and comprehensive research conducted by Robert Elliott and colleagues over many decades, from which this chapter draws heavily (Elliott et al., 2004, 2013, 2021). Specifically, his work has been a tour de force in both establishing humanistic and experiential therapies as having research support and maintaining their voices as relevant in a sea of growing conceptual frameworks. Following the theme of integrating EH therapies and experiential techniques, the following subsections will provide an overview of overlapping research areas between the two, which includes discussions of quantitative and qualitative support. Further research needs are elaborated later.

Quantitative Research

At the core of EH and experiential practice is the question of how clients and therapists experience a given context or interaction. Specifically, much early research tended to focus on change processes, which often attempted to delineate both client and therapist variables that contributed to successful therapeutic outcomes. As discussed previously, numerous early pioneers of both research approaches contended that the active exploration and facilitation of the client's perceptual field as a moment-to-moment phenomenological process is a primary method through which successful therapy occurs (Gendlin, 1969; Rogers, 1951). The way reported experiences were discussed and understood, rather than the content alone, was observed as most significant, which gave rise to research efforts aimed at understanding depth of in-session experiencing. One such effort was the development of the Client Experiencing Scale, which defines in-session experiencing as the holistic process of ongoing awareness, wherein methods that induce greater contact are used in the context of a connected therapeutic relationship (Klein et al., 1969). Utilizing scales such as the Client Experiencing Scale, researchers have consistently shown the efficacy of increased experiential processing and concluded that higher experiencing levels predict better psychotherapeutic outcomes (Hendricks, 2002) across every stage of the therapy (Pascual-Leone & Yeryomenko, 2017). Further, in controlled studies, approximately 80% of the pre–post gains reported by clients in therapies applying experiential techniques were attributable to the therapy, suggesting a strong causal relationship between such application and client change that was maintained over early and late follow-ups (Bohart & Watson, 2011).

Underscoring these process outcomes is the development of a strong alliance or therapeutic relationship. Indeed, a great deal of work has supported the conclusion that psychotherapeutic outcomes from all therapeutic stripes depend on strong relational conditions, such as therapist empathy, genuineness, positive regard, and a valued alliance (Norcross & Wampold, 2019a; see also Part II of this book). However, as Elliott and colleagues (2021) have noted, a consistent gap in the area of conventional outcome research is identifying what within the therapist–client relationship specifically mediates therapeutic outcomes, as greater nuance was required beyond the broad categories of Rogers's (1957) necessary and sufficient conditions of change. To address this concern, Watson and colleagues (2014) investigated mediating variables and found a significant direct relationship between therapist empathy and outcome, specifying the importance of perceived empathy from the therapist as attributable to significant improvement in client attachment insecurity and decreases in negative self-treatment. Continuing this effort, Malin and Pos (2015) found that client outcomes were mediated by therapist empathy, the working alliance, and client emotional processing during the initial session and middle stages of therapy. Additionally, the impact of clients' pretreatment characteristics and level of therapist responsiveness from the initial point of contact was strongly associated with the formation of a strong therapeutic alliance.

Specific to unique client presentations and specific therapeutic tasks, use of experiential methods has been studied extensively, utilizing pre–post, controlled, and comparative studies in six major domains: depression, relationship problems, coping with chronic medical problems, self-damaging behaviors (i.e., substance abuse and eating disorders), anxiety, and psychosis (Elliott et al., 2021). Except for anxiety, wherein more mixed but fewer studies were found, a great deal of evidentiary support exists for these presenting issues. Additionally, across the lifespan, there is a strong case for use of experiential therapies with children and adolescents, in particular for anxiety resulting from adjustment issues and traumatic events (Holldampf et al., 2010). Although several therapeutic tasks and methods were used to achieve the aforementioned outcomes, specific to experiential and EH therapies, narrative processes and assimilation were the most well-studied (Angus & Greenberg, 2011; Gonçalves et al., 2011). Within these central client change variables, their associated process measures include "emotional processing, including expression, deepening, transformation and regulation, the emergence of new client narratives, changes in clients' self-organization and the assimilation or problematic experiences" (Elliott et al., 2021, p. 41). Therein, these new conceptual frameworks and techniques provide greater nuance in how the client change process occurs.

Qualitative Research

Complementing quantitative research on EH and experiential therapies, qualitative research in these areas has provided flexibility and nuance in understanding what both clients and therapists experience as part of the therapy, along with the complexity inherent in the therapeutic change process (Hilton & Prior, 2018). Indeed, as a method, qualitative research has historically been favored by researchers in both EH and experiential camps due to philosophical compatibility and ease of conceptual integration through such methods as narrative accounts and case studies. Across qualitative studies, the most common data collection has been the posttherapy interview and follow-up, which frequently reflected positive outcomes related to increased emotional awareness, resilience, and feelings of empowerment (Greenberg, 2011).

As Elliott and colleagues (2021) have discussed, enough data from qualitative studies on experiential therapeutic applications now exist to allow for meta-analytic types of reviews, suggesting an increased interest and valuation in this type of methodology. Meeting that challenge, Timulak and Creaner (2010) began by creating a category system that summarized the qualitative experiences of 106 clients participating in several different EH and experiential therapies into 11 categories. This qualitative outcome was subsequently updated with an additional nine studies and 71 clients (Elliott et al., 2021), along with several comparison studies that highlighted nuances between those who reported the therapy as successful and those who reported it as unsuccessful (McElvaney & Timulak, 2013; Steinmann et al., 2017).

Regarding what factors may have helped or hindered these outcomes, qualitative research has revealed some of the complexities of both client and therapist's experience of therapy. By complexities, I mean differing agendas regarding the therapeutic work, client ambivalence, personality variables, and diversity characteristics, all of which can significantly affect the therapeutic outcome. More specifically, when therapists and clients were asked to provide feedback on their experiences in therapy and, in some instances, review prior transcripts or video recordings of sessions (Moerman & McLeod, 2006; Rennie et al., 1988), both therapists and clients reported a key factor in differentiating the quality of their experience as *therapeutic presence*, defined as engagement with both the in-session activities and relationship (Geller & Greenberg, 2002; Geller et al., 2010; see also Chapter 4 of this volume). When therapists were viewed as collaboratively present and engaged, their interventions were viewed as helpful; when viewed as distant or confusing, therapist interventions were viewed as hindering. Taken together, these findings underscore the importance of relational elements in therapy, such as the client's perception of being heard, validated, understood, and supported (MacLeod & Elliott, 2014; MacLeod et al., 2012), not only as indicative of developed rapport but as essential in client perception of personal change (Knox, 2008). In addition, related to qualitative change processes, clients viewed therapists' skills in clarification, guidance, awareness promotion, empathic understanding, and validation as playing an important role (Knox et al., 2012).

MULTICULTURAL CONSIDERATIONS

Of consistent import to the use of experiential techniques and integration into an EH framework is multicultural contextualization. At a social and cultural level, it is imperative for therapists to continually strive toward multicultural responsiveness in understanding and meeting the needs of an ever-expanding landscape of diverse clientele. Individually, if one is to take seriously the espoused values of EH and experiential therapies of helping clients find authentic expression and hear their own voices more clearly, then remaining open and present to each idiosyncratic encounter is essential (Davis et al., 2018; Vasquez, 2007). Regarding experiential techniques specifically, operating from a multicultural orientation enhances the therapist's awareness of the exquisite context dependence in how those techniques may be applied (Hook et al., 2017). In particular, there are three experiential practice areas that might benefit most strongly from continued multicultural development: case formulation, in-therapy experiencing, and process and meaning facilitation.

The umbrella term for the kind of relationship that is established between the client and therapist, along with mutual goals and expectations, is called the working alliance. Its articulation, which informs how the therapy is approached, is called the case formulation. Because EH and experiential therapies view the working alliance as constructively dialogic with an effort placed on articulating the client's lived experience, they are foundationally well-suited to address the needs of varying clients (see Hoffman & Cleare-Hoffman, 2025). As Felder and Robbins (2021) discuss, these therapies "maintain that cultural landscapes or interconnected world horizons of context and culture are inseparable from lived experience" (p. 4), wherein therapists attempt to attune "to a client's bodily or mooded way of being . . . as they relate to her, him, or them as a *sociocultural-being-in-the-world*" (p. 6, italics in original). Therefore, adapting experiential techniques to give maximal expression to the client's embodied "person–world dialogue" (p. 4) shares a close affinity to multicultural guidelines' focus on microlevel and macrolevel contexts that interact with sociocultural identities (Felder & Robbins, 2021; see also American Psychological Association, 2017; Vasquez, 2010).

Regarding in-therapy experiencing, Hoffman and colleagues (2015) state, "Embedded in much of Western psychology is an implicit theory of emotions that tends to impose upon clients without consideration being given pertaining to the client's view of emotions" (p. 16). Indeed, there are distinct divergences related to how clients experience emotions and the validity of their expression. Applied in a decontextualized manner, promotion of in-session experiencing of moment-to-moment emotional process may range from misattuned to injurious (Sue, 2015; Yeo & Torres-Harding, 2021). Sundararajan (2015) offers a contextual salve to these concerns through her elucidation of Chinese discourse on emotional experiencing, which de-emphasizes the typical East–West bifurcation in favor of a nuanced complementarity that finds resonance between traditional Chinese thinking and Western ideas. Though her commentary implicitly reflects some broad differences in worldview conceptualization, she explains these differences as context dependent rather than categorical (i.e., the *yin* and *yang* dialectic), similar to a phenomenological perspectivism offering multiple vantage points of the same object. To that end, in-therapy experiencing need not necessitate a particular way of experiencing or expressing emotions, and several authors have contributed ever-growing, valuable dialogues in working with emotional experiencing and expression in multitude of ways (Collins & Levitt, 2022; Hoffman & Cleare-Hoffman, 2011; Levitt et al., 2022).

Closely linked to in-session experience is how meaning is made from it in therapeutic or other contexts. Regardless of therapists' views regarding whether meaning is found or created, meaning structures require negotiation of both individual and cultural contexts. Similar techniques or strategies will undoubtedly be experienced differently when the cultural background between the therapist and client are recognized by each as varyingly similar or different. As one example, Hofstede (2011) contends that different cultures vary in how they engage in "uncertainty avoidance" (p. 10), a central area of EH exploration, which may influence how meaning interpretation may be understood or tolerated. Herein, experiential techniques such as Gendlin's (1996) focusing encourage therapists to attend and remain adaptive to meaning as it unfolds in the clinical encounter, being careful to not impose or prescribe a particular way of meaning making through overly interpretative statements or lack of self-awareness of one's stimulus value.

FUTURE RESEARCH NEEDS

Utilizing multiple research methods across a myriad of domains, a varied wealth of evidence exists, demonstrating experiential therapies as positively valuated and evidence based (Elliott et al., 2021). Therefore, continuing to refine and identify global and specific within-treatment variables in understanding client change processes remains an important priority. To that effect, while expanding (Elliott et al., 2021), a great deal of both quantitative and qualitative inquiry suffers from a paucity of cultural and clinical diversity regarding both researchers and study participants, which affects relevance and generalizability. This lack of clinical diversity also includes potential adverse or difficult experiences arising out of experiential and EH therapies (Elliott et al., 2021).

Specific to research from a quantitative perspective, many scales are observationally rated and do not ask clients about their own depth of experience. Creating questions or adding scales that more fully address this aspect may help contextualize and drive the data sets as a wholistic process. Additionally, as

Pascual-Leone and Yeryomenko (2017) have discussed, overlapping data sets in both single and meta-analytic studies, which are frequently unacknowledged by researchers, increase redundancy, which likely masks sample size and reduces the power of statistical analyses.

From a qualitative perspective, several limitations extend from the fact that, as a research framework, such methods are newer and therefore lessen the quality and number of studies conducted. While growing, more studies are needed to tease out consistency in understanding change processes, as most do not separate or compare by client issue or treatment orientation. In particular, despite complementary theoretical constructs, very few studies specifically discuss the treatment implications of using techniques across a variety of orientations (i.e. the use of experiential strategies in EH therapies). This not only affects treatment efficacy but, as a downstream effect, creates lack of focus and clarity in training future clinicians hoping to utilize these treatment orientations.

CONCLUSION

This chapter began with the express aim at meeting Gendlin's (1982) challenge to reconnect body and language—a unique return to embodied being-in-the-world. Together, EH and experiential therapies seem particularly well-suited to do so, as they are in many respects conceptual bedfellows that share strong evidence bases under the definitions of evidence-based practice. Additionally, with an increasing focus on commonalities among therapeutic orientations in general (Wampold, 2015) and the fluidity of each approach in particular, both approaches lend themselves well to discussions of integration (Schneider, 2008). Prior literature on EH and experiential therapy integration has tended to focus, importantly, on points of theoretical agreement; however, this often left interested practitioners with little pragmatic guidance. In an effort to fill that gap, this chapter will hopefully serve as a useful guide toward the complementary integration of experiential techniques within EH therapies.

REFERENCES

American Psychological Association. (2017). *Multicultural guidelines: An ecological approach to context, identity, and intersectionality, 2017*. https://www.apa.org/about/policy/multicultural-guidelines

Angus, L., & Greenberg, L. (2011). *Working with narrative in emotion-focused therapy: Changing stories, healing lives*. American Psychological Association. https://doi.org/10.1037/12325-000

Bigham, E., McDannel, L., Luciano, I., & Salgado-Lopez, G. (2014). Effect of a brief guided imagery on stress. *Biofeedback, 42*(1), 28–35. https://doi.org/10.5298/1081-5937-42.1.07

Bohart, A. C., & Watson, J. C. (2011). Person-centered psychotherapy and related experiential approaches. In S. B. Messer & A. S. Gurman (Eds.), *Essential psychotherapies: Theory and practice* (pp. 1–38). Guilford Press.

Buber, M., Cissna, K. N., Rogers, C. R., & Anderson, R. (1997). *The Martin Buber–Carl Rogers dialogue: A new transcript with commentary.* SUNY Press.

Collins, K. M., & Levitt, H. M. (2022). Healing from heterosexism: A discovery-oriented task analysis of emotion-focused writing. *Journal of Gay & Lesbian Mental Health, 26*(1), 2–23. https://doi.org/10.1080/19359705.2021.1876805

Cooper, M. (2003). *Existential therapies.* Sage.

Davis, D. E., DeBlaere, C., Owen, J., Hook, J. N., Rivera, D. P., Choe, E., Van Tongeren, D. R., Worthington, E. L., & Placeres, V. (2018). The multicultural orientation framework: A narrative review. *Psychotherapy, 55*(1), 89–100. https://doi.org/10.1037/pst0000160

DuBose, T. (2015). Engaged understanding for lived meaning. *Journal of Contemporary Psychotherapy, 45*(1), 25–35. https://doi.org/10.1007/s10879-014-9276-x

Elliott, R., & Greenberg, L. S. (2007). The essence of process–experiential/emotion-focused therapy. *American Journal of Psychotherapy, 61*(3), 241–254. https://doi.org/10.1176/appi.psychotherapy.2007.61.3.241

Elliott, R., Greenberg, L. S., & Germain, L. (2004). Research on experiential psychotherapies. In M. J. Lambert (Ed.), *Bergin & Garfield's handbook of psychotherapy and behavior change* (5th ed., pp. 493–539). John Wiley & Sons.

Elliott, R., Watson, J., Greenberg, L. S., Timulak, L., & Freire, E. (2013). Research on humanistic–experiential psychotherapies. In M. J. Lambert (Ed.), *Bergin & Garfield's handbook of psychotherapy and behavior change* (6th ed., pp. 495–538). John Wiley & Sons.

Elliott, R., Watson, J., Timulak, L., & Sharbanee, J. (2021). Research on humanistic–experiential psychotherapies: Updated review. In M. Barkham, W. Lutz, & L. G. Castonguay (Eds.), *Bergin & Garfield's handbook of psychotherapy and behavior change* (50th anniv. ed., pp. 421–467). John Wiley & Sons.

Felder, A. J., & Robbins, B. D. (2021). Approaching mindful multicultural case formulation: Rogers, Yalom, and existential phenomenology. *Person-Centered and Experiential Psychotherapies, 20*(1), 1–20. https://doi.org/10.1080/14779757.2020.1748697

Geller, S. M., & Greenberg, L. S. (2002). Therapeutic presence: Therapists' experience of presence in the psychotherapy encounter. *Person-Centered and Experiential Psychotherapies, 1*(1–2), 71–86. https://doi.org/10.1080/14779757.2002.9688279

Geller, S. M., Greenberg, L. S., & Watson, J. C. (2010). Therapist and client perceptions of therapeutic presence: The development of a measure. *Psychotherapy Research, 20*(5), 599–610. https://doi.org/10.1080/10503307.2010.495957

Gendlin, E. T. (1969). Focusing. *Psychotherapy, 6*(1), 4–15. https://doi.org/10.1037/h0088716

Gendlin, E. T. (1982). Two phenomenologists do not disagree. In R. Bruzina & B. Wilshire (Eds.), *Phenomenology: Dialogues and bridges* (pp. 321–335). State University of New York Press.

Gendlin, E. T. (1996). *Making concepts from experience.* Focusing Institute.

Gonçalves, M. M., Ribeiro, A. P., Mendes, I., Matos, M., & Santos, A. (2011). Tracking novelties in psychotherapy process research: The innovative moments coding system. *Psychotherapy Research, 21*(5), 497–509. https://doi.org/10.1080/10503307.2011.560207

Greenberg, L. S. (2002). *Emotion-focused therapy: Coaching clients to work through their feelings.* American Psychological Association. https://doi.org/10.1037/10447-000

Greenberg, L. S. (2011). *Emotion-focused therapy.* American Psychological Association.

Heller, M. C. (2012). *Body psychotherapy: History, concepts, methods.* W. W. Norton & Company.

Hendricks, M. N. (2002). Focusing-oriented/experiential psychotherapy. In D. J. Cain & J. Seeman (Eds.), *Humanistic psychotherapies: Handbook of research and practice* (pp. 221–251). American Psychological Association. https://doi.org/10.1037/10439-007

Hilton, J., & Prior, S. (2018). Re-visioning person-centred research. In *Re-Visioning Person-Centred Therapy* (pp. 277–288). Routledge. https://doi.org/10.4324/9781351186797-20

Hoffman, L. (2009). Introduction to existential–humanistic psychology in a cross-cultural context. In L. Hoffman, M. Yang, F. J. Kaklauskas, & A. Chan (Eds.), *Existential psychology East–West* (pp. 1–72). University of the Rockies Press.

Hoffman, L., & Cleare-Hoffman, H. P. (2011). Existential therapy and emotions: Lessons from cross-cultural exchange. *The Humanistic Psychologist, 39*(3), 261–267. https://doi.org/10.1080/08873267.2011.594342

Hoffman, L., & Cleare-Hoffman, H. P. (2025). *Case formulation in existential–humanistic therapy.* American Psychological Association. https://doi.org/10.1037/0000464-000

Hoffman, L., Vallejos, L., Cleare-Hoffman, H. P., & Rubin, S. (2015). Emotion, relationship, and meaning as core existential practice: Evidence-based foundations. *Journal of Contemporary Psychotherapy, 45*(1), 11–20. https://doi.org/10.1007/s10879-014-9277-9

Hofstede, G. (2011). Dimensionalizing cultures: The Hofstede model in context. *Online Readings in Psychology and Culture, 2*(1), 1–25. https://doi.org/10.9707/2307-0919.1014

Holldampf, D., Behr, M., & Crawford, I. (2010). Effectiveness of person-centered and experiential psychotherapies with children and young people: A review of outcome studies. In M. Cooper, J. C. Watson, & D. Holldampf (Eds.), *Person-centred and experiential therapies work: A review of the research on counseling, psychotherapy, and related practices* (pp. 16–44). PCCS Books.

Hook, J. N., Davis, D., Owen, J., & DeBlaere, C. (2017). *Cultural humility: Engaging diverse identities in therapy.* American Psychological Association. https://doi.org/10.1037/0000037-000

Klein, M. H., Mathieu, P., Gendlin, E. T., & Kiesler, D. J. (1969). *The experiencing scale: A research and training manual: Vol. 1.* Wisconsin Psychiatric Institute.

Knox, R. (2008). Clients' experiences of relational depth in person-centred counselling. *Counselling & Psychotherapy Research, 8*(3), 182–188. https://doi.org/10.1080/14733140802035005

Knox, R., Murphy, D., Wiggins, S., & Cooper, M. (2012). *Relational depth: New perspectives and developments.* Macmillan International Higher Education.

Levitt, H. M., Collins, K. M., Maroney, M. R., & Roberts, T. S. (2022). Healing from heterosexist experiences: A mixed method intervention study using expressive writing. *Psychology of Sexual Orientation and Gender Diversity, 9*(2), 152–164. https://doi.org/10.1037/sgd0000478

MacLeod, R., & Elliott, R. (2014). Nondirective person-centered therapy for social anxiety: A hermeneutic single-case efficacy design study of a good outcome case. *Person-Centered and Experiential Psychotherapies, 13*(4), 294–311. https://doi.org/10.1080/14779757.2014.910133

MacLeod, R., Elliott, R., & Rodgers, B. (2012). Process–experiential/emotion-focused therapy for social anxiety: A hermeneutic single-case efficacy design study. *Psychotherapy Research, 22*(1), 67–81. https://doi.org/10.1080/10503307.2011.626805

Madison, G. (2014a). Palpable existentialism: A focusing-oriented therapy. *Psychotherapy in Australia, 20*(2), 36–42.

Madison, G. (2014b). The palpable in existential counselling psychology. *Counselling Psychology Review, 29*(2), 25–33. https://doi.org/10.53841/bpscpr.2014.29.2.25

Madison, G., & Gendlin, E. (2012). Palpable existentialism: An interview with Eugene Gendlin. In L. Barnett & G. Madison (Eds.), *Existential therapy: Legacy, vibrancy and dialogue* (pp. 81–96). Routledge.

Malin, A. J., & Pos, A. E. (2015). The impact of early empathy on alliance building, emotional processing, and outcome during experiential treatment of depression. *Psychotherapy Research, 25*(4), 445–459. https://doi.org/10.1080/10503307.2014.901572

McElvaney, J., & Timulak, L. (2013). Clients' experience of therapy and its outcomes in quantitatively "good outcomes" and "poor outcomes" psychological therapy in a primary care setting: An exploratory study. *Counselling & Psychotherapy Research, 13*(4), 246–253. https://doi.org/10.1080/14733145.2012.761258

Merleau-Ponty, M. (1962). *Phenomenology of perception* (C. Smith, Trans.). Routledge & Kegan Paul.

Minuchin, S., & Fishman, H. C. (1981). *Family therapy techniques*. Harvard University Press. https://doi.org/10.4159/9780674041110

Moerman, M., & McLeod, J. (2006). Person-centered counseling for alcohol-related problems: The client's experience of self in the therapeutic relationship. *Person-Centered and Experiential Psychotherapies, 5*(1), 21–35. https://doi.org/10.1080/14779757.2006.9688390

Norcross, J. C., & Wampold, B. E. (Eds.). (2019a). *Psychotherapy relationships that work: Vol. 2. Evidence-based therapist responsiveness* (3rd ed.). Oxford Press. https://doi.org/10.1093/med-psych/9780190843960.001.0001

Norcross, J. C., & Wampold, B. E. (2019b). Relationships and responsiveness in the psychological treatment of trauma: The tragedy of the APA Clinical Practice Guideline. *Psychotherapy, 56*(3), 391–399. https://doi.org/10.1037/pst0000228

Paruzel-Czachura, M., & Konieczniak, B. (2020). *Let's introduce order into gestalt terminology: Method, concepts and techniques, and their development after 70 years of gestalt psychotherapy*. PsyArXiv Preprints. Advance online publication. https://doi.org/10.31234/osf.io/mxsd2

Pascual-Leone, A., & Yeryomenko, N. (2017). The client "experiencing" scale as a predictor of treatment outcomes: A meta-analysis on psychotherapy process. *Psychotherapy Research, 27*(6), 653–665. https://doi.org/10.1080/10503307.2016.1152409

Rennie, D. L., Phillips, J. R., & Quartaro, G. K. (1988). Grounded theory: A promising approach to conceptualization in psychology? *Canadian Psychology, 29*(2), 139–150. https://doi.org/10.1037/h0079765

Rogers, C. R. (1951). *Client-centered therapy: Its current practice, implications and theory*. Constable.

Rogers, C. R. (1957). The necessary and sufficient conditions of therapeutic personality change. *Journal of Consulting Psychology, 21*(2), 95–103. https://doi.org/10.1037/h0045357

Rogers, C. R. (1961). *On becoming a person*. Houghton Mifflin Company.

Rogers, C. R. (1980). *A way of being*. Houghton Mifflin Company.

Sandu, A. (2020). The importance and limits of experiential psychotherapy. *Logos Universality Mentality Education Novelty: Philosophy & Humanistic Sciences, 8*(2), 72–82. https://doi.org/10.18662/lumenphs/8.2/46

Schneider, K. J. (Ed.). (2008). *Existential integrative psychotherapy: Guideposts to the core of practice*. Routledge.

Schneider, K. J., Pierson, J. F., & Bugental, J. F. (Eds.). (2014). *The handbook of humanistic psychology: Theory, research, and practice*. Sage Publications.

Schoettle, U. C. (1980). Guided imagery—A tool in child psychotherapy. *American Journal of Psychotherapy, 34*(2), 220–227. https://doi.org/10.1176/appi.psychotherapy.1980.34.2.220

Serlin, I. A., & Shane, P. (1999). Laura Perls and gestalt therapy: Her life and values. In D. Moss (Ed.), *Humanistic and transpersonal psychology: A historical and biographical sourcebook* (pp. 374–384). Greenwood Press.

Spinelli, E. (2014a). Descriptive challenging in existential therapy. *Dasein, 3*(1), 11–27.

Spinelli, E. (2014b). *Practising existential therapy: The relational world*. Sage.

Steinmann, R., Gat, I., Nir-Gottlieb, O., Shahar, B., & Diamond, G. M. (2017). Attachment-based family therapy and individual emotion-focused therapy for unresolved anger: Qualitative analysis of treatment outcomes and change processes. *Psychotherapy, 54*(3), 281–291. https://doi.org/10.1037/pst0000116

Sue, D. W. (2015). Therapeutic harm and cultural oppression. *The Counseling Psychologist, 43*(3), 359–369. https://doi.org/10.1177/0011000014565713

Sundararajan, L. (2015). *Understanding emotion in Chinese culture: Thinking through psychology*. Springer International Publishing. https://doi.org/10.1007/978-3-319-18221-6

Timulak, L., & Creaner, M. (2010). Qualitative meta-analysis of outcomes of person-centred/experiential therapies. In M. Cooper, J. C. Watson, & D. Holledampf (Eds.), *Person-centred and experiential psychotherapies work*. PCCS Books.

Utay, J., & Miller, M. (2006). Guided imagery as an effective therapeutic technique: A brief review of its history and efficacy research. *Journal of Instructional Psychology, 33*(1), 40–43.

Van Kuiken, D. (2004). A meta-analysis of the effect of guided imagery practice on outcomes. *Journal of Holistic Nursing, 22*(2), 164–179. https://doi.org/10.1177/0898010104266066

Vasquez, M. J. T. (2007). Cultural difference and the therapeutic alliance: An evidence-based analysis. *American Psychologist, 62*(8), 878–885. https://doi.org/10.1037/0003-066X.62.8.878

Vasquez, M. J. T. (2010). Ethics in multicultural counseling practice. In J. G. Ponterotto, J. M. Casas, L. A. Suzuki, & C. M. Alexander (Eds.), *Handbook of multicultural counseling* (pp. 127–145). Sage.

Wade, J. (1996). *Changes of mind*. SUNY Press.

Wampold, B. E. (2015). How important are the common factors in psychotherapy? An update. *World Psychiatry, 14*(3), 270–277. https://doi.org/10.1002/wps.20238

Watson, J. C., Steckley, P. L., & McMullen, E. J. (2014). The role of empathy in promoting change. *Psychotherapy Research, 24*(3), 286–298. https://doi.org/10.1080/10503307.2013.802823

Yalom, I. D. (1980). *Existential psychotherapy*. Basic Books.

Yeo, E., & Torres-Harding, S. R. (2021). Rupture resolution strategies and the impact of rupture on the working alliance after racial microaggressions in therapy. *Psychotherapy, 58*(4), 460–471. https://doi.org/10.1037/pst0000372

Yontef, G. M., & Jacobs, J. (2008). Gestalt therapy. In R. Corsini & D. Wedding (Eds.), *Current psychotherapies* (pp. 328–367). Brooks/Cole-Thompson Learning.

17

An Existential–Humanistic Approach to Equine-Facilitated Psychotherapy

Aviva Vincent and Veronica Lac

Before considering equine-facilitated psychotherapy (EFP) as a model to provide an existential–humanistic (EH) mental health intervention, it is important to first consider the question, "Why horses?" If read sequentially, this text has offered a potentially new perspective to understanding EH within mental health practices. Moreover, the prior chapters intentionally discussed practice strategies including mindfulness and expressive arts. Humans have close-held bonds and relationships with a wide variety of mammals, so why then do horses rise from the herd to be the ideal partner for an EH intervention?

The emergence of therapeutic equestrianism dates differs based on whose narrative is prioritized: oral Indigenous histories or archaeological evidence. The latter tends to take precedent in Westernized history. Greek mythology tells of the powerful horses Pegasus, Chiron, and Iberia in 700 B.C.E. In 400 B.C.E., philosopher and Greek officer Xenophon noted that horses supported the rehabilitation of soldiers (Hallberg, 2008). However, "for Navajos, *the horse has always been here . . . since the beginning of time*" (John, 2023, italics in original). Although contemporary views of access and engagement in horseback riding tends to be framed with Eurocentric and White affluency, horses and humans have been working in partnership globally and toward mutual healing as far back as modern literature allows.

Reflecting on the multicultural impact of horses, they are unique in that they have a global presence as a means of transportation, an opportune pet, and a wild beast (Cross, 2019). Evidence of horses being harnessed and milked for human consumption dates back to 3500 B.C.E. in Kazakhstan and in 85%

https://doi.org/10.1037/0000446-018
The Evidence-Based Foundations of Existential–Humanistic Therapy, L. Hoffman and V. Lac (Editors)

of Asia (Williams, 2016). The transformational impact of the horse–human bond has helped individuals overcome physical and mental health challenges. The global equine industry has been referred to as "one of the biggest industries in plain sight" (Equine Business Association, 2023, para. 1). Since the mid-1900s, humans have made the vital connection that horses may also be conduits to healing of the self.

DEFINING EFP

EFP is a modality of mental health therapy that intentionally includes horses as cofacilitators in therapeutic sessions to address emotional, behavioral, and psychological challenges expressed by clients. This growing field of experiential therapy combines traditional psychotherapy techniques with interactions involving horses. Often, the connotation is that EFP is an alternative opportunity to talk therapy. Some clients have found their way to the stable when talk therapy is no longer serving them; however, EFP often includes talking and processing just the same. Hence, all professionals engaged in providing EFP must hold and maintain clinical licensure within a mental health field.

The inclusion of the horse is intended to achieve outcomes that otherwise would be more difficult or have been found ineffective in other environments (Nimer & Lundahl, 2007). There are a number of models and training options for conducting EFP (see Meola, 2023; Trotter & Baggerly, 2018); this chapter will not provide an overview of all of them but rather will emphasize one model that most closely aligns with EH therapy. Furthermore, all methods emphasize that clinicians are first and foremost mental health practitioners; however, the model discussed herein intentionally includes the horse as a cotherapist, not a canvas, metaphor, or other being. The horse is vital in the therapeutic process by nature of their fully sentient self.

The Horse

The horses are considered cotherapists because they are recognized as sentient beings involved in the therapeutic process. The horse is an active collaborator in the therapeutic process (Chandler, 2012; Matuszek, 2010) who aids in building social rapport, confidence, and introspective reflection for the client. The horse's nonjudgmental and intuitive nature is the foundation of the therapeutic environment wherein their innate behavior creates a safe and supportive environment for the client to explore and address their internalized and externalized challenges. The horse offers valuable feedback through behavioral responses during times of connection with the client. The interactions with horses can serve as a metaphor, mirror, or mimic for the client's emotions, thoughts, and patterns of behavior.

Since the focus is on the therapeutic interaction, the horse and client interact with feet on the ground in an effort to see and be with each other as two distinct and unique individuals. Physically getting onto a horse's back is infrequent in EFP sessions and is only included with clear and explicit parameters by the clinician.

Horses who engage in EFP have the right to choose not to work in sessions or with specific clients. Upholding choice is not only a fundamental equine welfare practice; within an EH framework of EFP, allowing the horses the explicit freedom of choice to engage in any interactions can be a powerful catalyst for change. In particular, for historically marginalized clients, witnessing the honoring of the horse's agency can lead to a deeper understanding of the systemic and existential freedoms they have been denied themselves.

The Client

Clients seek out EFP for a wide variety of reasons including past or current engagement with horses, lack of progress in traditional settings, referral from a trusted professional, or general curiosity (Chandler, 2012; Jegatheesan et al., 2015). Core outcomes of engaging in EFP are self-awareness, embodiment, emotional regulation, communication, trust and empathy, and growth. In pursuit of these outcomes, clients are encouraged to engage in a creative process. Creativity is more than manners of expression, though they can be a part of creativity. Instead, creativity is a deeper exploration of the self, or neuroplasticity. "The process of embodiment itself is a continuous, ever-changing, creative process" (Lac, 2023). Zinker (1978) states that "doing therapy is like making art. The medium is a human life" (p. 37). The psychotherapeutic process is a creative process wherein the clinician cultivates an attitude of experimentation that enlivens the therapeutic encounter (Lac, 2023). To make choices, derive meaning, and act on or express themselves through the choices they make is also a central tenant in EFP (Lac, 2017).

Horses provide clients with an opportunity to enhance self-awareness through practices of embodiment, and they provide opportunities to recognize, process, and understand their emotions, behaviors, and communication styles. Although this is a cognitive process at a surface level, the challenge is in the clinician supporting the client to experience and practice embodiment:

> Embodiment is about gaining, through the vehicle of awareness, the capacity to feel the ambient physical sensations of unfettered energy and aliveness as they pulse through our bodies. It is here that mind and body, thought and feeling, psyche and spirit, are held together, welded in an undifferentiated unity of experience. (Lac, 2017, p. 32)

This is the first core outcome because it is both the most complex and the most vital to authentically being with horses. Horses live and experience relationships in an embodied manner. To be fully present with horses means to live in the moment, fully embodied. Thus, embodiment is the "fluidity of intention through breath and movement" (Lac, 2017, p. 5) where two (or more) sentient beings—in this case, horse and human—find meaning in their connection. This connection is more than togetherness or joining, but a shift to an I-thou experience (Lac, 2017): "I am no longer only me, but me and thee make we" (Polster & Polster, 1974, p. 99).

It is important to note that the clinician must practice and experience embodiment in order to support the client. Doing so is fundamental to the practice of EH psychology (Schneider & Krug, 2010). "The more embodied we are, the more present we can be with ourselves and our clients" (Lac, 2014). This is not to state that clinicians must be embodied at all times, but rather that they excel at the process of practicing embodiment.

EFP facilitates opportunities to build skills in emotional and nervous system regulation by working with horses. Horses provide consistent opportunities for clients to practice managing stress, anxiety, and emotional reactivity. Regulation is a skill that requires practice for humans, whereas horses will naturally attune to their environment and respond through their body language, providing instant feedback to clients in sessions. They embody congruence and will often stay with clients as they recover and regulate (Lac, 2020). When regulation and congruence are present, horses will reengage based on prior expectations. This does not mean that horses are forgiving, as that would be anthropomorphizing; rather, horses embody their natural behaviors, which provides an active learning opportunity for the causation, impact, and repair of human actions and behaviors.

Since humans are working directly with horses, spoken language is only one of many methods of communication. Where humans prioritize spoken language with each other, the language of bodies becomes much more sensitive and attuned between horses and humans. Clients learn to develop more effective communication and refine their skills of communication through interactions with horses, as horses respond to nonverbal cues and body language.

Building relationships with horses can foster trust and empathy, which can be transferable to relationships with others. The relationships between horses can be just as important in the therapeutic process as those between horses and humans. This is an example where knowing the herd is important, as the clinician can facilitate conversation for the client to make meaning out of interactions and exchanges between horses. As a general modality, EFP can help clients process and heal from past traumatic experiences, which creates capacity for personal growth. The clinician and horse, as cotherapists, foster a safe environment that encourages practices of self-esteem and confidence as clients overcome challenges and achieve personal goals.

As with any therapeutic modality, EFP may not be appropriate for everyone. Individual preferences and needs should be considered. Past experiences with horses and other animals, cultural affiliation with horses, and other factors should be explored before connecting with the horses in session.

The Professional

In EFP, the mental health professional is a trained and licensed clinician in psychology, social work, or other aligned disciplines. Sessions may be between one clinician and client or may have a group of individuals. Similarly, there may be one horse or a herd of horses participating in a session. The clinician is responsible for practicing within their scope and having confidence in their knowledge of the herd or horse.

Again, the horse or herd is the cofacilitator of the therapeutic process; thus, there is an established relationship between the clinician and the horse prior to the session. Linking to the client's experience, the clinician is facilitating a creative process to build skills to bring about transformational change (Keeney, 2009; Yalom, 2001; Zinker, 1978). Acknowledging that the therapeutic process is a creative process aligns with the belief that "therapy is spontaneous, the relationship is dynamic and ever-evolving, and there is a continuous sequence of experiencing and then examining the process" (Yalom, 2001, p. 34). In fact, how one experiences themselves in their bodies is a culturally based phenomenon (Lac, 2023). This framework of an experiential, experimental, embodied creative process requires the therapist to take risks and be present with the client in their uncertainty of what might unfold or in the direction of where the therapy session is headed.

Another configuration of facilitating EFP is from the mental health clinician to partner with an equine specialist who is trained to recognize, respond to, and potentially reflect equine behavior and communication. This collaborative model is ideal when (a) working with a group of clients (i.e., less than five), (b) working with a dynamic herd of horses, or (c) having known concerns about human safety (i.e., clients who are not yet comfortable around horses). Additionally, for the safety of all involved, it is imperative that clinicians providing services are trained, qualified, and appropriately credentialed.

The issues of safety when working within EFP can bring profound awareness to clients who are experiencing psychological threats to emotional or physical safety. When entering into space with a herd of horses, practitioners are trained to provide a safety briefing to raise awareness of physical safety concerns when interacting with the horses. This often leads to discussions on how clients experience safety differently.

Case Example

The following is a case example[1] of an EFP safety issue in relation to everyday behavior. A teenage client with a history of risk-taking behavior repeatedly finds themselves standing in a corner against a wall or fence. Alternatively, they situate themself between two or more horses. By doing so, they are putting themself at risk of not being seen, being stepped on, or potentially being kicked or knocked over. When the practitioner shares their observation of this behavior as it is happening, the client begins to question how often they engage in this behavior. This conversation translates into their everyday life outside the barn. The practitioner mentions their observation, opening the possibility for introspection: How else might the client be putting themselves at risk—intentionally or otherwise?

---

[1]The case examples in this chapter have been modified to disguise the clients' identities and protect their confidentiality.

CONTEXTUALIZING EFP IN AN EH THERAPY CONTEXT

EH psychotherapy is inherently about being in relation with a sentient being other than oneself; hence, it is existential. Professionally, as a licensed mental health clinician, the priority of the clinical session is about the human. Thus, holding an existential relationship for humans to be in relation with others melds perfectly with the practice of EFP.

Horses experience their environment through the here-and-now, not what is coming for them in an hour or what just happened. That is not to say they are not critical thinkers with keen memory; in fact, they very much are (Lezama-García et al., 2019; Nakamura et al., 2018). Rather, they engage with their present environment by being present rather than reactionary. Thus, they require our presence to be in relationship with them.

The way that clinicians are trained to engage in EFP may differ greatly. Education and training are imperative to ensure a safe environment for the horse and human. At this time, there are more than six certificate programs accessible internationally (links to resources for further exploration will be listed at the end of the chapter). The human–equine relational development (HERD) model is the only method that centers EH at the core of education, training, and practice. Consistent with our practice and prioritization of equine welfare and EH therapy, the HERD model will be the foundation for the content herein.

The HERD Model

Western models of equestrianism often use pressure to seek compliance from horses. These pressure and release (i.e., negative and positive reinforcement), dominance, and hierarchy models view learned behavior, such as the horse turning toward the human, as connection (Rees, 2022). In contrast, the HERD model respects the horse as an independent, sentient being and allows for freedom, choice, and consent from horses during sessions.

Connection is inherent in sharing space regardless of physical contact. By starting at a place of mutual respect for space, the emphasis is on communication, presence, and patience. The HERD model is grounded in the experiential work of Schoen and Gordon (2015), who founded the 25 principles for embodying a compassionate equestrian. Engagement is a process in which both horse and human have a choice about their level of participation and engagement. A horse choosing not to make connection through physical contact is, in fact, part of the evolving relationship between the client and horse and provides an opportunity for a therapeutic connection, process, and conversation.

The HERD Model in Practice

Our whole self needs to be present in the here-and-now with the horse to foster an authentic relationship. This shift out of headspace and cognitive thought and into embodiment (into the body) increases opportunities for self-awareness and empathy for self and others. Thus, the answer for "Why horses?" lies in the prior chapters: presence, empathy, experiential learning, authenticity, self-awareness, the here-and-now, and the self. This existential, embodied, and relational approach is modeled by the horses in their way of being in the world. Thus, horses are indeed the ideal partner for an EH mental health intervention:

> The most meaningful therapy isn't about techniques or knowledge. As existential therapists, we bring ourselves fully into the moment and engage in relationships with our clients as fellow human beings. We share the moment, the space, and the air that we breathe as we connect with our clients and ourselves. There is mutuality in this connection that allows us to be not just a professional, but a living, breathing, sentient being with them. It is in this togetherness that healing occurs. As our clients find their place in the world, in their "herd," in their lives, we too find ourselves. This interconnectedness allows us to take ownership of the fact that our every action, or inaction, creates a ripple effect for those around us. Much like the horses in the herd, we cannot help but to make an impact on each other. (Lac, 2014, p. 5)

But What Happens in an EFP Session?

Clinicians, clients, and the community at large want to know what exactly is the activity that makes EFP impactful. The challenge is that EFP is not like a Western yoga class, that is, a designed series of movements with instruction and assistance. If yoga is the comparison, EFP is more like a free-form body movement session. Those in the session are aware of other humans in the environment; however, beyond knowing who is there, the session develops and unfolds organically. Transformational moments may even resonate with the client when driving home, the next day, or significantly later.

Though the emphasis of the session is not on the activity (see Lac, 2020), there are common methods used within EFP for facilitating horse and human engagement. Before the session, safety between humans and between horses and humans is explicitly discussed. Some sessions may be outside the pasture, where looking in on the horses holds meaning for the client. Other clients may seek out proximity to the horse. In this case, the clinician may welcome the client into a pasture or arena with the horses moving freely about. Contact may be facilitated through intentional grooming, mindful walking, navigating obstacle courses, and other movement-based collaborative activities (for session examples, see Hallberg, 2017; Lac, 2017).

There are uncountable opportunities to provide meaningful moments because it is not the activity that is important but the meaning the client attributes to the experiences. In the same grooming activity, for example, meaning may be found in the feeling of the horse's warmth and slow breath under the client's hands (regulation), the repetitive action of the brush along the horse's coat (mindfulness), or internalizing the joy of caring for another animal (empathy). Each has its own unique meaning to the client, and all outcomes stem from the same activity. The organic conversations that are generated through the sessions are the intention and core of the interaction; the horse is the facilitator of psychotherapy.

Case Study

The following case study explores an EFP session in regard to meaningful acceptance. During a session, the herd of three horses were grazing in the far corner of the pasture. The client, a combat veteran with posttraumatic stress, was commenting on the tranquility of the moment and how the horses were able to simply be in each other's presence without needing to be hypervigilant of their surroundings despite them being prey animals. He commented that it must be comforting to be surrounded by the herd and drew the parallel of being in combat, knowing that his fellow soldiers had his back. The session had started with the plan of walking out to the pasture to halter one of the horses and lead them back into the barn for a grooming activity, so I asked him if that was what he wanted to do now that he had named this feeling of comfort in being with the herd. He pondered my question for a moment and decided that he still wanted to connect with one of the horses that he had worked with previously. He had already formed a bond with my mare, Cheyenne, and was eager to continue developing a relationship with her.

As we approached the herd, Cheyenne lifted her head and watched us walking toward her. Simultaneously, the other two horses began to walk in the opposite direction, away from us, leaving Cheyenne standing in the middle. We stopped walking. She looked first at the other two horses and then at the two humans. I asked my client what he thought was happening. "It's like she's trying to decide who she wants to be with," he said. Cheyenne looked over her shoulder at her herd mates and then turned and looked at us again before slowly walking over and placing her head on my client's chest. I took a couple of steps back to give them space to sink into the moment. I noticed my client reaching up and stroking Cheyenne's neck as his eyes began to tear up.

In debriefing this experience during the session, my client talked about the profound acceptance he felt in Cheyenne choosing to be with him rather than rejoining the rest of the herd. To me, it felt like an I-thou moment of connection. However, it wasn't until a few weeks later that the real impact of the moment landed. In a subsequent session, the client commented that although he initially felt that the significance of that moment was that of being chosen, he realized later that it was actually a lesson to highlight that he had choices. The act of turning away from what was familiar and known and stepping toward the new and unknown became the central theme of the work that we did together.

EMPIRICAL EXPLORATION OF EFP

In an environmental scan of the literature, EBSCOhost was used to identify any peer-reviewed publications with the terms "existential–humanistic psychology" and "equine facilitated psychotherapy." This search yielded one result, from Lac (2017). Reducing the terms to "existential–humanistic" and "equine" yielded one additional text (Looman, 2012). Reducing the terms again, to "existential" and "equine," still with peer-review and full text available, yielded nine peer-reviewed texts.

Quantitative Research

Outside the scope of EH therapy, EFP has been investigated across populations including at-risk youth, veterans, and individuals with substance addictions. Veterans who experienced EFP self-reported higher levels of mindfulness post-session (Vincent et al., 2021). Shelef and colleagues (2019) utilized the Sheehan Disability Scale and the Short Post-Traumatic Stress Disorder Rating Interview assessments in a study with veterans that showed an improved ability to work and perform daily tasks and a reduction in the number of days of inefficiency. Machová and colleagues (2023) used the Assessment of Quality of Life scale and the Health of the Nation Outcome Scale and combined them with the Human–Animal Interaction Scale to assess clients with substance abuse disorders. They found that EFP interventions resulted in a significant increase in all three scales on clients' mood after every session and in the long-term perspective.

For adolescents with emotional and behavioral challenges, a comparison between EFP and traditional group therapy using the Positive and Negative Affect Scale revealed that EFP is statistically as effective as traditional group therapy at increasing positive affect scores and decreasing negative affect scores. Even more significant is that EFP resulted in higher positive affect before and after each session (Roberts & Honzel, 2020). Harvey and colleagues (2020) used the Behavior Assessment System for Children to collect data from parents and teachers of adolescent clients following participation in EFP sessions. Results indicated a significant improvement in behavior outcomes. The mechanisms by which bonding and intervention impacts clients vary by study, but overall studies cite the positive impact of the horse–human relationship.

Qualitative Research

Although there is still a paucity of qualitative research available, EFP as an experiential modality lends itself to a more holistic and qualitative lens. Felegy (2022) found that the quantitative assessment of their intervention offered no significant findings, but the qualitative data (i.e., clinical notes) were ripe with EH content: "transitions, resistance, openness to experience, willingness to engage, lack of engagement, connection, disconnection, thoughts/feelings/behaviors between students and horses, and meaninglessness" (p. iv). Related to feelings of safety and attachment as core elements of EH psychotherapy, Meyer and Sartori (2019) conducted in-depth interviews with Vietnam War veterans about their EFP experiences. Using the framework of attachment theory, qualitative themes emerged as positive changes in thoughts and behaviors, emotional regulation (including the alleviation of posttraumatic stress disorder symptoms), and interpersonal and interspecies relationships. This supports EH theory's focus on the importance of unconditional positive regard that is experienced as an embodied sense of belonging and acceptance (for more on acceptance, see Chapter 10 of this volume; Lac, 2023). This is further supported by Nieforth and Craig (2021) in their interviews with EFP practitioners to explore the role of equine communication as a model of client-centered communication that focuses on congruence, ongoing positive regard, and empathy. Lee and colleagues (2020) used a mixed methodology to study the impact of EFP on older adults experiencing functional and cognitive impairment. Findings suggest that clients found meaning in their interactions with horses, which led to improvements in social engagement and functioning.

The HERD model was developed from a phenomenological inquiry that focused on the embodied experience of EFP (Lac, 2016). Existential themes relating to isolation and belonging, freedom and choice, and meaning making became the foundation of the five-stage model. Participants described the process of beginning with an embodied sense of sharing space with the horses that allowed them to experience themselves in a way that felt like they were coming home to themselves, releasing internalized constraints, and expanding into authentic connection. This moment-to-moment unfolding of the fullness of one's bodily and emotional existence allowed for the revealing of a deeper capacity for relational being with others.

In the environmental scan of the literature, it was evident that qualitative findings make their way into books labeled as case studies and are therefore posited as less than. Qualitative research is what is needed to understand the complexity of lived experiences and being in relation with another sentient being. Here we find that the medical model and fixed categories of research are damaging to the opportunity of understanding EH therapy as a framework for EFP.

MULTICULTURAL CONSIDERATIONS

Awareness of dominant Western philosophies is imperative to ensure cultural humility within the practice of EH and EFP, as Western practices may not be applicable to non-Western societies (Argent & Vaught, 2022). By prioritizing authenticity and being present in interspecies relationships, clinicians and clients experience EH practices. Cultural humility includes a willingness to explore the client's values pertaining to sense of self, community, and generational relations and beliefs, especially in the context of addressing perceived interpersonal or internalized challenges (Lancia, 2022; Loue, 2022).

Practicing cultural humility includes the explicit spoken language by the clinician, as clients can be influenced by therapists' unintentional or intentional biases (Comas-Díaz, 2011). Day-Vines and colleagues (2007) provide a framework for how clinicians can competently and confidently talk about issues of race, ethnicity, and culture within the therapeutic dyad. Clinicians must also practice flexibility so as not to uphold stereotypes and biases that perpetuate marginalization. Humans do not fit into categories, which are inherently restrictive (Leung & Chen, 2009; Sue & Sue, 2008), and reliance on categories is problematic when translating experiences across multicultural communities (Leung & Chen, 2009). An alternative and inclusive practice is to center clients as experts of their lived experience. "Rather than positioning the client as being unable to do something, we are acknowledging their different way of operating and *our inability* to understand them" (Lac, 2020, p. 43, italics in original). Then, by becoming curious, we can reengage with clients authentically.

The importance of cultural humility has been expressed throughout the chapter. EFP and the HERD model use explicit practices of multiculturalism. The HERD Institute requires all participants to sign a Commitment of Belonging that outlines an expectation that they will commit to engaging in self-reflection and discussions about systemic inequalities; implicit bias; and ways to increase diversity, equity, and inclusion prior to starting education and certification. The HERD model shifts away from the Westernized model of equestrianism (inclusive of typical riding) and toward being in relationship with others, inclusive of the horse. The intentionality of the model has resulted in the highest number of diverse enrollments: racial and ethnic diversity; lesbian, gay, bisexual, transgender, and queer community involvement; body type inclusion; and neurodiverse practitioners.

Rather than reshaping prior multicultural theories (e.g., Allwood & Berry, 2006; Day-Vines et al., 2007; Hofstede, 1981), the HERD model encourages the use of field theory (see Lac, 2017), which is also consistent with EH therapy (Fernbacher & Plummer, 2005). Through increasing awareness of oneself in relation to others and the environment, we can create a "common communicative home, which is mutually constructed" (Parlett, 1991, p. 75).

Western clinicians must take active steps to cease the erasure of native and Indigenous experiences with horses. Intentional decolonization of horses from humans is needed. Researchers (see John, 2023) are shifting away from horses as a colonial tool, as horse histories need to be unfolded from "the American creation narrative" (p. 30). If effectively done, horses can be recognized as fully embodied beings within the process with humans, not for humans. This returns to the foundational concept of being in relation with each other as stated previously: "I am no longer only me, but me and thee make we" (Polster & Polster, 1974, p. 99).

FUTURE RESEARCH NEEDS

The critique and growth of research have run parallel for over a decade, with some critiquing the use of EFP interventions without rigorous research (i.e., Anestis et al., 2014) and others advocating that the steady growth of the research field demonstrates thoughtful research practices. As such, mixed methods research needs to continue in an effort to hear about lived experiences (qualitative) and quantify impact (quantitative). To date, the most comprehensive compendium of measures is by Anderson (2007); however, all measures are in relation to pets or companion animals. The Center for the Study of Animal Wellness Pet Bonding Scale by Johnson and Meadows (Anderson, 2007) was edited and applied in research with an equine assisted service program but did not yield meaningful cutoffs (Vincent et al., 2021). There has yet to be a mixed methods empirical study of the EFP landscape as well as outcomes and impact. Thus, there is a need for culturally relevant quantitative and qualitative data to support the benefits of the horse–human relationship within a therapy space.

CONCLUSION

Throughout this chapter, we have discussed a specific model of EFP for mental health that intentionally includes horses as cofacilitators in therapeutic sessions. EFP is often used by practitioners to address the emotional, behavioral, and psychological challenges of clients. The HERD model was discussed in depth as a framework to practice EFP. Within this model, there are core concepts that are foundational to EH psychology: being in the here-and-now, considering what and how, and the focus on I-thou ways of relating. A more nuanced look at the model emphasizes connection (sharing space regardless of physical contact), relationship, embodiment, regulation, and introspective reflection for the client.

Essentially, it is not possible to be with horses without being in relation with the horse and thereby the other humans in the session. Furthermore, horses encourage and challenge humans to be present in the here-and-now, which creates an opportunity to practice embodiment. It is impossible to be embodied with horses without being in relationship with them. Although the concept of anthropomorphism is sometimes seen to be not of therapeutic meaning, in EFP we must engage in a level of anthropomorphism because we are in relation with the horses. There must be some manner of seeing the horse's behavior as a form of communication to engage with the horse in a genuine interspecies relationship.

The HERD model provides an experiential, experimental, embodied, and creative process that requires the therapist to take risks and be present with the client in their uncertainty of what might unfold or in the direction of where the therapy session is headed. Clinicians must also practice and experience embodiment in order to support the client. Horses are cotherapists in the therapeutic process and create a team wherein the horses allow clients to access goals that would be more difficult without them present (Chandler, 2012; Matuszek, 2010). In pursuit of therapeutic outcomes, the horse, client, and clinician are encouraged to engage in a creative process involving their entire bodies and selves. Thus far, the research to support EH approaches to EFT is scant but promising.

This text offers many opportunities for merging EH psychology with alternative therapies, body movement, and relational practices. We began this chapter by asking, "Why horses?" but now we leave you with a new question: Why not horses?

REFERENCES

Allwood, C. M., & Berry, J. W. (2006). Origins and development of indigenous psychologies: An international analysis. *International Journal of psychology, 41*(4), 243–268.

Anderson, D. C. (2007). *Assessing the human–animal bond: A compendium of actual measures.* Purdue University Press.

Anestis, M. D., Anestis, J. C., Zawilinski, L. L., Hopkins, T. A., & Lilienfeld, S. O. (2014). Equine-related treatments for mental disorders lack empirical support: A systematic review of empirical investigations. *Journal of Clinical Psychology, 70*(12), 1115–1132. https://doi.org/10.1002/jclp.22113

Argent, G., & Vaught, J. (Eds.). (2022). *The relational horse: How frameworks of communication, care, politics and power reveal and conceal equine selves.* Brill. https://doi.org/10.1163/9789004514935

Chandler, C. K. (2012). *Animal assisted therapy in counseling.* Routledge. https://doi.org/10.4324/9780203956755

Comas-Díaz, L. (2011). Multicultural approaches to psychotherapy. In J. C. Norcross, G. R. VandenBos, & D. K. Freedheim (Eds.), *History of psychotherapy: Continuity and change* (2nd ed., pp. 243–267). *American Psychological Association.* https://doi.org/10.1037/12353-008

Cross, P. (2019, February). Global horse statistics internal 02 2019 [Paper presentation]. Global Horse Statistics Validation for HiPoint Agro Bedding Corp. Associates. https://www.researchgate.net/publication/331234705_Global_Horse_statistics_internal_02_2019

Day-Vines, N. L., Wood, S., Grothaus, T., Craigen, L., Holman, A., Dotson-Blake, K., & Douglass, M. J. (2007). Broaching the subjects of race, ethnicity and culture during the counseling process. *Journal of Counseling and Development, 85*(4), 401–409. https://doi.org/10.1002/j.1556-6678.2007.tb00608.x

Equine Business Association. (2023). *About the equine industry.* Retrieved April 12, 2024, from https://equinebusinessassociation.com/equine-industry-statistics/

Felegy, R. J. (2022). The effectiveness of equine-assisted psychotherapy on adolescents with mental health diagnoses: A mixed methods analysis (Publication No. 109497) [Master's thesis, Millersville University]. Millersville University Repository and Digital Archive. https://millersville.tind.io/record/109497?v=pdf

Fernbacher, S., & Plummer, D. (2005). Cultural influences and considerations in gestalt therapy. In A. Woldt & S. Toman (Eds.), *Gestalt therapy: History, theory and practice* (pp. 117–132). Sage Publications. https://doi.org/10.4135/9781452225661.n7

Hallberg, L. (2008). *Walking the way of the horse: Exploring the power of the horse-human relationship.* IUniverse.

Hallberg, L. (2017). *The clinical practice of equine-assisted therapy: Including horses in human healthcare.* Routledge. https://doi.org/10.4324/9781315545905

Harvey, C., Jedlicka, H., & Martinez, S. (2020). A program evaluation: Equine-assisted psychotherapy outcomes for children and adolescents. *Child & Adolescent Social Work Journal, 37*(6), 665–675. https://doi.org/10.1007/s10560-020-00705-0

Hofstede, G. (1981). *Culture's consequences: Comparing values, behaviors, institutions and organizations across nations.* Sage.

Jegatheesan, B., Beetz, A., Ormerod, E., Johnson, R., Fine, A. H., Yamazaki, K., Dudzik, C., Garcia, R. M., Winkle, M., & Choi, G. (2015). The IAHAIO definitions for animal assisted intervention and guidelines for wellness of animals involved. In A. H. Fine (Ed.), *Handbook on animal-assisted therapy* (4th ed., pp. 415–418). Academic Press.

John, K. D. (2023). The horse is indigenous to North America: Why silencing the horse is so important to the settler project. *Decolonising Animals, 19.*

Keeney, B. (2009). *The creative therapist: The art of awakening a session.* Routledge.

Lac, V. (2014). *A donkey's lips do not fit on a horse's mouth: Towards an embodied international psychology competency framework in China* [Unpublished manuscript].

Lac, V. (2016). *Coming home to relationship: Important embodied experiences in gestalt equine psychotherapy* [Unpublished doctoral dissertation]. Saybrook University.

Lac, V. (2017). *Equine-facilitated psychotherapy and learning: The human–equine relational development (HERD) approach.* Academic Press.

Lac, V. (2020). *It's not about the activity: Thinking outside the toolbox in equine-facilitated psychotherapy and learning.* University Professors Press.

Lac, V. (2023). *Obviously, I'm not from here: Embodying a sense of belonging with the help of horses.* University Professors Press.

Lancia, J. J. (2022). Ceremony and psychoanalytic thought: A theoretical framework for exploring horse–human relationships and connection. In G. Argent & J. Vaught (Eds.), *The relational horse: How frameworks of communication, care, politics and power reveal and conceal equine selves* (pp. 62–74). Brill. https://doi.org/10.1163/9789004514935_006

Lee, K., Dabelko-Schoeny, H., Jedlicka, H., & Burns, T. (2020). Older adults' perceived benefits of equine-assisted psychotherapy: Implications for social work. *Research on Social Work Practice, 30*(4), 399–407. https://doi.org/10.1177/1049731519890399

Leung, S. A., & Chen, P. H. (2009). Counseling psychology in Chinese communities in Asia: Indigenous, multicultural, and cross-cultural considerations. *The Counseling Psychologist, 37*(7), 944–966. https://doi.org/10.1177/0011000009339973

Lezama-García, K., Orihuela, A., Olmos-Hernández, A., Reyes-Long, S., & Mota-Rojas, D. (2019). Facial expressions and emotions in domestic animals. *CABI Reviews,* 1–12. https://doi.org/10.1079/PAVSNNR201914028

Looman, M. (2012). Grounded strategies that improve self-efficacy. In K. S. Trotter (Ed.), *Harnessing the power of equine-assisted counseling: Adding animal assisted therapy to your practice.* (pp. 253–263). Routledge/Taylor & Francis Group.

Loue, S. (2022). *Diversity, cultural humility, and the helping professions: Building bridges across difference.* Springer. https://doi.org/10.1007/978-3-031-11381-9

Machová, K., Juríčková, V., Kasparová, A., Petrová, K., Sládková, B., & Svobodová, I. (2023). An evaluation of the effect of equine-facilitated psychotherapy on patients with substance use disorders. *PLOS One, 18*(6), Article e0286867. https://doi.org/10.1371/journal.pone.0286867

Matuszek, S. (2010). Animal-facilitated therapy in various patient populations: Systematic literature review. *Holistic Nursing Practice, 24*(4), 187–203. https://doi.org/10.1097/HNP.0b013e3181e90197

Meola, C. (2023). *Integrating horses into healing.* Elsevier.

Meyer, L., & Sartori, A. (2019). Attachment theory and equine-facilitated psychotherapy for Vietnam veterans. *Society & Animals, 27*(3), 288–306. https://doi.org/10.1163/15685306-12341510

Nakamura, K., Takimoto-Inose, A., & Hasegawa, T. (2018). Cross-modal perception of human emotion in domestic horses (*Equus caballus*). *Scientific Reports, 8*(1), 8660. https://doi.org/10.1038/s41598-018-26892-6

Nieforth, L. O., & Craig, E. A. (2021). Patient-centered communication (PCC) in equine assisted mental health. *Health Communication, 36*(13), 1656–1665. https://doi.org/10.1080/10410236.2020.1785376

Nimer, J., & Lundahl, B. (2007). Animal-assisted therapy: A meta-analysis. *Anthrozoös, 20*(3), 225–238. https://doi.org/10.2752/089279307X224773

Parlett, M. (1991). Reflections on field theory. *British Gestalt Journal, 1*(2), 69–81.

Polster, E., & Polster, M. (1974). *Gestalt therapy integrated: Contours of theory & practice.* Vintage Books.

Rees, L. (2022). Synchrony or dominance? Social relations in feral and domestic horses. In G. Argent & J. Vaught (Eds.), *The relational horse: How frameworks of communication, care, politics and power reveal and conceal equine selves* (pp. 21–33). Brill. https://doi.org/10.1163/9789004514935_003

Roberts, H., & Honzel, N. (2020). The effectiveness of equine-facilitated psychotherapy in adolescents with serious emotional disturbances. *Anthrozoos, 33*(1), 133–144. https://doi.org/10.1080/08927936.2020.1694317

Schoen, A., & Gordon, S. (2015). *The compassionate equestrian: 25 principles to live by when caring for and working with horses.* Trafalgar Square Books.

Schneider, K. J., & Krug, O. T. (2010). *Existential–humanistic therapy.* American Psychological Association. https://doi.org/10.1037/12050-000

Shelef, A., Brafman, D., Rosing, T., Weizman, A., Stryjer, R., & Barak, Y. (2019). Equine assisted therapy for patients with post traumatic stress disorder: A case series study. *Military Medicine, 184*(9–10), 394–399. https://doi.org/10.1093/milmed/usz036

Sue, D. W., & Sue, D. (2008). Culturally appropriate intervention strategies. In D. W. Sue & D. Sue (Eds.), *Counseling the culturally diverse* (5th ed., pp. 157–182). John Wiley & Sons.

Trotter, K. S., & Baggerly, J. N. (Eds.). (2018). *Equine-assisted mental health for healing trauma.* Routledge. https://doi.org/10.4324/9780429456107

Vincent, A., Ballard, I., & Farkas, K. J. (2021). Mind full or mindful? A cohort study of equine-facilitated therapy for women veterans. *Journal of Creativity in Mental Health, 18*(3), 367–382. https://doi.org/10.1080/15401383.2021.1984353

Williams, W. (2016). *The horse: The epic history of our noble companion.* Scientific American/Farrar, Straus and Giroux.

Yalom, I. D. (2001). *The gift of therapy: Reflections on being a therapist.* Piatkus Books.

Zinker, J. (1978). *Creative process in Gestalt therapy.* First Vintage Books.

INDEX

ABOUT THE EDITORS

Louis Hoffman, PhD, is a licensed psychologist in private practice and the executive director of the Rocky Mountain Humansitic Counseling and Psychological Association. An avid writer, Dr. Hoffman has published over 20 books and 100 journal articles and book chapters. His books include the *APA Handbook of Humansitic and Existential Psychology* (Volumes 1 & 2), *Eros & Psyche: Existential Perspectives on Sexuality* (Volumes 1 & 2), *Existential Psychology East–West* (Volumes 1 & 2), and *Becoming an Existential–Humanistic Therapist*. He has been recognized as a fellow of the American Psychological Association and six of its divisions (1: The Society for General Psychology & Interdisciplinary Inquiry; 10: Society for the Psychology of Aesthetics, Creativity, & the Arts; 32: Society for Humanistic Psychology; 36: Society for Psychology of Religion and Spirituality; 48: Society for the Study of Peace, Conflict and Violence: Peace Psychology Division; & 52: International Psychology) and is a recipient of the Rollo May Award of the Society for Humanistic Psychology. He serves on the editorial boards of the *Journal of Humanistic Psychology* (senior international editor), *The Humanistic Psychologist*, and the *Journal of Constructivist Psychology*.

Veronica Lac, PhD, is the founder and executive director of the Human–Equine Relational Development Institute. Existential–humanistic values and principles are embedded in her way of being in the world as an educator and mental health practitioner. Lac holds master's degrees in both Training and Performance Management and Gestalt Psychotherapy as well as a PhD in Psychology (with an Existential, Humanistic, and Transpersonal specialization). She is passionate about bringing a cultural competence framework into her practice and teaching. Dr. Lac specializes in working with eating disorders, trauma, and attachment and has developed equine and canine-assisted programs for at-risk adolescents in collaboration with residential treatment centers and eating disorder clinics. She is also a Professional Association of Therapeutic Horsemanship International certified therapeutic riding instructor for clients with cognitive, physical, and emotional disabilities and a certified equine specialist in mental health and learning. She believes that research is the key to supporting evidence-based practice for equine-facilitated psychotherapy and has multiple publications published internationally in peer-reviewed journals. Lac currently serves on the Board of Trustees for the Professional Association of Therapeutic Horsemanship International and as a Governance Committee member, as well as a founding member of their Diversity, Equality and Inclusion Committee. She serves or has served on the Executive Board of a number of professional organizations including as secretary of the American Psychological Association Division 32 (Society for Humanistic Psychology), as an editor for the University Professors Press, as chair for the Gestalt Psychotherapy Training Institute, and The Humanitarian Alliance. She is also a peer reviewer for *The Journal of Humanistic Psychology* and *The Humanistic Psychologist*. Dr. Lac is the recipient of the 2022 American Psychological Association Division 32 Camri Harari Early Career Award.